THE MERCK MANUAL GO-TO HOME GUIDE FOR SYMPTOMS

ROBERT S. PORTER, MD, *EDITOR-IN-CHIEF*

Executive Director, Merck & Co., Inc.; Clinical Assistant Professor, Department of Emergency Medicine, Jefferson Medical College

JUSTIN L. KAPLAN, MD, *DEPUTY EDITOR-IN-CHIEF*

Director, Merck & Co., Inc.; Clinical Associate Professor, Department of Emergency Medicine, Jefferson Medical College

Published by
MERCK SHARP & DOHME CORP., A SUBSIDIARY OF MERCK & CO., INC.
Whitehouse Station, NJ
2013

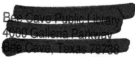

EDITORIAL AND PRODUCTION STAFF

Executive Editor: Keryn A.G. Lane
Senior Staff Writers: Susan T. Schindler
                          Susan C. Short
Staff Editor: Michelle A. Steigerwald
Operations Supervisor: Jennifer A. Doyle
Executive Assistant: Jean Perry
Designer: Jerilyn Bockorick
Illustrator: Michael Reingold

Publisher: Gary Zelko
Associate Director, Digital Publications: Michael A. DeFerrari
Manager, Social Media: Ryan D. Billings
Advertising and Promotions Supervisor: Pamela J. Barnes
Sales and Service Specialist: Leta S. Bracy

Library of Congress Catalog Card Number 2013942601
ISBN (13 digit) 978-0-911910-98-8
ISBN (10 digit) 0-911910-99-9
ISSN 2329-6216

PREFACE

For over a century, *The Merck Manual* has been widely used by people looking for medical information about diseases. However, people who have a disease first develop *symptoms*, which of course are what actually brings them to see a doctor. For that reason, several years ago, we created *The Merck Manual of Patient Symptoms*, a book to help medical students and doctors diagnose the cause of many common symptoms. *The Merck Manual Go-to Home Guide for Symptoms* is a lay-friendly version of that professional reference. Of course, unlike our professional version, the *Home Guide for Symptoms* does not intend to enable readers to diagnose themselves. Making a diagnosis can be challenging even for experienced physicians who have obtained a whole battery of test results. Instead, this book provides a framework for understanding a symptom, particularly its possible causes and what doctors might do to evaluate it, including the questions they ask, the physical findings they look for during their examination, and what tests they might order.

In addition to the framework for understanding a symptom, we provide a list of warning signs, which, if present, warrant a higher degree of concern. We also provide advice on when to see the doctor and then outline what to expect when seeing the doctor.

Typically, the best way to treat a symptom is to treat its cause. However, because most symptoms have a large number of possible causes, this book cannot cover treatment of the specific diseases that may be responsible for a symptom (please see *The Merck Manual Home Health Handbook* for such information, which can be accessed online free of charge at www.merckmanuals.com). But we do discuss ways that doctors, and sometimes people at home, can relieve many symptoms.

Doctors often avoid telling people all the possible causes of their symptoms. This is not to keep people in ignorance but simply to avoid needless worry—after all, most headaches are just headaches and not meningitis or a brain tumor—and some people have trouble resisting the tendency to think the worst. However, in the internet age, where anxiety-producing information is only a few clicks away, we feel that people need truthful, complete medical facts that are presented in a way that is neither alarming nor sensationalistic and is accompanied by information on what is truly worrisome and what is not.

We hope that *The Merck Manual Go-to Home Guide for Symptoms* will serve as an aid to you, our readers, compatible with your needs and worthy of frequent use. We thank the dozens of contributors who have poured their knowledge into this volume. Suggestions for improvements will be warmly welcomed and carefully considered.

Robert S. Porter, MD
Editor-in-Chief

Important: Even a book this size cannot cover all the possible ways that diseases can affect people. Nor can we take into account each person's unique characteristics, circumstances, and medical conditions. Thus, although we are confident that our list of warning signs and recommendations on when to see the doctor cover many situations, we encourage all readers who feel that they need to see a doctor to do so. Do not let us override your judgment about the urgency of your symptoms.

CONTENTS

ADVISORY BOARD REVIEWERS

Parswa Ansari, MD

Program Director, Department of Surgery, Lenox Hill Hospital, New York

Itching, Anal

David H. Barad, MD, MS

Associate Clinical Professor, Department of Obstetrics, Gynecology and Women's Health, Albert Einstein College of Medicine; Director, Assisted Reproductive Technology, Center for Human Reproduction

Pelvic Pain; Vaginal Bleeding; Vaginal Discharge; Vaginal Itching

Alfred J. Cianflocco, MD

Director, Primary Care Sports Medicine, Cleveland Clinic Sports Health, Department of Orthopaedic Surgery, Cleveland Clinic

Back Pain; Neck Pain

Kathryn Colby, MD, PhD

Associate Professor of Ophthalmology, Harvard Medical School; Surgeon in Ophthalmology, Cornea Service, Massachusetts Eye and Ear Infirmary

Eye Floaters; Eye Pain; Eye Redness; Eyelid Swelling; Eyes, Bulging, Eyes, Watery; Pupils, Unequal; Vision, Blurred; Vision, Double; Vision Loss, Sudden

Deborah M. Consolini, MD

Assistant Professor of Pediatrics, Jefferson Medical College; Staff Physician, Diagnostic Referral Division, Nemours/Alfred I. duPont Hospital for Children

Constipation in Children; Cough in Children; Crying in Infants, Excessive; Diarrhea in Children; Fever in Infants and Children; Nausea and Vomiting in Infants and Children

Caroline Carney Doebbeling, MD, MSc

Chief Medical Officer, MDWise, Inc; Chief Executive Officer; Cetan Health Consultants LLC

Personality and Behavior Changes

Karl Doghramji, MD

Professor of Psychiatry, Neurology, and Medicine; Medical Director, Jefferson Sleep Disorders Center; and Program Director, Fellowship in Sleep Medicine, Thomas Jefferson University

Insomnia and Excessive Daytime Sleepiness; Snoring

James D. Douketis, MD

Professor, Department of Medicine, Division of General Internal Medicine, McMaster University; Associate Director, Clinical Teaching Unit, and Staff Physician, Clinical Thromboembolism and General Internal Medicine Services, St. Joseph's Hospital

Swollen Lymph Nodes

Alberto J. Espay, MD

Associate Professor and Clinical Research Director of the James J. and Joan A. Gardner Center for Parkinson's Disease and Movement Disorders, University of Cincinnati

Tremor

T. Ernesto Figueroa, MD

Chief, Division of Pediatric Urology, Nemours/Alfred I. duPont Hospital for Children; Clinical Associate Professor of Urology, Thomas Jefferson University

Urinary Incontinence in Children

Marvin P. Fried, MD

Professor and University Chairman, Department of Otorhinolaryngology—Head and Neck Surgery, Montefiore Medical Center and Albert Einstein College of Medicine

Nasal Congestion and Discharge; Neck Lump; Nosebleeds; Smell, Loss of; Sore Throat

Eric Gibson, MD

Associate Professor, Neonatal-Perinatal Medicine, Nemours/Alfred I. duPont Hospital for Children, Thomas Jefferson University

Jaundice in Newborns

Hector Alberto Gonzalez Usigli, MD

Assistant Professor in Neurology, Department of Internal Medicine, Instituto Mexicano del Seguro Social, Guadalajara

Tremor

Norton J. Greenberger, MD

Clinical Professor of Medicine, Harvard Medical School; Senior Physician, Brigham and Women's Hospital

Abdominal Pain, Acute; Abdominal Pain, Chronic; Constipation in Adults; Diarrhea in Adults; Gas; Gastrointestinal Bleeding; Heartburn and Indigestion; Hiccups; Lump in Throat; Nausea and Vomiting in Adults; Swallowing Difficulty

R. Phillips Heine, MD

Associate Professor and Director, Division of Maternal-Fetal Medicine, Department of Obstetrics and Gynecology, Duke University Medical Center

Nausea and Vomiting During Early Pregnancy; Pelvic Pain During Early Pregnancy; Swelling During Late Pregnancy; Vaginal Bleeding During Early Pregnancy; Vaginal Bleeding During Late Pregnancy

Steven K. Herrine, MD

Professor of Medicine, Division of Gastroenterology and Hepatology, Thomas Jefferson University; Assistant Dean for Academic Affairs, Jefferson Medical College

Jaundice in Adults

Lyall A. J. Higginson, MD

Professor of Medicine, University of Ottawa Heart Institute

Chest Pain; Dizziness When Standing Up; Fainting and Light-headedness; Limb Pain; Palpitations; Swelling

Irvin H. Hirsch, MD

Clinical Professor, Department of Urology, Thomas Jefferson University

Erectile Dysfunction

Mary Ann Kosir, MD

Associate Professor of Surgery and Oncology, Wayne State University School of Medicine; Walt Breast Center, Karmanos Cancer Institute

Breast Lumps; Nipple Discharge

Noah Lechtzin, MD, MHS

Associate Professor, Department of Medicine, Division of Pulmonary and Critical Care Medicine, Johns Hopkins University School of Medicine

Cough in Adults; Coughing Up Blood; Shortness of Breath; Wheezing

Michael C. Levin, MD

Professor of Neurology, University of Tennessee Health Science Center

Memory Loss; Muscle Cramps; Numbness; Weakness

Wendy S. Levinbook, MD

Private Practice, Hartford Dermatology Associates

Hair Loss; Hairiness

Karen McKoy, MD, MPH

Senior Staff, Department of Dermatology, Lahey Clinic Medical Center

Hives; Itching

Joel L. Moake, MD

Professor of Medicine (Emeritus), Baylor College of Medicine; Associate Director, Biomedical Engineering Laboratory, Rice University

Bruising and Bleeding

David F. Murchison, DDS, MMS

Clinical Professor, Texas A&M Health Science Center, Baylor College of Dentistry; Senior Lecturer, University of Texas at Dallas

Bad Breath; Mouth, Dry; Mouth Growths; Mouth Sores; Toothache

Ursula Nawab, MD

Assistant Professor, Department of Pediatrics, Division of Neonatology, Nemours/Alfred I. duPont Hospital for Children, Thomas Jefferson University

Jaundice in Newborns

John K. Niparko, MD

Associate Professor, Department of Otolaryngology–Head & Neck Surgery, Johns Hopkins University School of Medicine

Hearing Loss; Hearing Loss: Sudden Deafness

JoAnn V. Pinkerton, MD

Professor of Obstetrics and Gynecology and Director, Division of Midlife Health, University of Virginia Health System

Menstrual Periods, Absence of; Menstrual Periods, Painful

Anuja P. Shah, MD

Assistant Professor, David Geffen School of Medicine at UCLA; Faculty, Division of Nephrology, Harbor-UCLA Medical Center

Erection, Persistent; Scrotal Pain; Scrotal Swelling; Semen, Blood in; Urination, Excessive or Frequent; Urination, Pain or Burning With; Urine, Blood in

Patrick J. Shenot, MD

Associate Professor, Department of Urology, Thomas Jefferson University

Urinary Incontinence in Adults

Stephen D. Silberstein, MD

Professor of Neurology, Thomas Jefferson University; Director, Jefferson Headache Center, Thomas Jefferson University Hospital

Headache

Geeta K. Swamy, MD

Associate Professor, Division of Maternal-Fetal Medicine, Department of Obstetrics and Gynecology, Duke University Medical Center

Nausea and Vomiting During Early Pregnancy; Pelvic Pain During Early Pregnancy; Swelling During Late Pregnancy; Vaginal Bleeding During Early Pregnancy; Vaginal Bleeding During Late Pregnancy

Debara L. Tucci, MD, MS

Associate Professor of Surgery, Division of Otolaryngology—Head and Neck Surgery, Duke University Medical Center

Dizziness and Vertigo; Earache; Ear Discharge; Ear, Ringing or Buzzing in

Allan R. Tunkel, MD, PhD

Professor of Medicine, Drexel University College of Medicine; Chair, Department of Medicine, Monmouth Medical Center

Fever in Adults

Alexandra Villa-Forte, MD, MPH

Staff Physician, Center for Vasculitis Care and Research, Department of Rheumatic and Immunologic Diseases, Cleveland Clinic

Joint Pain: Many Joints; Joint Pain: Single Joint

Michael R. Wasserman, MD

Assistant Clinical Professor, University of Colorado Denver School of Medicine

Fatigue; Weight Loss

A GUIDE FOR READERS

The Merck Manual Go-to Home Guide for Symptoms is organized alphabetically, and each symptom follows a structured format. Understanding this structure will help the reader navigate the topics. Topics of interest may be quickly located by consulting the Contents or Index.

TOPIC STRUCTURE

Each symptom follows a set structure: Causes, Evaluation, and Treatment. Under Causes, the most common and least common causes are usually listed. Under Evaluation, Warning Signs are always listed first, followed by When to See a Doctor, What the Doctor Does, and Testing. Nearly every topic has a table that covers many causes and features of that particular symptom. Many topics contain "Essentials for Older People" to address specific aging-related information. All topics conclude with boxed Key Points.

MEDICAL TERMS

Medical terms are often provided, usually in parentheses after the common term. On the next page is a list of prefixes, roots, and suffixes used in medical terminology. This list can help take the mystery out of medicine's multisyllabic vocabulary.

DIAGNOSTIC TESTS

Diagnostic tests are mentioned throughout the book. Usually, an explanation is provided the first time a test is mentioned in a topic. On page 475, an Appendix on Common Medical Tests gives many common diagnostic tests and procedures and explains what they are used for.

SPECIAL NOTE TO READERS

The authors, reviewers, and editors have made extensive efforts to ensure that the information is accurate and conforms to the standards accepted at the time of publication. However, constant changes in information resulting from continuing research and clinical experience, reasonable differences in opinions among authorities, unique aspects of individual situations, and the possibility of human error in preparing an extensive text require that the reader exercise judgment when making decisions and consult and compare information from other sources. In particular, the reader is advised to discuss information obtained in this book with a doctor, pharmacist, nurse, or other health care practitioner.

UNDERSTANDING MEDICAL TERMS

At first glance, medical terminology can seem like a foreign language. But often the key to understanding medical terms is focusing on their components (prefixes, roots, and suffixes). For example, spondylolysis is a combination of "spondylo, "which means vertebra, and "lysis," which means dissolve, and so means dissolution of a vertebra.

The same components are used in many medical terms. "Spondylo" plus "itis," which means inflammation, forms spondylitis, an inflammation of the vertebrae. The same prefix plus "malacia," which means soft, forms spondylomalacia, a softening of the vertebrae.

Knowing the meaning of a small number of components can help with interpretation of a large number of medical terms. The following list defines many commonly used medical prefixes, roots, and suffixes.

a(n)	absence of	cry(o)	cold
acou, acu	hear	cut	skin
aden(o)	gland	cyan(o)	blue
aer(o)	air	cyst(o)	bladder
alg	pain	cyt(o)	cell
andr(o)	man	dactyl(o)	finger or toe
angi(o)	vessel	dent	tooth
ankyl(o)	crooked, curved	derm(ato)	skin
ante	before	dipl(o)	double
anter(i)	front, forward	dors	back
anti	against	dys	bad, faulty, abnormal
arteri(o)	artery	ectomy	excision (removal by cutting)
arthr(o)	joint	emia	blood
articul	joint	encephal(o)	brain
ather(o)	fatty	end(o)	inside
audi(o)	hearing	enter(o)	intestine
aur(i)	ear	epi	outer, superficial, upon
aut(o)	self	erythr(o)	red
bi, bis	double, twice, two	eu	normal
brachy	short	extra	outside
brady	slow	gastr(o)	stomach
bucc(o)	cheek	gen	become, originate
carcin(o)	cancer	gloss(o)	tongue
cardi(o)	heart	glyc(o)	sweet, or referring to glucose
cephal(o)	head	gram, graph	write, record
cerebr(o)	brain	gyn	woman
cervic	neck	hem(ato)	blood
chol(e)	bile, or referring to gallbladder	hemi	half
chondr(o)	cartilage	hepat(o)	liver
circum	around, about	hist(o)	tissue
contra	against, counter	hydr(o)	water
corpor	body	hyper	excessive, high
cost(o)	rib	hypo	deficient, low
crani(o)	skull	hyster(o)	uterus

iatr(o)	doctor	pharyng(o)	throat
infra	beneath	phleb(o)	vein
inter	among, between	phob(ia)	fear
intra	inside	plasty	repair
itis	inflammation	pleg(ia)	paralysis
lact(o)	milk	pnea	breathing
lapar(o)	flank, abdomen	pneum(ato)	breath, air
latero	side	pneumon(o)	lung
leuk(o)	white	pod(o)	foot
lingu(o)	tongue	poie	make, produce
lip(o)	fat	poly	much, many
lys(is)	dissolve	post	after
mal	bad, abnormal	poster(i)	back, behind
malac	soft	presby	elder
mamm(o)	breast	proct(o)	anus
mast(o)	breast	pseud(o)	false
megal(o)	large	psych(o)	mind
melan(o)	black	pulmon(o)	lung
mening(o)	membranes	pyel(o)	pelvis of kidney
my(o)	muscle	pyr(o)	fever, fire
myc(o)	fungus	rachi(o)	spine
myel(o)	marrow	ren(o)	kidneys
nas(o)	nose	rhag	break, burst
necr(o)	death	rhe	flow
nephr(o)	kidney	rhin(o)	nose
neur(o)	nerve	scler(o)	hard
nutri	nourish	scope	instrument
ocul(o)	eye	scopy	examination
odyn(o)	pain	somat(o)	body
oma	tumor	spondyl(o)	vertebra
onc(o)	tumor	steat(o)	fat
oophor(o)	ovaries	sten(o)	narrow, compressed
ophthalm(o)	eye	steth(o)	chest
opia	vision	stom	mouth, opening
opsy	examination	supra	above
orchi(o)	testes	tachy	fast, quick
osis	condition	therap	treatment
osse(o)	bone	therm(o)	heat
oste(o)	bone	thorac(o)	chest
ot(o)	ear	thromb(o)	clot, lump
path(o)	disease	tomy	incision (operation by cutting)
ped(o)	child	tox(i)	poison
penia	deficient, deficiency	uria	urine
peps, pept	digest	vas(o)	vessel
peri	around	ven(o)	vein
phag(o)	eat, destroy	vesic(o)	bladder
pharmaco	drug	xer(o)	dry

ABDOMINAL PAIN, ACUTE

Abdominal pain is common and often minor. Severe abdominal pain that comes on quickly, however, almost always indicates a significant problem. The pain may be the only sign of the need for surgery and must be attended to swiftly. Abdominal pain is of particular concern in people who are very young or very old and those who have human immunodeficiency virus (HIV) infection or are taking drugs that suppress the immune system. Older adults may have less abdominal pain than younger adults with a similar disorder, and, even if the condition is serious, the pain may develop more gradually. Abdominal pain also affects children, including newborns and infants—who cannot communicate the reason for their distress.

TYPES OF ABDOMINAL PAIN

There are different types of abdominal pain depending on the structures involved.

Visceral pain comes from the organs within the abdominal cavity (which are called the viscera). The viscera's nerves do not respond to cutting, tearing, or inflammation. Instead, the nerves respond to the organ being stretched (as when the intestine is expanded by gas) or surrounding muscles contract. Visceral pain is typically vague, dull, and nauseating. It is hard to pinpoint. Upper abdominal pain results from disorders in organs such as the stomach, duodenum, liver, and pancreas. Midabdominal pain (near the navel) results from disorders of structures such as the small intestine, upper part of the colon, and appendix. Lower abdominal pain results from disorders of the lower part of the colon and organs in the genitourinary tract.

Somatic pain comes from the membrane (peritoneum) that lines the abdominal cavity (peritoneal cavity). Unlike nerves in the visceral organs, nerves in the peritoneum respond to cutting and irritation (such as from blood, infection, chemicals, or inflammation). Somatic pain is sharp and fairly easy to pinpoint.

Referred pain is pain perceived distant from its source (see art box on page 32). Examples of referred pain are groin pain caused by kidney stones and shoulder pain caused by blood or infection irritating the diaphragm.

PERITONITIS

Peritonitis is inflammation of the peritoneal cavity. It is very painful and almost always signals a very serious or life-threatening disorder. It can result from any abdominal problem in which the organs are inflamed or infected. Common examples include appendicitis, diverticulitis, and pancreatitis. Also, blood and body fluids (such as intestinal contents or urine) are very irritating when they leak into the peritoneal cavity and can cause peritonitis. Disorders that cause blood and body fluids to leak include spontaneous organ rupture (such as a perforated intestine or ruptured ectopic pregnancy) and severe abdominal injury.

Once peritonitis has been present for a number of hours, the inflammation causes fluid to leak into the abdominal cavity. The person may then develop dehydration and go into shock. Inflammatory substances released into the bloodstream may affect various organs, causing severe lung inflammation, kidney failure, liver failure, and other problems. Without treatment, people may die.

CAUSES

Pain can arise from any of many causes, including infection, inflammation, ulcers, perforation or rupture of organs, muscle contractions that are uncoordinated or blocked by an obstruction, and blockage of blood flow to organs.

Immediately life-threatening disorders, which require rapid diagnosis and surgery, include

- Ruptured abdominal aortic aneurysm
- Perforated stomach or intestine
- Blockage of blood flow to the intestine (mesenteric ischemia)
- Ruptured ectopic pregnancy

Serious disorders that are nearly as urgent include

- Intestinal obstruction
- Appendicitis
- Sudden (acute) inflammation of the pancreas (pancreatitis)

Sometimes, disorders outside the abdomen cause abdominal pain. Examples include heart attack, pneumonia, and twisting of a testis (testicular torsion). Less common problems outside the abdomen that cause abdominal pain include

1

ABDOMINAL PAIN IN NEWBORNS, INFANTS, AND YOUNG CHILDREN

Cause of Pain	Description	Comments
Meconium peritonitis	Inflammation and sometimes infection of the abdominal cavity and its lining (peritonitis) caused by a perforation in the intestine and leakage of meconium (the dark green fecal material that is produced in the intestines before birth)	Occurs while infants are still in the womb or shortly after birth
Hypertrophic pyloric stenosis	A blockage at the stomach outlet (duodenum)	Forceful (projectile) vomiting occurs after feedings Usually begins between birth and 4 months of age
Esophageal webs	Thin membranes that grow across the inside of the upper one third of the esophagus from its lining (mucosa)	Solids are difficult to swallow
Volvulus	Twisting of a loop of the intestines	Causes intestinal obstruction and cuts off the blood supply to intestines Commonly, vomiting, diarrhea, abdominal swelling, and episodic and excessive crying (colic)
Imperforate anus (anal atresia)	Narrowing or blockage of the anal opening	Normally detected by doctors when infants are examined after birth and usually requires immediate surgery
Intussusception	The condensing and overlapping (telescoping) of one portion of the intestine into another	Causes intestinal obstruction and cuts off the blood supply to the intestine Causes sudden pain, vomiting, bloody stools, and fever Typically affects children between the ages of 6 months and 2 years
Intestinal obstruction	A blockage that completely stops or seriously impairs the passage of intestinal contents	Commonly caused by a birth defect, meconium, or volvulus in newborns and infants Various symptoms depending on the type of obstruction but may include cramping pain in the abdomen, bloating, disinterest in eating, vomiting, severe constipation, diarrhea, and fever

diabetic ketoacidosis, porphyria, sickle cell disease, and certain bites and poisons (such as a black widow spider bite, heavy metal or methanol poisoning, and some scorpion stings).

Abdominal pain in newborns, infants, and young children has numerous causes not encountered in adults (see Table, above).

EVALUATION

The following information can help people decide when a doctor's evaluation is needed and help them know what to expect during the evaluation.

WARNING SIGNS

In people with acute abdominal pain, certain symptoms and characteristics are cause for concern. They include

- Severe pain
- Signs of shock (for example, a rapid heart rate, low blood pressure, sweating, and confusion)
- Signs of peritonitis (for example, constant pain that doubles the person over and/or pain that worsens with gentle touching or with bumping the bed)
- Swelling of the abdomen

People who have warning signs should go to the hospital right away. People who have no warning signs should see a doctor within the day.

Doctors ask questions about the person's symptoms and medical history and do a physical examination. What doctors find during the history and physical examination helps them decide what, if any, tests need to be done. Doctors follow the same process whether they are evaluating mild or severe pain, although a surgeon may be involved early on in the evaluation of severe abdominal pain.

When taking the medical history (see Table, below), doctors ask questions about the pain's location (see art box on page 5) and characteristics, whether the person has had similar symptoms in the past, and what other symptoms the person has along with the abdominal pain. Symptoms such as reflux, nausea, vomiting, diarrhea, constipation, jaundice, blood in the stool or urine, coughing up blood, and weight loss help guide the doctor's evaluation. Doctors ask questions about drugs taken, including prescription and illicit drugs as well as alcohol.

HISTORY IN PEOPLE WITH ACUTE ABDOMINAL PAIN

Questions That Doctors Ask	Possible Responses	Possible Causes or Source
Where is the pain?	See art box on page 5	See art box on page 5
What is the pain like?	Waves of sharp pain that "take the breath away"	Renal or biliary colic (episodes of intense pain in the affected area)
	Waves of dull pain with vomiting	Intestinal obstruction
	Colicky pain that becomes steady	Appendicitis
		Strangulating intestinal obstruction (blockage that cuts of the blood supply to the intestines)
		Mesenteric ischemia (blockage of blood flow to part of the intestines due to a blood clot or buildup of fatty materials in an artery)
	Sharp, constant pain, worsened by movement	Peritonitis
	Tearing pain	Aortic dissection (a tear in the inner layer of the aorta)
	Dull ache	Appendicitis
		Diverticulitis
		Kidney infection
Have you had it before?	Yes	Recurring problems such as ulcer disease, gallstones, diverticulitis, or mittelschmerz (pain during ovulation, usually the middle of the menstrual cycle)
Did the pain begin suddenly?	Sudden ("like a light switching on")	Perforated ulcer
		Kidney stone
		Ruptured ectopic (abnormally located) pregnancy
		Twisting of ovary or testis
		Some ruptured aneurysms
	Less sudden	Most other causes

(continued)

HISTORY IN PEOPLE WITH ACUTE ABDOMINAL PAIN (continued)

Questions That Doctors Ask	Possible Responses	Possible Causes or Source
How severe is the pain?	Severe pain	A tear (perforation) in an organ
		Kidney stone
		Peritonitis
		Pancreatitis
	Severe pain but a comparatively normal physical examination	Mesenteric ischemia
Does the pain travel to any other part of your body?	Right shoulder blade	Gallbladder pain
	Left shoulder region	Ruptured spleen
		Pancreatitis
	Pubic bone or vagina	Kidney pain
	Back	Ruptured aortic aneurysm
What relieves the pain?	Antacids	Peptic ulcer disease
	Lying as quietly as possible	Peritonitis
What other symptoms occur with the pain?	Vomiting that precedes the pain and is followed by diarrhea	Gastroenteritis
	Delayed vomiting, no bowel movements, and no passing of gas (flatulence)	Sudden (acute) intestinal obstruction
	Severe vomiting that precedes intense pain in the upper middle of the abdomen, left chest, or shoulder	Perforation of the esophagus

Doctors ask questions about known medical conditions and previous abdominal surgeries. Women are asked whether they are or could be pregnant.

When conducting a physical examination, doctors first note the person's general appearance. A comfortable-appearing person rarely has a serious problem, unlike one who is anxious, pale, sweating, or in obvious pain. The focus of the examination is the abdomen, and doctors inspect, tap, and touch (a process called palpation) the abdominal area. They examine the rectum and pelvis (for women) to locate tenderness, masses, and blood.

Doctors touch the whole abdomen gently to detect areas of particular tenderness, as well as the presence of guarding, rigidity, rebound, and any masses. Guarding is when a person involuntary contracts the abdominal muscles when the doctor touches the abdomen. Rigidity is when the abdominal muscles stay firmly contracted even when the doctor is not touching them. Rebound is when a person flinches in pain as the doctor's hand is briskly withdrawn. Guarding, rigidity, and rebound are signs of peritonitis.

TESTING

Sometimes, people have findings so significant that doctors realize right away that they need surgery. Doctors try not to delay surgery on such people by doing tests. However, more often, doctors must do tests to help choose among several different causes suggested by the person's symptoms and physical examination results. Doctors select tests based on what they suspect.

- Urine pregnancy test for all girls and women of childbearing age
- Imaging tests based on suspected diagnosis

An abdominal computed tomography (CT) scan helps identify many, but not all, causes of abdominal pain. Urine tests (for example, urinalysis) are frequently done to look for signs of a urinary tract infection or a kidney stone. Blood tests are often done but rarely identify a specific cause (although blood tests can be used to diagnose pancreatitis). An ultrasound is helpful if doctors suspect a gynecologic disorder.

CAUSES OF ABDOMINAL PAIN BY LOCATION

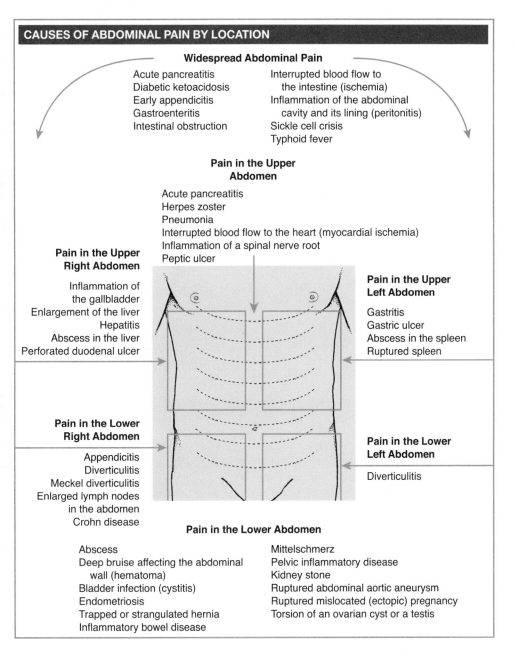

Widespread Abdominal Pain

Acute pancreatitis
Diabetic ketoacidosis
Early appendicitis
Gastroenteritis
Intestinal obstruction

Interrupted blood flow to
  the intestine (ischemia)
Inflammation of the abdominal
  cavity and its lining (peritonitis)
Sickle cell crisis
Typhoid fever

**Pain in the Upper
Abdomen**

Acute pancreatitis
Herpes zoster
Pneumonia
Interrupted blood flow to the heart (myocardial ischemia)
Inflammation of a spinal nerve root
Peptic ulcer

**Pain in the Upper
Right Abdomen**

Inflammation of
  the gallbladder
Enlargement of the liver
Hepatitis
Abscess in the liver
Perforated duodenal ulcer

**Pain in the Upper
Left Abdomen**

Gastritis
Gastric ulcer
Abscess in the spleen
Ruptured spleen

**Pain in the Lower
Right Abdomen**

Appendicitis
Diverticulitis
Meckel diverticulitis
Enlarged lymph nodes
  in the abdomen
Crohn disease

**Pain in the Lower
Left Abdomen**

Diverticulitis

Pain in the Lower Abdomen

Abscess
Deep bruise affecting the abdominal
  wall (hematoma)
Bladder infection (cystitis)
Endometriosis
Trapped or strangulated hernia
Inflammatory bowel disease

Mittelschmerz
Pelvic inflammatory disease
Kidney stone
Ruptured abdominal aortic aneurysm
Ruptured mislocated (ectopic) pregnancy
Torsion of an ovarian cyst or a testis

TREATMENT

The specific cause of the pain is treated. Until recently, doctors thought that it was not wise to give pain relievers to people with severe abdominal pain until a diagnosis was made because the pain reliever might mask important symptoms. However, pain relievers are now often given while tests are in progress.

KEY POINTS

- Doctors look first for any life-threatening causes for the pain.
- Doctors rule out pregnancy in girls and women of childbearing age.
- Blood tests rarely identify a specific cause of acute abdominal pain.

ABDOMINAL PAIN, CHRONIC

Chronic abdominal pain is pain that is present for more than 3 months. It may be present all the time or come and go (recurring). Chronic abdominal pain usually occurs in children beginning after age 5 years. About 10 to 15% of children aged 5 to 16 years, particularly those aged 8 to 12 years, have chronic or recurring abdominal pain. It is somewhat more common among girls. About 2% of adults, mainly women, have chronic abdominal pain.

People with chronic abdominal pain may also have other symptoms, depending on the cause.

CAUSES

Usually by the time abdominal pain has been present for 3 months or more, people have been evaluated by a doctor, and typical disorders that cause abdominal pain (see Abdominal Pain, Acute on page 1) have already been identified. If people have been evaluated and the cause has not been identified by this time, only about 10% of them have a specific physical disorder (see Table on pages 7 to 10). The remaining 90% have what is called functional abdominal pain.

Functional pain is real pain that occurs with no evidence of a specific physical disorder (such as peptic ulcer disease). It is also not related to body functions (such as menstrual periods, bowel movements, or eating), a drug, or a toxin. Functional pain can be severe and typically interferes with the person's life. Exactly what causes the pain is unknown. But the nerves of the digestive tract may become oversensitive to sensations (such as normal movements of the digestive tract), which do not bother most people. Genetic factors, life stresses, personality, social situations, and underlying mental disorders (such as depression or anxiety) may all contribute to functional pain. Chronic abdominal pain in children may be related to a need for attention (as when a sibling is born or the family moves), the stress of starting school, lactose intolerance, or sometimes child abuse.

COMMON PHYSICAL CAUSES

Many physical disorders cause chronic abdominal pain (see Table on pages 7 to 10). The most common causes vary by age.

In **children,** the most common causes are

- Lactose intolerance (lactose is a sugar in dairy products)
- Constipation
- Gastroesophageal reflux disease

In **young adults,** common causes include

- Indigestion (dyspepsia) due to peptic ulcer or another problem
- Stomach irritation (caused by aspirin or nonsteroidal anti-inflammatory drugs [NSAIDs], cola beverages [acidity], and spicy foods)
- Liver disorders, such as hepatitis
- Gallbladder disorders, such as cholecystitis
- Pancreatic disorders, such as pancreatitis
- Parasitic infections, such as giardiasis
- Inflammatory bowel disease, such as Crohn disease
- Irritable bowel syndrome

In **older adults,** cancer (such as stomach, pancreatic, colon, or ovarian cancer) becomes more common.

EVALUATION

Doctors first focus on whether the pain is functional pain or is caused by a disorder, drug, or toxin. Making this distinction may be difficult. However, if warning signs are present, functional pain is unlikely (but not impossible).

WARNING SIGNS

The following symptoms are cause for concern:

- Fever
- Loss of appetite and weight
- Pain that awakens the person during the night
- Blood in vomit, stool, or urine
- Severe or frequent vomiting or diarrhea
- Jaundice
- Swelling of the abdomen and/or legs
- Difficulty swallowing

WHEN TO SEE A DOCTOR

If people with chronic abdominal pain develop warning signs, they should see a doctor right away unless the only warning signs are loss of appetite, jaundice, and/or swelling. People with loss of appetite, jaundice, and/or swelling or with steady, worsening pain should see a doctor within a few days to a week. When these warning signs are present, a physical cause is very likely. People without warning signs should see a doctor at some point, but a delay of a few days or so is not harmful.

WHAT THE DOCTOR DOES

Doctors first ask questions about the person's symptoms and medical history. Doctors then do a physical examination. What they find during the history and physical examination often suggests a cause of the pain and the tests that may need to be done (see Table, below).

Doctors ask particularly about activities (such as eating, urinating, or having a bowel movement) that relieve or worsen the pain. Whether the pain or other digestive upset occurs after eating or drinking dairy products is important

because lactose intolerance is common, especially among blacks. Doctors also ask about other symptoms (such as vomiting, diarrhea, or constipation), about diet, and about any surgery involving the abdomen, drugs used, and previous tests and treatments for the pain. Whether any family members have disorders that cause abdominal pain is also important.

The physical examination focuses particularly on the abdomen to identify any tender areas, masses, or enlarged organs. Usually, a rectal examination is done, and the doctor tests the stool for blood. A pelvic examination is done in women. Doctors note whether the skin looks yellow (jaundice) and whether people have a rash or swelling in the legs.

Between the initial visit and follow-up visits, people are often asked to record information about the pain, bowel movements, diet, any activities that seem to trigger pain, any remedies tried, and the effects of the remedies.

PHYSICAL CAUSES AND FEATURES OF CHRONIC ABDOMINAL PAIN

Cause*	Common Features†	Tests‡
Disorders of the digestive tract		
Celiac disease	In children, not growing as expected (failure to thrive) Abdominal bloating and often diarrhea or light-colored, bulky, and unusually foul-smelling stools that may appear oily Symptoms that worsen when people eat foods containing wheat products (which contain gluten)	Blood tests to measure levels of antibodies produced when people with celiac disease eat foods containing gluten Often biopsy of the upper small intestine
Cholecystitis (inflammation of the gallbladder), if chronic	Recurring crampy pain in the upper right part of the abdomen	Ultrasonography to look for gallstones Imaging of the gallbladder after a radioactive substance (radionuclide) is injected intravenously (cholescintigraphy)
Colon cancer	Usually no discomfort, but if the colon is partially blocked, possibly crampy discomfort Sometimes blood in stool (blood may be visible or detected during a doctor's examination)	Colonoscopy Imaging tests such as CT or x-rays after barium is inserted in the rectum (barium enema)
Constipation	Hard, less frequent bowel movements that are difficult to pass Crampy pain in the lower abdomen that decreases after a bowel movement Sometimes pain during a bowel movement	A doctor's examination, including thorough dietary history

(continued)

PHYSICAL CAUSES AND FEATURES OF CHRONIC ABDOMINAL PAIN *(continued)*

Cause*	Common Features†	Tests‡
Crohn disease	Recurring episodes of severe pain with fever, loss of appetite, weight loss, and diarrhea	CT and/or colonoscopy X-rays of the small intestine
Gastroesophageal reflux disease (sometimes related to a hiatus hernia)	Heartburn (burning pain that begins in the upper abdomen and travels up to the throat, sometimes with an acid taste in the mouth) Sometimes chest pain Sometimes a cough, hoarseness, or both Symptoms sometimes relieved by lying down Relief with antacids	Often only a doctor's examination plus trying treatment with drugs to suppress acid production (if symptoms are relieved, the cause is probably gastroesophageal reflux disease) Sometimes endoscopy of the upper digestive tract (examination of the esophagus and stomach using a flexible viewing tube) or x-rays of the upper digestive tract after barium is given by mouth (barium swallow)
Hepatitis, if chronic	Discomfort in the upper right part of the abdomen A general feeling of illness (malaise) Loss of appetite Jaundice (uncommon) Sometimes in people known to have had acute hepatitis	Blood tests to evaluate liver function and to check for hepatitis viruses
Lactose intolerance	Bloating, cramps, passing of gas (flatulence), and diarrhea after consuming milk products	Sometimes a breath test to detect hydrogen, indicating undigested food A diet that excludes foods containing lactose (elimination diet) to determine whether those foods trigger the symptoms
Pancreatic cancer	Severe, constant pain in the upper abdomen, often radiating to the back Weight loss Sometimes jaundice	CT MRI (magnetic resonance cholangiopancreatography, or MRCP)
Pancreatitis, if chronic or accompanied by a pancreatic pseudocyst	Episodes of severe pain in the upper middle of the abdomen Sometimes diarrhea and fat in stool Usually in people known to have had acute pancreatitis	Blood tests to measure levels of an enzyme produced by the pancreas Imaging tests such as CT or MRI
Parasitic infections (particularly giardiasis)	Recent travel to developing countries, ingestion of water from streams or lakes, or contact with people with the infection Cramps, flatulence, and diarrhea	Examination of stool to check for parasites or their eggs
Peptic ulcers	Stomach pain relieved by eating food and taking antacids May awaken people at night	Endoscopy and biopsy for *Helicobacter (H.) pylori* (bacteria that can cause peptic ulcers) Sometimes an *H. pylori* breath test

(continued)

PHYSICAL CAUSES AND FEATURES OF CHRONIC ABDOMINAL PAIN *(continued)*

Cause*	Common Features†	Tests‡
Scar tissue that develops around the intestines (adhesions) in people who have had abdominal surgery	Crampy discomfort accompanied by nausea and sometimes vomiting	Barium swallow
Stomach cancer	Indigestion or mild pain Often tiny amounts of blood in stool (detectable only during a doctor's examination) Typically in older adults	Endoscopy of the esophagus and stomach
Ulcerative colitis	Crampy pain with several separate episodes of bloody diarrhea Typically in young adults	Sigmoidoscopy or colonoscopy Biopsy of the rectum or colon
Kidney and urinary tract disorders		
Birth defects of the urinary tract	Frequent urinary tract infections Typically in children	Intravenous urography Ultrasonography
Kidney stones	Pain in the side (flank) that comes and goes, often in people known to have stones Sometimes fever Dark or bloody urine	Urinalysis CT or intravenous urography
Reproductive system disorders (in women)		
Endometriosis	Discomfort mainly before or during menstrual periods	Laparoscopy
Ovarian cyst	Vague discomfort in the lower abdomen	Ultrasonography of the pelvis
Ovarian cancer	Bloating Sometimes a mass in the pelvis detected during a doctor's examination	Ultrasonography of the pelvis
Systemic disorders		
Familial Mediterranean fever	Family members who have the disorder Episodes of abdominal pain lasting 48 to 72 hours and often accompanied by fever Starting during childhood or adolescence	Genetic testing
A food allergy	Symptoms that develop only after eating certain foods such as seafood	An elimination diet
Immunoglobulin A–associated vasculitis (Henoch-Schönlein purpura)	A reddish-purple rash of tiny dots (petechiae) or larger splotches (purpura) on the arms, legs, buttocks, and top of the feet Achy, tender, swollen joints Nausea, vomiting, and diarrhea Blood in stool detected during a doctor's examination	Biopsy of affected skin

(continued)

PHYSICAL CAUSES AND FEATURES OF CHRONIC ABDOMINAL PAIN *(continued)*

Cause*	Common Features†	Tests‡
Lead poisoning	Crampy abdominal pain	Blood tests to measure the lead level
	Mental changes such as a reduced attention span, confusion, and altered behavior	
	Loss of appetite, vomiting, and constipation	
	Achy joints	
	Usually only in workers exposed to lead	
	More often in young children who live in houses over 30 years old, in which lead-based paint may have been used	
Porphyria	Recurring attacks of severe abdominal pain and vomiting	Urine and blood tests to check for substances (porphyrins) produced during the attacks
	Sometimes muscle weakness, seizures, and mental disturbances (such as irritation or agitation)	
	In some types of porphyria, blistering of the skin when exposed to sunlight	
Sickle cell disease	Severe episodes of abdominal pain lasting over a day	Blood tests to check for sickle-shaped red blood cells and for the abnormal hemoglobin that characterizes sickle cell disease
	Recurring pain in places other than the abdomen, such as the back, chest, arms, and/or legs	
	In black children who typically have family members with the disorder	

*Physical causes are responsible for only about 10% of cases of chronic abdominal pain. Most cases are functional abdominal pain.

†Features include symptoms and the results of the doctor's examination. Features mentioned are typical but not always present.

‡For most people with chronic abdominal pain, doctors typically do basic blood and urine tests such as a complete blood cell count, blood tests to evaluate how the liver and pancreas are functioning, and urinalysis. Other tests are done based on results of these tests and the examination.

CT = computed tomography; MRI = magnetic resonance imaging.

TESTING

Usually, doctors do certain tests. These tests include urinalysis, a complete blood cell count, blood tests to evaluate how the liver and pancreas are functioning, and a blood test to measure the erythrocyte sedimentation rate (ESR). The ESR is a general test to check for inflammation somewhere in the body. Usually if people are over 50, a colonoscopy is also recommended. Some doctors recommend computed tomography (CT) of the abdomen if people are under 50, but other doctors wait for specific symptoms to develop. Other tests are done depending on results of the history and physical examination (see Table on pages 7 to 10).

Additional tests are done if any test results are abnormal, if people develop new symptoms, or if new abnormalities are detected during the examination.

TREATMENT

Treatment depends on the cause. For example, if people have lactose intolerance, a lactose-free diet (eliminating milk and other dairy products) can help. If people are constipated, using a laxative for a few days plus adding fiber to the diet can help.

FUNCTIONAL PAIN

Treatment focuses on helping people return to normal daily activities and lessening the discomfort. Usually, treatment involves a combination of strategies. Several visits to the doctor may be needed to develop the best combination. Doctors often arrange follow-up visits every week, month, or 2 months, depending on people's needs. Visits are continued until well after the problem has resolved.

After functional pain is diagnosed, doctors emphasize that the pain, although real, does not have a serious cause and that stress and other psychologic factors can affect the body. Doctors try to avoid repeating tests after thorough testing has failed to show a physical cause of the symptoms.

Although there are no treatments to cure functional chronic abdominal pain, many helpful measures are available. These measures depend on a trusting, empathic relationship between the doctor, person, and person's family members. Doctors explain how the laboratory and other test results show that the person is not in danger. The doctor also explains how functional abdominal pain develops and how people perceive it. For example, they tend to feel pain when they are under stress. Doctors encourage people to participate in work, school, and social activities. Such participation does not worsen the condition but instead encourages independence and self-reliance. People who withdraw from their daily activities risk having their symptoms control their life rather than having their life control their symptoms.

Doctors recommend acetaminophen or other mild pain relievers to relieve the pain. A high-fiber diet and fiber supplements can also help. Many drugs have been tried with varying success. They include drugs that reduce or stop muscle spasms in the digestive tract (antispasmodics), peppermint oil, cyproheptadine (an antihistamine), and drugs that suppress acid production in the stomach.

Sources of stress or anxiety are minimized as much as possible. Parents and other family members should avoid reinforcing the pain by giving it too much attention. If people continue to feel anxious, doctors may prescribe antidepressants or drugs to reduce anxiety. Therapies that help people modify their behavior, such as relaxation training, biofeedback, and hypnosis, may also help reduce anxiety and help people better tolerate their pain.

For children, help from parents is essential. Parents are advised to encourage the child to become independent and to fulfill the child's normal responsibilities, particularly attending school. Allowing the child to avoid activities may actually increase the child's anxiety. Parents can help the child manage pain during daily activities by praising and rewarding the child's independent and responsible behaviors. For example, parents could reward the child by scheduling special time with the child or a special outing. Involving school personnel can help. Arrangements can be made to let the child rest briefly in the nurse's office during the school day, then return to class after 15 to 30 minutes. The school nurse can be authorized to give the child a mild pain reliever such as acetaminophen. The nurse can sometimes allow the child to call a parent, who should encourage the child to stay in school.

KEY POINTS

- Usually, chronic or recurring abdominal pain is functional pain, often related to stress, anxiety, or diet.
- Symptoms that require a doctor's immediate attention include a high fever, loss of appetite or weight, pain that awakens the person, blood in stool or urine, jaundice, and swelling of the legs and/or abdomen.
- Blood and urine tests are usually done to check for disorders that may cause the pain.
- Additional tests are needed only if people have abnormal test results, warning signs, or symptoms of a specific disorder.
- For functional pain, treatment involves learning to minimize stress, participating in normal daily activities, relieving pain (with mild pain relievers), sometimes taking drugs or using behavioral modification therapies to relieve anxiety, and/or altering the diet.

BACK PAIN

Low back pain is very common and becomes more common as people age, affecting more than half of people over 60. It is one of the most common reasons for health care visits. Low back pain is very costly in terms of health care payments, disability payments, and missed work. However, the number of back injuries in the workplace is decreasing, perhaps because people are more aware of the problem and preventive measures have improved.

The spine (spinal column) consists of back bones (vertebrae). The vertebrae are covered by a thin layer of cartilage and separated and cushioned by shock-absorbing disks made of jelly-like material and cartilage. They are held in place by ligaments and muscles, which include the following:

- Two iliopsoas muscles, which run along both sides of the spine
- Two erector spinae muscles, which run along the length of the spine behind it
- Many short paraspinal muscles, which run between the vertebrae

These muscles help stabilize the spine. The abdominal muscles, which run from the bottom of the rib cage to the pelvis, also help stabilize the spine by supporting the abdominal contents.

Enclosed in the spine is the spinal cord. Along the length of the spinal cord, the spinal nerves emerge through spaces between the vertebrae to connect with nerves throughout the body. The part of the spinal nerve nearest the spinal cord is called the spinal nerve root. Because of their position, spinal nerve roots can be squeezed (compressed) when the spine is injured, resulting in pain.

The lower (lumbar) spine connects the chest to the pelvis and legs, providing mobility—for turning, twisting, and bending. It also provides strength—for standing, walking, and lifting. Thus, the lower back is involved in almost all activities of daily living. Low back pain can limit many activities and reduce the quality of life.

TYPES

Common types of back pain include local, radiating, and referred pain.

Local pain occurs in a specific area of the lower back. It is the most common type of back pain. The cause is usually a muscle sprain, a strain, or another injury. The pain may be constant and aching or, at times, intermittent and sharp. Sudden pain may be felt when the cause is an injury. Local pain can be aggravated or relieved by changes in position. The lower back may be sore when touched. Muscle spasms may occur.

Radiating pain is dull, aching pain that travels from the lower back down the leg. It may be accompanied by sharp, intense pain. It typically involves only the side or back of the leg rather than the entire leg. The pain may travel all the way to the foot or only to the knee. Radiating pain typically indicates compression of a nerve root caused by disorders such as a herniated disk, osteoarthritis, or spinal stenosis. Coughing, sneezing, straining, or bending over while keeping the legs straight may trigger the pain. If pressure on the nerve root is great or if the spinal cord is also compressed, the pain may be accompanied by muscle weakness in the leg, a pins-and-needles sensation, or even loss of sensation and loss of bladder or bowel control (incontinence).

Referred pain is felt in a different location from the actual cause of the pain (see art box on page 32). For example, some people who have a heart attack feel pain in their left arm. Referred pain in the lower back tends to be deep and aching, and its exact location is hard to pinpoint. Typically, movement does not worsen it, unlike pain from a musculoskeletal disorder.

CAUSES

Most back pain is caused by disorders of the spine and the muscles, ligaments, and nerve roots around it or the disks between vertebrae. Often in such cases, no single specific cause can be identified. Whatever the cause, many factors such as fatigue, obesity, and lack of exercise can worsen back pain. Also, any painful disorder of the spine may cause reflex tightening (spasm) of muscles around the spine. This spasm worsens the existing pain. Stress may worsen low back pain, but how it does so is unclear.

Occasionally, back pain is due to disorders outside the spine, such as those of the kidneys and urinary tract, digestive tract, and blood vessels.

COMMON CAUSES

The most common cause of low back pain is

- Muscle strains and ligament sprains

Muscle strains and ligament sprains may result from lifting, exercising, or moving in an unexpected way (such as when falling or when in a car accident). In addition to snatching a heavy weight from the ground, strains and sprains may be caused by pushing against an opposing lineman in football, suddenly turning to dribble after a rebound in basketball, swinging a bat in baseball, or swinging a club in golf. The lower back is more likely to be injured when a person's physical conditioning is poor and the supporting muscles of the back are weak. Having poor posture, lifting incorrectly, being overweight, and being tired also contribute.

Other common causes of low back pain include

- Osteoarthritis
- Compression fractures
- A ruptured or herniated disk
- Lumbar spinal stenosis
- Spondylolisthesis
- Fibromyalgia

Osteoarthritis (degenerative arthritis) causes the cartilage that covers and protects the vertebrae to deteriorate. This disorder is thought to be due, at least in part, to the wear and tear of years of use. People who repetitively stress one joint or a group of joints are more likely to develop osteoarthritis. The disks between the vertebrae deteriorate, narrowing the spaces between them and often compressing spinal nerve roots. Irregular projections of bone (spurs) may develop on the vertebrae and compress spinal nerve roots. All of these changes can cause low back pain as well as stiffness.

Compression (crush) fractures commonly develop when bone density decreases because of osteoporosis, which typically develops as people age. Vertebrae are particularly susceptible to the effects of osteoporosis. Compression fractures (which sometimes cause sudden, severe back pain) can be accompanied by compression of spinal nerve roots (which may cause chronic back pain). However, most fractures

due to osteoporosis occur in the upper and middle back and cause upper and middle rather than low back pain.

A **ruptured or herniated disk** (see art box on page 14) can cause low back pain. A disk has a tough covering and a soft, jelly-like interior. If a disk is suddenly squeezed by the vertebrae above and below it (as when lifting a heavy object), the covering may tear (rupture), causing pain. The interior of the disk can squeeze through the tear in the covering, so that part of the interior bulges out (herniates). This bulge can compress, irritate, and even damage the spinal nerve root next to it, causing more pain. A ruptured or herniated disk also commonly causes sciatica (see art box on page 15).

Lumbar spinal stenosis is narrowing of the spinal canal (which runs through the center of the spine and contains the spinal cord) in the lower back. It is a common cause of low back pain in older people. Spinal stenosis also develops in middle-aged people who were born with a narrow spinal canal. It is caused by such disorders as osteoarthritis, spondylolisthesis, rheumatoid arthritis, ankylosing spondylitis, and Paget disease of bone. Spinal stenosis may cause sciatica as well as low back pain.

Spondylolisthesis is partial displacement of a vertebra in the lower back. It usually occurs in people who have a common bone birth defect (spondylolysis) that weakens part of the vertebrae. Usually, during adolescence or young adulthood (often in athletes), a minor injury causes a part of the vertebra to fracture. The vertebra then slips forward over the one below it. If it slips far, pain can result. Spondylolisthesis can also occur in older adults. People with spondylolisthesis are at risk of developing lumbar spinal stenosis.

Fibromyalgia is a common cause of body pain, sometimes including low back pain. This disorder causes chronic widespread (diffuse) pain in muscles and other soft tissues in areas outside the lower back.

LESS COMMON CAUSES

Less common causes that are serious include

- Spinal infections
- Spinal tumors
- A bulge (aneurysm) in the large artery in the abdomen (abdominal aortic aneurysm)
- Certain digestive disorders, such as a perforated peptic ulcer, diverticulitis, and pancreatitis

A HERNIATED DISK

The tough covering of a disk in the spine can tear (rupture), causing pain. The soft, jelly-like interior may then bulge out (herniate) through the covering, causing more pain. Pain occurs because the bulge puts pressure on the spinal nerve root next to it. Sometimes the nerve root becomes inflamed or is damaged.

More than 80% of herniated disks occur in the lower back. They are most common among people aged 30 to 50 years. Between these ages, the covering weakens. The jelly-like interior, which is under high pressure, may squeeze through a tear or a weakened spot in the covering and bulge out. After age 50, the interior of the disk begins to harden, making herniation less likely.

A disk may herniate because of a sudden, traumatic injury or repeated minor injuries. Being overweight or lifting heavy objects, particularly lifting incorrectly, increases the risk.

Often, herniated disks, even ones that appear obviously bulging or herniated on imaging tests such as magnetic resonance imaging (MRI) or computed tomography (CT), cause no symptoms. Herniated discs that do not cause symptoms are more common as people age. However, herniated disks may cause slight to debilitating pain. Movement often intensifies the pain.

Where the pain occurs depends on which disk is herniated and which spinal nerve root is affected. The pain may be felt along the pathway of the nerve compressed by the herniated disk. For example, a herniated disk commonly causes sciatica—pain along the sciatic nerve, down the back of the leg.

A herniated disk can also cause numbness and muscle weakness. If pressure on the nerve root is great, a leg may be paralyzed. Rarely, the disk can put pressure on the spinal cord itself, possibly causing weakness or paralysis of both legs. If the cauda equina (the bundle of nerves extending from the bottom of the cord) is affected, control of bladder and bowels can be lost. If these serious symptoms develop, medical attention is required immediately.

Most people recover without any treatment, usually within 3 months, but often much faster. Applying cold (such as ice packs) or heat (such as a heating pad) or using over-the-counter analgesics may help relieve the pain. Sometimes surgery to remove part or all the disk and part of a vertebra is necessary. In 10 to 20% of people who have surgery for sciatica due to a herniated disk, another disk ruptures.

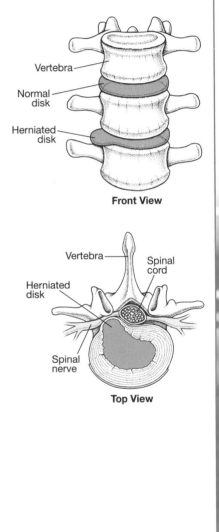

Front View

Top View

- Certain urinary tract disorders, such as kidney infections, kidney stones, and prostate infections
- Certain disorders involving the pelvis, such as ectopic pregnancy, pelvic inflammatory disease, and cancer of the ovaries or other reproductive organs

Less common causes that are not as serious include shingles and several types of inflammatory arthritis, such as ankylosing spondylitis.

WHAT IS SCIATICA?

The two sciatic nerves are the widest and longest nerves in the body. Each is almost as wide as a finger. On each side of the body, the sciatic nerve runs from the lower spine, behind the hip joint, down the buttock and back of the knee. There the sciatic nerve divides into several branches and continues to the foot. When the sciatic nerve is pinched, inflamed, or damaged, pain—sciatica—may radiate along the length of the sciatic nerve to the foot. Sciatica occurs in about 5% of people who have back pain.

In some people, no cause can be detected. In others, the cause may be a herniated disk, irregular projections of bone due to osteoarthritis, spinal stenosis, or swelling due to a sprained ligament. Rarely, Paget disease of bone, nerve damage due to diabetes (diabetic neuropathy), a tumor, or an accumulation of blood (hematoma) or pus (abscess) causes sciatica. Some people seem to be prone to sciatica.

Sciatica usually affects only one side. It may cause a pins-and-needles sensation, a nagging ache, or shooting pain. Numbness may be felt in the leg or foot. Walking, running, climbing stairs, straightening the leg, and sometimes coughing or straining worsens the pain, which is relieved by straightening the back or standing.

Often, the pain goes away on its own. Resting, sleeping on a firm mattress, taking over-the-counter acetaminophen or nonsteroidal anti-inflammatory drugs (NSAIDs), and applying heat and cold may be sufficient treatment. For many people, sleeping on their side with the knees bent and a pillow between the knees provides relief. Stretching the hamstring muscles gently after warming up may help.

Occasionally, other treatments are used, depending on the cause of sciatica. Treatments may include physical therapy, corticosteroids injected into the back, anticonvulsants, tricyclic depressants, and, for severe and persistent pain, surgery.

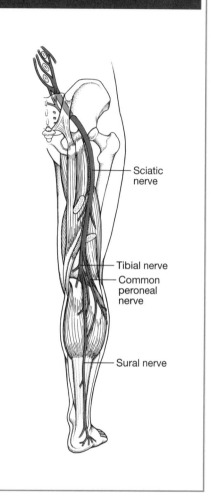

Sciatic nerve

Tibial nerve

Common peroneal nerve

Sural nerve

EVALUATION

The doctor aims to identify any serious disorders. Because low back pain is often caused by several problems, diagnosing a single cause may not be possible. Doctors may only be able to tell that the cause is a musculoskeletal disorder and is not serious.

WARNING SIGNS

In people with low back pain, certain symptoms and characteristics are cause for concern. They include

- A history of cancer
- Pain for more than 6 weeks

- Numbness, weakness in one or both legs, difficulty emptying the bladder (retention of urine), or loss of bladder or bowel control (incontinence)—symptoms that suggest nerve damage
- Fever
- Weight loss
- Severe pain at night
- Pain in people aged 55 or older without an obvious explanation (such as an injury)
- Use of drugs that suppress the immune system, HIV infection or AIDS, use of injected drugs, recent surgery, or a wound—conditions that increase the risk of infection

- Difficulty breathing, paleness, light-headedness, sudden sweating, a racing heartbeat, or loss of consciousness—symptoms that suggest an abdominal aortic aneurysm
- Vomiting, severe abdominal pain, or stool that is black or bloody—symptoms that suggest a digestive disorder
- Difficulty urinating, blood in the urine, or severe crampy pain on one side radiating into the groin—symptoms that suggest a urinary tract disorder

WHEN TO SEE A DOCTOR

People should see a doctor immediately if they have fever or symptoms suggesting nerve damage, an abdominal aortic aneurysm, a digestive disorder, or a urinary tract disorder. People with most other warning signs should see a doctor within a day. If pain is not severe and people have no warning signs other than pain for more than 6 weeks, they can wait several days to see a doctor.

WHAT THE DOCTOR DOES

Doctors first ask questions about the person's symptoms and medical history. Doctors then do a physical examination. What they find during the history and physical examination often suggests a cause and the tests that may need to be done (see Table on pages 17 to 18).

Doctors ask questions about the pain:

- What is the pain like?
- How severe is it?
- Where is it and where does it radiate?
- What relieves or worsens it (for example, changes in position or weight bearing)?
- When and how did it start?
- Are there other symptoms (such as numbness, weakness, retention of urine, or incontinence)?

Certain characteristics of the pain can give clues to possible causes:

- Pain in an area that is tender to the touch and is worsened by changes in position or weight bearing is usually local pain.
- Pain on only one side of the back probably does not involve the spine.
- Pain that radiates down the leg, such as sciatica (see art box on page 15), is usually caused by compression of a spinal nerve root.
- Pain that is moderate or severe, is not affected by changes in position of the back,

and is not accompanied by tenderness may be referred pain.

- Pain that is constant, severe, progressively worse, and unrelieved by rest, particularly if it keeps the person awake at night, may indicate cancer or an infection.

The physical examination focuses on the spine and on evaluation of the nerves to the groin and legs to look for signs of nerve root compression. Signs of nerve root compression include weakness of one of the muscle groups in a leg, abnormal reflexes (tested by tapping the tendons below the knee and behind the ankle), decreased sensation in the groin area, retention of urine, and incontinence of urine or stool.

Doctors may ask the person to move in certain ways to determine the type of pain. For example, they may ask the person to lie flat, then lift the leg without bending the knee, and then stand and bend over. Doctors may also check a person's abdomen for tenderness or a mass, particularly in people over 55, who may have an aortic aneurysm. They examine the prostate in men by doing a digital rectal examination and the internal reproductive organs in women by doing a pelvic examination.

With information about the pain, the person's medical history, and results of a physical examination, doctors may be able to determine as much as is necessary about the cause.

TESTING

Usually, no tests are needed because most back pain results from strains and sprains or other minor musculoskeletal disorders and resolves within 6 weeks. Imaging tests are often needed if

- Another cause is suspected.
- Warning signs are present.
- Back pain persists.

X-rays of the lower back show only the bones. They can help detect degenerative changes due to osteoarthritis, compression fractures, spondylolisthesis, and ankylosing spondylitis. However, magnetic resonance imaging (MRI) or computed tomography (CT) provides clearer images of bones and, particularly MRI, can show soft tissues (including disks and some nerves). MRI or CT is usually necessary when doctors are checking for disorders that cause subtle changes in

SOME CAUSES AND FEATURES OF LOW BACK PAIN

Cause	Common Features*	Tests†
Common causes		
Sprains and strains	Pain that ■ Often occurs on one or both sides of the spine ■ Worsens with movement and lessens with rest ■ Typically develops while lifting, bending, or twisting	A doctor's examination
Osteoarthritis, sometimes with compression of a spinal nerve root	Pain in the middle of the back that sometimes ■ Travels down a leg ■ Is accompanied by numbness and/or weakness ■ Is worsened by coughing, sneezing, or straining Usually in older people with pain and/or deformities in other joints	X-rays
Compression fractures	Pain in the middle of the back, sometimes starting suddenly Usually in people who are older or who have osteoporosis	X-rays
A herniated disk, usually with compression of a spinal nerve root	Pain in the middle of the back that usually ■ Travels down a leg ■ Is accompanied by numbness and/or weakness ■ Is worsened by coughing, sneezing, straining, or leaning forward	A doctor's examination Sometimes MRI or CT
Lumbar spinal stenosis	Pain in the middle of the back that ■ Is worsened by straightening the back (as when walking or leaning back) ■ Is relieved by leaning forward ■ May travel down one leg or both legs Usually in older adults	A doctor's examination Sometimes MRI
Spondylolisthesis, sometimes with compression of a spinal nerve root	Pain in the middle of the back that sometimes ■ Travels down a leg ■ Is accompanied by numbness and/or weakness ■ Is worsened by coughing, sneezing, or straining Often in adolescent or young adult athletes after a minor injury or in older adults	X-rays
Fibromyalgia	Aching and stiffness in many areas of the body (not just the lower back) Sore areas that are tender to the touch Often poor sleep Most common among women aged 20 to 50	A doctor's examination

(continued)

SOME CAUSES AND FEATURES OF LOW BACK PAIN *(continued)*

Cause	Common Features*	Tests†
Less common causes		
Ankylosing spondylitis (inflammation of the spine and large joints)	Stiffness, often worse immediately after awakening	X-rays
	Progressive loss of back flexibility, often causing the back to hunch forward	Blood tests
	Sometimes a painful red eye and/or pain in other joints	
	Often in young men	
Compression of the spinal cord	Pain in the middle of the back	MRI
	Numbness and weakness of usually both legs	
Cauda equina syndrome	Numbness in the groin and around the anus	MRI
	Loss of bladder and/or bowel control (incontinence)	
Shingles	Pain in a strip of skin on either the right or left side, but not both	A doctor's examination
	Usually blisters that develop on the painful strip of skin a few days after the pain starts	
Cancer	Progressively worsening pain, regardless of position or activity	Usually x-rays
	Sometimes loss of appetite and/or weight	MRI or CT
Infection	Progressively worsening, constant pain, regardless of position or activity	Usually x-rays
■ In the vertebrae (osteomyelitis)	Sometimes fever and/or night sweats	MRI or CT
■ In the disk (diskitis)	Often in people who have had back surgery, who have an immune disorder, who take drugs that suppress the immune system, or who use IV drugs	Blood tests
■ Around the spinal cord (spinal epidural abscess)		

*Features include symptoms and results of the doctor's examination. Features mentioned are typical but not always present.
†If pain resolves without treatment and no warning signs are present, testing may not be necessary.
CT = computed tomography; IV = intravenous; MRI = magnetic resonance imaging.

bone and disorders of soft tissue. For example, MRI or CT can confirm or exclude the diagnosis of a herniated disk, spinal stenosis, cancer, and usually infection. These tests can also indicate whether nerves are being compressed.

If compression of the spinal cord is suspected, MRI is done immediately. Rarely, when results of MRI are unclear, myelography with CT is required. Rarely, if cancer or infection is suspected, removal of tissue (biopsy) is necessary. Occasionally, electromyography and nerve conduction studies are done to confirm the presence, location, and sometimes duration and severity of nerve root compression.

PREVENTION

The most effective way to prevent low back pain is to exercise regularly. Aerobic exercise and specific muscle-strengthening and stretching exercises can help.

Aerobic exercise, such as swimming and walking, improves general fitness and generally strengthens muscles.

Specific exercises to strengthen and stretch the muscles in the abdomen, buttocks, and back (core muscles) can help stabilize the spine and decrease strain on the disks that cushion the spine and the ligaments that hold it in place.

Muscle-strengthening exercises include pelvic tilts and abdominal curls. Stretching exercises include the sitting leg stretch and knee-to-chest stretch. Stretching exercises can increase back pain in some people and therefore should be done carefully. As a general rule, any exercise that causes or increases back pain should be stopped. Exercises should be repeated until the muscles feel mildly but not completely fatigued. Breathing during each exercise is important. People who have back pain should consult a doctor before beginning to exercise.

Exercise can also help people maintain a desirable weight. Weight-bearing exercise can help people maintain bone density. Thus, exercise may reduce the risk of developing two conditions that can lead to low back pain—obesity and osteoporosis.

Maintaining good posture when standing and sitting reduces stress on the back. Slouching should be avoided. Chair seats can be adjusted to a height that allows the feet to be flat on the floor, with the knees bent up slightly and the lower back flat against the back of the chair. If a chair does not support the lower back, a pillow can be used behind the lower back. Sitting with the feet on the floor rather than with the legs crossed is advised. People should avoid standing or sitting for long periods. If prolonged standing or sitting

---

EXERCISES TO PREVENT LOW BACK PAIN

Pelvic Tilts

Lie on the back with the knees bent, the heels on the floor, and the weight on the heels. Press the small of the back against the floor, contract the buttocks (raising them about half an inch from the floor), and contract the abdominal muscles. Hold this position for a count of 10. Repeat 20 times.

Abdominal Curls

Lie on the back with the knees bent and feet on the floor. Place the hands across the chest. Contract the abdominal muscles, slowly raising the shoulders about 10 inches from the floor while keeping the head back (the chin should not touch the chest). Then release the abdominal muscles, slowly lowering the shoulders. Do 3 sets of 10.

Knee-to-Chest Stretch

Lie flat on the back. Place both hands behind one knee and bring it to the chest. Hold for a count of 10. Slowly lower that leg and repeat with the other leg. Do this exercise 10 times.

Sitting Leg Stretch

Sit on the floor with the knees straight but slightly flexed (not locked) and the legs as far apart as possible. Place both hands on the same knee. Slowly slide both hands toward the ankle. Stop if pain is felt, and go no farther than a position that can be held comfortably for 10 seconds. Slowly return to a sitting position. Repeat with the other leg. Do this exercise 10 times for each leg.

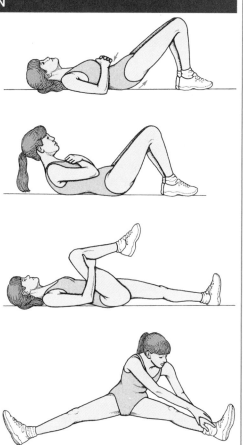

is unavoidable, changing positions frequently may reduce stress on the back.

Sleeping in a comfortable position on a firm mattress is recommended. People who sleep on their back can place a pillow under their knees. People who sleep on their side should use a pillow to support their head in a neutral position (not tilted down toward the bed or up toward the ceiling). They should place another pillow between their knees with their hips and knees bent slightly.

Learning to lift correctly helps prevent back injury. The hips should be aligned with the shoulders (that is, not rotated to one side or the other). People should not bend over with their legs nearly straight and reach out with their arms to pick up an object. Instead, they should bend at the hips and knees. Bending this way keeps the back straighter and brings the arms down to the object with the elbows at the side. Then, keeping the object close to the body, they lift the object by straightening their legs. This way, the legs, not the back, lift the object. Lifting an object over the head or twisting while lifting increases the risk of back injury.

Stopping smoking is also recommended.

TREATMENT

If a specific cause can be diagnosed, that disorder is treated. For example, antibiotics are used to treat a prostate infection. However, there is no specific treatment for musculoskeletal pain due to sprains or strains nor for many other musculoskeletal causes. But many general measures can help. Usually, these general measures are also used when a spinal nerve root is compressed.

GENERAL MEASURES

Measures include

- Modifying activities
- Taking drugs that relieve pain
- Applying heat or cold to the painful area
- Doing exercises

For low back pain that has recently developed, treatment begins with avoiding activities that stress the spine and cause pain—such as lifting heavy objects and bending. Bed rest does not hasten the resolution of the pain, and most experts recommend continued light activity.

Bed rest, if required to relieve severe pain, should last no more than 1 or 2 days. Longer bed rest weakens the core muscles and increases stiffness, thus worsening back pain and prolonging recovery. Spinal corsets and traction are not helpful. Traction may delay recovery.

Acetaminophen is usually recommended for pain relief unless inflammation is present. If inflammation is present, over-the-counter or prescription nonsteroidal anti-inflammatory drugs (NSAIDs) can relieve pain and reduce inflammation. If acetaminophen or NSAIDs do not provide sufficient pain relief, opioid analgesics may be required.

Muscle relaxants, such as carisoprodol, cyclobenzaprine, diazepam, metaxalone, or methocarbamol, are sometimes given to relieve muscle spasms, but their usefulness is controversial. These drugs are not recommended for older people, who are more likely to have side effects.

Application of heat or cold may help. Cold is usually preferred to heat during the first 2 days after an injury. Ice and cold packs should not be applied directly to the skin. They should be enclosed (for example, in plastic) and placed over a towel or cloth. The ice is removed after 20 minutes, then reapplied for 20 minutes over a period of 60 to 90 minutes. This process can be repeated several times during the first 24 hours. Heat, using a heating pad, can be applied for the same periods of time. Because the skin on the back may be insensitive to heat, heating pads must be used cautiously to prevent burns. People should not use a heating pad at bedtime to avoid the risk of falling asleep with the pad still on their back.

Massage may speed the resolution of musculoskeletal pain due to muscle spasm, strains, or sprains. Some studies suggest that acupuncture may have similar benefits, but others suggest little or no benefit. Spinal manipulation, done by chiropractors or some other doctors (such as osteopathic doctors), may also speed the resolution of pain due to muscle spasm, strains, or sprains. However, it may have risks for people with osteoporosis or a herniated disk.

After the pain has subsided, light activity, as recommended by a doctor or physical therapist, can speed healing and recovery. Specific exercises to strengthen and stretch the back and to strengthen core muscles are usually recommended to help prevent low back pain from becoming chronic or recurring.

Other preventive measures (maintaining good posture, using a firm mattress with appropriately placed pillows, lifting correctly, and stopping smoking) should be continued or started. In response to these measures, most episodes of back pain resolve in several days to 2 weeks. Regardless of treatment, 80 to 90% of such episodes resolve within 6 weeks.

TREATMENT OF CHRONIC PAIN

Additional measures are needed for chronic low back pain. Aerobic exercise may help, and weight reduction, if necessary, is advised. If analgesics are ineffective, other treatments can be considered.

Transcutaneous electrical nerve stimulation (TENS) may be used. The TENS device produces a gentle tingling sensation by generating a low oscillating current. This current can block transmission of some pain sensation from the spinal cord to the brain. The current can be applied to the painful area several times a day for 20 minutes to several hours at a time, depending on the severity of the pain.

Sometimes a corticosteroid (such as dexamethasone or methylprednisolone) plus a local anesthetic (such as lidocaine) can be periodically injected into the epidural space—between the spine and the outer layer of tissue covering the spinal cord. These injections are more effective for sciatica caused by a herniated disk than for lumbar spinal stenosis. However, they are usually effective only for several days to weeks. Their main use is to relieve pain enough that an exercise program, which can provide long-term pain relief, can be started.

SURGERY FOR BACK PAIN

If a herniated disk is causing relentless or chronic sciatica, weakness, loss of sensation, or loss of bladder and bowel control, surgical removal of the disk (diskectomy) and sometimes part of the vertebra (laminectomy) may be necessary. A general anesthetic is usually required. The hospital stay is usually 1 or 2 days. Often, microsurgical techniques, with a small incision and regional spinal anesthesia (which numbs only a specific part of the body), can be used to remove the herniated portion of the disk. Hospitalization is not required. However, when the incision is small, the surgeon may not be able to see and therefore may not remove all fragments of the herniated disk. After either procedure, most people can resume all of their activities in a few weeks. More than 90% of people recover fully.

For severe spinal stenosis, a large part of a vertebra may be surgically removed to widen the spinal canal. A general anesthetic is usually required. The hospital stay is usually 4 or 5 days. People may need 3 to 4 months before they can resume all of their activities. About two thirds of people have a good or full recovery. For most of the rest, such surgery prevents symptoms from worsening.

When the spine is unstable (as may result from severe osteoarthritis), surgery can be done to fuse vertebrae together. However, fusion decreases mobility and may put additional stress on the rest of the spine.

O—π KEY POINTS

- Low back pain is very common and usually caused by a musculoskeletal disorder of the spine plus other factors, such as fatigue, obesity, and lack of exercise.
- In young people, low back pain is rarely serious, and testing is usually unnecessary unless symptoms persist for weeks.
- People who have warning signs or who are older than age 55 should see a doctor without delay.
- Strengthening abdominal and back muscles can help prevent the most common types of low back pain.
- For most low back pain, avoiding activities that stress the back, taking pain relievers, and sometimes applying ice or heat are sufficient treatment.
- Prolonged bed rest and traction can delay recovery.

BAD BREATH
(HALITOSIS)

Bad breath (halitosis) is a frequent or persistent unpleasant odor to the breath.

Certain diseases produce substances that are detectable on the breath, but these odors are typically mild and not considered bad breath. Liver failure gives the breath a mousy or sometimes faintly rotten egg–like (sulfurous) odor. Kidney failure makes the breath smell like urine or ammonia. Severe, uncontrolled diabetes makes the breath smell like nail polish remover (acetone).

CAUSES

Most bad breath is caused by problems in the mouth. Causes that contribute to bad breath are listed in the Table on page 23).

COMMON CAUSES

The most common causes of bad breath are

- Periodontal diseases
- Odor-causing bacteria on the tongue
- Certain foods and alcoholic beverages
- Tobacco use

Bad breath is most often caused by the action of certain mouth bacteria on food particles in the mouth. These bacteria break down (ferment) the food particles into foul-smelling substances. These bacteria are more common among people with periodontal diseases (such as gingivitis and periodontitis) and poor oral hygiene.

Periodontal diseases inflame and destroy the structures surrounding and supporting the teeth, such as the gums and the outer layer of the tooth root, and are caused mainly by an accumulation of certain bacteria. These bacteria grow in deep pockets that surround the teeth. These bacteria can also grow on the back of the tongue, even in people who do not have periodontal disease.

These bacteria can also overgrow due to a decrease in the flow of saliva (caused by some diseases or the use of certain drugs—see Mouth, Dry on page 270) or a decrease in the acidity of saliva.

After digestion, odors caused by certain foods or spices, such as onions or garlic, pass from the bloodstream into the lungs. The odors are then exhaled and may be unpleasant to others. For example, the odor of garlic can be smelled on the breath by others 2 or 3 hours after it is eaten, long after it is gone from the mouth and stomach. Oral hygiene cannot remove these odors.

Bad breath is more common among smokers than nonsmokers.

LESS COMMON CAUSES

Less common causes of bad breath include

- Infections in the sinuses or lungs
- Cancer of the nasal passages, mouth, or throat
- Foreign object in the nose (typically in children)
- Imagined halitosis (psychogenic halitosis)

Although people commonly think that gastrointestinal (GI) disorders cause bad breath, they rarely do because the muscular channel that connects the throat with the stomach (esophagus) is normally collapsed. Bad breath is not caused by poor digestion, nor does it indicate how a person's digestive system or bowels are functioning. However, rarely, a pouch in the esophagus (Zenker diverticulum), present at birth, can collect food particles. The food particles can decompose and create a foul odor.

Bad breath that is imagined is called psychogenic halitosis. People believe that their breath smells bad when it actually does not. This problem may occur in people who tend to exaggerate normal body sensations or in people who have a serious mental disorder, such as schizophrenia. Some people with obsessive thoughts have an overwhelming sense of feeling dirty and believe that their breath smells bad.

EVALUATION

Bad breath rarely requires an immediate evaluation by a doctor or dentist. The following information can help people decide whether an evaluation is needed and help them know what to expect during the evaluation.

WARNING SIGNS

Certain symptoms and characteristics are cause for concern. They include

- Fever

SOME CAUSES AND FEATURES OF BAD BREATH

Cause	Common Features*	Tests
Disorders in the mouth (oral)		
Bacteria on the back of the tongue	Unpleasant-smelling tongue scrapings Healthy gums and teeth	A doctor's or dentist's examination
Periodontal disorders, such as gingivitis and periodontitis	Affected gums and teeth noted during the examination In people with a history of poor oral hygiene	A dentist's examination
Cancers of the mouth (most are identified during a doctor's or dentist's examination long before they cause bad odors)	Usually identified during the examination More common among older people, who often have an extensive history of using alcohol and/or tobacco	Biopsy, CT, or MRI
Disorders outside the mouth (extraoral)		
A foreign object (body) in the nose†	Often a pus-filled or bloody discharge from the nose Seen during the examination Usually in children	A doctor's examination Sometimes imaging
Cancer of the nasal passages and upper throat†	Discomfort when swallowing	A doctor's examination
Lung infections, such as a lung abscess, bronchiectasis, or an infection caused by an inhaled foreign object	Cough that produces blood or sputum (phlegm) Fevers	Chest x-ray Cultures of sputum Sometimes CT or bronchoscopy
Imagined halitosis (psychogenic halitosis)	Unpleasant smell not detected by others Often in people known to exaggerate other normal body sensations	A doctor's examination Sometimes a consultation with a psychologist
Sinus infection†	A pus-filled discharge from the nose Face pain, headache, or both	A doctor's examination Sometimes CT
Zenker diverticulum	Spitting up of undigested food (regurgitation) when lying down or bending over	Video of the upper digestive tract after barium is given by mouth (barium swallow)
Swallowed or inhaled substances		
Alcoholic beverages, garlic, onions, tobacco	Apparent based on the person's history Diagnosed after the doctor's examination rules out other causes	A doctor's examination Avoidance of the substance to see if symptoms go away

*Features include symptoms and the results of a doctor's or dentist's examination. Features mentioned are typical but not always present.
†The odor is typically more noticeable from the nose than from the mouth.
CT = computed tomography; MRI = magnetic resonance imaging.

- Pus-filled (purulent) sputum or discharge from the nose
- Visible or touchable lesions in the mouth

People who have fever or purulent sputum or nasal discharge or who may have inhaled a foreign body should see a doctor right away. Those who discover a lesion in their mouth should see a doctor within several days.

People with bad breath but no warning signs and who otherwise feel well should see a dentist nonurgently.

Doctors first ask questions about the person's symptoms and medical history. Doctors then do a physical examination. What they find during the history and physical examination often suggests a cause of the bad breath and the tests that may need to be done (see Table on page 23).

The sniff test is a helpful part of the examination that can help tell whether the bad odor is coming from a nose or sinus disorder versus a mouth or lung disorder. The person exhales about 4 inches (about 10 centimeters) away from the doctor's nose, first through the mouth with the nose pinched shut and then through the nose with the mouth closed. If the odor is worse through the mouth, the cause most likely originates in the mouth. If the odor is worse through the nose, the cause most likely originates in the nose or sinuses. If the odor is similar from both the nose and the mouth, the cause most likely originates from another part of the body or the lungs. If the examiner is unable to tell where the cause originates, the back of the tongue is scraped with a plastic spoon. After 5 seconds, the spoon is sniffed. A bad odor on the spoon shows that the likely problem is bacteria on the tongue.

The need for testing depends on what the doctor finds during the history and physical examination, particularly whether warning signs are present. Some specialists who focus on bad breath have unusual testing equipment such as portable sulfur monitors, gas chromatography, and chemical tests for tongue scrapings. Such testing is rarely needed except for medical research.

The doctor may suggest that people whose symptoms seem to be related to ingested or inhaled substances avoid the suspected substances for a period of time to see whether the symptoms go away (trial of avoidance).

Once diagnosed, any causes of bad breath are treated.

Physical causes can be removed or corrected. For example, people can stop eating garlic, onions, and other odor-producing food and stop smoking. If the cause is oral, people should see a dentist for professional cleaning and treatment of periodontal diseases and cavities. At home, people should improve their daily oral hygiene routine, including thorough flossing, toothbrushing, and brushing of the top and back of the tongue with the toothbrush or a tongue scraper. Many deodorant mouthwashes and sprays are available, but these are of limited benefit. The effects of most of these products do not last more than 20 minutes.

People with psychogenic halitosis may need to see a psychologist.

Older people are more likely to take drugs that cause dry mouth, which leads to difficulties with oral hygiene and hence to bad breath, but are otherwise not more likely to have halitosis. Also, oral cancers are more common with aging and are more of a concern among older than younger people.

- Most bad breath is caused by fermentation of food particles by bacteria in the mouth.
- Disorders outside the mouth may cause bad breath but are often recognizable based on findings during a doctor's or dentist's examination.
- Bad breath is not caused by poor digestion, nor does it indicate how a person's digestive system or bowels are functioning.
- The effects of mouthwashes do not last very long.

BREAST LUMPS

A breast lump is a thickening or bump that feels different from surrounding breast tissue. A lump may be discovered in a breast incidentally, during a breast self-examination, or during a routine physical examination by a doctor.

Lumps in the breasts are relatively common and usually not cancerous.

Lumps may be painless or painful. They are sometimes accompanied by nipple discharge (see Nipple Discharge on page 308) or changes in the skin, such as irregularities, redness, a dimpled texture (called peau d'orange, or skin of an orange), or tightened skin. Lumps may be fluid-filled sacs (cysts) or solid masses, which are usually fibroadenomas. Fibroadenomas are not cancerous, and cysts usually are not.

CAUSES

COMMON CAUSES

The most common causes include

- Fibroadenomas
- Fibrocystic changes

Fibroadenomas are typically painless lumps that feel like small, slippery marbles. They usually develop in young women, especially adolescents. These lumps may be mistaken for cancer, but they are not.

Fibrocystic changes include pain, cysts, and general lumpiness (including fibroadenomas) in the breast. Women may have one or more of these symptoms. Breasts feel lumpy and dense and are often tender when touched.

In most women, fibrocystic changes are related to the monthly fluctuations in levels of the female hormones estrogen and progesterone. These hormones stimulate breast tissue.

Most fibrocystic changes do not increase the risk of breast cancer. A few of them do, but only slightly.

OTHER CAUSES

Lumps sometimes result from

- Breast infections, including collections of pus (abscesses)

- A clogged milk gland (galactocele), which usually occurs 6 to 10 months after breast-feeding stops
- Injuries, which can result in the formation of scar tissue
- Cancer

Infections, galactoceles, and scar tissue formation do not increase the risk of breast cancer.

EVALUATION

The following information can help people decide whether a doctor's evaluation is needed and help them know what to expect during the evaluation.

WARNING SIGNS

Certain symptoms and characteristics are cause for concern:

- A lump that is stuck to the skin or chest wall
- A lump that is hard and irregular in texture
- Dimpling of skin near the lump
- Lymph nodes in the armpit that are matted together or stuck to the skin or chest wall
- A bloody nipple discharge

WHEN TO SEE A DOCTOR

Because breast lumps may be cancerous (although they seldom are), they should be evaluated by a doctor within about 3 to 7 days.

Delay of a week or so is not harmful unless there are signs of infection such as redness, swelling, and/or a discharge of pus. Women with such symptoms should see a doctor within 1 or 2 days.

WHAT THE DOCTOR DOES

Doctors ask the woman questions about the lump and other symptoms, including general symptoms such as weight loss, fatigue, and bone pain (which may indicate advanced cancer). Doctors also ask the woman about her medical and family history, including risk factors for breast cancer.

Doctors then do a physical examination, focusing on the breasts and areas near it. Painful, rubbery lumps in younger women are usually fibrocystic changes, particularly if the woman has had similar lumps before. Doctors determine whether the breasts are similar in shape and size and check each breast for abnormalities, particularly warning signs. Cancer is more likely if warning signs are present.

TESTING

Usually, testing is needed because determining whether breast lumps are cancerous or not during a physical examination is difficult and because failing to identify cancer has serious consequences.

Ultrasonography is typically done first to try to differentiate solid lumps from cysts, which are rarely cancerous.

If the lump appears to be a cyst, a needle with a syringe is often inserted into the cyst, and the fluid is removed (called aspiration) and examined. The fluid is tested for cancer cells if it is bloody, if little fluid is obtained, or if the lump remains after aspiration. Otherwise, the woman is checked again in 4 to 8 weeks. If the cyst cannot be felt, it is considered noncancerous. If it recurs, aspiration is done again, and the fluid is sent for analysis regardless of appearance. If the fluid in the cyst suggests cancer or if the cyst recurs a third time, biopsy is done.

If the lump appears to be solid, mammography is typically done, followed by a biopsy. Most women do not need to be hospitalized for these procedures. Usually, only a local anesthetic is needed.

TREATMENT

Treatment depends on the cause. For fibrocystic changes, wearing a soft, supportive bra and taking pain relievers, such as acetaminophen or a nonsteroidal anti-inflammatory drug (NSAID), may help relieve symptoms.

Sometimes cysts are drained. Fibroadenomas can usually be removed. However, they may recur.

KEY POINTS

- Most breast lumps are not cancer.
- Because noncancerous and cancerous lumps are hard to tell apart during an examination, testing is usually done.

BRUISING AND BLEEDING

Bruising or bleeding after an injury is normal. However, some people have disorders that cause them to bruise or bleed too easily. Sometimes people bleed without any obvious triggering event or injury. Spontaneous bleeding may occur in almost any part of the body, but it is most common in the nose and mouth and the digestive tract. People with hemophilia often bleed into their joints or muscles. Most often, bleeding is minor, but it can be severe enough to be life-threatening. However, even minor bleeding is dangerous if it occurs in the brain.

Several symptoms may suggest that a person has a bleeding disorder:

- Unexplained nosebleeds (epistaxis)
- Excessive or prolonged menstrual blood flow (menorrhagia)
- Prolonged bleeding after minor cuts, blood drawing, minor surgical or dental procedures, or tooth brushing or flossing
- Unexplained skin marks, including tiny red or purple dots (petechiae), red or purple patches (purpura), bruises (ecchymoses), or small blood vessels that are widened and therefore visible in the skin or mucous membranes (telangiectasias)

Sometimes a laboratory test done for some other reason shows the person has a susceptibility to bleeding.

CAUSES

Three things are needed to help injured blood vessels stop bleeding: platelets (cell-like blood particles that help in blood clotting), blood clotting factors (proteins largely produced by the liver that are required for blood clotting), and blood vessel narrowing (constriction). An abnormality in any of these factors can lead to excessive bleeding or bruising:

- Platelet disorders, including too few platelets (thrombocytopenia), too many platelets, and defective platelet function
- Decreased activity of blood clotting factors (for example, due to hemophilia, liver

disorders, or vitamin K deficiency or to the use of certain drugs)
- Defects in blood vessels

Platelet disorders first cause small red or purple dots on the skin. Later, if the disorder becomes severe, bleeding may occur. A decrease in blood clotting factors usually causes bleeding and bruising. Defects in blood vessels usually cause red or purple spots and patches on the skin, rather than bleeding.

COMMON CAUSES

Overall, the most common causes of easy bleeding include

- Severe platelet deficiency
- Use of drugs that inhibit clotting (anticoagulants) such as warfarin or heparin
- Liver disease (causing inadequate production of clotting factors)

Platelet deficiency can be due to inadequate production of platelets by the bone marrow or excessive destruction of platelets (for example, by an enlarged spleen or certain drugs or infections). People who have a tendency to form blood clots may take drugs such as heparin or warfarin to decrease that tendency. However, sometimes these drugs decrease the body's clotting ability too much, and people have bleeding and/or bruising. Because the liver helps to regulate blood clotting, people with liver disease (for example, hepatitis or cirrhosis) also have a tendency to bleed easily.

Most commonly, easy or excessive bruising occurs because the skin and blood vessels are fragile. Women and older people of both sexes are more commonly affected. Bruises tend to develop on the thighs, buttocks, and upper arms. However, people have no other symptoms of excessive bleeding, and blood test results are normal. This condition is not serious, and no treatment is needed.

LESS COMMON CAUSES

Hemophilia A and hemophilia B are hereditary disorders in which the body does not make enough of one of the clotting factors. People have excessive bleeding into deep tissues such as muscles, joints, and the back of the abdominal cavity, usually following minor trauma. Bleeding may occur in the brain, which can be fatal.

Uncommonly, certain disorders trigger the clotting system throughout the body. Instead of causing blood clots everywhere, platelets and clotting factors are quickly used up and bleeding occurs. This disorder, called disseminated intravascular coagulation (DIC), can be triggered by many conditions, including severe infections, severe injury, labor and delivery, and certain cancers. People with DIC are usually already in a hospital. They bleed excessively from needle punctures and often have significant digestive tract bleeding.

SOME CAUSES OF EXCESSIVE BLEEDING

Cause	Examples
Platelet disorders	
Decreased number of platelets	Aplastic anemia
	Cirrhosis if the spleen is enlarged
	DIC if it progresses rapidly
	Drugs that can trigger destruction of platelets (such as heparin, quinidine, quinine, sulfonamides, sulfonylureas, or rifampin)
	Hemolytic-uremic syndrome
	HIV infection
	Immune thrombocytopenia
	Leukemia
	Thrombotic thrombocytopenic purpura
Increased number of platelets (which often causes excessive clotting but sometimes causes excessive bleeding)	Primary thrombocythemia
Inadequate platelet function	Drugs that can cause platelets to malfunction (such as aspirin or other NSAIDs)
	Kidney failure
	Multiple myeloma
	Von Willebrand disease
Clotting disorders	
Acquired	Anticoagulants (drugs that inhibit clotting) such as warfarin or heparin
	DIC if it progresses slowly
	Liver disease
	Vitamin K deficiency
Hereditary	Hemophilia
Blood vessel disorders	
Acquired	Immunoglobulin A–associated vasculitis (Henoch-Schönlein purpura)
	Vitamin C deficiency
Hereditary	Connective tissue disorders (such as Marfan syndrome)
	Hereditary hemorrhagic telangiectasia

DIC = disseminated intravascular coagulation; HIV = human immunodeficiency virus; NSAIDs = nonsteroidal anti-inflammatory drugs.

EVALUATION

Doctors first try to establish whether the person's symptoms actually represent easy or excessive bleeding. If so, they look for possible causes. The following information can help people know when to see a doctor and help them know what to expect during the evaluation.

WARNING SIGNS

In people with easy bruising or bleeding, certain symptoms and characteristics are cause for concern. They include

- Symptoms of serious blood loss, such as sweating, weakness, faintness or dizziness, nausea, or extreme thirst
- Pregnancy or recent delivery
- Signs of infection, such as fever, chills, diarrhea, or feeling ill all over
- Headache, confusion, or other sudden symptoms related to the brain or nervous system

WHEN TO SEE A DOCTOR

People with warning signs should see a doctor right away, as should those who are still bleeding and those who have lost more than a small amount of blood. People without warning signs who notice that they bleed or bruise easily should call their doctor. The doctor determines how quickly to evaluate people based on their symptoms and other factors. Typically, people who do not feel well or have risk factors for bleeding, such as liver disease or use of certain drugs, or who have a family history of a bleeding disorder should be seen within a day or two. People who feel well but had a few nosebleeds that stopped on their own or who have bruises or spots on their skin can be seen when practical. A delay of a week or so is unlikely to be harmful.

WHAT THE DOCTOR DOES

Doctors first ask questions about the person's symptoms and medical history. Doctors then do a physical examination. What they find during the history and physical examination sometimes suggests a cause of the bleeding or bruising, but typically tests need to be done.

Doctors ask about types of bleeding, including frequent nosebleeds, gum bleeding while tooth brushing, coughing up blood (hemoptysis),

blood in stool or urine, or dark tarry stool (melena). They also ask about other symptoms, including abdominal pain and diarrhea (suggesting a digestive disorder), joint pain (suggesting a connective tissue disorder), and lack of menstrual periods and morning sickness (suggesting pregnancy). They ask about whether the person is taking drugs (such as heparin or warfarin) that are known to increase the risk of bleeding. Easy bleeding in a person taking warfarin, especially if the dose has recently increased, is likely due to the drug. Doctors also ask if the person has a condition that is likely to cause a problem with blood clotting, such as

- Severe infection, cancer, liver disease (such as cirrhosis or hepatitis), human immunodeficiency virus (HIV) infection, pregnancy, systemic lupus erythematosus (lupus), or kidney failure
- Prior excessive or unusual bleeding or transfusions
- Family history of excessive bleeding

People are asked about use of alcohol or intravenous (IV) drugs. Heavy alcohol use is a risk factor for liver disease, and IV drug use is a risk factor for HIV infection.

People with a family history of excessive bleeding are likely to have an inherited bleeding disorder such as hereditary hemorrhagic telangiectasia, hemophilia, or von Willebrand disease. However, not all people with these disorders know about a family history of the disorder.

During the physical examination, doctors check vital signs (temperature, blood pressure, and heart rate). These signs can give an early indication of serious disorders, especially low blood volume or an infection.

They examine the skin and mucous membranes (nose, mouth, and vagina) looking for signs of bleeding. A digital rectal examination is done to look for bleeding from the digestive tract. Doctors also look for signs, such as tenderness during movement and local swelling, that may indicate bleeding in deeper tissues. A person with bleeding inside the head may have confusion, a stiff neck, or neurologic abnormalities. The sites of bleeding may offer a clue to the cause. Bleeding from superficial sites, including skin and mucous membranes, suggests a problem with platelets or blood vessels. On the other hand, bleeding into deep tissues suggests a problem with clotting.

Additional findings may help doctors narrow the cause. Accumulation of fluid in the abdomen (ascites), an enlarged spleen (splenomegaly), and yellow color of the skin and/or eyes (jaundice) suggest bleeding caused by liver disease. A woman who is pregnant or has recently delivered or a person who is in shock or has a fever, chills, and other signs of serious infection is at risk of disseminated intravascular coagulation. In children, fever and digestive upset, especially bloody diarrhea, suggest hemolytic-uremic syndrome. A rash on the legs, joint pain, and digestive upset suggest immunoglobulin A–associated vasculitis.

TESTING

Most people require blood tests. The initial tests are

- Complete blood count (including platelet count), which evaluates all the cellular components of a blood sample
- Peripheral blood smear (examination of a sample of blood under a microscope to see whether blood cells are damaged, abnormal, or immature)
- Prothrombin time (PT) and partial thromboplastin time (PTT), which measure the activity of blood clotting factors

These tests are considered screening tests. They are done to determine whether the clotting system is normal. If one of these tests reveals an abnormality, additional tests are usually needed to identify the cause.

Other blood tests may be needed to confirm bleeding caused by HIV infection or hepatitis. A bone marrow biopsy may be needed if doctors suspect a bone marrow disorder.

Imaging tests are often done to detect internal bleeding in people with bleeding disorders. For example, computed tomography (CT) of the head should be done in people with severe headaches, head injuries, or impairment of consciousness. Abdominal CT is done in people with abdominal pain.

TREATMENT

The specific treatment for easy bruising and bleeding depends on the cause. For example, cancers and infections are treated, causative drugs are stopped, vitamins are given for vitamin deficiency, and people with liver disease are sometimes given vitamin K or fresh frozen plasma transfusions.

People with more serious bleeding need intravenous fluids and sometimes blood transfusions. Those with a very low platelet count often need platelet transfusions. Doctors may give fresh frozen plasma, which contains all clotting factors, to a person with a clotting disorder until the specific deficiency has been identified. Once the deficient factor is identified, the person can be given that factor.

People with easy bruising due to skin and blood vessel fragility do not need to be treated, although doctors sometimes suggest that people avoid taking aspirin and nonsteroidal anti-inflammatory drugs (NSAIDs).

ESSENTIALS FOR OLDER PEOPLE

Older people may be more prone to easy bruising. As people age, the skin thins and people lose some of the protective layer of fat below the skin surface. So a minor bump is more likely to cause blood vessels to break, leading to bruising. Also, the small blood vessels themselves become less elastic and more fragile, leading to easier bruising. Older people also are more likely to take drugs such as warfarin and aspirin, which make bruising and bleeding more likely.

KEY POINTS

- Excessive bleeding may occur on its own or after minor injury.
- Bleeding can range from minimal to massive and is very dangerous if it occurs within the brain.
- Liver disease, low platelet count, and certain drugs (especially warfarin, heparin, aspirin, and NSAIDs) are common causes.
- Disseminated intravascular coagulation is an uncommon but serious cause that most often develops in people who are already ill or in the hospital.
- Easy bruising is common and is rarely a cause for concern if people feel well and have no other signs of easy bleeding.

CHEST PAIN

Chest pain is a very common complaint. Pain may be sharp or dull, although some people with a chest disorder describe their sensation as discomfort, tightness, pressure, gas, indigestion, burning, or aching. Sometimes, people also have pain in the back, neck, jaw, upper part of the abdomen, or arm. Other symptoms, such as nausea, cough, or difficulty breathing, may be present depending on the cause of the chest pain.

Many people are well aware that chest pain is a warning of potential life-threatening disorders and seek evaluation for minimal symptoms. Other people, including many with serious disease, minimize or ignore its warnings.

CAUSES

Many disorders cause chest pain or discomfort. Not all of these disorders involve the heart. Chest pain may also be caused by disorders of the digestive system, lungs, muscles, nerves, or bones.

COMMON CAUSES

Overall, the most common causes of chest pain are

- Disorders of the ribs, rib cartilage, chest muscles (musculoskeletal chest wall pain), or nerves in the chest
- Inflammation of the membrane that covers the lungs (pleuritis)
- Inflammation of the membrane that covers the heart (pericarditis)
- Digestive disorders (such as esophageal reflux or spasm, ulcer disease, or gallstones)
- Heart attack or angina (acute coronary syndromes and stable angina)
- Undiagnosed causes that go away on their own

Acute coronary syndromes involve a sudden blockage of an artery in the heart (coronary artery) that cuts off the blood supply to an area of the heart muscle. If some of the heart muscle dies because it does not get enough blood, that effect is termed a heart attack (myocardial infarction). In stable angina, long-term narrowing of a coronary artery (for example by atherosclerosis) limits blood flow through that artery. This limited blood flow causes chest pain when people exert themselves.

LIFE-THREATENING CAUSES

Some causes of chest pain are immediately life threatening but, except for acute coronary syndromes, are less common:

- Heart attack or unstable angina
- A tear in the wall of the aorta (thoracic aortic dissection)
- A type of collapsed lung in which pressure builds up enough to obstruct blood flow returning to the heart (tension pneumothorax)
- A tear of the esophagus
- Blockage of an artery to the lungs by a blood clot (pulmonary embolism)

Other causes range from serious, potential threats to disorders that are simply uncomfortable.

EVALUATION

People with chest pain should be evaluated by a doctor. The following information can help people decide when evaluation is needed and help them know what to expect during the evaluation.

WARNING SIGNS

In people with chest pain or discomfort, certain symptoms and characteristics are cause for concern. They include

- Crushing or squeezing pain
- Shortness of breath
- Sweating
- Nausea or vomiting
- Pain in the back, neck, jaw, upper abdomen, or one of the shoulders or arms
- Light-headedness or fainting
- Sensation of rapid or irregular heartbeat

WHEN TO SEE A DOCTOR

Although not all causes of chest pain are serious, because some causes are life threatening, people with new chest pain (within several days), who have a warning sign, or who suspect that a heart attack is occurring (for example, because symptoms resemble a previous heart attack) should see a doctor right away. They should call emergency services (911) or be taken to an emergency department as quickly as possible. People should not try to drive themselves to the hospital.

Chest pain that lasts for seconds (less than 30 seconds) is rarely caused by a heart disorder. People with very brief chest pain need to see a doctor, but emergency services are usually not needed.

People who have had chest pain for a longer time (a week or more) should see a doctor within several days unless they develop warning signs or the pain has steadily been getting worse

or coming more often, in which case they should go to the hospital right away.

WHAT THE DOCTOR DOES

Doctors first ask questions about the person's symptoms and medical history and then do a physical examination. What they find during the history and physical examination often suggests a cause of the chest pain and the tests that may need to be done. However, symptoms due to dangerous and not dangerous chest disorders overlap and vary greatly. For example, although a typical heart attack causes dull, crushing chest pain, some people with a heart attack have only mild chest discomfort or complain only of

WHAT IS REFERRED PAIN?

Pain felt in one area of the body does not always represent where the problem is because the pain may be referred there from another area. For example, pain produced by a heart attack may feel as if it is coming from the arm because sensory information from the heart and the arm converge on the same nerve pathways in the spinal cord.

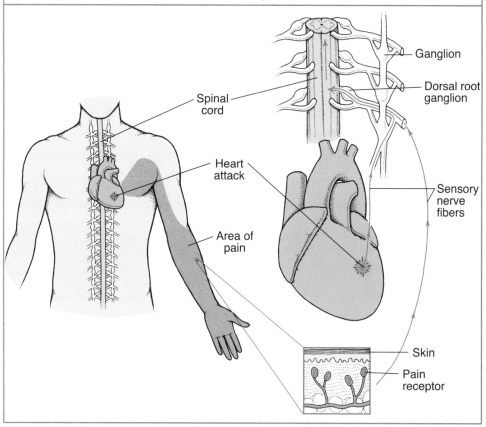

SOME CAUSES AND FEATURES OF CHEST PAIN

Causes	Common Features*	Tests†
Heart disorders		
Heart attack (myocardial infarction) or unstable angina, which are acute coronary syndromes	Immediately life threatening Sudden, crushing pain that ■ Spreads to the jaw or arm ■ May be constant or come and go Sometimes shortness of breath or nausea Pain that occurs during exertion and is relieved by rest (angina pectoris) Certain abnormal heart sounds, heard through a stethoscope Often warning signs‡	ECG, done several times over a period of time Blood tests to measure substances that indicate heart damage (cardiac markers) If ECG and cardiac marker levels are normal, CT of heart arteries or a stress test If ECG or cardiac marker levels are abnormal, heart catheterization
Thoracic aortic dissection (a tear in the wall of the part of aorta in the chest)	Immediately life threatening Sudden, tearing pain that spreads to or starts in the middle of the back Sometimes light-headedness, stroke, or pain, coldness, or numbness in a leg (indicating inadequate blood flow to the leg) Sometimes a pulse or blood pressure in one limb that differs from that in the other limb Usually in people who are over 55 and have a history of high blood pressure Warning signs‡	Chest x-ray CT of the aorta Transesophageal echocardiography (ultrasonography of the heart with the ultrasound device passed down the throat)
Pericarditis (inflammation of the membrane around the heart)	Potentially life threatening Sharp pain that ■ Is constant or comes and goes ■ Is often worsened by breathing, swallowing food, or lying on the back ■ Is relieved by leaning forward An abnormal heart sound, heard through a stethoscope	ECG Echocardiography
Digestive tract disorders		
Esophageal rupture	Immediately life threatening Sudden, severe pain immediately after vomiting or after a medical procedure involving the esophagus (such as endoscopy of the esophagus and stomach or transesophageal echocardiography) Several warning signs‡	Chest x-ray X-rays of the esophagus taken after the person swallows water-soluble contrast (esophagography)

(continued)

SOME CAUSES AND FEATURES OF CHEST PAIN *(continued)*

Causes	Common Features*	Tests†
Pancreatitis	Potentially life threatening Severe, constant pain that ▪ Occurs in the upper middle of the abdomen or in the lower chest ▪ Is often worse when lying flat ▪ Is relieved by leaning forward Vomiting Upper abdominal tenderness Shock Often in people who abuse alcohol or who have gallstones	Blood tests to measure an enzyme (lipase) produced by the pancreas Sometimes CT of the abdomen
Peptic ulcer§	Recurring, vague discomfort that ▪ Occurs in the upper middle of the abdomen or lower chest ▪ Is relieved by food, antacids, or both Often in people who smoke, drink alcohol, or do both No warning signs‡	A doctor's examination Sometimes endoscopy
Gastroesophageal reflux (GERD)§	Recurring, burning pain that ▪ Spreads from the upper middle of the abdomen to the throat ▪ Is worsened by bending over or lying down ▪ Is relieved by antacids	A doctor's examination Sometimes endoscopy
Gallbladder and bile duct disorders (biliary tract disease)§	Recurring discomfort that ▪ Occurs in the upper right of the abdomen or the lower middle of the chest ▪ Occurs after meals (but not after exertion)	Ultrasonography of the gallbladder
Swallowing disorders in which there is abnormal movement (propulsion) of food through the esophagus	Pain that ▪ Has developed gradually over a long period of time ▪ May or may not occur during swallowing Usually difficulty swallowing	Sometimes x-rays of the upper digestive tract after barium is given by mouth (barium swallow)
Lung disorders		
Pulmonary embolism (blockage of an artery in the lungs by a blood clot)	Immediately life threatening Often sharp pain when breathing in, shortness of breath, rapid breathing, and a rapid heart rate Sometimes mild fever, coughing up blood, or shock More likely in people with risk factors for pulmonary embolism (such as previous blood clots, recent surgery especially surgery on the legs, prolonged bed rest, a cast or splint on a leg, older age, smoking, or cancer)	CT or nuclear scanning of the lungs Sometimes a blood test to detect blood clots (D-dimer test)

(continued)

SOME CAUSES AND FEATURES OF CHEST PAIN *(continued)*

Causes	Common Features*	Tests†
Tension pneumothorax (a collapsed lung with a high-pressure buildup of air in the chest)	Immediately life threatening Significant shortness of breath Low blood pressure, swollen neck veins, and weak breath sounds on one side, heard through a stethoscope Typically occurs only after a severe chest injury	Usually only a doctor's examination Sometimes chest x-ray
Pneumonia	Potentially life threatening Fever, chills, cough, and usually yellow or green phlegm Often shortness of breath Sometimes pain when breathing in A rapid heart rate and congested lungs, detected during the examination	Chest x-ray
Pneumothorax (a collapsed lung)	Potentially life threatening Sudden, sharp pain, usually on one side of the chest Sometimes shortness of breath Sometimes weak breath sounds on one side, heard through a stethoscope	Chest x-ray
Pleuritis (inflammation of the membrane around the lung)§	Sharp pain when breathing Usually in people who have recently had pneumonia or a viral respiratory infection Sometimes cough No warning signs‡	Usually only a doctor's examination
Other disorders		
Pain in the chest wall,§ including the muscles, ligaments, nerves, and ribs (musculoskeletal chest wall pain)	Pain that ■ Is typically persistent (lasting days or longer) ■ Is worsened by movement and/or breathing ■ May have no apparent cause or may result from coughing or overuse Tenderness in one spot on the chest No warning signs‡	Only a doctor's examination
Herpes zoster infection§	Sharp pain in a band around the middle of the chest but only on one side	Only a doctor's examination

(continued)

SOME CAUSES AND FEATURES OF CHEST PAIN (continued)

Causes	Common Features*	Tests†
Herpes zoster infection§ (continued)	A rash of many small blisters. sometimes filled with pus, in the painful area and sometimes appearing only after the pain	

*Features include symptoms and the results of the doctor's examination. Features mentioned are typical but not always present.

†For most people with chest pain, the oxygen level in blood is measured with a sensor placed on a finger (pulse oximetry), ECG is done, and a chest x-ray is taken.

‡Warning signs include
- Abnormal vital signs (an abnormally slow or fast heart rate, rapid breathing, and abnormally low blood pressure)
- Signs of decreased blood flow (such as confusion, pale or gray skin color, and excessive sweating)
- Shortness of breath
- Abnormal breath sounds or pulses
- New heart murmurs

§Unless otherwise described, causes are usually not dangerous, although they are uncomfortable.

CT = computed tomography; ECG = electrocardiography.

---

indigestion or arm or shoulder pain (referred pain—see art box on page 32). On the other hand, people with indigestion may simply have an upset stomach, and those with shoulder pain may have only sore muscles. Similarly, although the chest is tender when touched in people with musculoskeletal chest wall pain, the chest can also be tender in people who are having a heart attack. Thus, doctors usually do tests on people with chest pain.

TESTING

For adults with sudden chest pain, tests are done to rule out dangerous causes. For most people, initial tests include

- Measurement of oxygen levels with a sensor placed on a finger (pulse oximetry)
- Electrocardiography (ECG)
- Chest x-ray

If symptoms suggest an acute coronary syndrome or if no other cause is clear (particularly in people who are at high risk), doctors usually measure levels of substances that indicate heart damage (cardiac markers) in the blood (at least two separate times over a few hours) and do several ECGs. If these tests do not show an acute coronary syndrome, doctors often then do a stress test before people go home or within a few days. For a stress test, ECG or an imaging test (such as echocardiography) is done during exercise (often on a treadmill) or after a drug is given to make the heart beat fast.

If pulmonary embolism is suspected, computed tomography (CT) of the lungs or a lung scan is done. If pulmonary embolism is considered only somewhat possible, a blood test to detect clots (D-dimer test) is often done. If this test is negative, pulmonary embolism is unlikely, but if the test is positive, other tests, such as ultrasonography of the legs or CT of the chest, are often done.

In people who have had chest pain for a long time, immediate threats to life are unlikely. Most doctors initially do only a chest x-ray and then do other tests based on the person's symptoms and examination findings.

TREATMENT

Specific identified disorders are treated. If the cause is not clearly benign, people are usually admitted to the hospital or an observation unit for heart monitoring and more extensive evaluation. Symptoms are treated with acetaminophen or opioids as needed until a diagnosis is made.

KEY POINTS

- Chest pain may be caused by serious life-threatening disorders, so people with new chest pain (within a few days) should get immediate medical attention.
- The symptoms of life-threatening and non–life-threatening disorders overlap, so testing is needed to determine a cause.

CONSTIPATION IN ADULTS

Constipation is difficult or infrequent bowel movements, hard stool, or a feeling that the rectum is not totally empty after a bowel movement (incomplete evacuation). Constipation in children is discussed on page 44.

Constipation may be acute or chronic. Acute constipation begins suddenly and noticeably. Chronic constipation may begin gradually and persists for months or years.

Many people believe they are constipated if they do not have a bowel movement every day. However, daily bowel movements are not normal for everyone. Having less frequent bowel movements does not necessarily indicate a problem unless there has been a substantial change from previous patterns. The same is true of the color, size, and consistency of stool. People often blame constipation for many symptoms (such as abdominal discomfort, nausea, fatigue, and poor appetite) that are actually the result of other disorders (such as irritable bowel syndrome [IBS] and depression). People should not expect all symptoms to be relieved by a daily bowel movement, and measures to aid bowel habits, such as laxatives and enemas, should not be overused. However, people may harmlessly help relieve their symptoms by eating more fruits, vegetables, fiber, and cereals.

COMPLICATIONS

The complications of constipation include

- Hemorrhoids
- Rectal prolapse
- Anal fissure
- Diverticular disease
- Fecal impaction

Excessive straining during bowel movements increases pressure on the veins around the anus and can lead to hemorrhoids and, rarely, protrusion of the rectum through the anus (rectal prolapse). Passing hard stool can cause a split in the skin of the anus (anal fissure). Each of these complications can make having a bowel movement uncomfortable and make people reluctant to move their bowels. Putting off bowel movements can cause a vicious circle of worsening constipation and complications.

Diverticular disease can develop if the walls of the large intestine are damaged by the increased pressure required to move small, hard stools. Damage to the walls of the large intestine leads to the formation of balloon-like sacs or outpocketings (diverticula), which can become clogged and inflamed (diverticulitis). Diverticula sometimes bleed and rarely rupture (causing peritonitis).

Fecal impaction, in which stool in the rectum and last part of the large intestine hardens and completely blocks the passage of other stool, sometimes develops in people with constipation. Fecal impaction leads to cramps, rectal pain, and strong but futile efforts to defecate. Sometimes, watery mucus or liquid stool oozes around the blockage, which gives the false impression of diarrhea (paradoxic diarrhea). Fecal impaction is particularly common among older people, especially those who are bedridden or have decreased physical activity, pregnant women, and people who have been given barium by mouth or as an enema for certain types of x-ray tests.

Overconcern with regular bowel movements causes many people to abuse their bowels with laxatives, suppositories, and enemas. Overusing these treatments can actually inhibit the bowel's normal contractions and worsen constipation. People with obsessive-compulsive disorder (OCD) often feel the need to rid their body daily of "unclean" wastes or "toxins." Such people often spend excessive time on the toilet or become chronic users of laxatives.

CAUSES

The **most common causes** of constipation include

- Changes in diet (such as decreased fluid intake, low-fiber diet, and/or constipating foods)
- Drugs that slow the bowels
- Disordered defecation
- Laxative overuse

Dietary causes are very common. Dehydration causes constipation because the body tries to conserve water in the blood by removing additional water from the stool. Stool that contains less water is harder to pass. Fruits, vegetables, cereals, and other fiber-containing foods are the natural laxatives of the digestive tract. People who do not eat enough of these foods can become constipated. Lack of fiber (the indigestible part of food) in the diet can lead to constipation because fiber helps hold water in the stool and increases its bulk, making it easier to pass.

The most common drugs that can slow the bowels include opioids, iron salts, and drugs with anticholinergic effects (such as many antihistamines and tricyclic antidepressants). Other drugs include aluminum hydroxide (common in over-the-counter antacids), bismuth subsalicylate, certain drugs that lower blood pressure (antihypertensives), and many sedatives.

Disordered defecation (dyschezia) refers to a problem with the bowels generating enough force to propel stool from the rectum and/or difficulty relaxing the muscle fibers around the rectum and the external anal sphincter during defecation. People with dyschezia sense the need to have a bowel movement but cannot. Even stool that is not hard may be difficult to pass. People with irritable bowel syndrome (IBS) may have IBS-disordered defecation.

People who frequently use laxatives and/or enemas often lose the ability to move their bowels without such aids. A vicious circle can result with constipation leading to more laxative use and thus more constipation.

Less common causes of constipation include specific medical disorders (see Table on pages 39 to 40), such as intestinal obstruction, and certain metabolic disorders and neurologic disorders. Constipation also can occur during any major illness that requires prolonged bed rest (because physical activity helps the intestines move stool along), with decreased food intake, with use of drugs that can cause constipation, and after a head or spinal cord injury. In many cases, however, the cause of constipation is unknown.

Constipation is sometimes caused by obstruction of the large intestine. Obstruction can be caused by a large cancer, especially in the last portion of the large intestine, that blocks the movement of stool. People who previously had abdominal surgery may develop obstruction, usually of the small intestine, because bands of fibrous tissues (adhesions) can form around the intestines and impede the flow of stool.

Disorders and diseases that often cause constipation include an underactive thyroid gland (hypothyroidism), high blood calcium levels (hypercalcemia), and Parkinson disease. People with diabetes often develop nerve damage (neuropathy). If the neuropathy affects nerves to the digestive tract, the intestines may slow down, resulting in constipation. Spinal cord injury can also interfere with the nerves to the intestines and cause constipation.

EVALUATION

Not every episode of constipation requires immediate evaluation by a doctor. The following information can help people decide whether a doctor's evaluation is needed and help them know what to expect during the evaluation.

WARNING SIGNS

In people with constipation, certain symptoms and characteristics are cause for concern. They include

- Distended, swollen abdomen
- Vomiting
- Blood in stool
- Weight loss
- New/worsening severe constipation in older people

WHEN TO SEE A DOCTOR

People who have warning signs should see a doctor right away, unless the only warning signs are weight loss and/or new constipation in older people. In such cases, a delay of a few days to a week is not harmful.

People who have constipation but no warning signs should call their doctor, who can help decide how quickly they need to be seen. Depending on the person's other symptoms and known disorders, doctors may wish to see the person within a few days or may simply recommend trying changes in diet and/or a mild laxative.

WHAT THE DOCTOR DOES

Doctors first ask questions about the person's symptoms and medical history. Doctors then do a physical examination. What they find during the history and physical examination often suggests a cause of the constipation and the tests that may need to be done (see Table).

SOME CAUSES AND FEATURES OF CONSTIPATION

Cause	Examples/Common Features*	Tests
Acute constipation†		
Acute intestinal obstruction	Twisting of a loop of intestine (volvulus), hernia, adhesions, and fecal impaction Usually vomiting and a distended abdomen	Abdominal x-rays Sometimes CT
Ileus (temporary absence of the contractile movements of the intestine)	Major acute illness, such as sepsis (a severe infection of the bloodstream) Immediately after abdominal surgery Recent head or spinal cord injury Prolonged bed rest	Abdominal x-rays
Drugs	Drugs with anticholinergic effects, such as antihistamines, some antidepressants, antipsychotic drugs, drugs used to treat Parkinson disease, and drugs that reduce or stop muscle spasms in the digestive tract (antispasmodic drugs) Drugs containing certain metals (iron, aluminum, calcium, barium, or bismuth) Opioids Calcium channel blockers Usually constipation that begins shortly after starting a new drug	A doctor's examination to exclude other causes of constipation Sometimes stopping the drug to see whether constipation resolves
Chronic constipation†		
Colon cancer	Often constipation that has recently developed, persists for weeks, and gradually worsens as the tumor grows Sometimes blood in stool (blood may be visible or detected during a doctor's examination)	Colonoscopy with biopsy
Metabolic disorders	Diabetes mellitus, an underactive thyroid gland (hypothyroidism), high levels of calcium in the blood (hypercalcemia), kidney failure, or pregnancy	Blood tests
Central nervous system disorders (affecting the brain or spinal cord)	Parkinson disease, multiple sclerosis, stroke, or spinal cord injury or disorders	MRI and/or CT
Peripheral nervous system disorders (affecting nerves outside the brain and spinal cord)	Hirschsprung disease, neurofibromatosis, or autonomic neuropathy	A doctor's examination Sometimes x-rays after barium is inserted in the rectum (barium enema) and/or biopsy
Systemic disorders	Systemic sclerosis, amyloidosis, skin inflammation plus muscle inflammation and muscle degeneration (dermatomyositis), or weakness and stiff muscles (myotonic dystrophy)	A doctor's examination Sometimes biopsy and/or blood tests

(continued)

SOME CAUSES AND FEATURES OF CONSTIPATION *(continued)*

Cause	Examples/Common Features*	Tests
Functional disorders	Inactive colon (colonic inertia), irritable bowel syndrome, or disordered defecation	A doctor's examination

Sometimes sigmoidoscopy |
| | Often a sense of a blockage in the anus and/or rectum, prolonged or difficult defecation, or excessive straining | |
| Dietary factors | Low-fiber diet or chronic laxative abuse | A doctor's examination |

*Features include symptoms and the results of the doctor's examination. Features mentioned are typical but not always present.
†There is some overlap between causes of acute and chronic constipation. In particular, drugs are common causes of both.
CT = computed tomography; MRI = magnetic resonance imaging.

During the history, doctors ask about the following:

- Stool frequency, consistency, and the need to strain or use maneuvers (such as pushing on the area between the scrotum or vagina and the anus [perineum]) during defecation)
- Satisfaction after defecation, including how often and how long people have used laxatives or enemas
- Diet and physical activity level, particularly any change in these factors
- Prescription and nonprescription drug use (particularly those known to cause constipation)

Doctors also ask about symptoms of metabolic (such as hypothyroidism and diabetes) and neurologic (such as spinal cord injury) disorders.

During the physical examination, doctors look at the following:

- Signs of bodywide (systemic) disease, including weight loss, fever, and severe wasting away of muscle and fat tissue (cachexia)
- The abdomen for distention and masses
- The rectum for fissures, hemorrhoids, blood, or masses (including fecal impaction) and also anal muscle tone and sensation

TESTING

The need for tests depends on what doctors find during the history and physical examination, particularly whether warning signs are present. When the cause of the constipation is clear (such as due to drugs, injury, or bed rest), doctors often treat the person's symptoms and do no testing.

People with symptoms of intestinal obstruction undergo abdominal x-rays and possibly a computed tomography (CT) scan. Most people with no clear cause or whose symptoms have not been relieved with treatment should have tests. Typically, doctors do a colonoscopy (to detect cancer) and blood tests to check for an underactive thyroid gland (hypothyroidism) or high calcium levels in the blood (hypercalcemia).

TREATMENT

Any underlying disorder causing constipation must be treated. When possible, drugs that cause constipation are stopped or changed.

Constipation is best prevented with a combination of exercise, a high-fiber diet, and an adequate intake of fluids. When a potentially constipating drug is prescribed and/or people are placed on bed rest, doctors often give a laxative and recommend increased intake of dietary fiber and fluids rather than waiting for constipation to develop.

There are three approaches to treating people with constipation:

- Diet and behavior
- Laxatives
- Enemas

Doctors are cautious with use of laxatives, suppositories, and enemas, because they can cause diarrhea, dehydration, cramps, and/or dependence on laxatives. People with sudden abdominal pain of unknown cause, inflammatory bowel disorders, intestinal obstruction, gastrointestinal bleeding, or fecal impaction should not use laxatives or enemas.

DIET AND BEHAVIOR

People need to ingest enough fiber in their diet (typically 15 to 20 grams per day) to ensure adequate stool bulk. Vegetables, fruits, and bran are excellent sources of fiber. Many people find it convenient to sprinkle 2 or 3 teaspoons of unrefined miller's bran on high-fiber cereal or fruit 2 or 3 times a day. To work well, fiber must be consumed with plenty of fluids.

People should try to make changes to their behavior. For example, people should try to move their bowels at the same time every day, preferably 15 to 45 minutes after breakfast, because eating food stimulates movement in the colon. Glycerin suppositories may also help people have regular, unhurried bowel movements.

Doctors explain to people why diet and behavior modification are important in treating constipation. Doctors also explain that daily bowel movements are not necessary, that the bowel must be given a chance to function, and that frequent use of laxatives or enemas (more than once every 3 days) denies the bowel that chance.

LAXATIVES

Some laxatives are safe for long-term use. Other laxatives should be used only occasionally. Some laxatives are good for preventing constipation, others for treating it. There are several classes of laxatives, including the following:

- Bulking agents
- Stool softeners
- Osmotic agents
- Stimulants

Bulking agents, such as bran and psyllium (also available in the fiber of many vegetables), add bulk to the stool and absorb water. The increased bulk stimulates the natural contractions of the intestine, and bulkier stools that contain more water are softer and easier to pass. Bulking agents act slowly and gently and are among the safest ways to promote regular bowel movements. These agents generally are taken in small amounts at first. The dose is increased gradually until regularity is achieved. People who use bulking agents should always drink plenty of fluids. These agents may cause problems with increased gas (flatulence) and bloating.

Stool softeners, such as docusate or mineral oil, act slowly to soften stools, making them easier to pass. In addition, the slightly increased bulk that results from these drugs stimulates the natural contractions of the large intestine and thus promotes easier elimination. Some people, however, find the softened nature of the stool unpleasant. Stool softeners are best reserved for people who must avoid straining, such as people who have hemorrhoids or have recently had abdominal surgery.

Osmotic agents pull large amounts of water into the large intestine, making the stool soft and loose. The excess fluid also stretches the walls of the large intestine, stimulating contractions. These laxatives consist of salts or sugars that are poorly absorbed. They may cause fluid retention in people who have kidney disease or heart failure, especially when given in large or frequent doses. In general, osmotic laxatives are reasonably safe even when used regularly. However, osmotic agents that contain magnesium and phosphate are partially absorbed into the bloodstream and can be harmful to older people, people who have kidney failure or kidney disease, and people who take drugs that affect kidney function (such as diuretics, angiotensin-converting enzyme [ACE] inhibitors, and angiotensin II receptor blockers). Although a rare occurrence, some people have developed kidney failure from taking sodium phosphate laxatives by mouth to clear stool from the intestine before x-rays of the digestive tract are taken or before a colonoscopy is done.

Stimulant laxatives (such as phenolphthalein, bisacodyl, and anthraquinones) contain irritating substances, such as senna and cascara. These substances stimulate the walls of the large intestine, causing them to contract and move the stool. They are useful for preventing constipation in people who are taking drugs that will almost certainly cause constipation, such as opioids. Stimulant laxatives are also often used to empty the large intestine before diagnostic tests are done.

Taken by mouth, stimulant laxatives usually cause a semisolid bowel movement in 6 to 8 hours, but they often cause cramping as well. As suppositories, stimulant laxatives often work in 15 to 60 minutes. Prolonged use of stimulant laxatives can create abnormal deposits of a dark pigment in the lining of the large intestine (a condition called melanosis coli). Other side effects include allergic reactions and loss of electrolytes from the blood. Also, the large intestine can become dependent on stimulant laxatives, leading to lazy bowel syndrome. Therefore, stimulant laxatives should be used only for brief periods.

Bisacodyl is an effective drug for chronic constipation. Anthraquinones are found in senna, cascara sagrada, aloe, and rhubarb and are common components of herbal and over-the-counter laxatives. Lubiprostone works by making the large intestine secrete extra fluid, which makes stool easier to pass. Unlike other stimulant laxatives, lubiprostone is safe for prolonged use.

ENEMAS

Enemas mechanically flush stool from the rectum and lower part of the large intestine. Small-volume enemas can be purchased in squeeze bottles at a pharmacy. They can also be

AGENTS USED TO PREVENT OR TREAT CONSTIPATION

Agent	Some Side Effects	Comments
Bulking agents (fiber)*		
Bran	Bloating, passing of gas (flatulence), and poor absorption of iron and calcium	Bulking agents generally are used to prevent or control chronic constipation
Polycarbophil	Bloating and flatulence	
Methylcellulose	Less bloating than with other fiber agents	
Psyllium	Bloating and flatulence	
Stool softeners		
Docusate	—	Stool softeners may be used to treat constipation and are often used to help prevent it.
Glycerin	Rectal irritation	
Mineral oil	Lung inflammation caused by fats in the lungs (lipid pneumonia), poor absorption of fat-soluble vitamins, dehydration, and loss of control over bowel movements (fecal incontinence)	Docusate is not effective for severe constipation.
Osmotic agents		
Lactulose	Abdominal cramps and flatulence	Osmotic agents are better for treating constipation than for preventing it.
Magnesium salts (magnesium hydroxide and magnesium citrate)	Too much magnesium in the body (magnesium toxicity), dehydration, abdominal cramps, and fecal incontinence	
Polyethylene glycol	Fecal incontinence (related to dosage)	
Sodium phosphate	Rare cases of sudden kidney failure	
Sorbitol	Abdominal cramps and flatulence	
Stimulant laxatives		
Anthraquinones (found in senna, cascara, and castor oil)	Abdominal cramps and dehydration	Stimulant laxatives are not used if there is a possibility of an intestinal obstruction.
Bisacodyl	Fecal incontinence, a low level of potassium in the blood (hypokalemia), abdominal cramps, and rectal burning with daily use of the suppository form	Prolonged use of anthraquinones can damage the large intestine.
Lubiprostone†	Nausea, particularly when the drug is taken on an empty stomach	Lubiprostone can be used for chronic constipation. It has been approved for long-term use.

(continued)

AGENTS USED TO PREVENT OR TREAT CONSTIPATION *(continued)*

Agent	Some Side Effects	Comments
Tegaserod‡	Diarrhea, headache, heart attack, and stroke	
Enemas		
Mineral oil or olive oil retention	Fecal incontinence	Although rare, giving an enema can injure the rectum if the procedure is done roughly.
Tap water	Fluid overload if a lot of water is absorbed	
Phosphate	A high level of phosphate in the blood (hyperphosphatemia)	
Soapsuds	Cramps	

*The dose of fiber supplements should be gradually increased over several weeks to the recommended dose.
†Lubiprostone is available only by prescription.
‡Tegaserod is available in a restricted-use program.

given with a reusable squeeze-ball device. However, small-volume enemas are often inadequate, especially for older people, whose rectal capacity increases with age, thus making the rectum more easily stretched. Larger-volume enemas are given with an enema bag.

Plain water is often the best fluid to be used as an enema. The water should be room temperature to slightly warm, not hot or cold. About 5 to 10 fluid ounces (150 to 300 milliliters) is gently directed into the rectum. (CAUTION: *Additional force is dangerous.*) People then expel the water, washing stool out with it.

Various ingredients are sometimes added to enemas. Prepackaged enemas often contain small amounts of salts, often phosphates. Other enemas contain small amounts of soap (soapsuds enema), which has a stimulant laxative effect, or mineral oil. These enemas offer little advantage, however, to plain water.

Very large-volume enemas, called colonic enemas, are rarely used in medical practice. Doctors use colonic enemas in people with very severe constipation (obstipation). Some practitioners of alternative medicine use colonic enemas in the belief that cleansing the large intestine is beneficial. Tea, coffee, and other substances are often added to colonic enemas but have no proven health value and may be dangerous.

FECAL IMPACTION

Fecal impaction cannot be treated by modifying the diet or taking laxatives. Fecal impaction is first treated with enemas of tap water followed by small enemas of commercially prepared solutions. If these enemas do not work,

the hard stool must be removed by a doctor or nurse using a gloved finger. This procedure is painful, so an anesthetic (such as lidocaine 5% ointment) is often applied. Some people need to be sedated. Typically, an enema is given after the hard stool is removed.

ESSENTIALS FOR OLDER PEOPLE

The rectum enlarges as people age, and increased storage of stool in the rectum means that older people often need to have larger volumes of stool in their rectum in order to feel the urge to defecate. The increased rectal volume also allows hard stool to become impacted.

Other common factors in older people that lead to constipation include increased use of constipating drugs, a low-fiber diet, coexisting medical conditions (such as diabetes), and reduced physical activity. Many older people also have misconceptions about normal bowel habits and use laxatives too often.

KEY POINTS

- Drug causes (such as chronic laxative abuse or use of anticholinergic or opioid drugs) are common.
- Doctors look for intestinal obstruction when constipation is sudden and severe.
- Symptoms may be treated if no warning signs are found and doctors find no evidence of disordered defecation.

CONSTIPATION IN CHILDREN

Constipation refers to delay or difficulty in passing stool for a period of at least 1 month in infants and toddlers and a period of 2 months in older children. Stools are harder and sometimes larger than usual and may be painful to pass. Constipation is very common among children. It accounts for up to 5% of children's visits to the doctor. Infants and children are particularly prone to developing constipation at three periods of time. The first period is when cereals and solid food are introduced into the infant's diet, the second period is during toilet training, and the third period is around the start of school.

The frequency and consistency of bowel movements (BMs) vary throughout childhood, and there is no single definition of what is normal. Newborns typically have four or more loose, yellow, seedy stools per day. During the first year, infants have 2 to 4 a day. Breastfed infants typically have more BMs than formula-fed infants and may have one after each breastfeeding. After a month or two, some breastfed infants have BMs less frequently, but the stools remain mushy or loose. After 1 year of age, most children have one or sometimes two soft but formed stools a day. However, some infants and young children typically have BMs only once every 3 to 4 days. Guidelines for identifying constipation in infants and children include no BMs for 2 or 3 more days than usual, hard or painful BMs, large-diameter stools that may clog the toilet, or drops of blood on the outside of the stool.

In infants, signs of effort such as straining and crying before successfully passing a soft stool usually do not indicate constipation. These symptoms are usually caused by failure to relax the pelvic floor muscles during passage of stool and typically resolve spontaneously.

Parents often worry about their child's BMs, but constipation usually has no serious consequences. Some children with constipation regularly complain of abdominal pain, particularly after meals. Occasionally, passing large, hard stools may cause a small tear in the anus (anal fissure). Anal fissures are painful and may result in streaks of bright red blood on the outside of the stool or on toilet paper. Rarely, chronic constipation can contribute to urinary problems such as urinary tract infections and bed wetting.

CAUSES

COMMON CAUSES

In 95% of children, constipation results from

- Dietary issues
- Behavioral issues

Constipation that results from dietary or behavioral issues is called functional constipation.

Dietary issues that cause constipation include a diet that is low in fluids and/or fiber (as occurs in fruits, vegetables, and whole grains).

Behavioral issues that may be associated with constipation include stress (as may be felt when a sibling is born), resistance to toilet training, and a desire for control. Also, children may intentionally put off having BMs (called stool withholding) because they have a painful anal fissure or because they do not want to stop playing. Sexual abuse may result in stress or injury that causes children to withhold stool. If children do not move their bowels when the natural urge comes, the rectum eventually stretches to accommodate the stool. When the rectum has stretched, the urge to have a BM lessens, and more and more stool accumulates and hardens. A vicious circle of worsening constipation may result. If the accumulated stool hardens, it sometimes blocks the passage of other stool—a condition called fecal impaction. Looser stool from above the hardened stool may leak around the impaction into the child's underwear. Parents may then think that the child has diarrhea when the actual problem is constipation.

LESS COMMON CAUSES

In about 5% of children, constipation results from a physical disorder, drug, or toxin. Disorders may be apparent at birth or develop later. Constipation that results from a disorder, drug, or toxin is called organic constipation.

In newborns and infants, the most common disorder that causes constipation is

- Hirschsprung disease (an inadequate nerve supply to the large intestine)

Other causes of organic constipation include

- Birth defects of the anus
- Cystic fibrosis
- Metabolic and electrolyte disorders, such as an abnormally high level of calcium (hypercalcemia) or low level of potassium (hypokalemia)
- Spinal cord problems
- Hormonal disorders, such as an underactive thyroid gland (hypothyroidism)
- Intestinal disorders, such as a cow's milk protein allergy or celiac disease
- Drugs, such as powerful pain relievers called opioids (for example, codeine and morphine)
- Toxins, such as infant botulism or lead

Children with serious abdominal disorders (such as appendicitis or a blockage in the intestine) often do not have BMs. However, these children typically have other, more prominent symptoms, such as abdominal pain, swelling, and/or vomiting. These symptoms typically lead parents to seek medical care before the number of BMs decreases.

EVALUATION

Doctors first try to determine whether constipation results from dietary or behavioral issues (functional) or from a disorder, toxin, or drug (organic).

WARNING SIGNS

Certain symptoms are cause for concern and should raise suspicion for an organic cause of constipation:

- No BMs during the first 24 to 48 hours after birth
- Weight loss or poor growth
- Decreased appetite
- Blood in the stools
- Fever
- Vomiting
- Abdominal swelling
- Abdominal pain (in children old enough to communicate this)

- In infants, loss of muscle tone (the infant appears floppy or weak) and reduced ability to suck
- In older children, an involuntary release of urine (urinary incontinence—see Urinary Incontinence in Children on page 405), back pain, leg weakness, or problems with walking

WHEN TO SEE A DOCTOR

Children should be evaluated by a doctor right away if they have any warning signs. If no warning signs are present but the child is passing infrequent, hard, or painful BMs, then the doctor should be called. Depending on the child's other symptoms (if any), the doctor may advise trying simple home treatments (see Treatment on page 48) or ask the parents to bring the child for an examination.

WHAT THE DOCTOR DOES

Doctors first ask questions about the child's symptoms and medical history. Doctors then do a physical examination. What they find during the history and physical examination often suggests a cause of the constipation and the tests that may need to be done (see Table on pages 46 to 48).

Doctors determine whether newborns have ever had a BM (the first BM is called meconium). Newborns who have not had a BM within 24 to 48 hours after birth should have a thorough examination to rule out the possibility of Hirschsprung disease, imperforate anus, or other serious disorder.

For infants and older children, doctors ask whether constipation began after a specific event, such as introducing cereal or other solid foods, eating honey, beginning toilet training, or starting school. For all age groups, doctors ask about diet and about disorders, toxins, and drugs that can cause constipation.

For the physical examination, doctors first look at the child overall for signs of illness and measure height and weight to check for signs of delayed growth. Doctors then focus on the abdomen, the anus (including examination of the rectum using a gloved finger), and nerve function (which can affect how the digestive tract functions).

TESTING

If the cause appears to be functional, no tests are needed unless children do not respond to

SOME PHYSICAL CAUSES AND FEATURES OF CONSTIPATION IN INFANTS AND CHILDREN

Cause	Common Features*	Tests
Birth defects of the anus		
Abnormal position of the anus	Opening of the anus that appears closer than normal to the genitals	Measurements to determine the exact location of the anus's opening
Anal stenosis (a narrowed anus)	Delayed passage of the first BM (called meconium) during the first 24–48 hours of life Explosive and painful BMs A swollen abdomen Abnormal appearance or position of the anus	A doctor's examination
Blockage of the opening of the anus (imperforate anus, or anal atresia)	A swollen abdomen No BMs A blockage of the anus detected during a doctor's examination	A doctor's examination done soon after birth
Spinal cord problems		
Meningomyelocele (the most severe form of spina bifida)	A raw, red area on the back where the spinal cord protrudes, seen at birth A decrease in reflexes of the legs or in muscle tone Absence of the normal reflex of the anus (a tightening when lightly touched, called anal wink)	Plain x-rays of the lower spine MRI of the spine
Occult spina bifida (incomplete formation of the bones of the spine)	A tuft of hair or dimpling on the skin over the defect, seen at birth	MRI of the spine
A tethered spinal cord (during fetal development, the spinal cord is stuck at the lower end of the spinal column and cannot move up to its normal position)	Problems with walking, pain or weakness in the legs, and back pain Urinary incontinence	MRI of the spine
A tumor near the tailbone (sacral teratoma) or other spinal cord tumor	Back pain, problems with walking, and pain or weakness in the legs Urinary incontinence	MRI of the spine
Infection of the spine or spinal cord	Back pain, problems with walking, and pain or weakness in the legs Fever Urinary incontinence	MRI of the spine
Hormonal, metabolic, or electrolyte disorders		
Diabetes insipidus (due to problems with antidiuretic hormone, which helps regulate the amount of water in the body)	Excessive thirst and excessive crying that is quieted by giving children water Excessive urination of dilute urine Weight loss and vomiting	Urine and blood tests to measure how dilute urine and blood are (osmolality) Blood tests to measure antidiuretic hormone levels

(continued)

SOME PHYSICAL CAUSES AND FEATURES OF CONSTIPATION IN INFANTS AND CHILDREN *(continued)*

Cause	Common Features*	Tests
Hypercalcemia (an abnormally high calcium level)	Nausea and vomiting, loss of appetite, weight loss, muscle weakness, and abdominal pain Excessive thirst and excessive urination	Blood tests to measure the calcium level
Hypokalemia (an abnormally low potassium level)	Muscular weakness Excessive urination and dehydration Not growing as expected (failure to thrive) Possibly use of diuretics or certain antibiotics	Blood tests to measure levels of electrolytes
Hypothyroidism (an underactive thyroid gland)	Poor feeding A slow heart rate In newborns, large soft spots (fontanelles) between the skull bones and slack muscle tone Dry skin, intolerance of cold, fatigue, and jaundice	Blood tests to measure thyroid hormone levels

Intestinal disorders		
Cystic fibrosis	Delayed passage of the first BM Poor weight gain or failure to thrive Frequent bouts of pneumonia	A sweat test Possibly genetic testing to confirm the diagnosis
Hirschsprung disease	Delayed passage of the first BM A swollen abdomen Green or yellow vomit, indicating that it contains bile A narrowed anus detected during a doctor's examination	X-rays of the lower digestive tract after barium is inserted in the rectum (barium enema) Measurement of pressure inside the anus and rectum (manometry) Biopsy of the rectum
Allergy to cow's milk protein	Vomiting Poor feeding Weight loss, poor growth, or both Blood in stools	Stool tests Symptoms that lessen when the formula is changed Possibly endoscopy, colonoscopy, or both
Celiac disease	Abdominal pain Bloating Weight loss Fatigue	Blood tests Endoscopy
Irritable bowel syndrome	Long-standing (chronic) abdominal pain Diarrhea and constipation that come and go A feeling of incomplete emptying after a BM	Evaluation of BM patterns and the timing and characteristics of pain Exclusion of other disorders by history, physical examination, and possibly blood tests, stool tests, imaging, or colonoscopy

(continued)

SOME PHYSICAL CAUSES AND FEATURES OF CONSTIPATION IN INFANTS AND CHILDREN (continued)

Cause	Common Features*	Tests
Pseudo-obstruction (which causes symptoms of a blockage but no blockage is detected)	Nausea and vomiting Abdominal pain and a swollen abdomen	X-ray of the abdomen Tests to assess how well the bowel functions (bowel motility studies)
A tumor in the abdomen	Weight loss, night sweats, and fever Abdominal swelling or pain An abdominal mass detected during a doctor's examination	MRI
Drug side effects		
Use of drugs with anticholinergic effects (such as antihistamines), antidepressants, chemotherapy drugs, or opioids	Use of drugs that can cause constipation	A doctor's examination
Toxins		
Infant botulism	A sudden reduction in the ability to suck Loss of muscle tone Sometimes consumption of honey before age 12 months	A test for botulinum toxin in stool
Lead poisoning	Usually no symptoms Possibly abdominal pain, fatigue, and irritability Regression in development	Blood tests to measure the lead level

*Features include symptoms and results of the doctor's examination. Features mentioned are typical but not always present.
BM = bowel movement; MRI = magnetic resonance imaging.

treatment. If children do not respond or if doctors suspect that the cause is another disorder, an x-ray of the abdomen is taken, and tests for other disorders are done based on the results of the examination.

TREATMENT

Treatment depends on the cause. When constipation results from a specific disorder, a drug, or a toxin, that cause is treated or corrected. For functional constipation, measures include

- Changing the diet
- Modifying behavior
- Sometimes using stool softeners or laxatives

CHANGING THE DIET

Dietary changes for infants include giving them 1 to 4 ounces (30 to 120 milliliters [mL]) of prune, pear, or apple juice each day. For infants younger than 2 months, 1 teaspoon (5 mL) of light corn syrup can be added to their formula in the morning and evening.

Older infants and children should increase their consumption of fruits, vegetables, and high-fiber cereals and decrease consumption of constipating foods, such as milk and cheese.

MODIFYING BEHAVIOR

Behavioral modification can help older children. Measures include

- Encouraging children who are toilet trained to sit on the toilet for 5 to 10 minutes after meals and encouraging them when they make progress (for example, noting progress on a wall chart)

- Giving children who are being toilet trained a break from toilet training until constipation resolves

Sitting on the toilet after a meal can help because eating a meal triggers a reflex to have a BM. Frequently, children ignore the signals from this reflex and put off having a BM. This technique uses the reflex to help retrain the digestive tract, establish a toilet routine, and encourage more regular BMs.

STOOL SOFTENERS AND LAXATIVES

If constipation does not respond to behavioral modification and changes in diet, doctors may recommend certain drugs that help soften stool (stool softeners) and/or increase the spontaneous movement of the digestive tract (laxatives). Such drugs include polyethylene glycol, lactulose, mineral oil, milk of magnesia (magnesium hydroxide), senna, and bisacodyl. Many of these drugs are now available over the counter. However, doses should be based on the age and body weight of the child as well as the severity of constipation. Thus, parents should consult a doctor regarding the appropriate dose and number of doses per day before using these treatments. The goal of treatment is the passage of one soft stool per day.

If children have a fecal impaction, options include gentle enemas and agents (such as mineral oil or polyethylene glycol) taken by mouth with large amounts of fluid. If these treatments are ineffective, children may need to be hospitalized to have the impaction removed.

Infants do not usually require any of these treatments. Typically, a glycerin suppository is adequate.

To maintain regular BMs, some children may require fiber supplements (such as psyllium), which may be obtained without a prescription. For these supplements to be effective, children must drink 32 to 64 ounces of water a day.

KEY POINTS

- Usually, constipation is caused by behavioral or dietary issues (functional constipation).
- Children should be evaluated by a doctor if the interval between BMs has been 2 or 3 days more than usual, if their stools are hard or large, if stools cause pain or bleeding, or if children have other symptoms.
- If a newborn does not have a BM within 24 to 48 hours after birth, a thorough evaluation should be done to rule out the presence of Hirschsprung disease or another serious disorder.
- Addition of fiber to the diet or behavioral modification can help when dietary or behavioral issues are the cause.

COUGH IN ADULTS

Cough is a sudden, forceful expulsion of air from the lungs. It is the fifth most common reason people see a doctor. The function of a cough is to clear material from the airways and to protect the lungs from particles that have been inhaled. People may cough on purpose (voluntarily) or spontaneously (involuntarily).

Coughs vary considerably. A cough may be dry (unproductive) or it may be productive, bringing up blood or sputum (also called phlegm). Sputum is a mixture of mucus, debris, and cells expelled by the lungs. It may be clear, yellow, green, or streaked with blood.

People who cough very hard may strain their rib muscles or cartilage, causing pain in the chest, particularly when they breathe in, move, or cough again. Cough may be very distressing and interfere with sleep. However, if coughing increases slowly over decades, as it may in smokers, people may hardly be aware of it.

CAUSES

Cough occurs when the airways are irritated. Likely causes of cough depend on whether the cough has lasted less than 3 weeks (acute) or 3 weeks or longer (chronic).

COMMON CAUSES

For acute cough, the most common causes are

- An upper respiratory infection (URI), including acute bronchitis
- Postnasal drip (drainage of secretions from the nose down the throat, or pharynx)
- A flare-up of chronic obstructive pulmonary disease (COPD)
- Pneumonia

For chronic cough, the most common causes are

- Chronic bronchitis
- Postnasal drip
- Airway irritation that remains after a respiratory infection resolves
- Gastroesophageal reflux

LESS COMMON CAUSES

For acute cough, less common causes include

- A blood clot in the lungs (pulmonary embolism)
- Heart failure
- A foreign object (such as a piece of food) that has been inhaled (aspirated)

However, people who accidentally inhale something typically know why they are coughing and tell their doctor unless they have dementia, stroke, or another disorder that causes difficulty communicating.

For chronic cough, less common causes include

- Use of blood pressure drugs called angiotensin-converting enzyme (ACE) inhibitors
- Lung cancer
- Tuberculosis
- Fungal infections of the lungs

People who have dementia or stroke often have trouble swallowing. As a result, they may aspirate small amounts of food and drink, saliva, or stomach contents into their windpipe (trachea). These people may repeatedly aspirate small amounts of these materials without their caregiver's knowledge and may then develop a chronic cough.

Asthma may cause cough. Rarely, the main symptom of asthma is cough rather than wheezing. This type of asthma is called cough-variant asthma.

EVALUATION

Not every cough requires immediate evaluation by a doctor. The following information can help people decide whether a doctor's evaluation is needed and help them know what to expect during the evaluation.

WARNING SIGNS

In people with a cough, certain symptoms and characteristics are cause for concern. They include

- Shortness of breath
- Coughing up blood

- Weight loss
- Fever that lasts longer than about 1 week
- Risk factors for tuberculosis, such as being exposed to tuberculosis, having HIV infection, or taking corticosteroids
- Risk factors for HIV infection, such as high-risk sexual activities or use of street drugs by injection

WHEN TO SEE A DOCTOR

People who have warning signs should see a doctor right away unless the only warning sign is weight loss. Then, a delay of a week or so is not harmful. People who may have inhaled something should also see a doctor right away.

People with an acute cough but no warning signs can wait a few days to see whether the cough stops or becomes less severe, particularly if they also have a congested nose and sore throat, which suggest that the cause may be a URI.

People who have had a chronic cough but no warning signs should see a doctor at some point, but a delay of a week or so is unlikely to be harmful.

WHAT THE DOCTOR DOES

Doctors first ask questions about the person's symptoms and medical history. Doctors then do a physical examination. What they find during the history and physical examination often suggests a cause of the cough and the tests that may need to be done (see Table, below).

Some obvious findings are less helpful in making a diagnosis because they can occur in several disorders that cause cough. For example, whether sputum is yellow or green or thick or thin does not help distinguish bacterial infection from other possible causes. Wheezing may occur with bronchitis, asthma, or other disorders. A cough that brings up blood may be caused by bronchitis, tuberculosis, or lung cancer.

SOME CAUSES AND FEATURES OF COUGH

Cause	Common Features*	Tests
Acute (lasting less than 3 weeks)		
Upper respiratory infections, including acute bronchitis	A runny, congested nose with red mucosa (the tissues that line the nose) Sore throat	A doctor's examination
Pneumonia	Fever, a feeling of illness, a cough that produces sputum (productive cough), and shortness of breath Sudden onset of sharp chest pain that worsens when taking deep breaths Certain abnormal breath sounds, heard through a stethoscope	A chest x-ray For people who are seriously ill or who become ill while in the hospital, cultures of sputum and blood
Postnasal drip (due to an allergy, a virus, or bacteria)	Headache, sore throat, and a congested nose with pale, swollen mucosa Nausea Sometimes a drip visible at the back of the throat	Usually only a doctor's examination Sometimes use of antihistamines and decongestant drugs to see whether symptoms go away
A chronic obstructive pulmonary disease (COPD) flare-up	Wheezing, shortness of breath, and breathing through pursed lips Cough often produces sputum In people who already have COPD	A doctor's examination Sometimes a chest x-ray
A foreign object[†]	A cough that begins suddenly in people who have a disorder that interferes with communication, swallowing, or both	A chest x-ray Bronchoscopy

(continued)

SOME CAUSES AND FEATURES OF COUGH (continued)

Cause	Common Features*	Tests
A foreign object† (continued)	No symptoms of an upper respiratory infection In people who otherwise are feeling well	
Pulmonary embolism† (sudden blockage of an artery in a lung, usually by a blood clot)	Sudden appearance of sharp chest pain that usually worsens when inhaling Shortness of breath A rapid heart rate and a rapid breathing rate Often risk factors for pulmonary embolism, such as cancer, immobility (as results from being bedbound), blood clots in the legs, pregnancy, use of birth control pills (oral contraceptives) or other drugs that contain estrogen, recent surgery or hospitalization, or a family history of the disorder	Specialized lung imaging tests, such as CT angiography or ventilation-perfusion (V/Q) scanning
Heart failure†	Shortness of breath that worsens while lying flat or that appears 1–2 hours after falling asleep Sounds suggesting fluid in the lungs, heard through a stethoscope Usually swelling (edema) in the legs	A chest x-ray Sometimes a blood test to measure a substance that is produced when the heart is strained called brain natriuretic peptide (BNP) Sometimes echocardiography
Chronic (lasting 3 weeks or longer)		
Chronic bronchitis (in smokers)	A productive cough on most days of the month or for 3 months of the year for 2 successive years Frequent clearing of the throat and shortness of breath No congested nose or sore throat In people known to have COPD	A chest x-ray Tests to evaluate how well the lungs are functioning (pulmonary function testing)
Postnasal drip (typically due to an allergy)	Headache, sore throat, and a congested nose with pale, swollen mucosa Sometimes a drip visible at the back of the throat	Sometimes only a doctor's examination Sometimes use of antihistamines and decongestants to see whether symptoms go away Sometimes allergy testing
Gastroesophageal reflux	Burning pain in the chest (heartburn) or abdomen that tends to worsen after eating certain foods, while exercising, or while lying flat A sour taste, particularly after awakening Hoarseness Wheezing A cough that occurs in the middle of the night or early morning Sometimes no symptoms other than cough	Sometimes only a doctor's examination Sometimes use of drugs that suppress acid, such as a histamine-2 (H_2) blocker or proton pump inhibitor, to see whether symptoms go away Sometimes insertion of a flexible viewing tube into the esophagus and stomach (endoscopy) Sometimes placement of a sensor in the esophagus to monitor acidity (pH) for 24 hours (continued)

SOME CAUSES AND FEATURES OF COUGH *(continued)*

Cause	Common Features*	Tests
Asthma (cough-variant)	A cough that seems to occur after various triggers, such as exposure to pollen or another allergen, cold, or exercise Possibly wheezing and shortness of breath	Pulmonary function testing Sometimes use of bronchodilators (drugs that widen airways), such as albuterol, to see whether symptoms go away
Airway irritation that remains after a respiratory tract infection resolves	A dry, nonproductive cough that occurs immediately after a respiratory tract infection No congested nose or sore throat	A chest x-ray
Angiotensin-converting enzyme (ACE) inhibitors	A dry, persistent cough Use of an ACE inhibitor (cough may develop within days or months after starting the drug)	Stopping the ACE inhibitor to see whether symptoms go away
Aspiration	A wet-sounding cough after eating or drinking, visible difficulty swallowing, or both In people who have had a stroke or another disorder that causes difficulty communicating (such as dementia)	A chest x-ray Sometimes x-ray tests of swallowing (modified barium pharyngography) Bronchoscopy
A lung tumor†	A cough that sometimes produces blood Weight loss, fever, and night sweats Enlarged, firm, painless lymph nodes in the neck	A chest x-ray Often CT of the chest Often bronchoscopy
Tuberculosis or fungal infections†	A cough that sometimes produces blood Weight loss, fever, and night sweats Exposure to someone with tuberculosis Residence in or travel to an area where tuberculosis or fungal lung infections are common Presence of HIV infection or risk factors for HIV infection	A chest x-ray Skin testing and, if positive, examination and culture of sputum Sometimes CT of the chest

*Features include symptoms and results of the doctor's examination. Features mentioned are typical but not always present.
†These causes are rare.
CT = computed tomography.

TESTING

The need for tests depends on what doctors find during the history and physical examination, particularly whether warning signs are present.

If people have any warning signs, tests usually include

- Measurement of oxygen levels in the blood with a sensor placed on a finger (pulse oximetry)
- A chest x-ray

Skin tests, chest x-ray, and sometimes computed tomography (CT) of the chest for tuberculosis and blood tests for HIV infection are also done if people have lost weight or have risk factors for these disorders.

If no warning signs are present, doctors can often make a diagnosis based on the history and physical examination and begin treatment without doing tests. In some people, the examination suggests a diagnosis, but tests are done to confirm it (see Table on pages 51 to 53).

If the examination does not suggest a cause of a cough and no warning signs are present, many doctors try giving people a drug to treat one of two common causes of cough:

- An antihistamine/decongestant combination or a nasal corticosteroid spray (for postnasal drip)
- A proton pump inhibitor or histamine-2 (H_2) blocker (for gastroesophageal reflux disease)

If these drugs relieve cough, further testing is usually unnecessary. If cough is not relieved, doctors typically do tests in the following order until a test suggests a diagnosis:

- A chest x-ray
- Pulmonary function tests to check for asthma
- CT of the sinuses to check for sinus disorders
- Placement of an acid sensor in the esophagus to check for gastroesophageal reflux disease

If people have a chronic cough, doctors usually do a chest x-ray. If the cough produces blood, doctors typically send a sputum sample to the laboratory. There, technicians try to grow bacteria in the sample (sputum culture) and use a microscope to check the sample for cancer cells (cytology). Often, if doctors suspect lung cancer (for example, in middle-aged or older people who have smoked for a long time and who have lost weight or have other general symptoms), they also do CT of the chest and sometimes bronchoscopy.

TREATMENT

The best way to treat cough is to treat the underlying disorder. For example, antibiotics can be used for pneumonia, and inhalers containing drugs that widen airways (bronchodilators) or corticosteroids can be used for COPD or asthma. Generally, because coughing plays an important role in bringing up sputum and clearing the airways, a cough should not be suppressed. However, if the cough is severe, interferes with sleep, or has certain causes, various treatments may be tried.

There are two basic approaches to people who are coughing:

- Cough suppressants (antitussive therapy), which reduce the urge to cough

- Expectorants, which are meant to thin the mucus blocking the airways to the lungs and make mucus easier to cough up (but evidence of effectiveness is lacking)

COUGH SUPPRESSANTS

Cough suppressants include the following.

All **opioids** suppress cough because they reduce the responsiveness of the cough center in the brain. Codeine is the opioid used most often for cough. Codeine and other opioid cough suppressants may cause nausea, vomiting, and constipation and may be addictive. They can also cause drowsiness, particularly when a person is taking other drugs that reduce concentration (such as alcohol, sedatives, sleep aids, antidepressants, or certain antihistamines). Thus, opioids are not always safe, and doctors usually reserve them for special situations, such as cough that persists despite other treatments and that interferes with sleep.

Dextromethorphan is related to codeine but is technically not an opioid. It also suppresses the cough center in the brain. Dextromethorphan is the active ingredient in many over-the-counter (OTC) and prescription cough preparations. It is not addictive and, when used correctly, causes little drowsiness. However, it is frequently abused by people, particularly adolescents, because in high doses, it causes euphoria. Overdose causes hallucinations, agitation, and sometimes coma. Overdose is particularly dangerous for people who are taking drugs for depression called serotonin reuptake inhibitors.

Benzonatate is a local anesthetic taken by mouth. It numbs receptors in the lungs that respond to stretching and thus makes the lungs less sensitive to irritation that triggers cough.

Certain people, especially those who are coughing up a large amount of sputum, should limit their use of drugs that suppress cough.

EXPECTORANTS

Some doctors recommend expectorants (sometimes called mucolytics) to help loosen mucus by making bronchial secretions thinner and easier to cough up. Expectorants do not suppress a cough, and the effectiveness of these drugs is lacking. The most commonly used expectorants are OTC preparations that contain guaifenesin. Doctors may prescribe a saturated solution of potassium iodide to loosen mucus. A small dose of syrup of ipecac may help children, especially those who have croup.

In people with cystic fibrosis, dornase alfa (inhaled recombinant human deoxyribonuclease I) can be used to help thin the pus-filled mucus that results from chronic respiratory infections.

Also, inhaling a saline (salt) solution or inhaling acetylcysteine (for up to a few days) sometimes helps thin excessively thick and troublesome mucus.

OTHER DRUGS

Antihistamines, which dry the respiratory tract, have little or no value in treating a cough, except when it is caused by an allergy involving the nose, throat, and windpipe. When coughs have other causes, such as bronchitis, the drying action of antihistamines can be harmful, thickening respiratory secretions and making them difficult to cough up.

Decongestants (such as phenylephrine) that relieve a stuffy nose are only useful for relieving a cough that is caused by postnasal drip.

OTHER TREATMENTS

Steam inhalation (for example, using a vaporizer) is commonly thought to reduce cough. Other topical treatments, such as cough drops, are also popular, but there is no convincing evidence that these other treatments are effective.

O—ᴛᴛ KEY POINTS

- Most coughs are caused by minor respiratory infections or postnasal drip.
- Warning signs in people with a cough include shortness of breath, coughing up blood, weight loss, and fever that lasts longer than about 1 week.
- Doctors can usually make a diagnosis based on results of the medical history and physical examination.
- Drugs (cough suppressants and expectorants) should be used to treat cough only they are when appropriate—cough suppressants only when cough is severe, expectorants only when thick mucus is difficult to cough up, or either type when a doctor recommends it.

COUGH IN CHILDREN

Cough helps clear materials from the airways and prevent them from going to the lungs. The materials may be particles that have been inhaled or substances from the lungs and/or airways. Most commonly, material coughed up from the lungs and airways is sputum (also called phlegm—a mixture of mucus, debris, and cells ejected from the lungs). But sometimes a cough brings up blood (see Coughing Up Blood on page 61). A cough that brings up either is considered productive. Older children (and adults) typically cough material out, but younger children usually swallow it. Some coughs do not bring anything up. They are considered dry or nonproductive.

Cough is one of the most common reasons parents bring their children to a health care practitioner.

CAUSES

Likely causes of cough depend on whether the cough has lasted less than 4 weeks (acute) or 4 weeks or more (chronic).

COMMON CAUSES

For **acute cough,** the most common cause is

- An upper respiratory infection due to a virus

For **chronic cough,** the most common causes are

- Asthma (the most common)
- Gastroesophageal reflux
- Postnasal drip (drainage of fluid from the nose down the throat)

LESS COMMON CAUSES

Acute cough may also result from a foreign body (such as a piece of food or a piece of a toy) inhaled into the lungs (aspiration) or less common respiratory infections such as pneumonia, whooping cough, or tuberculosis.

Chronic cough may also result from aspiration of a foreign body, hereditary disorders such as cystic fibrosis or primary ciliary dyskinesia, a birth defect of the airways or lungs, inflammatory disorders involving the airways or lungs, or may be stress-related (also known as a habit or psychogenic cough).

EVALUATION

Not every cough requires immediate evaluation by a doctor. Knowing which symptoms may indicate a serious cause can help parents decide whether contacting a doctor is needed.

WARNING SIGNS

The following symptoms are of particular concern:

- A blue tint to the lips and/or skin (cyanosis)
- A loud squeaking noise (stridor) when the child breathes in
- Difficulty breathing
- An ill appearance
- Spasms of uncontrollable, repetitive coughing followed by a high-pitched intake of air (sounds like a whoop)

WHEN TO SEE A DOCTOR

Children who have warning signs should be taken to a doctor right away, as should those whose parents think they may have inhaled a foreign body. If children have no warning signs but have a frequent harsh or barking cough, parents should call the doctor. Doctors typically want to see such children within a day or so, depending on their age, other symptoms (such as fever), and medical history (particularly a history of lung disorders, such as asthma or cystic fibrosis). Otherwise healthy children who have a cough occasionally and have typical cold symptoms (such as a runny nose) may not need to be seen by a doctor.

Children with a chronic cough and no warning signs should be seen by a doctor, but a delay of a few days to a week is not harmful.

WHAT THE DOCTOR DOES

Doctors first ask questions about the child's symptoms and medical history. Doctors then do a physical examination. What they find during the history and physical examination often suggests a cause of the cough and the tests that may need to be done (see Table on pages 57 to 59).

Information about the cough helps a doctor determine its cause. Therefore, a doctor may ask:

- What time of day does the cough occur?

- What factors—such as cold air, body position, talking, eating, drinking, or exercise—trigger or relieve the cough?
- What does the cough sound like?
- Did symptoms begin suddenly or gradually?
- What are the child's other symptoms?
- Does the cough bring up sputum or blood?

A nighttime cough can be caused by asthma or postnasal drip. A barky cough suggests croup or sometimes a cough that is left over from a viral upper respiratory infection. A cough that started suddenly in a child with no other symptoms suggests possible inhalation of a foreign body. Contrary to what many people think, whether sputum is yellow or green or thick or thin does not help distinguish bacterial infection from other causes.

When children are 6 months to 4 years old, parents are asked about the possibility of swallowing a foreign body (such as a small toy) or small, smooth, firm foods (such as peanuts or grapes). Doctors also ask whether the child has had any recent respiratory infections, frequent bouts of pneumonia, allergies, or asthma or has been exposed to tuberculosis or other infections, as may occur during travel to certain countries.

A physical examination is done. To check for breathing problems, doctors observe the child's chest, listen to it with a stethoscope, and tap (percuss) it. Doctors also check for cold symptoms, swollen lymph nodes, and abdominal pain.

SOME CAUSES AND FEATURES OF COUGH IN CHILDREN

Cause	Common Features*	Tests
Acute (lasting less than 4 weeks)		
Bronchiolitis	At first, symptoms of a cold	A doctor's examination
	Wheezing and, if bronchiolitis is severe, rapid breathing, with flared nostrils, and difficulty breathing	Sometimes a chest x-ray and culture of mucus from the nose (taken with a swab) to identify the virus
	Possibly vomiting after coughing	
	Typically in infants up to 24 months old, most often in those 3–6 months old	
Croup	At first, symptoms of a cold	A doctor's examination
	Then a frequent, barky cough (worse at night) and, when croup is severe, a loud squeaking noise when the child breathes in (stridor) and rapid breathing, with flared nostrils	Sometimes a neck and chest x-ray
	Typically in children 6 months to 3 years old	
A foreign object in the windpipe (trachea) or larger airways of the lungs (bronchi)	Cough and choking that begin suddenly	A chest x-ray
	No fever initially	Sometimes bronchoscopy
	No symptoms of a cold	
	Typically in children 6 months to 4 years old	
Pertussis (whooping cough)	Mild coldlike symptoms for 1–2 weeks, followed by coughing fits	Culture of a sample of mucus taken from the nose
	Infants: Coughing fits that may be associated with a blue tint to the lips or skin (cyanosis), vomiting after coughing, or pauses in breathing (apnea)	
	Older children: Coughing fits that may be followed by a prolonged, high-pitched sound (called the whoop)	
	Cough that may persist for several weeks	

(continued)

SOME CAUSES AND FEATURES OF COUGH IN CHILDREN *(continued)*

Cause	Common Features*	Tests
Pneumonia	Typically fever	A doctor's examination
	Sometimes wheezing, shortness of breath, and chest pain	Often a chest x-ray
	Cough that is sometimes productive	
Upper respiratory infections (most common)	A runny nose and nasal congestion	A doctor's examination
	Possibly fever and sore throat	
	Possibly small, nontender, swollen lymph nodes in the neck	
Chronic† (lasting 4 weeks or more)		
Asthma	Periodic attacks of coughing in response to a trigger (such as pollen or other allergens), exposure to cold air, or exercise	A doctor's examination
		Treatment with asthma drugs to see whether symptoms are relieved
	Coughing during the night	Breathing tests to evaluate lung function (pulmonary function tests)
	Sometimes family members who have asthma	
Birth defects affecting the lungs	Several episodes of pneumonia in the same part of the lungs	Chest x-ray
		Sometimes CT or MRI
Birth defects affecting the windpipe (trachea), esophagus, or both	Vary by defect	Chest x-ray
	Typically in newborns or infants	Sometimes bronchoscopy and endoscopy
	If the trachea has not developed normally, possibly a loud squeaking noise when the child breathes in (stridor) or a barky cough and difficulty breathing	If an abnormal trachea is suspected, also CT or MRI
	If there is an abnormal connection between the trachea and esophagus (tracheoesophageal fistula), a cough or difficulty breathing when the child is fed and frequent bouts of pneumonia	
Cystic fibrosis	A blockage in the intestine by thick secretions (meconium ileus) detected shortly after birth	A sweat test
		Possibly genetic testing to confirm the diagnosis
	Frequent bouts of pneumonia, sinusitis, or both	
	Not growing as expected (failure to thrive)	
	Enlargement of the fingertips or a change in the angle of the nail bed (clubbing) and nail beds that are tinted blue	
A foreign object in the lung or airways	Cough and choking that began suddenly	Chest x-rays while breathing out and breathing in
	Resolution of choking but cough that persists or progressively worsens over several weeks	Bronchoscopy
	Possibly a fever	
	No symptoms of a cold	
	Typically in children 6 months to 4 years old	*(continued)*

SOME CAUSES AND FEATURES OF COUGH IN CHILDREN *(continued)*

Cause	Common Features*	Tests
Gastroesophageal reflux	**Infants:** Fussiness, spitting up after feedings, arching of the back, or crying after feedings and a cough when lying down Poor weight gain **Older children and adolescents:** Chest pain or heartburn after meals and when lying down and possibly wheezing, hoarseness, nausea, and regurgitation Cough that is often worse at night	A doctor's examination **Infants:** Sometimes an x-ray of the upper digestive tract after barium is given by mouth to determine whether anatomy is normal Treatment with histamine-2 (H$_2$) blockers (if symptoms are relieved, the cause is probably gastroesophageal reflux disease) Sometimes a test to measure acidity or reflux episodes in the esophagus (called a pH probe or an impedance probe) or x-rays taken after formula is given by mouth (gastric emptying scan) to determine the frequency and severity of reflux episodes **Older children:** Treatment with H$_2$ blockers or proton pump inhibitors to see whether symptoms are relieved Possibly endoscopy
Postnasal drip	Headache, itchy eyes, a mild sore throat particularly in the morning, and coughing at night and when waking up A history of allergies	Treatment with an antihistamine or a corticosteroid nasal spray (if symptoms are relieved, the cause is an allergy) Possibly x-rays or CT of the sinuses
Psychogenic or habit cough	May develop in children after a cold or other airway irritant Frequent (may be up to every 2–3 seconds), harsh, or honking cough when awake, possibly lasting for weeks to months Cough that stops completely when the child falls asleep Lack of fever or other symptoms	A doctor's examination Sometimes chest x-rays to look for other causes
Tuberculosis	Recent contact with an infected person Usually a weakened immune system (immunocompromise) Sometimes fever, night sweats, chills, and weight loss	A chest x-ray A tuberculin skin test

*Features include symptoms and the results of the doctor's examination. Features mentioned are typical but not always present.

†Children with disorders that cause chronic cough may also be brought to a doctor before 4 weeks. A chest x-ray is always done when children with a chronic cough are first evaluated.

CT = computed tomography; MRI = magnetic resonance imaging.

TESTING

Tests may or may not be needed depending on symptoms and the causes that doctors suspect. For children with warning signs, doctors typically measure the oxygen concentration in blood using a clip-on sensor (pulse oximetry) and take a chest x-ray. These tests are also done if children have a chronic cough or if a cough is worsening. Doctors may also do other tests depending on what they find during the history and physical examination (see Table on pages 57 to 59).

For children without warning signs, tests are rarely done if the cough has lasted 4 weeks or less and cold symptoms are present. In such cases, the cause is usually a viral infection.

Tests also may not be needed if symptoms strongly suggest a cause. In such cases, doctors may simply start treatment for the presumed cause. However, if symptoms persist despite treatment, tests are often done.

TREATMENT

Treatment focuses on treating the cause (for example, antibiotics for bacterial pneumonia or antihistamines for allergic postnasal drip).

To relieve cough symptoms, parents have often been advised to use home remedies such as having the child inhale moist air (as from a vaporizer or in a hot shower) and drink extra fluids. Although these remedies are harmless, there is little scientific evidence that they make any difference in how children feel.

Cough suppressant drugs (such as dextromethorphan and codeine) are rarely recommended for children. Cough is an important way for the body to clear secretions from the airways. Also, these drugs may have side effects, such as confusion and sedation, and there is very little evidence that they help children feel better or recover more quickly. Expectorants, which are supposed to thin and loosen mucus (making it easier to cough up), are also usually discouraged in children.

O—ᴨ KEY POINTS

- Usually, the cause can be identified based on results of the doctor's examination.
- In children aged 6 months to 4 years, a foreign body in the airways must be considered.
- Chest x-rays are taken if children have warning signs or a cough that has lasted more than 4 weeks.
- Usually, cough suppressants and expectorants are not recommended.

COUGHING UP BLOOD

Coughing up blood from the respiratory tract is called hemoptysis. The amount of blood produced can vary from a few streaks of blood mixed with normal sputum to large amounts of pure blood. Other symptoms, such as fever and difficulty breathing, may be present depending on the cause of hemoptysis.

CAUSES

Although hemoptysis can be frightening, most causes turn out not to be serious. Blood-streaked sputum is common in many minor respiratory illnesses, such as upper respiratory infections and viral bronchitis. Sometimes the cause is blood from the nose that has traveled down the throat and then is coughed up. Such blood is not considered hemoptysis.

COMMON CAUSES

Infection is the most common cause (see Table on pages 63 to 64). In adults, 70 to 90% of cases are caused by

- Bronchitis
- Bronchiectasis, which is an abnormal, irreversible widening of part of the breathing tubes or airways (called bronchi)
- Tuberculosis
- Pneumonia

In children, common causes are

- A lower respiratory tract infection
- A foreign object that has been inhaled (aspirated)

LESS COMMON CAUSES

Lung cancer that starts in the lungs is an important cause in smokers over age 40. However, cancer that has spread to the lungs from elsewhere in the body rarely causes hemoptysis. Fungal infection with *Aspergillus* is increasingly recognized as a cause but is not as common as cancer.

Other causes include a blood clot in an artery in a lung (pulmonary embolism) and inflammation of blood vessels (vasculitis) in the lung, such as Goodpasture syndrome.

MASSIVE HEMOPTYSIS

Massive hemoptysis is the production of more than a pint (about 600 milliliters) of blood within 24 hours. The most common causes include the following:

- Lung cancer
- Bronchiectasis
- Some pneumonias, including that from tuberculosis

RISK FACTORS

Some conditions increase the risk that hemoptysis is caused by a serious disorder:

- Human immunodeficiency virus infection (for Kaposi sarcoma, tuberculosis, and fungal infections)
- Use of drugs that suppress the immune system called immunosuppressants (for tuberculosis and fungal infections)
- Exposure to tuberculosis
- A long history of smoking (for cancer)
- Recent bed rest or surgery, cancer, a previous occurrence of or a family history of clotting, pregnancy, use of drugs that contain estrogen, and recent long-distance travel (for pulmonary embolism)

EVALUATION

The following information can help people decide whether a doctor's evaluation is needed and help them know what to expect during the evaluation.

WARNING SIGNS

In people with hemoptysis, the following symptoms are of particular concern:

- Massive amounts of blood coughed up
- Shortness of breath
- Signs of significant blood loss (weakness, dizziness when standing up, thirst, sweating, and a rapid heart rate)

WHEN TO SEE A DOCTOR

People with warning signs should go the hospital immediately. People without warning signs who have risk factors for serious disorders and those with more than just blood-streaked sputum should see a doctor in a day or two.

If people have only blood-streaked sputum (which is usually caused by an upper respiratory infection), a doctor's evaluation is not as urgent. People can call a doctor, who can decide whether and how rapidly they need to be seen based on their symptoms, medical history, and other factors. Typically, a delay of a few days or so is not harmful.

WHAT THE DOCTOR DOES

Doctors first ask questions about the person's symptoms and medical history and then do a physical examination. What doctors find during the history and physical examination often suggests a cause and the tests that may need to be done (see Table on pages 63 to 64).

Doctors ask

- When the person started coughing up blood
- How long the coughing has been going on
- Whether anything specific triggers it (such as cold, exertion, or lying down)
- About how much blood is coughed up (such as streaks, a teaspoonful, or a cupful)
- Whether the person has other symptoms, such as fever, weight loss, chest pain, or leg pain

Doctors determine whether blood was actually coughed (and not vomited or dripped down the back of the throat from a nosebleed).

Doctors ask people about their medical history (if not already known) and their risk factors for causes. A history of frequent nosebleeds, easy bruising, or liver disease suggests a possible blood clotting disorder. Doctors review the drugs the person is taking to check for drugs that inhibit clotting (anticoagulants).

During the physical examination, doctors review vital signs to check for fever, rapid heart or breathing rates, and a low oxygen level in the blood. They do a full heart and lung examination, inspect the neck veins for signs of fullness such as bulging, and check the legs for puffiness. Puffiness in one leg may indicate deep vein thrombosis. Puffiness in both legs may indicate heart failure. Doctors also examine the abdomen, skin, and mucous membranes. The person is asked to cough during the examination. If any blood is coughed up, the doctor notes its color and the amount of blood. Doctors also check the nose and mouth for bleeding sites.

Clues from the history and examination help doctors determine the cause. A sensation of postnasal drip or any bleeding from the nose, particularly without coughing, may mean that the blood being coughed up has dripped down the back of the throat from the nose. Nausea and vomiting of black, brown, or coffee-ground–colored material usually means that the blood is from the stomach or intestine and is being vomited and not coughed. Frothy sputum, bright red blood, and, if the amount is massive, a sensation of choking usually mean that the blood is from the trachea or lungs (called true hemoptysis).

If cough has just begun and if the person is otherwise in good health and has no risk factors for tuberculosis, fungal infection, or pulmonary embolism, the cause is usually an acute respiratory infection, such as bronchitis. If coughing up blood is caused by a heart or lung disorder, the person has almost always already been diagnosed with that heart or lung disorder. That is, coughing up blood is usually not the first symptom of a heart or lung disorder.

TESTING

If hemoptysis is severe, persistent, or unexplained, testing is needed. If people have coughed up massive amounts of blood, they are treated and stabilized before testing is done.

A chest x-ray is taken routinely. If the chest x-ray is abnormal or if the person has symptoms of or risk factors for a particular disorder, computed tomography (CT) and bronchoscopy are done. In bronchoscopy, a flexible viewing tube is inserted into the windpipe and bronchi to identify the bleeding site. Occasionally, bronchoscopy is necessary to confirm that blood is being coughed up from the lower airways and not from the nose, stomach, or intestine.

If pulmonary embolism seems possible, doctors do CT using a radiopaque dye to show blood vessels (called CT angiography) or a scan using a radioactive marker (called a lung perfusion scan).

Doctors often check for lung cancer, especially in smokers over age 40 (and even in younger smokers if they started smoking during adolescence), even if the sputum is only blood-streaked.

In most people, a complete blood count and blood tests that assess the blood's ability to clot are done to detect blood clotting problems.

SOME CAUSES AND FEATURES OF HEMOPTYSIS

Cause	Common Features*	Tests†
A blood clotting disorder Use of anticoagulants (as used to treat pulmonary embolism, blood clots in the legs, or atrial fibrillation or to reduce the risk of clots after certain heart procedures) Use of drugs that dissolve clots (thrombolytic drugs, as used to treat a heart attack or stroke)	Sometimes bleeding from other sites, such as the nose or digestive tract (seen in stool) In people taking anticoagulants or thrombolytic drugs Sometimes a family history of a blood clotting disorder	Blood tests that assess the blood's ability to clot
Bronchiectasis	A chronic cough and mucus production in people with a history of recurring infections	High-resolution CT of the chest Sometimes bronchoscopy
Bronchitis	*Acute:* A cough that may or may not produce sputum (productive or nonproductive) and sometimes symptoms of an upper respiratory infection (such as a stuffy nose) *Chronic:* A productive cough on most days of the month or for 3 months of the year for 2 successive years in smokers or in people known to have chronic obstructive pulmonary disease	*Acute:* A doctor's examination *Chronic:* A chest x-ray Tests to evaluate how well the lungs are functioning (pulmonary function tests)
Certain long-lasting lung infections (tuberculosis, fungal infections, parasitic infections, or syphilis that affects the lungs)	Fever, cough, night sweats, and weight loss in people known to be exposed to the infection Often a history of a weakened immune system (immunosuppression) due to a disorder or drug	A chest x-ray CT of the chest Testing of sputum samples or samples of fluid from the lungs obtained with a bronchoscope
A foreign object that has been present a long time and has not been identified	A chronic cough (typically in infants or young children) without symptoms of an upper respiratory infection Sometimes a fever	A chest x-ray Sometimes bronchoscopy
Goodpasture syndrome	Fatigue and weight loss Often blood in the urine Sometimes shortness of breath Sometimes swelling (edema) of the legs	A biopsy of kidney tissue Blood tests to check for antibodies characteristic of the disorder (anti–glomerular basement membrane antibodies)
Heart failure	Frothy, pink sputum, sometimes with blood streaks Shortness of breath that worsens while lying flat or that appears 1–2 hours after falling asleep Sounds suggesting fluid in the lungs, heard through a stethoscope Usually swelling (edema) of the legs	A chest x-ray Sometimes a blood test to measure a substance that is produced when the heart is strained (called brain natriuretic peptide, or BNP) Sometimes echocardiography

(continued)

SOME CAUSES AND FEATURES OF HEMOPTYSIS *(continued)*

Cause	Common Features*	Tests†
Lung abscess	Fever, usually for one or more weeks A cough, night sweats, loss of appetite, and weight loss	A chest x-ray Sometimes CT or bronchoscopy
Lung cancer	Night sweats and weight loss Usually in middle-aged or older people with a history of heavy smoking	A chest x-ray CT Bronchoscopy
Pneumonia	Fever, a feeling of illness, a productive cough, and shortness of breath Sudden appearance of chest pain when taking deep breaths Certain abnormal breath sounds, heard through a stethoscope	A chest x-ray
Pulmonary embolism (sudden blockage of an artery in a lung, usually by a blood clot)	Sudden appearance of sharp chest pain that usually worsens when inhaling Shortness of breath A rapid heart rate and a rapid breathing rate Often risk factors for pulmonary embolism, such as cancer, immobility (as results from being bedbound), blood clots in the legs, pregnancy, use of birth control pills (oral contraceptives) or other drugs that contain estrogen, recent surgery or hospitalization, or a family history of the disorder	Specialized lung imaging tests, such as CT angiography or ventilation/perfusion (V/Q) scanning

*Features include symptoms and results of the doctor's examination. Features mentioned are typical but not always present.
†If people have hemoptysis, doctors always take a chest x-ray and measure oxygen levels in the blood with a sensor placed on a finger (pulse oximetry).
CT = computed tomography.

Despite testing, the cause of hemoptysis is not identified in 30 to 40% of people. However, when hemoptysis is severe, the cause is usually identified.

TREATMENT

Bleeding may produce clots that block the airways and lead to further breathing problems. Therefore, coughing is important to keep the airways clear and should not be suppressed with cough suppressants (antitussive drugs).

Hemoptysis may be mild and may stop by itself or when the disorder causing the bleeding (such as heart failure or infection) is successfully treated.

If a large clot blocks a major airway, doctors may have to remove the clot using bronchoscopy.

Rarely, hemoptysis is severe or does not stop by itself. If so, a tube may need to be inserted through the mouth or nose into the windpipe or lower into the airways to help keep the airways open.

If the source of bleeding is a major blood vessel, a doctor may try to close off the bleeding vessel using a procedure called bronchial artery embolization. Using x-rays for guidance, the doctor passes a catheter into the vessel and then injects a chemical, fragments of a gelatin sponge, or a wire coil to block the blood vessel and thereby stop the bleeding. Sometimes bronchoscopy or surgery may be needed to stop severe or continuing bleeding, or surgery may be needed to remove a diseased or cancerous portion of the lung. These high-risk procedures are used only as last resorts.

If clotting abnormalities are contributing to the bleeding, a person may need a transfusion of plasma, clotting factors, or platelets.

O—π KEY POINTS

- Blood-streaked sputum is usually caused by a respiratory infection and, if it resolves, is not usually cause for worry.
- A lower respiratory tract infection and inhalation of a foreign object are the most common causes in children.
- Doctors must distinguish hemoptysis from bleeding that comes from the mouth, nose, or throat and from blood that is vomited.
- Blood-streaked sputum in people who smoke usually requires further evaluation.
- People who cough up massive amounts of blood must be treated and stabilized before testing can be done.

CRYING IN INFANTS, EXCESSIVE

All infants and young children cry as a form of communication. It is the only way they have to express a need. Thus, most crying is in response to hunger, discomfort (such as that due to a wet diaper), fear, or separation from parents. Such crying is normal and typically stops when the needs are met—for example, when infants are fed, burped, changed, or cuddled. This crying tends to occur less often and for shorter times after children are 3 months old.

Excessive crying refers to crying that continues after caregivers have attempted to meet routine needs or crying that continues for longer than usual for a given child.

CAUSES

More than 95% of the time, there is no specific medical disorder responsible for excessive crying. Although such crying is stressful for parents, children eventually settle down and stop crying on their own. Fatigue is a common cause of crying in infants. Between 6 months and 3 years of age, crying at night is often due to difficulty falling back to sleep after normal night awakenings. Falling back to sleep on their own is especially difficult for children who are used to falling asleep under certain conditions such as while being rocked or with a pacifier. Nighttime fears are common after age 3 years. The particular fears usually depend on the child's age and stage of emotional and physical development. Sometimes children aged 3 to 8 years cry fearfully in the middle of the night and do not seem to be awake or able to be comforted. They also have no memory of a dream or of the crying when they wake in the morning. These episodes of crying are called night terrors.

MEDICAL DISORDERS

Less than 5% of the time, excessive crying is caused by a medical disorder. Some disorders are uncomfortable but not immediately dangerous. Such less serious causes of crying include gastroesophageal reflux, hair wrapped around a

finger or toe (hair tourniquet), a scratch on the surface of the eye (corneal abrasion), an anal fissure, and a middle ear infection.

Less commonly, a serious disorder is the cause. Such disorders include a blocked intestine caused by intussusception (sliding of one segment of intestine into another) and volvulus (twisting of the intestine), as well as heart failure, meningitis, and head injuries that cause bleeding within the skull. Infants with such severe disorders often have other symptoms (such as vomiting or fever), which alert parents to the presence of a more serious problem. However, sometimes excessive crying is the first sign.

Colic refers to excessive crying that has no identifiable cause and that occurs at least 3 hours a day for more than 3 days a week for more than 3 weeks. Colic typically occurs in infants about 6 weeks to 3 or 4 months old.

EVALUATION

Doctors try to identify any medical disorder that may be causing an infant's persistent crying.

WARNING SIGNS

Certain symptoms are cause for concern and suggest that a medical disorder is causing the crying:

- Difficulty breathing
- Bruises or swelling over the head or other parts of the body
- Abnormal movements or twitching of any body part
- Extreme irritability (normal handling or movement causes crying or distress)
- Continuous crying, especially if it is accompanied by a fever
- Fever in an infant under 8 weeks old

WHEN TO SEE A DOCTOR

Children should be evaluated by a doctor right away if they have any warning signs, if they are vomiting, if they have stopped eating, or if parents notice swelling of the abdomen, a red and/or swollen scrotum, or any unusual behavior (in addition to the crying).

If children without such signs appear well otherwise, parents can try typical measures such as feeding, burping, changing, and cuddling. If crying continues after such measures, parents should call the doctor. The doctor can help parents determine how quickly the child needs to be evaluated.

WHAT THE DOCTOR DOES

Doctors first ask questions about the child's symptoms and medical history. Doctors then do a physical examination. What they find during the history and physical examination often suggests a cause of the crying and the tests that may need to be done (see Table, below). Infants with fever often have an infection, those with difficulty breathing may have a heart or lung disorder, and those with vomiting, diarrhea, or constipation may have a digestive disorder.

Doctors ask about the crying:

- When it started
- How long it lasts
- How often it happens
- Whether it is related to feeding or bowel movements
- How infants respond to efforts to soothe them

Parents are asked about recent events that may explain the crying (such as recent immunizations, injuries, and illnesses), and about drugs given to the infant. Doctors also ask questions to learn how well the parents are bonding with the infant and managing the infant's needs.

A physical examination is done to check for symptoms of disorders that can cause discomfort or pain. Doctors look particularly at the child's eyes for a corneal abrasion and at fingers, toes, and the penis for a hair tourniquet.

TESTING

Tests may or may not be needed depending on the infant's symptoms and the causes that doctors suspect. If the doctor's examination does not suggest a serious disorder, tests are not usually done, but doctors may schedule a follow-up visit to reevaluate the infant.

SOME MEDICAL DISORDERS THAT CAUSE EXCESSIVE CRYING IN INFANTS AND YOUNG CHILDREN

Cause*	Common Features†	Tests
Heart disorders		
Heart failure or an abnormal heart rhythm	Difficulty breathing, difficulty feeding, and excessive sweating	Chest x-ray
		ECG
	Often an abnormal heart sound detected during a doctor's examination	Echocardiography
Digestive disorders		
Allergy to cow's milk protein	Vomiting	Stool tests
	Diarrhea or constipation	Symptoms that lessen when the formula is changed
	Poor feeding	
	Weight loss, poor growth, or both	Possibly endoscopy, colonoscopy, or both
	Blood in stools	
Constipation	Hard, less frequent bowel movements that are difficult to pass	A doctor's examination
	Sometimes apparent pain during a bowel movement	
	Sometimes tears (fissures) in the anus	*(continued)*

SOME MEDICAL DISORDERS THAT CAUSE EXCESSIVE CRYING IN INFANTS AND YOUNG CHILDREN *(continued)*

Cause*	Common Features†	Tests
Gastroesophageal reflux	Symptoms that occur after feeding, including fussiness or crying, spitting up, or arching of the back Sometimes a cough when lying down or poor weight gain	A doctor's examination Sometimes treatment with drugs to suppress acid production (if symptoms are relieved, the cause is probably gastroesophageal reflux disease) Sometimes x-rays of the upper digestive tract after barium is given by mouth or a test to measure acidity or reflux episodes in the esophagus (called a pH probe or an impedance probe) or endoscopy
Incarcerated hernia	Red, swollen, tender bulge in the groin	A doctor's examination
Intussusception (sliding of one segment of intestine into another)	Crying that occurs in bouts every 15 to 20 minutes with children often drawing their legs up to their chest Later, tenderness of the abdomen when it is touched and bowel movements that look like currant jelly (because they contain blood) Typically in children 3 to 36 months old	Ultrasonography of the abdomen Insertion of air into the rectum (air enema)
Volvulus (twisting of the intestine)	Vomiting, a swollen abdomen, and/or tenderness of the abdomen when it is touched Possibly blood in stools or no stools	An x-ray of the abdomen Barium or air enema
Infections		
Ear infection (otitis media)	Often cold symptoms (such as a runny nose and cough) Sometimes fever Ear pain	A doctor's examination
Meningitis	Fever and lethargy or listlessness Bulging of the soft spots (fontanelles) between the skull bones Fussiness and irritability (especially when held), inconsolability, and poor feeding	A spinal tap (lumbar puncture)
Urinary tract infections (UTIs)	Often fever Crying or complaints of pain with urination	Examination (urinalysis) and culture of urine
Injury		
Broken bone	Swelling or bruising Unwillingness to use a limb Pain during bathing, changing, or a doctor's examination	X-rays

(continued)

SOME MEDICAL DISORDERS THAT CAUSE EXCESSIVE CRYING IN INFANTS AND YOUNG CHILDREN *(continued)*

Cause*	Common Features†	Tests
Corneal abrasion (a scratch on the surface of the eye)	No other symptoms	Examination of the eye after applying an eye drop that makes abrasions visible (fluorescein test)
Hair tourniquet	Swollen tip of a toe, a finger, or the penis with a hair wrapped below the swelling	A doctor's examination
A head injury	An inconsolable, high-pitched cry Sometimes a swollen area on the head	CT of the head
Other causes		
Drugs used to treat colds	Recent drug treatment for a cold	A doctor's examination
Teething	A tooth erupting or about ready to erupt, drooling Sometimes sleeplessness or restless sleep at night Sometimes mild fever	Symptoms that resolve after tooth erupts
Testicular torsion (twisting of a testis)	A swollen, painful, red scrotum	Doppler ultrasonography of the scrotum
A vaccine reaction	Recent vaccination (within 24–48 hours)	A doctor's examination

*Medical disorders cause fewer than 5% of cases of excessive crying.
†Features include symptoms and results of the doctor's examination. Features mentioned are typical but not always present.
CT = computed tomography; ECG = electrocardiography.

TREATMENT

Any specific disorder is treated. For example, a hair tourniquet is removed, or a corneal abrasion is treated with antibiotic ointment.

For infants who have no specific disorder, parents or caregivers should continue to look for obvious causes of crying, such as a wet diaper or clothing that is too hot, and meet those needs. They can try various other strategies. For example, an infant may be soothed by

- Being held, gently rocked, or patted
- Listening to white noise, such as the sound of rain or the electronically produced sounds made by a fan, washing machine, vacuum, or hair dryer
- Riding in a car
- Sucking on a pacifier
- Using nipples with a smaller hole if infants are feeding too quickly
- Being snugly wrapped (swaddled)
- Being burped
- Being fed (but parents should avoid overfeeding in an attempt to stop the crying)

When the cause of the crying is fatigue, many of the above interventions only briefly console infants and the crying returns as soon as the stimulation or activity stops, leaving infants even more fatigued. Sometimes it is more effective to encourage self-soothing and sleep by routinely laying infants in their crib awake so they do not depend on their parents or certain motions, objects, or sounds to fall asleep.

Mothers who are breastfeeding may notice that after they eat certain foods, their infant cries. They should then avoid eating those foods.

Teething eventually passes, and the crying it causes usually lessens with time. Mild pain relievers and teething rings can help in the meantime.

SUPPORT FOR PARENTS

When an infant cries excessively for no apparent reason, parents may feel exhausted and stressed. Sometimes they become so frustrated that child abuse occurs. Emotional support from friends, family members, neighbors, and doctors can help parents cope. Parents should ask for whatever help they need (with siblings, errands, or child care) and share their feelings and fears with each other and with other support people. If parents are feeling frustrated, they should take a break from the crying infant or child and put the infant or child in a safe environment for a few minutes. Such a strategy can help parents cope and help prevent abuse.

Doctors can provide information about support services to parents who feel overwhelmed.

KEY POINTS

- Crying is a way to communicate and is part of normal development.
- Often, identifying and meeting the infant's need stops the crying.
- Crying typically decreases after infants are 3 months old.
- Less than 5% of crying is caused by a medical disorder.
- If parents are concerned about an infant's crying, they can call a doctor, who can advise them about bringing the infant in for evaluation.
- Parents may need support when infants cry excessively for no apparent reason and cannot by soothed.

DIARRHEA IN ADULTS

Diarrhea is an increase in the volume, wateriness, or frequency of bowel movements. However, the frequency of bowel movements alone is not the defining feature of diarrhea. Some people normally move their bowels 3 to 5 times a day. People who eat large amounts of vegetable fiber may produce more than a pound (1/2 kilogram) of stool a day, but the stool in such cases is well formed and not watery. Diarrhea is often accompanied by gas, cramping, an urgency to defecate, and, if the diarrhea is caused by an infectious organism or a toxic substance, nausea and vomiting.

COMPLICATIONS

Diarrhea can lead to dehydration and a loss of electrolytes, such as sodium, potassium, magnesium, chloride, and bicarbonate, from the blood. If large amounts of fluid and electrolytes are lost, the person feels weak, and blood pressure can drop enough to cause fainting (syncope), heart rhythm abnormalities (arrhythmias), and other serious disorders. At particular risk are the very young, the very old, the debilitated, and people with very severe diarrhea.

CAUSES

There are many different causes, depending on how long the diarrhea has lasted (see Table on pages 74 to 75).

The most common causes of acute diarrhea (lasting less than a week) are

- Infection with viruses, bacteria, or parasites (gastroenteritis)
- Food poisoning
- Drug side effects

The most common causes of chronic diarrhea (lasting more than 4 weeks) are

- Irritable bowel syndrome
- Inflammatory bowel disease
- Drug side effects
- Recent antibiotic use (causing *Clostridium difficile* infection)

Diarrhea that has been present for 1 to 4 weeks may be a lingering case of acute diarrhea or the early stage of a disorder that causes chronic diarrhea.

CLASSIFICATION

Normally, stool is 60 to 90% water. Diarrhea occurs when not enough water is removed from the stool, making the stool loose and poorly formed. Stool may contain too much water if it

- Passes too quickly through the digestive tract
- Contains certain substances that prevent the large intestine from absorbing water
- Contains excess water secreted by the intestines

Rapid passage (transit) of stool is one of the most common general causes of diarrhea. For stool to have normal consistency, it must remain in the large intestine for a certain amount of time. Stool that leaves the large intestine too quickly is watery. Many medical conditions and treatments can decrease the amount of time that stool stays in the large intestine. These conditions include an overactive thyroid (hyperthyroidism); Zollinger-Ellison syndrome (a condition of over-production of acid by a tumor); surgical removal of part of the stomach, small intestine, or large intestine; surgical bypass of part of the intestine; inflammatory bowel disease (such as ulcerative colitis); and use of drugs such as antacids containing magnesium, laxatives, prostaglandins, serotonin, and even caffeine. Many foods, especially those that are acidic or have a very high amount of sugar (such as waffle or maple syrup), can increase the rate of transit. Some people are intolerant of specific foods and always develop diarrhea after eating them. Stress and anxiety are also common causes.

Osmotic diarrhea occurs when certain substances that cannot be absorbed through the colon wall remain in the intestine. These substances cause excessive amounts of water to remain in the stool, leading to diarrhea. Certain foods (such as some fruits and beans) and sugar substitutes in dietetic foods, candy, and chewing gum (for example, hexitols, sorbitol, and mannitol—see Table on page 72) can cause osmotic diarrhea. Also, lactase deficiency can lead to osmotic diarrhea. Lactase is an enzyme

FOODS AND BEVERAGES THAT CAN CAUSE DIARRHEA	
Food or Beverage	**Ingredient Causing Diarrhea**
Sugar-free gum, mints, sweet cherries, or prunes	Hexitols, sorbitol, or mannitol
Apple juice, pear juice, grapes, honey, dates, nuts, figs, soft drinks (especially fruit flavors), prunes, or waffle or maple syrup	Fructose
Milk, ice cream, yogurt, or soft cheese	Lactose
Coffee, tea, cola drinks, or some over-the-counter headache remedies	Caffeine
Certain fat-free potato chips or fat-free ice cream	Olestra

normally found in the small intestine that converts lactose (milk sugar) to glucose and galactose, so that it can be absorbed into the bloodstream. When people with lactase deficiency drink milk or eat dairy products, lactose is not digested. As lactose accumulates in the intestine, it causes osmotic diarrhea—a condition known as lactose intolerance. The severity of osmotic diarrhea depends on how much of the osmotic substance is consumed. Diarrhea stops soon after the person stops eating or drinking the substance. Blood in the digestive tract also acts as an osmotic agent and results in black, tarry stools (melena). Another cause of osmotic diarrhea is an overgrowth of normal intestinal bacteria or the growth of bacteria normally not found in the intestines. Antibiotics can cause osmotic diarrhea by destroying the normal intestinal bacteria.

Secretory diarrhea occurs when the small and large intestines secrete salts (especially sodium chloride) and water into the stool. Certain toxins—such as the toxin produced by a cholera infection or during some viral infections—can cause these secretions. Infections by certain bacteria (for example, *Campylobacter*) and parasites (for example, *Cryptosporidium*) can also stimulate secretions. The diarrhea can be massive—more than a quart (1 liter) of stool an hour in cholera. Other substances that cause salt and water secretion include certain laxatives, such as castor oil, and bile acids (which may build up after surgery to remove part of the small intestine). Certain rare tumors—such as carcinoid, gastrinoma, and vipoma—also can cause secretory diarrhea, as can some polyps.

Inflammatory diarrhea occurs when the lining of the large intestine becomes inflamed, ulcerated, or engorged and releases proteins,

blood, mucus, and other fluids, which increase the bulk and fluid content of the stool. This type of diarrhea can be caused by many diseases, including ulcerative colitis, Crohn disease, tuberculosis, and cancers such as lymphoma and adenocarcinoma. When the lining of the rectum is affected, people often feel an urgent need to move their bowels and have frequent bowel movements because the inflamed rectum is more sensitive to expansion (distention) by stool.

EVALUATION

Not every episode of diarrhea requires immediate evaluation by a doctor. The following information can help people decide whether a doctor's evaluation is needed and help them know what to expect during the evaluation.

WARNING SIGNS

Certain findings raise suspicion of a more serious cause of diarrhea.

- Blood or pus in the stool
- Fever
- Signs of dehydration (such as decreased urination, lethargy or listlessness, extreme thirst, and a dry mouth)
- Chronic diarrhea
- Diarrhea at night
- Weight loss

WHEN TO SEE A DOCTOR

People who have warning signs of blood or pus in the stool, fever, or signs of dehydration should see a doctor right away, as should those with significant abdominal pain. Such people may need immediate testing, treatment, and sometimes admission to a hospital. If the only warning signs are chronic or nighttime diarrhea or weight loss, people should see a doctor within a week or so. People without warning signs should call a doctor if diarrhea lasts for more than 72 hours. Depending on the person's other symptoms, age, and medical history, the doctor may recommend the person have an examination or try at-home or over-the-counter treatments (see Treatment, below).

WHAT THE DOCTOR DOES

Doctors first ask questions about the person's symptoms and medical history. Doctors then do a physical examination. What they find during the history and physical examination often suggests a cause of the diarrhea and the tests that may need to be done (see Table on pages 74 to 75).

A doctor begins by asking how long the diarrhea has been going on and how severe it has been. Simultaneous occurrence of diarrhea in friends, family members, or other personal contacts is sought. Other important questions focus on

- Circumstances around when it started (including recent travel, food ingested, and source of water)
- Drug use (including any antibiotics within the previous 3 months)
- Abdominal pain or vomiting
- Frequency and timing of bowel movements
- Changes in stool characteristics (for example, presence of blood, pus, or mucus and changes in color or consistency)
- Changes in weight or appetite
- Feeling an urgent need to defecate or to defecate constantly

The physical examination begins with the doctor's evaluation of the person's fluid and hydration status. A full examination of the abdomen is done, as is a digital rectal examination to check for the presence of blood.

TESTING

The need for testing depends on what the doctor finds during the history and physical examination (see Table on pages 74 to 75). Acute watery diarrhea (lasting less than about 4 days) without warning signs is usually caused by a viral infection, and people who otherwise appear well do not require testing.

People with warning signs of dehydration, bloody stool, fever, or severe abdominal pain typically need testing—particularly those who are very young or very old. In these people, doctors do blood tests to detect blood and electrolyte abnormalities and stool tests to detect blood, white blood cells, and the presence of infectious organisms (such as *Campylobacter*, *Yersinia*, amebas, *Giardia*, and *Cryptosporidium*). Some causes of infection are detected by looking under the microscope, whereas others require a culture (growing the organism in the laboratory) or special enzyme tests (for example, *Shigella* or *Giardia*). If the person has taken antibiotics within the past 2 to 3 months, the doctor may test the stool for *Clostridium difficile* toxin. A colonoscopy is usually not necessary.

For diarrhea lasting more than 4 weeks (more than 1 week for people who have a weakened immune system or who appear seriously ill), similar tests are done. In addition, the doctor may test the stool for fat (indicating malabsorption) and do a colonoscopy to examine the lining of the rectum and colon and to gather samples to test for infection. People whose symptoms seem related to diet may have a breath test to look for hydrogen, which suggests they are not absorbing carbohydrates. Sometimes a biopsy (removal of a tissue specimen for examination under a microscope) of the rectal lining is done to look for inflammatory bowel disease. Sometimes the volume of stool over a 24-hour period is determined. Imaging tests, such as computed tomography (CT) enterography, may be needed if the doctor suspects certain tumors. If doctors are still uncertain about the diagnosis, they may need to assess the function of the pancreas. Depending on the person's symptoms, doctors may also conduct tests for thyroid or adrenal disease.

TREATMENT

Treatment is directed at the cause of diarrhea, when possible. For example, dietary and drug causes are avoided, tumors are removed, and drugs are given to eradicate a parasitic infection. However, in many cases, the body heals itself. A viral cause usually resolves by itself in 24 to 48 hours.

SOME CAUSES AND FEATURES OF DIARRHEA

Cause	Common Features*	Tests
Acute (less than 1 week)†		
Gastroenteritis due to viruses, bacteria, or parasites‡	Often vomiting	A doctor's examination
	Rarely fever or blood in stool	Sometimes examination and testing of stool
	Little or no abdominal pain (except during vomiting)	
	Sometimes recent contact with infected people (such as those at a day care center, at a camp, or on a cruise), with animals at a petting zoo (where *Escherichia* [*E.*] *coli* may be acquired), or with reptiles (where *Salmonella* bacteria may be acquired)	
	Sometimes recent consumption of undercooked, contaminated food or contaminated water	
Food poisoning	Diarrhea that started suddenly, often with vomiting, within 4 to 8 hours of eating contaminated food	A doctor's examination
	Often present in other people	
	Typically lasting 12 to 24 hours	
Side effects of drugs‡ (including antibiotics, many cancer chemotherapy drugs, colchicine, and quinine/quinidine)	Recent use of a drug that causes diarrhea	A doctor's examination
	Often no other symptoms	Sometimes tests for *Clostridium difficile* toxin in stool
Chronic (4 weeks or more)		
Dietary factors such as	Diarrhea only after consuming a substance that could cause diarrhea	A doctor's examination
■ Intolerance of cow's milk		Sometimes a breath test to detect hydrogen, indicating undigested food
■ Overeating of certain fruits or juices (such as pear, apple, or prune)	Abdominal bloating and passing of gas (flatulence)	Examination and analysis of stool to check for unabsorbed carbohydrates
	Explosive diarrhea	
Irritable bowel syndrome	Intermittent diarrhea usually preceded by abdominal discomfort, bloating, or pain	A doctor's examination
	Often diarrhea alternating with constipation	Sometimes blood tests and colonoscopy
	No bleeding, weight loss, or fever	
	Usually begins during the teens or 20s	
	Symptoms usually present for more than 12 weeks	
	Changes in the frequency of bowel movements or consistency of stool	

(continued)

SOME CAUSES AND FEATURES OF DIARRHEA *(continued)*

Cause	Common Features*	Tests
Inflammatory bowel disease such as ■ Crohn disease ■ Ulcerative colitis	Blood in stool, crampy abdominal pain, weight loss, and loss of appetite Sometimes arthritis, rashes, sores in the mouth, and tears in the rectum	Colonoscopy Sometimes CT or x-rays after barium is inserted in the rectum (barium enema)
Malabsorption disorders such as ■ Celiac disease ■ Tropical sprue ■ Pancreatic insufficiency	Light-colored, soft, bulky, and unusually foul-smelling stool that may appear oily Abdominal bloating and flatulence Weight loss For tropical sprue, long-term (over 1 month) residence in a tropical country For pancreatic insufficiency, usually in a person known to have a disorder of the pancreas (such as chronic pancreatitis or cystic fibrosis)	Tests to measure the amount of fat in stool samples collected over several days If celiac disease is suspected, blood tests to measure the antibodies produced when people with celiac disease eat foods containing gluten For both celiac disease and tropical sprue, especially celiac disease, biopsy of the small intestine
Certain tumors ■ Colon cancer or villous adenoma ■ Endocrine tumors (such as vipoma, gastrinoma, carcinoid, mastocytosis, or medullary carcinoma of the thyroid) ■ Lymphoma	For colon cancer, sometimes blood in stool, decreased stool diameter, and weight loss For endocrine tumors, various symptoms, including abdominal pain or cramping, flushing, and massive watery diarrhea	Blood tests Colonoscopy
Hyperthyroidism	Often nervousness, fatigue, palpitations, weight loss, and rapid heart rate	Blood tests
Surgery on the stomach or intestines (such as gastric bypass for weight loss or removal of a significant length of intestine)	Obvious recent surgery	A doctor's examination

*Features include symptoms and the results of the doctor's examination. Features mentioned are typical but not always present.

†Diarrhea that has been present for 1 to 4 weeks may be a lingering case of acute diarrhea or the early stage of a disorder that causes chronic diarrhea.

‡Certain infections and certain drugs can also cause chronic diarrhea.

CT = computed tomography; HIV = human immunodeficiency virus.

DEHYDRATION

Extra fluids containing a balance of water, sugars, and salts are needed for people who are dehydrated. As long as the person is not vomiting excessively, these fluids can be given by mouth. Seriously ill people and those with significant electrolyte abnormalities require intravenous fluid and sometimes hospitalization.

DRUGS

Drugs that relax intestinal muscles (antidiarrheal drugs) can help slow diarrhea. Loperamide

is available over-the-counter. Opioid drugs, such as codeine, diphenoxylate, and paregoric (tincture of opium), are available by prescription and also can help. However, certain bacterial causes of gastroenteritis, particularly *Salmonella, Shigella,* and *Clostridium difficile,* can be worsened by antidiarrheal drugs. Doctors typically recommend antidiarrheal drugs only for people with watery diarrhea and no warning signs because such people are unlikely to have such bacterial infections.

Over-the-counter drugs include adsorbents (for example, kaolin-pectin), which adhere to chemicals, toxins, and infectious organisms. Some adsorbents also help firm up the stool. Bismuth helps many people with diarrhea. It has a normal side effect of turning the stool black.

Bulking agents used for chronic constipation, such as psyllium or methylcellulose, can sometimes help relieve chronic diarrhea as well.

KEY POINTS

- In people with acute diarrhea, doctors examine the stool only if they suspect people have an acute infection or if people have prolonged symptoms (that is, more than 1 week) or warning signs.
- Doctors avoid using antidiarrheal drugs if there is a possibility that the person has *Clostridium difficile, Salmonella,* or *Shigella.*

DIARRHEA IN CHILDREN

Diarrhea is a very common problem in children. Diarrhea is frequent, loose, or watery bowel movements (BMs) that differ from a child's normal pattern. Sometimes diarrhea contains blood or mucus. Identifying mild diarrhea may be difficult because in healthy children, the number and consistency of BMs vary with age and diet. For example, breastfed infants who are not yet receiving solid food often have frequent, loose stools that are considered normal. A sudden increase in number and looseness may indicate diarrhea in these infants. However, having watery stools for more than 24 hours is never normal.

Children with diarrhea may lose their appetite, vomit, lose weight, or have a fever. If diarrhea is severe or lasts a long time, dehydration is likely. Infants and young children can become dehydrated more quickly, sometimes in less than 1 day. Severe dehydration can cause seizures, brain damage, and death.

Worldwide, diarrhea causes 2 to 3 million deaths a year mostly in underdeveloped countries. In the United States, diarrhea accounts for about 9% of hospitalizations for children under 5 years old.

CAUSES

Likely causes of diarrhea depend on whether it lasts less than 2 weeks (acute) or more than 2 weeks (chronic). Most cases of diarrhea are acute.

COMMON CAUSES

Acute diarrhea is usually caused by

- Infectious gastroenteritis
- Food poisoning
- Use of antibiotics
- Food allergies

Gastroenteritis is usually caused by a virus, but it can be caused by bacteria or a parasite.

Food poisoning usually refers to diarrhea, vomiting, or both caused by eating food contaminated by toxins produced by certain bacteria, such as staphylococci or clostridia.

Certain antibiotics can alter the types and number of bacteria in the intestine. As a result,

diarrhea can occur. Sometimes using antibiotics enables a particularly dangerous bacteria, *Clostridium difficile,* to multiply. *Clostridium difficile* releases toxins that can cause inflammation of the lining of the large intestine (colitis).

Chronic diarrhea is usually caused by

- Dietary factors, such as lactose intolerance or overconsumption of certain foods
- Infections (particularly those caused by parasites)
- Celiac disease
- Inflammatory bowel disease

LESS COMMON CAUSES

Acute diarrhea can also result from more serious disorders such as appendicitis, intussusception, and hemolytic-uremic syndrome (a complication of certain types of bacterial infection). These serious disorders are usually associated with other worrisome symptoms besides diarrhea, such as severe abdominal pain or swelling, bloody stools, fever, and ill appearance.

Chronic diarrhea can also result from disorders that interfere with the absorption of food (malabsorption disorders), such as cystic fibrosis, and a weakened immune system (due to a disorder such as AIDS or use of certain drugs).

Diarrhea sometimes results from constipation. When hardened stool accumulates in the rectum, soft stool may leak around it and into the child's underwear.

EVALUATION

WARNING SIGNS

Certain symptoms are cause for concern. They include

- Signs of dehydration, such as decreased urination, lethargy or listlessness, crying without tears, extreme thirst, and a dry mouth
- Ill appearance
- Blood in stool

- Pain in the abdomen and, when touched, extreme tenderness
- Bleeding in the skin (seen as tiny reddish purple dots [petechiae] or splotches [purpura])

WHEN TO SEE A DOCTOR

Children with any warning signs should be evaluated by a doctor right away, as should those who have had more than 3 or 4 episodes of diarrhea and are not drinking or are drinking very little.

If children have no warning signs and are drinking and urinating normally, the doctor should be called if diarrhea lasts 2 days or more or if there are more than 6 to 8 episodes of diarrhea a day. If diarrhea is mild, a doctor's visit is unnecessary. Children with diarrhea for 14 days or more should be seen by a doctor.

WHAT THE DOCTOR DOES

Doctors first ask questions about symptoms and medical history. Doctors then do a physical examination. What they find during the history and physical examination often suggests a cause and the tests that may need to be done (see Table, below).

Doctors ask what the BMs look like, how frequent they are, how long they last, and whether the child has other symptoms, such as fever, vomiting, or abdominal pain.

Doctors also ask about potential causes, such as diet, use of antibiotics, consumption of possibly contaminated food, recent contact with animals, and recent travel.

A physical examination is done, looking for symptoms of dehydration and disorders that can cause diarrhea. The abdomen is checked for swelling and tenderness. Doctors also evaluate growth.

SOME CAUSES AND FEATURES OF DIARRHEA

Cause	Common Features*	Tests
Acute (lasting less than 2 weeks)		
Antibiotic use	Recent use of antibiotics	A doctor's examination
	Often no other symptoms	Sometimes tests for *Clostridium difficile* toxin in stool
Gastroenteritis due to viruses, bacteria, or parasites†	Often with vomiting	A doctor's examination
	Dehydration common especially among infants and young children	Sometimes examination and testing of stool
	Sometimes fever and abdominal pain	
	Rarely blood in stool	
	Sometimes recent contact with infected people (such as those at a day care center, at a camp, or on a cruise), with animals at a petting zoo (where *Escherichia [E.] coli* may be acquired), or with reptiles (which may be infected with *Salmonella* bacteria) or recent consumption of undercooked, contaminated food or contaminated water	
Food allergy	Hives, swelling of the lips, and difficulty breathing within minutes to several hours after eating	A doctor's examination
	Sometimes vomiting	
	Often an already identified food allergy	
Hemolytic-uremic syndrome	Abdominal pain, vomiting, and usually bloody diarrhea for a few days, followed by development of pale skin and decreased urination	Blood tests
		Examination and testing of stool
	Sometimes bleeding in the skin (seen as tiny reddish purple dots or splotches)	

(continued)

SOME CAUSES AND FEATURES OF DIARRHEA (continued)

Cause	Common Features*	Tests
Chronic (lasting 2 weeks or more)		
Allergy to cow's milk protein	Vomiting Poor feeding Weight loss, poor growth, or both Blood in stools	Stool tests Symptoms that lessen when the formula is changed Possibly endoscopy, colonoscopy, or both
Excessive consumption of fruit juices (especially apple, pear, and prune)	Drinking more than 4–8 ounces of fruit juice a day Often no other symptoms except diarrhea	A doctor's examination Resolution of diarrhea after decreasing consumption of fruit juices
Inflammatory bowel disease such as ■ Crohn disease ■ Ulcerative colitis	Blood in stool, crampy abdominal pain, weight loss, loss of appetite, and poor growth Sometimes arthritis, rashes, sores in the mouth, and tears in the rectum	Colonoscopy Sometimes CT or x-rays after barium is inserted in the rectum (barium enema)
Lactose intolerance (inability to digest lactose, the sugar in milk and dairy products)	Abdominal bloating, passing of gas (flatulence), and explosive diarrhea Diarrhea after consumption of milk and dairy products	A doctor's examination Sometimes a breath test to detect hydrogen (indicates undigested carbohydrates) Examination and analysis of stool to check for unabsorbed carbohydrates
Malabsorption disorders such as ■ Celiac disease ■ Cystic fibrosis ■ Acrodermatitis enteropathica	Light-colored, soft, bulky, and unusually foul-smelling stool that may appear oily Abdominal bloating and flatulence Poor weight gain With cystic fibrosis, frequent respiratory infections With acrodermatitis enteropathica, rash and cracks in the corners of the mouth	Examination and testing of stool If celiac disease is suspected, blood tests to measure antibodies against gluten (a protein in wheat) and biopsy of the small intestine If cystic fibrosis is suspected, a sweat test and possibly genetic testing If acrodermatitis enteropathica is suspected, a blood test for zinc deficiency
A weakened immune system due to ■ HIV infection or an immunodeficiency disorder ■ Use of drugs that suppress the immune system	Frequent infections Weight loss or poor weight gain Sometimes an already identified HIV infection	Blood tests for HIV A complete blood cell count and other blood tests to evaluate the immune system

*Features include symptoms and results of the doctor's examination. Features mentioned are typical but not always present.
†Infections by bacteria, parasites, or viruses can also cause chronic diarrhea.
CT = computed tomography; HIV = human immunodeficiency virus.

TESTING

If diarrhea lasts less than 2 weeks, the cause is probably gastroenteritis due to a virus, and testing is usually unnecessary. However, if doctors suspect another cause, tests are done to check for it.

Tests are also done when children have warning signs. If they have signs of dehydration, blood tests are done to measure levels of electrolytes (calcium and other minerals necessary to maintain the fluid balance in the body). If other warning signs are present, tests may include a complete blood cell count, urine tests, examination and analysis of stool, abdominal x-rays, or a combination.

TREATMENT

Specific causes are treated. For example, if children have celiac disease, gluten is removed from their diet. Antibiotics that cause diarrhea are stopped if a doctor recommends it. Gastroenteritis due to a virus usually disappears without treatment.

Drugs to stop diarrhea, such as loperamide, are not recommended for infants and young children.

DEHYDRATION

Because the main concern in children is dehydration, treatment focuses on giving fluids and electrolytes. Most children with diarrhea are successfully treated with fluids given by mouth (orally). Fluids are given by vein (intravenously) only if children are not drinking or are severely dehydrated. Oral rehydration solutions that contain the right balance of carbohydrates and sodium are used. In the United States, these solutions are widely available without a prescription from pharmacies and most supermarkets. *Sports drinks, sodas, juices, and similar drinks have too little sodium and too much carbohydrate and should not be used.*

If children are also vomiting, small, frequent amounts of fluid are given at first. Typically, 1 teaspoon (5 milliliters) is given every 5 minutes. If children keep this amount down, the amount is gradually increased. With patience and encouragement, most children can take enough fluid by mouth to avoid the need for intravenous fluid. However, children with severe dehydration may need intravenous fluids.

DIET

As soon as children have received sufficient fluids and are not vomiting, they should be given an age-appropriate diet. Infants may resume breast milk or formula.

In children with chronic diarrhea, the treatment depends on the cause, but providing and maintaining adequate nutrition and monitoring for possible vitamin or mineral deficiencies is most important.

KEY POINTS

- Diarrhea is common among children.
- Gastroenteritis, usually due to a virus, is the most common cause.
- Children should be evaluated by a doctor if they have any warning sign (such as signs of dehydration, severe abdominal pain, fever, or blood or pus in stool).
- Testing is rarely necessary when diarrhea lasts less than 2 weeks.
- Dehydration is likely if diarrhea is severe or lasts a long time.
- Giving fluids by mouth effectively treats dehydration in most children.
- Drugs to stop diarrhea, such as loperamide, are not recommended for infants and young children.

DIZZINESS AND VERTIGO

Dizziness is an inexact term people often use to describe various related sensations, including

- Faintness (feeling about to pass out)
- Light-headedness
- Feeling off balance or unsteady
- A vague spaced-out or swimmy-headed feeling

For dizziness that occurs only on standing up, see page 87.

Vertigo is

- A false sensation of movement

With vertigo, people usually feel that they, their environment, or both are spinning. The feeling is similar to that produced by the childhood game of spinning round and round, then suddenly stopping and feeling the surroundings spin. Occasionally, people simply feel pulled to one side. Vertigo is not a diagnosis—it is a description of a sensation.

People with dizziness or vertigo may also have nausea and vomiting, difficulty with balance, and/or trouble walking. Some people have a rhythmic jerking movement of the eyes (nystagmus) during an episode of vertigo.

Different people often use the terms "dizziness" and "vertigo" differently, perhaps because these sensations are hard to describe in words. Also, people may describe their sensations differently at different times. For example, the sensations might feel like light-headedness one time and like vertigo the next. Because of this inconsistency, many doctors prefer to consider the two symptoms together.

However they are described, dizziness and vertigo can be disturbing and even incapacitating, particularly when accompanied by nausea and vomiting. Symptoms cause particular problems for people doing an exacting or dangerous task, such as driving, flying, or operating heavy machinery.

Dizziness accounts for about 5 to 6% of doctor visits. It may occur at any age but becomes more common as people age. It affects about 40% of people older than 40 at some time.

Dizziness may be temporary or chronic. Dizziness is considered chronic if it lasts more than a month. Chronic dizziness is more common among older people.

CAUSES

Dizziness and vertigo are usually caused by disorders of the parts of the ear and brain that are involved in maintaining balance:

- Inner ear
- Brain stem and cerebellum
- Nerve tracts connecting the brain stem and cerebellum or within the brain stem

The inner ear contains structures (the semicircular canals, saccule, and utricle) that enable the body to sense position and motion. Information from these structures is sent to the brain through the vestibulocochlear nerve (8th cranial nerve, which is also involved in hearing). This information is processed in the brain stem, which adjusts posture, and the cerebellum, which coordinates movements, to provide a sense of balance. A disorder in any of these structures can cause dizziness, vertigo, or both. Disorders of the inner ear sometimes also cause decreased hearing and/or ringing in the ear (tinnitus—see Ear, Ringing or Buzzing in on page 98).

Also, any disorder that affects brain function in general (for example, low blood sugar, low blood pressure, severe anemia, or many drugs) can make people feel dizzy. Although symptoms may be disturbing and even incapacitating, only about 5% of cases result from a serious disorder.

COMMON CAUSES

Although there is some overlap, causes can roughly be divided into those with and without vertigo.

The most common causes of dizziness with vertigo include the following:

- Benign paroxysmal positional vertigo
- Meniere disease
- Vestibular neuronitis

- Labyrinthitis
- Vestibular migraine headache

Vestibular migraine headache is an increasingly common cause of dizziness with vertigo. This type of migraine most often occurs in people who have a history or family history of migraines. People often have headache with the vertigo or dizziness. Some have other migraine-like symptoms, such as seeing flashing lights, having temporary blind spots, or being very sensitive to light and sound. People may also have hearing loss, but it is not a common symptom.

The **most common causes of dizziness** *without* vertigo include the following:

- Drug effects
- Multifactorial causes

Several kinds of drugs can cause dizziness. Some drugs are directly toxic to the nerves of the ears and/or balance organs (ototoxic drugs). Other drugs, for example, sedatives, affect the brain as a whole. In older people, dizziness often is due to several factors, usually a combination of drug side effects plus an age-related decrease in sensory function.

Very often, no particular cause is found, and symptoms go away without treatment.

LESS COMMON CAUSES

Less common causes include a tumor of the vestibulocochlear nerve (acoustic neuroma); a tumor, stroke, or transient ischemic attack (TIA) affecting the brain stem; an injury to the eardrum, inner ear, or base of the skull; multiple sclerosis; low blood sugar; and pregnancy.

EVALUATION

The following information can help people decide whether a doctor's evaluation is needed and help them know what to expect during the evaluation.

WARNING SIGNS

In people with dizziness or vertigo, certain symptoms and characteristics are cause for concern. They include

- Headache
- Neck pain

- Difficulty walking
- Loss of consciousness (fainting)
- Other neurologic symptoms (such as trouble hearing, seeing, speaking, or swallowing or difficulty moving an arm or leg)

WHEN TO SEE A DOCTOR

People who have warning signs, those whose symptoms are severe or have been continuous for over an hour, and those with vomiting should go to a hospital right away. Other people may see their doctor within several days. People who had a single, brief (less than 1 minute), mild episode with no other symptoms may choose to wait and see whether they have another episode.

WHAT THE DOCTOR DOES

Doctors first ask questions about the person's symptoms and medical history. Doctors then do a physical examination. What they find during the history and physical examination often suggests a cause of the dizziness or vertigo and the tests that may need to be done (see Table on pages 83 to 84).

In addition to warning signs, important features that doctors ask about include severity of the symptoms (has the person fallen or missed work), presence of vomiting and/or ringing in the ears, whether symptoms come and go or have been continuous, and possible triggers of the symptoms (for example, changing position of the head or taking a new drug).

Doctors then do a physical examination. The ear, eye, and neurologic examinations are particularly important. Hearing is tested, and the ears are examined for abnormalities of the ear canal and eardrum. The eyes are checked for abnormal movements, such as nystagmus.

Nystagmus suggests a disorder affecting the inner ear or various nerve connections in the brain stem. With nystagmus, the eyes rapidly and repeatedly jerk in one direction and then return more slowly to their original position. Doctors deliberately try to trigger nystagmus if people do not have it spontaneously because the direction in which the eyes move and how long the nystagmus lasts help doctors diagnose the cause of vertigo. To trigger nystagmus, doctors first lay people on their back and gently roll them from side to side while watching their eyes. Specialists sometimes have the person wear thick, one-way, magnifying glasses called Frenzel lenses. Doctors can easily see the person's magnified eyes through the lenses, but the person sees a blur and cannot visually fixate on anything (visual fixation makes it harder to trigger nystagmus). During the maneuver to induce nystagmus, eye movements may be recorded by using electrodes (sensors that stick to the skin)

SOME CAUSES AND FEATURES OF DIZZINESS AND VERTIGO

Cause	Common Features*	Tests
Common causes		
Benign paroxysmal positional vertigo (BPPV)	Severe, brief (lasting less than 1 minute) spinning episodes triggered by moving the head in a specific direction, especially while lying down Sometimes nausea and vomiting Normal hearing and neurologic function	A doctor's examination, typically including the Dix-Hallpike maneuver
Meniere disease	Multiple separate episodes of vertigo accompanied by ringing, hearing loss, and ear fullness/pressure usually in 1 ear only	Audiometry and gadolinium-enhanced MRI
Vestibular neuronitis (probably caused by a virus)	Sudden, severe vertigo with no hearing loss or other findings Severe vertigo may last several days, with gradual lessening of symptoms and possible development of positional vertigo	A doctor's examination Sometimes gadolinium-enhanced MRI
Labyrinthitis (viral or bacterial cause)	Sudden hearing loss with severe dizziness, often with tinnitus	Temporal bone CT scan if doctors suspect a bacterial infection Gadolinium-enhanced MRI for people with hearing loss and ringing in ear
Drugs that affect the inner ear (particularly aminoglycoside antibiotics, chloroquine, furosemide, and quinine)	Usually hearing loss in both ears Possible causative drug recently started	A doctor's examination Sometimes electronystagmography and rotary chair tests
Drugs that affect the brain overall (particularly drugs for anxiety, depression, and seizures, as well as sedative drugs in general)	Symptoms unrelated to movement or position No hearing loss or other symptoms Possible causative drug recently started	Measuring blood levels of certain causative drugs Stopping the drug to see whether symptoms stop
Migraine	Multiple, separate episodes of vertigo, or chronic dizziness, sometimes accompanied by nausea Headache or other migraine symptoms such as visual or other aura (altered sensations that come before the headache such as flashing lights) and sensitivity to light and/or noise Often history or family history of migraine	Often MRI to rule out other causes Trial of drugs to prevent migraine *(continued)*

SOME CAUSES AND FEATURES OF DIZZINESS AND VERTIGO (continued)

Cause	Common Features*	Tests
Less common causes, typically *with* ear symptoms (hearing loss and/or ringing in the ear)		
Middle ear infection (acute or chronic)	Ear pain, sometimes discharge from the ear	A doctor's examination
	Abnormal appearance of the eardrum during examination	Sometimes CT scan (for people with chronic infection)
Trauma (such as ruptured eardrum, skull fracture, or concussion)	Obvious recent trauma	Usually CT, depending on cause and doctor's findings
	Other findings depending on location and extent of damage	
Acoustic neuroma	Slowly progressive hearing loss and/or ringing in one ear	Audiometry
	Rarely, numbness and/or weakness of the face	Gadolinium-enhanced MRI if hearing loss or tinnitus
Defect of the bone around a semicircular canal	Dizziness triggered by sound, low tone hearing loss	Usually a CT scan, vestibular testing, and tympanometry
Less common causes, typically *without* ear symptoms		
Brain stem stroke	Sudden onset, continuous symptoms	Immediate gadolinium-enhanced MRI
Bleeding in the cerebellum	Sudden onset, with continuous symptoms	Immediate gadolinium-enhanced MRI
	Difficulty walking and with tests of coordination	
	Often headache	
	Symptoms worsen rapidly	
Multiple sclerosis	Multiple, separate episodes of neurologic symptoms such as weakness or numbness with different episodes affecting different parts of the body	Gadolinium-enhanced MRI of brain and spine
Low blood sugar (usually caused by drugs for diabetes)	Recent dose increase	Finger-stick glucose test (during symptoms if possible)
	Sometimes sweating	
Low blood pressure (such as caused by heart disorders, blood pressure drugs, blood loss, or dehydration)	Symptoms when rising, but not with head motion or while lying flat	Testing directed at suspected cause
	Symptoms of the cause often obvious (such as severe blood loss or diarrhea)	
Pregnancy (often not known by the person)	Sometimes late menstrual period and/or morning sickness	Pregnancy test
	No ear symptoms	
Syphilis	Chronic symptoms with on and off hearing loss in both ears and episodes of vertigo	Syphilis blood test
Thyroid disorders	Weight change	Thyroid function blood tests
	Heat or cold intolerance	

*Features include symptoms and the results of the doctor's examination. Features mentioned are typical but not always present.
CT = computed tomography; MRI = magnetic resonance imaging.

placed around each eye (electronystagmography) or by a video camera attached to the Frenzel lenses (video electronystagmography). If no nystagmus occurs with rolling side to side, doctors try other maneuvers. These other maneuvers include putting ice-cold water into the ear canal (caloric testing) and rapidly changing the position of the person's head (Dix-Hallpike maneuver). Doctors also do a complete neurologic examination, paying particular attention to tests of walking, balance, and coordination.

There is some overlap. However, generally people with disorders of the inner ear often have hearing symptoms (such as hearing loss or ringing in the ear), but people with other disorders do not.

TESTING

The need for tests depends on what doctors find during the history and physical examination, particularly whether warning signs are present.

For people with a sudden attack that is still going on, doctors usually apply a fingertip oxygen sensor, measure blood glucose from a drop of blood from the fingertip, and, for women, do a urine pregnancy test.

People with warning signs typically require gadolinium-enhanced magnetic resonance imaging (MRI), as do people without warning signs who have had symptoms for a long time.

Several tests can be used to evaluate balance and gait, such as the Romberg test. Another test of balance has the person walking a straight line with one foot behind the other. If the doctor's examination shows possible hearing loss, people are usually sent to a specialist for a formal hearing test (audiometry).

Comprehensive vestibular testing is sometimes done. This testing includes video electronystagmography, rotary chair testing, and vestibular-evoked myogenic potential testing. These tests are typically done by doctors who specialize in the care of the ear (otolaryngologists).

Electrocardiography (ECG), Holter monitoring for heart rhythm abnormalities, echocardiography, and exercise stress testing may be done to evaluate heart function. For dizziness that occurs only when standing up (see page 87), specific tests may be needed.

Blood tests are usually not helpful unless the person's symptoms suggest possible syphilis or a thyroid disorder.

TREATMENT

The cause is treated whenever possible. Treatment includes stopping or reducing the dose of any drug that is the cause or switching to an alternative drug.

Nausea and vomiting can be treated with drugs such as meclizine or promethazine.

Vertigo caused by disorders of the inner ear, such as Meniere disease, labyrinthitis, or vestibular neuronitis, can often be relieved by benzodiazepine drugs such as diazepam or lorazepam. Antihistamine drugs such as meclizine are an alternative.

If vertigo persists for a long time, some people benefit from physical therapy to help them cope with their disturbed sense of balance. Therapists may also recommend such strategies as

- Avoiding movements that may trigger dizziness, such as looking up or bending down
- Storing items at levels that are easy to reach
- Getting up slowly after sitting or lying down
- Clenching hands and flexing feet before standing
- Learning exercises that combine eye, head, and body movements to help prevent dizziness
- Doing physical therapy and exercises to strengthen muscles and maintain independent gait as long as possible
- Undergoing vestibular rehabilitation therapy (a specialized form of physical therapy that targets symptoms of peripheral and central vestibular dysfunction)

ESSENTIALS FOR OLDER PEOPLE

As people grow older, many factors make dizziness and vertigo more common. The organs involved in balance, particularly the structures of the inner ear, function less well. It becomes harder to see in dim light. The body's mechanisms that control blood pressure respond more slowly (for example, to standing up). Older people are also more likely to be taking drugs that can cause dizziness.

Although dizziness and vertigo are unpleasant at any age, they cause particular problems for older people. Frail people have a much higher risk of falling when they are dizzy. Even if they do not fall, their fear of falling often significantly affects their ability to do daily activities.

The drugs that help relieve vertigo can make people feel sleepy. This effect is more common and sometimes more severe in older people.

Even more so than younger people, older people with dizziness or vertigo may benefit from general physical therapy and exercises to strengthen their muscles to help them maintain their independence. Physical therapists can also provide important safety information for older or disabled people to help prevent falls.

KEY POINTS

- Dizziness and vertigo often result from disorders that affect the inner ear or the parts of the brain involved in balance or from use of certain prescription drugs.
- Severe headache and any sign of difficulty with brain function (such as difficulty walking, talking, seeing, speaking, or swallowing) are warning signs.
- People with warning signs should see a doctor right away, and they often need an MRI.
- Drugs, such as diazepam or meclizine, often help relieve vertigo, and prochlorperazine can help relieve nausea.
- Thorough evaluation by a specialist is needed if drugs are used long term.

DIZZINESS WHEN STANDING UP

In some people, particularly older people, blood pressure drops excessively when they sit or stand up (a condition called orthostatic or postural hypotension). Symptoms of faintness, light-headedness, dizziness, confusion, or blurred vision occur within seconds to a few minutes of standing (particularly after lying in bed or sitting for a long time) and resolve rapidly when the person lies down. However, some people fall, faint, or very rarely have a brief seizure. Symptoms are often more common and worse after people exercise or have consumed alcohol and/or a heavy meal.

Some younger people experience similar symptoms upon standing but without having a drop in blood pressure. Often, their heart rate increases (tachycardia) more than normal upon standing, so this condition is called postural orthostatic tachycardia syndrome (POTS). The reason why such people feel dizzy despite having normal blood pressure is not yet clear.

CAUSES

Dizziness or light-headedness when standing up occurs as a result of abnormal blood pressure regulation. Normally, when people stand, gravity causes blood to pool in the veins of the legs and trunk. This pooling lowers the blood pressure and the amount of blood the heart pumps to the brain. Low blood flow to the brain causes the dizziness and other symptoms. To compensate, the nervous system quickly increases the heart rate and constricts blood vessels, which rapidly returns blood pressure to normal before symptoms can develop. The part of the nervous system responsible for this compensation is the autonomic nervous system.

Many disorders can cause problems with blood pressure regulation and lead to dizziness when standing up. Categories of causes include

- Malfunction of the autonomic nervous system due to disorders or drugs
- Decreased ability of the heart to pump blood
- Decreased blood volume (hypovolemia)
- Faulty hormonal responses

Causes differ depending on whether symptoms are new or have been present for some time.

COMMON CAUSES

The most common causes of new dizziness when standing up include

- Decreased blood volume (as may result from dehydration or blood loss)
- Drugs
- Prolonged bed rest
- An underactive adrenal gland (adrenal insufficiency)

The most common causes of dizziness when standing up that has been present for a long time (chronic) include

- Age-related changes in blood pressure regulation
- Drugs
- Malfunction of the autonomic nervous system

EVALUATION

People who become dizzy or light-headed when standing up often recover quickly when they sit down and then slowly stand again. However, it is usually important to determine what is causing the dizziness. The following information can help people decide when to see a doctor and help them know what to expect during the evaluation.

WARNING SIGNS

In people who become dizzy or light-headed when standing up, certain symptoms and characteristics are cause for concern. They include

- Blood in the stool or black, tarry stool
- Nervous system symptoms such as difficulty walking and/or poor coordination or balance

WHEN TO SEE A DOCTOR

People who have warning signs and those who have fallen or fainted should see a doctor right away. Other people who have frequent or ongoing episodes of dizziness upon standing should see a doctor when practical. Typically a delay of a week or so is not harmful. People who have only an occasional episode of dizziness upon standing should call their doctor. The doctor will decide whether and how quickly to see the person depending on the other symptoms and medical history.

WHAT THE DOCTOR DOES

The doctor first asks questions about the person's symptoms and medical history. Doctors then do a physical examination. What they find during the history and physical examination often suggests a cause of the dizziness and the tests that may need to be done.

Doctors ask

- How long the dizziness has been occurring
- Whether the person has fainted or fallen during an episode of dizziness
- Whether the person has experienced conditions that are known to cause dizziness (such as bed rest or fluid loss)

- Whether the person has a disorder (such as diabetes, Parkinson disease, or a cancer) that may cause dizziness
- Whether the person is taking a drug (for example, an antihypertensive) that may cause dizziness

The doctor then does a physical examination. The person lies down for 5 minutes, and then the doctor measures the blood pressure and heart rate. Blood pressure and heart rate are measured again after the person stands or sits up for 1 minute and again after standing or sitting for 3 minutes. The doctor may do a digital rectal examination to see whether the person might have some bleeding in the digestive tract. A neurologic examination to test strength, sensation, reflexes, balance, and gait is important.

The most common causes of sudden dizziness—drugs, bed rest, and decreased blood volume—are usually obvious. In people with long-term symptoms, findings such as movement problems may indicate Parkinson disease. Numbness, tingling, or weakness may indicate a nervous system disorder.

SOME CAUSES AND FEATURES OF DIZZINESS OR LIGHT-HEADEDNESS WHEN STANDING UP

Cause	Common Features*	Tests
Central nervous system† disorders		
Multiple system atrophy (previously called Shy-Drager syndrome)	Muscle stiffness Slow, shaky movements Loss of coordination and/or balance Incontinence or inability to urinate	A doctor's examination Sometimes MRI
Parkinson disease	Muscle stiffness Tremor Slow, shaky movements and a shuffling gait Difficulty walking	Only a doctor's examination
Strokes if several have occurred	In people who are known to have had strokes	Only a doctor's examination
Spinal cord disorders		
Syphilis that affects the spinal cord (tabes dorsalis)	Intense, stabbing pains in the legs that come and go Unsteady walking Decreased sensation in the legs and numbness or tingling	Blood tests and sometimes a spinal tap (to obtain cerebrospinal fluid) to check for syphilis

(continued)

SOME CAUSES AND FEATURES OF DIZZINESS OR LIGHT-HEADEDNESS WHEN STANDING UP *(continued)*

Cause	Common Features*	Tests
Tumors	Back pain Muscle weakness and decreased sensation in the legs	MRI
Peripheral nerve† disorders		
Amyloidosis	Numbness, tingling, and weakness	Biopsy
Nerve damage caused by diabetes, excessive alcohol use, or nutritional deficiencies	Often burning pain and/or numbness in the feet and hands Sometimes weakness Usually in people who are known to have a disorder that can cause nerve damage	Nerve conduction testing and electromyography
Pure autonomic failure (formerly called idiopathic orthostatic hypotension)	Sometimes decreased sweating and intolerance of heat Constipation or loss of control over bowel movements (fecal incontinence) Difficulty emptying the bladder	A doctor's examination Blood tests
A decreased volume of blood (hypovolemia)		
Dehydration	Thirst, decreased urination, and confusion	Only a doctor's examination
Excessive loss of blood	Usually in people who have had an injury or surgery Blood in stool or black, tarry stool	A doctor's examination, including testing stool for blood A complete blood count
An underactive adrenal gland	Weakness and fatigue	Blood tests
Heart and blood vessel disorders		
Chronic venous insufficiency (causing blood to pool in the legs)	Long-lasting, nonpitting swelling in one or both legs Chronic mild discomfort or aching in the ankles or legs but no pain Sometimes reddish brown, leathery areas on the skin and shallow sores, usually on the lower legs Often varicose veins	A doctor's examination
Heart failure	Shortness of breath and fatigue	A doctor's examination Sometimes echocardiography (ultrasonography of the heart)
Heart attack (myocardial infarction)	Chest pain or pressure Shortness of breath or fatigue Sometimes in people who are known to have had a recent heart attack	ECG and blood tests to measure substances that indicate heart damage (cardiac markers)
High levels of the hormone aldosterone (hyperaldosteronism, usually caused by a tumor in the adrenal gland)	Weakness, tingling, and muscle spasms	Blood tests

(continued)

SOME CAUSES AND FEATURES OF DIZZINESS OR LIGHT-HEADEDNESS WHEN STANDING UP *(continued)*

Cause	Common Features*	Tests
Drugs		
Drugs for high blood pressure or angina: Calcium channel blockers, clonidine, diuretics (such as furosemide), methyldopa, nitrates, prazosin, or rarely beta-blockers	In people known to use one of these drugs	A doctor's examination Sometimes stopping the drug to see if symptoms go away
Drugs that affect the central nervous system: Antipsychotics (particularly phenothiazines), monoamine oxidase inhibitors, or tricyclic or tetracyclic antidepressants	In people known to use one of these drugs	Only a doctor's examination
Sedatives: Alcohol or barbiturates	In people known to use one of these drugs	Only a doctor's examination
Other drugs: Quinidine or vincristine	In people known to use one of these drugs	Only a doctor's examination
Other problems		
Age-related changes in blood pressure regulation	In older people No other symptoms	Only a doctor's examination
Bed rest if prolonged	In people who have been at bed rest for a long time	Only a doctor's examination
A low level of potassium in the blood	Muscle weakness and cramping Pins-and-needles sensation	Blood tests

*Features include symptoms and the results of the doctor's examination. Features mentioned are typical but not always present.

†The central nervous system includes the brain and spinal cord. The peripheral nervous system includes the nerves outside the brain and spinal cord.

CT = computed tomography; ECG = electrocardiography; MRI = magnetic resonance imaging.

TESTING

Unless the cause is obvious (for example, bed rest), testing is usually needed. The doctor usually does electrocardiography (ECG), a complete blood count, and other blood tests (for example, measuring levels of electrolytes). Other tests are done based on what doctors find during the examination, especially if the person's symptoms suggest a heart or nerve problem.

If doctors suspect a drug is causing the dizziness, they may ask the person to stop taking the drug and observe whether the dizziness also stops, thus confirming the cause.

Tilt table testing may be done when doctors suspect malfunction of the autonomic nervous system. The person lies flat on a special motorized table for several minutes. Then the table is tilted up at a 60° to 80° angle for 15 to 20 minutes while blood pressure and heart rate are continuously monitored. If blood pressure does not decrease, the person is given isoproterenol (a drug that stimulates the heart) intravenously in a dose large enough to accelerate the heart rate by 20 beats per minute, and the test is repeated. This procedure takes 30 to 60 minutes and is very safe.

TREATMENT

Any causes are treated when possible, including changing or stopping any causative drugs. However, many causes cannot be cured, and people must take measures to decrease their symptoms. Measures include lifestyle changes and drugs.

People requiring prolonged bed rest should sit up each day and exercise in bed when possible. People who are lying down or sitting should rise slowly and carefully. In general, it is helpful to consume adequate fluids, limit or avoid alcohol, and exercise regularly when feasible. Regular exercise of modest intensity increases the muscle tone in blood vessel walls, which reduces pooling of blood in the legs. Sleeping with the head of the bed raised may help relieve symptoms. For some people, increasing salt intake may increase water retention and lessen symptoms. Doctors may recommend that people increase their salt intake by liberally salting food or taking sodium chloride tablets. However, increasing salt intake may not be recommended for people with heart disorders.

Doctors may give fludrocortisone, a drug that helps the body retain salt and water and thus prevent blood pressure from dropping when a person stands. However, this drug may cause high blood pressure when people are lying down, heart failure, and low levels of potassium in the blood. Sometimes doctors combine propranolol or another beta-blocker with fludrocortisone. Midodrine is a drug that narrows both arteries and veins, helping prevent blood pooling. Side effects include tingling or numbness and itching. This drug is not recommended for people with coronary artery or peripheral arterial disease.

Other drugs such as nonsteroidal anti-inflammatory drugs (NSAIDs) and L-dihydroxyphenylserine may help in some cases.

ESSENTIALS FOR OLDER PEOPLE

Dizziness or light-headedness when standing occurs in about 20% of older people. It is more common among people with coexisting disorders, especially high blood pressure, and among residents of long-term care facilities. Many falls may result from dizziness when standing. Older people should avoid prolonged standing.

The increased incidence in older people is due to decreases in the responsiveness of the receptors that manage blood pressure plus increases in arterial wall stiffness, which make it more difficult for arteries to move more blood to increase blood pressure. Decreases in receptor responsiveness delay the normal heart and blood vessel responses to standing. Paradoxically, high blood pressure, which is more common among older people, may contribute to poor receptor sensitivity, increasing vulnerability to dizziness when standing.

KEY POINTS

- Dizziness or light-headedness when standing typically involves a decrease in body fluid volume or autonomic nervous system dysfunction.
- Aging often causes some degree of autonomic nervous system dysfunction, but doctors examine all affected people to ensure that no nervous system disorders are present.
- Tilt table testing is a common test of autonomic function.
- Treatment involves physical measures to reduce venous pooling, regular exercise, increased salt intake, and sometimes fludrocortisone or midodrine.

EARACHE

Earache (otalgia) usually occurs in only one ear. Some people also have ear discharge (see page 95) or, rarely, hearing loss (see page 188).

CAUSES

Pain may be due to a disorder within the ear itself or a disorder in a nearby body part that shares the same nerves to the brain as the ear. Such body parts include the nose, sinuses, throat, and temporomandibular joint (TMJ).

With **acute pain** (pain for less than 2 weeks), the most common causes are

- Middle ear infection (otitis media)
- External ear infection (otitis externa)
- Sudden pressure change (barotrauma)

Middle and external ear infections cause painful inflammation. A middle ear infection also causes a build up of pressure behind the eardrum (tympanic membrane [TM]). This build up of pressure is painful and also causes the eardrum to bulge. After the eardrum bulges, it occasionally bursts and releases a small amount of pus from the ear. Rarely, a middle ear infection spreads to the mastoid bone behind the ear (causing mastoiditis).

People with diabetes and those who have a compromised immune system (due to HIV infection or chemotherapy for cancer) may develop a particularly severe form of external otitis termed malignant or necrotizing external otitis.

Pressure changes during airplane flights and underwater diving can cause ear pain. Such ear pain occurs when the tube that connects the middle ear and the back of the nose (eustachian tube) is blocked or fails to function normally. The blockage or dysfunction keeps pressure in the middle ear from equalizing with outside pressure. The pressure difference pushes or pulls on the eardrum, causing pain. Pressure changes can also cause the TM to rupture.

With **chronic pain** (pain for more than 2 to 3 weeks), the most common causes are

- TMJ disorders
- Chronic eustachian tube dysfunction
- Chronic external ear infection

A less common cause of chronic pain is cancer, mainly in older people.

EVALUATION

The following information can help people decide when a doctor's evaluation is needed and help them know what to expect during the evaluation.

WARNING SIGNS

In people with earache, certain symptoms and characteristics are cause for concern:

- Diabetes or a compromised immune system
- Redness and swelling behind the ear
- Severe swelling at the opening of the ear canal
- Fluid draining from the ear
- Chronic pain, especially in people who have other head/neck symptoms (such as hoarseness, difficulty swallowing, or nasal obstruction)

WHEN TO SEE A DOCTOR

People with warning signs or ear discharge should see a doctor as soon as possible, unless the only warning sign is chronic pain. Then, a delay of a week or so is not harmful. People with acute pain should see a doctor within a few days (or sooner if pain is severe).

WHAT THE DOCTOR DOES

Doctors first ask questions about the person's symptoms and medical history. Doctors then do a physical examination that is focused on the ears, nose, and throat. What they find during the history and physical examination often suggests a cause of the earache and the tests that may need to be done (see Table on pages 93 to 94).

In addition to the presence of warning signs, an important feature is whether the ear examination is normal. Middle and external ear disorders cause abnormalities, which, when combined with the person's symptoms and other medical history, usually suggest a cause.

People with a normal ear examination may have a visible cause, such as tonsillitis, for their ear pain. If no abnormalities are found during the ear examination but the person has chronic pain, doctors suspect the ear pain might be due to a TMJ disorder. However, people should have a thorough head and neck examination (including fiberoptic examination) to rule out cancer or a tumor in the nasal passages and upper throat (nasopharynx).

SOME CAUSES AND FEATURES OF EARACHE

Cause	Common Features*†	Tests
Middle ear		
Acute eustachian tube obstruction (for example, due to a cold or allergies)	Mild to moderate discomfort	A doctor's examination
	Gurgling, crackling, or popping noises, with or without nasal congestion	
	Decreased hearing in affected ear	
Pressure changes (barotrauma)	Severe pain	A doctor's examination
	History of recent rapid change in air pressure (such as air travel or scuba diving)	
	Often blood visible on or behind eardrum	
Mastoiditis	Recent middle ear infection	A doctor's examination
	Redness and tenderness behind the ear	Sometimes CT scan
	Often fever and/or ear discharge	
Otitis media (acute or chronic)	Severe pain, often with cold symptoms	A doctor's examination
	Bulging, red eardrum	
	More common among children	
	Sometimes ear discharge	
Infectious myringitis (eardrum infection)	Severe pain	A doctor's examination
	Inflamed eardrum	
	Small blisters on surface of eardrum	
Herpes zoster oticus	Severe pain	A doctor's examination
	Blisters or pustules on the outer ear	
	May be accompanied by hearing loss or facial weakness	
External ear		
Impacted wax or foreign object	Visible during a doctor's examination	A doctor's examination
	Foreign objects almost always in children	
Injury	Usually in people who were attempting to clean their ear	A doctor's examination
	Visible during a doctor's examination	
Otitis externa (acute or chronic)	Itching and pain (more itching and only mild discomfort in chronic otitis externa)	A doctor's examination
	Often history of swimming or recurrent water exposure	CT scan if malignant external otitis suspected
	Sometimes foul-smelling discharge	
	Red, swollen external ear canal filled with pus-like material	*(continued)*

SOME CAUSES AND FEATURES OF EARACHE *(continued)*

Cause	Common Features*	Tests
Causes due to structures near the ear‡		
Cancer of the throat, tonsils, base of tongue, voice box (larynx), or nasal passages and upper throat (nasopharynx)	Chronic discomfort	Gadolinium-enhanced MRI
	Often long history of tobacco and/or alcohol use	Removal and examination (biopsy) of visible lesions
	Sometimes enlarged, nontender lymph nodes in the neck	
	Usually in older people	
Infection (tonsils, peritonsillar abscess)	Pain much worse with swallowing	A doctor's examination
	Visible redness of throat and/or tonsils	
Neuralgia (inflamed nerve)	Very severe, frequent, sharp pains lasting less than 1 second	A doctor's examination
TMJ disorders	Pain worsens with jaw movement	A doctor's examination
	Lack of smooth TMJ movement	

*Features include symptoms and the results of the doctor's examination. Features mentioned are typical but not always present.
†Many people with middle and external ear disorders have some hearing loss.
‡A common feature is a normal ear examination.
CT = computed tomography; MRI = magnetic resonance imaging; TMJ = temporomandibular joint.

TESTING

Most often, the doctor's examination provides a diagnosis, and tests are not needed. However, people with a normal ear examination, particularly those with chronic or recurrent pain, may need tests to look for cancer. Such tests usually include examination of the nose, throat, and voice box (larynx) with a flexible viewing scope (endoscope) and magnetic resonance imaging (MRI) of the head and neck.

TREATMENT

The best way to treat earache is to treat the underlying disorder.

People may take a pain-relieving drug by mouth. Usually a nonsteroidal anti-inflammatory drug (NSAID) or acetaminophen is adequate. However, some people, particularly those who have a severe external ear infection, need to take an opioid such as oxycodone or hydrocodone for a few days. For a severe external ear infection, doctors also often suction pus or other discharge from the ear canal and insert a small foam wick. The wick can be soaked with antibiotic and/or corticosteroid ear drops.

Ear drops that contain pain relievers (such as antipyrine/benzocaine combinations) are generally not very effective but can be used for a few days. These drops (and any other ear drops, such as those to remove earwax) should not be used by people who might have a perforated eardrum, so a doctor should be consulted before drops are used.

People should avoid digging in their ears with any objects (no matter how soft the object or how careful people think they are). Also, people should not try to flush out their ears unless instructed by a doctor to do so, and then only gently. An oral irrigator (such as used for teeth cleaning) should never be used in the ear.

O—π KEY POINTS

- Most earaches are due to infection of the middle or external ear.
- A doctor's examination is usually all that is needed for diagnosis.
- If the ear appears normal during the examination, doctors look for a disorder in the structures near the ear.

EAR DISCHARGE

Ear discharge (otorrhea) is drainage from the ear. The drainage may be watery, bloody, or thick and whitish, like pus (purulent). Depending on the cause of the discharge, people may also have ear pain (see page 92), fever, itching, vertigo (see page 81), ringing in the ear (tinnitus—see page 98), and/or hearing loss (see page 188). Symptoms range from sudden and severe to slowly developing and mild.

CAUSES

Discharge may originate from the ear canal, the middle ear, or, rarely, from inside the skull.

Overall, the **most common causes** are

- Acute (sudden and severe) middle ear infection (otitis media) with perforation (puncture) of the eardrum
- Chronic otitis media (with perforation of the eardrum, cholesteatoma, or both)
- External ear infection (otitis externa)

In some people with otitis media (usually children), the eardrum ruptures, releasing the infected material collected behind the eardrum. The hole in the eardrum almost always heals, but sometimes a small perforation remains. A perforation may also result from injury or surgery to the eardrum. When a perforation is present, people are at risk of chronic middle ear infections, which can cause ear discharge.

SOME CAUSES AND FEATURES OF EAR DISCHARGE		
Cause	Common Features*	Tests
Acute discharge (lasting less than 6 weeks)		
Acute otitis media with perforated eardrum	Severe ear pain significantly relieved when a thick, whitish discharge starts	A doctor's examination
Chronic otitis media (acute flare up)	History of eardrum perforation and/or cholesteatoma (a noncancerous growth of skin cells in the middle ear), and previous discharge Eardrum appears abnormal during doctor's examination	A doctor's examination Sometimes high-resolution temporal bone CT scan
Cerebrospinal fluid leak caused by severe head injury or recent neurosurgery	Obvious recent head injury or neurosurgery Fluid ranges from crystal clear to blood	Head CT, including skull base
Otitis externa (infectious or allergic)	*Infectious*: Often after swimming or injury; severe pain, worse with pulling on ear *Allergic*: Often after use of ear drops; more itching and redness, and less pain than with infectious cause Typically a rash on the earlobe, where drops trickled out of ear canal *Both*: Ear canal very red, swollen, and filled with debris; eardrum appears normal	A doctor's examination
Chronic discharge (lasting more than 6 weeks)		
Cancer of ear canal	Discharge often bloody, mild pain Sometimes doctor can see a growth in ear canal Typically in older people	Removal and examination (biopsy) of ear tissue Usually CT or MRI *(continued)*

SOME CAUSES AND FEATURES OF EAR DISCHARGE (continued)

Cause	Common Features*	Tests
Chronic otitis media	History of ear infections and typically eardrum perforation and/or cholesteatoma	A doctor's examination
	Less pain than with external otitis	Usually growth and examination of a sample of the ear discharge (culture)
	Eardrum appears abnormal during doctor's examination	
Foreign object	Usually in children	A doctor's examination
	Drainage foul-smelling, pus-filled (purulent)	
	Foreign object often visible during examination unless visibility blocked by swelling and/or discharge	
Mastoiditis	Often fever, history of untreated or unresolved otitis media	A doctor's examination
	Redness, tenderness over mastoid	Sometimes CT
Necrotizing external otitis	Usually people have an immune deficiency or diabetes	CT or MRI
	Chronic severe pain	
	Swelling and tenderness around ear, abnormal tissue in ear canal	
	Sometimes weakness of facial muscles on affected side	

*Features include symptoms and the results of the doctor's examination. Features mentioned are typical but not always present.

CT = computed tomography; MRI = magnetic resonance imaging.

Serious, but rare, causes include

- Cancer of the ear canal
- Fracture of the base of the skull
- Necrotizing external otitis
- Cholesteatoma

The ear canal passes through the base of the skull. If a skull fracture (from a severe head injury) involves that part of the skull, blood and/or cerebrospinal fluid may leak from the ear.

Necrotizing, or malignant, external otitis is a particularly severe form of external ear infection that typically occurs only in people with diabetes or those who have a compromised immune system (due to HIV infection or chemotherapy for cancer).

Some people with chronic otitis media develop a noncancerous (benign) growth of skin cells in the middle ear (cholesteatoma) that can cause discharge. Although a cholesteatoma is noncancerous, it can cause significant damage to the ear and nearby structures. In severe cases, a cholesteatoma may lead to deafness, facial weakness or paralysis, and complications with the brain such as an abscess and other infections.

EVALUATION

The following information can help people decide when a doctor's evaluation is needed and help them know what to expect during the evaluation.

WARNING SIGNS

In people with ear discharge, certain symptoms and characteristics are cause for concern:

- Recent major head injury
- Any neurologic symptoms (such as vertigo or difficulty seeing, speaking, swallowing, and/or talking)
- Hearing loss in the affected ear

- Fever
- Redness and/or swelling of the ear or area around the ear
- Diabetes or a compromised immune system

WHEN TO SEE A DOCTOR

People with warning signs should see a doctor right away. People without warning signs should see a doctor within several days and avoid getting water in the ear until it can be evaluated.

WHAT THE DOCTOR DOES

Doctors first ask questions about the person's symptoms and medical history. Doctors then do a physical examination. What they find during the history and physical examination often suggests a cause of the ear discharge and the tests that may need to be done (see Table on pages 95 to 96).

During the medical history, doctors ask about the following:

- Activities that can affect the ear canal or eardrum (for example, swimming; insertion of objects, including cotton swabs; and use of ear drops)
- Whether people have had repeated ear infections
- Any severe head injury

During the physical examination, doctors focus on examining the ears, nose, throat, and neurologic system. By examining the ear canal with a light, doctors can usually diagnose perforated eardrum, external otitis, foreign object, and other common causes of ear discharge. Other findings (see Table) suggest the diagnosis.

TESTING

Many causes are clear after the doctor's examination. Possible tests include

- Audiometry
- CT or MRI

If the cause is not clear, doctors usually do a formal hearing test (audiometry) and computed tomography (CT) or gadolinium-enhanced magnetic resonance imaging (MRI). If abnormal tissue is present in the ear canal, a tissue sample (biopsy) may be taken. Sometimes culture swabs are taken of the drainage to identify infection.

TREATMENT

Treatment is directed at the cause. People who have a large perforation of the eardrum are advised to keep water out of the ear. People can keep water out of the ear while showering or washing their hair by coating a cotton ball with petroleum jelly and placing it at the opening of the ear canal. Doctors can also make plugs out of silicone and place them in the canal. Such plugs are carefully sized and shaped so that they do not get lodged deep in the ear canal and cannot be removed. People who have a small perforation, such as that caused by a ventilation tube, should ask a doctor whether they need to keep water out of the ear. A cholesteatoma is treated surgically.

KEY POINTS

- Acute discharge in people without longstanding ear problems or a weakened immune system is usually not dangerous and is typically due to an external ear infection or a perforated eardrum resulting from a middle ear infection.
- People who have chronic ear symptoms or any symptoms besides ear discharge (particularly any neurologic symptoms) should be evaluated by a specialist.

EAR, RINGING OR BUZZING IN (TINNITUS)

Ringing in the ears (tinnitus) is noise originating in the ear rather than in the environment. It is a symptom and not a specific disease. Tinnitus is very common—10 to 15% of people experience it to some degree.

The noise heard by people with tinnitus may be a buzzing, ringing, roaring, whistling, or hissing sound and is often associated with hearing loss. Some people hear more complex sounds that may be different at different times. These sounds are more noticeable in a quiet environment and when people are not concentrating on something else. Thus, tinnitus tends to be most disturbing to people when they are trying to sleep. However, the experience of tinnitus is highly individual. Some people are very disturbed by their symptoms, whereas others find them quite bearable.

Subjective tinnitus is by far the most common type. It is caused by abnormal activity in the part of the brain responsible for processing sound (auditory cortex). Doctors do not fully understand how this abnormal activity develops.

Objective tinnitus is much less common. It represents actual noise created by structures near the ear. Other people can sometimes hear the sounds of objective tinnitus if they listen closely.

CAUSES

SUBJECTIVE TINNITUS

More than 75% of ear-related disorders include tinnitus as a symptom. The most common causes include

- Exposure to loud noises or explosions (acoustic trauma)
- Aging
- Certain drugs that damage the ear (ototoxic drugs)
- Meniere disease

Other causes include middle ear infections, disorders that block the ear canal (such as an external ear infection [external otitis], excessive ear wax, or foreign bodies), problems with the eustachian tube (which connects the middle ear and the back of the nose) due to allergies or other causes of obstruction, and otosclerosis (a disorder of excess bone growth in the middle ear). An uncommon but serious cause is an acoustic neuroma, a noncancerous (benign) tumor of part of the nerve leading from the inner ear.

OBJECTIVE TINNITUS

Objective tinnitus usually involves noise from blood vessels near the ear. In such cases, the sound comes with each beat of the pulse (pulsatile). Causes include

- Turbulent flow through the carotid artery or jugular vein
- Certain middle ear tumors that are rich in blood vessels
- Malformed blood vessels of the membrane covering the brain

The most common noise is the sound of rapid or turbulent blood flow in major vessels of the neck. This abnormal blood flow may occur because of a reduced red blood cell count (anemia) or a blockage of the arteries (atherosclerosis) and may be worsened in people with poorly controlled high blood pressure (hypertension). Some small tumors of the middle ear called glomus tumors are rich in blood vessels. Although the tumors are small, they are very near the sound-receiving structures of the ear, and blood flow through them can sometimes be heard (only in one ear). Sometimes, blood vessel malformations that involve abnormal connections between arteries and veins (arteriovenous malformations) develop in the membrane covering the brain (the dura). If these malformations are near the ear, the person sometimes can hear blood flowing through them.

Less commonly, spasms of muscles of the palate or the small muscles of the middle ear cause clicking sounds. These sounds do not follow the beat of the pulse. Such spasms often have no known cause but may be due to tumors, head injury, or diseases that affect the covering of nerves (for example, multiple sclerosis).

EVALUATION

Not all tinnitus requires evaluation by a doctor. The following information can help people decide whether a doctor's evaluation is needed and help them know what to expect during the evaluation.

WARNING SIGNS

Certain symptoms and characteristics are cause for concern. They include

- Tinnitus in only one ear
- Any neurologic symptoms (other than hearing loss), particularly difficulty with balance or walking, but also vertigo or difficulty seeing, speaking, swallowing, and/or talking

WHEN TO SEE A DOCTOR

People with warning signs should see a doctor right away. People without warning signs in whom tinnitus recently developed should call their doctor, as should people with pulsatile tinnitus. Most people with tinnitus and no warning signs have had tinnitus for a long time.

They can discuss the matter with their doctor and be seen at a mutually convenient time.

WHAT THE DOCTOR DOES

Doctors first ask questions about the person's symptoms and medical history. Doctors then do a physical examination. What they find during the history and physical examination may suggest a cause of the tinnitus and the tests that may need to be done (see Table, below).

During the medical history, doctors ask about the following:

- The nature of the tinnitus, including whether it is in one or both ears and whether it is constant or pulsatile
- Whether the person has any neurologic symptoms
- Whether the person has been exposed to loud noise or to drugs that can affect the ears

During the physical examination, doctors focus on examining the ears (including hearing) and the neurologic system. They also listen with a stethoscope over and near the person's ear and on the neck for sounds of objective tinnitus. The findings often suggest a cause.

SOME CAUSES AND FEATURES OF TINNITUS

Cause	Common Features*	Tests
Subjective tinnitus (typically a constant tone and accompanied by some degree of hearing loss)		
Acoustic trauma (noise-induced hearing loss)	History of occupational or recreational exposure to noise Hearing loss	A doctor's examination[†]
Aging (presbycusis)	Progressive hearing loss, often with family history	A doctor's examination[†]
Barotrauma (ear damage due to sudden pressure change)	Clear history of ear damage	A doctor's examination[†]
Brain tumors (such as acoustic neuroma or meningioma)	Tinnitus and often hearing loss in only one ear Sometimes other neurologic abnormalities	Gadolinium-enhanced MRI Audiometry
Drugs (particularly aspirin, aminoglycoside antibiotics, certain diuretics, and some chemotherapy drugs, including cisplatin)	Tinnitus beginning in both ears shortly after starting use of drug Except with aspirin, hearing loss also possible With aminoglycoside antibiotics, possible dizziness and problems with balance	A doctor's examination[†] *(continued)*

SOME CAUSES AND FEATURES OF TINNITUS *(continued)*

Cause	Common Features*	Tests
Eustachian tube dysfunction	Often a long history of decreased hearing and frequent colds, and problems clearing ears with air travel or other pressure change May be in one or both ears (often one ear more of a problem than the other)	Audiometry Tympanometry
Infections (such as otitis media, labyrinthitis, meningitis, or syphilis)	History of such infection	A doctor's examination[†]
Meniere disease	Repeated episodes of hearing loss, tinnitus, and/or fullness in one ear and severe vertigo	Audiometry Vestibular testing Gadolinium-enhanced MRI to rule out acoustic neuroma
Obstruction of ear canal (due to wax, foreign object, or external otitis)	Only one ear affected Visible abnormalities seen during ear examination, including discharge with external otitis	A doctor's examination[†]

Objective tinnitus (typically pulsatile or intermittent)

Artery and vein (arteriovenous) malformations of the dura	Constant, pulsatile tinnitus in only one ear Usually no other symptoms Possible humming or pulsing noise over the skull heard during examination	Magnetic resonance angiography (MRA) or angiography
Spasm of muscles of the palate or of the middle ear	Irregular clicking or mechanical-sounding noise Possibly other neurologic symptoms (when the cause of the spasm is a neurologic disease such as multiple sclerosis) Possible movement of the palate and/or eardrum when symptoms occur	MRI
Turbulent blood flow in carotid artery or jugular vein	Possible humming or pulsing noise heard over the neck during examination The noise may stop when the doctor pushes on the jugular vein and/or has people turn their head to the side	A doctor's examination[†]
Vascular middle ear tumors (such as glomus tumors)	Constant, pulsatile tinnitus in only one ear Possible pulsing noise heard over the affected ear during examination Sometimes doctors can see the tumor behind the eardrum when they look in the ear canal with a light	CT MRI Angiography (usually done before surgery)

*Features include symptoms and results of the doctor's examination. Features mentioned are typical but not always present.
[†]Most doctors routinely do a full hearing test (audiometry).
CT = computed tomography; MRI = magnetic resonance imaging.

TESTING

Possible tests include

- Formal hearing test (including tympanometry)

Most people should have a formal hearing test done by either the doctor or a hearing specialist (audiologist). People with tinnitus in only one ear and hearing loss should have gadolinium-enhanced magnetic resonance imaging (MRI). People with tinnitus in only one ear and normal hearing should have an MRI if tinnitus lasts more than 6 months. People with pulsatile tinnitus often require magnetic resonance angiography (MRA) and sometimes angiography.

TREATMENT

Attempts to identify and treat the disorder causing tinnitus are often unsuccessful. However, correcting any hearing loss (for example, with a hearing aid) relieves tinnitus in some people.

Various techniques can help make tinnitus tolerable, although the ability to tolerate it varies from person to person. Many people find that background sound helps mask the tinnitus and helps them fall asleep. Some people play background music. Other people use a tinnitus masker, which is a device worn like a hearing aid that produces a constant level of neutral sounds. For the profoundly deaf, an implant in the cochlea (the organ of hearing) may reduce tinnitus but is only done for people with severe to profound hearing loss in both ears. If these standard techniques are not helpful, people may want to seek treatment in clinics that specialize in the treatment of tinnitus.

KEY POINTS

- Most tinnitus is due to causes that are not dangerous, for example, exposure to loud noise, aging, Meniere disease, and use of certain drugs.
- In many cases, the cause is unknown.
- Findings that are of concern include tinnitus accompanied by any neurologic symptoms and tinnitus in only one ear (particularly when accompanied by hearing loss, dizziness, and/or balance difficulty).
- Tinnitus rarely can be stopped, but certain techniques help people manage their symptoms effectively.

ERECTILE DYSFUNCTION (IMPOTENCE)

Every man occasionally has a problem achieving an erection, and such occurrences are considered normal. Erectile dysfunction (ED) occurs when a man is

- Never able to achieve an erection
- Achieves erection briefly but not long enough for intercourse
- Achieves effective erection inconsistently

In the United States, about 50% of men aged 40 to 70 are affected somewhat, and the percentage increases with aging. However, ED is not considered a normal part of aging and can be successfully treated at any age.

CAUSES

To achieve an erection, the penis needs an adequate amount of blood flowing in, a slowing of blood flowing out, proper function of nerves leading to and from the penis, adequate amounts of the male sex hormone testosterone, and sufficient sex drive (libido), so a disorder of any of these systems may lead to ED.

Most cases of ED are caused by abnormalities of the blood vessels or nerves of the penis. Other possible causes include hormonal disorders, structural disorders of the penis, use of certain drugs (see Table on page 103), and psychologic problems (see Table on pages 104 to 105). The most common specific causes are

- Hardening of the arteries (atherosclerosis) that affects the arteries to the penis
- Diabetes mellitus
- Complications of prostate surgery

BLOOD VESSEL DISORDERS

Atherosclerosis may partially block blood flow to the legs (peripheral vascular disease). Usually, arteries to the penis are also blocked, decreasing the amount of blood flow to the penis and causing ED. Diabetes, high cholesterol levels, high blood pressure, and smoking contribute to atherosclerosis and therefore to ED.

Sometimes blood leaks out of the veins in the penis too fast, decreasing blood pressure in the penis and thus interfering with achieving or maintaining an erection (called veno-occlusive dysfunction).

Prolonged, painful erection (priapism—see page 109) may damage the erectile tissue of the penis, leading to ED.

NERVE DISORDERS

If the nerves sending messages to the penis are damaged, ED can occur. In addition to causing atherosclerosis, diabetes can also affect the nerves that supply the penis. Because nerves to the penis run along the prostate gland, prostate surgery (such as for cancer or an enlarged prostate) often causes ED.

Less common nerve disorders that cause ED include spinal cord injury, multiple sclerosis, and stroke. Also, prolonged pressure on the nerves in the buttocks and genital area (the so-called saddle area), as may occur during long-distance bicycle riding, can cause temporary ED.

OTHER DISORDERS

Hormonal disturbances (such as abnormally low levels of testosterone) tend to decrease sex drive but can also result in ED. In Peyronie disease, scar tissue develops inside the penis, resulting in curved and often painful erections and causing ED. Certain prescription drugs, alcohol, and illicit drugs such as cocaine and amphetamines can also cause or contribute to ED.

Sometimes psychologic problems (such as performance anxiety or depression) or factors that decrease a man's energy level (such as illness, fatigue, or stress) cause or contribute to ED. ED may be situational, involving a particular place, time, or partner.

Often several factors contribute to ED. For example, a man with a slight decrease in erectile function caused by diabetes or peripheral vascular disease can develop severe ED after starting a new drug or if stress increases.

EVALUATION

An occasional episode of ED is not uncommon, but men who are consistently unable to

SOME COMMONLY USED DRUGS THAT CAN CAUSE ERECTILE DYSFUNCTION

Class	Drugs
Drugs to treat high blood pressure (antihypertensives)	Beta-blockers (such as atenolol, carvedilol, metoprolol, and propranolol)
	Clonidine
	Diuretics (such as furosemide, hydrochlorothiazide, and chlorthalidone)
	Methyldopa
	Spironolactone
Drugs to treat prostate enlargement	Alpha-adrenergic blockers (such as terazosin, doxazosin, tamsulosin, and silodosin)
	5-Alpha-reductase inhibitors (such as finasteride and dutasteride)
Drugs to treat prostate cancer	Hormonal drugs (such as leuprolide, triptorelin, and goserelin)
	Abiraterone
	Bicalutamide
	Ketoconazole
Drugs that affect the central nervous system	Alcohol
	Benzodiazepines (such as alprazolam, chlordiazepoxide, diazepam, and lorazepam)
	Cocaine or amphetamines, with chronic use
	Monoamine oxidase inhibitors (such as phenelzine, selegiline, and tranylcypromine)
	Opioids (such as codeine, heroin, hydromorphone, methadone, morphine, or oxycodone), if used chronically
	Selective serotonin reuptake inhibitors (such as citalopram, escitalopram, fluoxetine, paroxetine, and sertraline)
	Tricyclic antidepressants (such as amitriptyline, desipramine, imipramine, and nortriptyline)
Other	Androgen antagonists (such as megestrol)
	Anticancer drugs (most cancer chemotherapy drugs)
	Cimetidine
	Drugs with anticholinergic effects (such as many antihistamines and some antidepressants)
	Estrogens

achieve or maintain an erection should see their doctor because ED may be a sign of a serious health problem, such as atherosclerosis or a nerve disorder. Most causes of ED are treatable. The following information can help men know when to see a doctor and what to expect during the evaluation.

WARNING SIGNS

In men with ED, certain symptoms and characteristics are cause for concern. They include

- Absence of erections during the night or upon awakening in the morning

- Numbness in the area between and around the buttocks and genital area (called the saddle area)
- Painful cramping in the muscles of the legs that occurs during physical activity but is relieved promptly by rest (claudication)

WHEN TO SEE A DOCTOR

Although ED may diminish a man's quality of life, it is not itself a dangerous condition. However, ED may be a symptom of a serious medical disorder. Because numbness in the groin or leg can be a sign of spinal cord damage, men who

COMMON CAUSES AND FEATURES OF ERECTILE DYSFUNCTION

Cause	Common Features*	Tests†
Blood vessel disorders		
Blockage of arteries (peripheral vascular disease)	Claudication (painful, aching, cramping, or tired feeling in the muscles of the legs that occurs regularly and predictably during physical activity but is relieved promptly by rest)	Comparison of blood pressures measured in the ankle and arm at the same time (called the ankle-brachial index)
	Usually risk factors (for example, high blood pressure, diabetes, or abnormal blood levels of cholesterol and lipids)	Testing for risk factors (for example, elevated blood sugar and blood lipid levels)
Venous leak (when the veins in the penis cannot prevent blood from leaving the penis during an erection, as they normally do)	Erections that occur but cannot be sustained	Ultrasonographic testing
Nerve disorders		
Nerve damage caused by diabetes (diabetic neuropathy)	Known diabetes	A doctor's examination
	Sometimes numbness, burning, or other pains of the feet	Sometimes electromyography and nerve conduction studies
	Sometimes urinary incontinence	
Multiple sclerosis	Intermittent episodes of weakness or numbness in different parts of the body at different times	MRI
		Sometimes spinal tap (lumbar puncture) and tests of spinal fluid
Nerve injury during prostate surgery	Known surgery	Only a doctor's examination
Spinal cord disorders (such as tumors or injuries)	Numbness in the area between the penis and anus	MRI
	Usually other symptoms of spinal cord disorder (for example, numbness and weakness of legs and incontinence)	
Prolonged pressure in the buttocks and genital area (the so-called saddle area), as occurs when riding a bicycle or a horse	Usually competitive athletes who bicycle for long periods	Only a doctor's examination
	Symptoms occur shortly afterward	
Prostatitis (inflammation of the prostate)	Pain in the pelvic or groin area and bothersome urinary symptoms, such as pain, a burning sensation, blood in the urine, having to urinate frequently, or having difficulty starting to urinate	Only a doctor's examination
Stroke	Known stroke	Only a doctor's examination
Hormonal disorders		
Hypogonadism (testosterone deficiency)	Loss of sex drive, sleep disturbances, and depression or mood changes	Measurement of the testosterone level in the blood
	Eventually, decreases in the size of muscles and testes, bone density, and body hair	
	Eventually, an increase in body fat and breast size	

(continued)

COMMON CAUSES AND FEATURES OF ERECTILE DYSFUNCTION (continued)

Cause	Common Features*	Tests†
Cushing syndrome	Round face, increased body fat in the trunk, purple streaks on the abdomen, high blood pressure, and mood changes	Measurement of levels of cortisol in the urine
		Sometimes blood tests
Severe hyperthyroidism (thyroid hormone excess)	Restlessness, increased heart rate and blood pressure, tremor, weight loss, and inability to tolerate heat	Measurement of levels of thyroid hormone in the blood
Severe hypothyroidism (thyroid hormone deficiency)	Sluggishness, decreased heart rate and blood pressure, thickened skin, decreased appetite, weight gain, and inability to tolerate cold	Measurement of levels of thyroid hormone in the blood
Structural disorders		
Peyronie disease (formation of scar tissue in the erectile tissue of the penis)	Firm tissue in the penis Often severe curving of the penis Often pain during intercourse	Only a doctor's examination
Hypospadias (a birth defect)	Urethra located on the underside of the penis	Only a doctor's examination
Microphallus (a birth defect)	Abnormally small penis	Only a doctor's examination
Psychologic disorders		
Depression	Sadness, helplessness, hopelessness, loss of appetite, and problems sleeping	Only a doctor's examination
Performance anxiety or stress	Full erections during sleep and when masturbating Concern about sexual performance Sometimes ED occurring only with certain partners or in certain situations	Only a doctor's examination
Other		
Drugs (see Table on page 103)	History of taking a drug known to cause ED	Only a doctor's examination
Hypoxemia (chronically low blood oxygen levels)	Usually a chronic lung disorder (for example, chronic obstructive pulmonary disease)	Pulse oximetry (measurement of the level of oxygen in the blood)

*Features include symptoms and the results of the doctor's examination. Features mentioned are typical but not always present.

†Testosterone level is usually measured. If the level is low, doctors measure levels of other hormones.

ED = erectile dysfunction; MRI = magnetic resonance imaging.

suddenly develop such numbness should see a doctor right away. Men who have other warning signs should call their doctor and ask how soon they need to be seen and examined.

WHAT THE DOCTOR DOES

Doctors first ask questions about the man's symptoms and medical history. Doctors then do a physical examination. What they find during the history and physical examination often suggests a cause for ED and additional tests that may need to be done (see Table on pages 104 to 105).

Doctors ask about

- Drug and alcohol use
- Smoking history

- History of diabetes
- History of high blood pressure
- History of atherosclerosis
- History of surgery (for example, for prostate enlargement, prostate or rectal cancer, or blood vessel disorders)
- History of injury (for example, a broken pelvic bone or a back injury)
- Symptoms of disorders of the blood vessels (for example, pain in the calves when walking or coolness, numbness, or blue color of the feet)
- Symptoms of nerve disorders (for example, numbness, tingling, weakness, incontinence, or falling)
- Symptoms of hormonal disorders (for example, loss of sex drive, increased size of breasts, decreased size of testes, loss of body hair, tremor, changes in weight or appetite, or difficulty tolerating heat or cold)
- Symptoms of psychologic disorders, particularly depression
- Satisfaction with sexual relationships
- Sexual dysfunction (for example, vaginitis or depression) in the man's partner

Even though men may be embarrassed to talk to their doctors about some of these subjects, the information is important in determining the cause of ED.

The physical examination focuses on the genitals and prostate, but doctors also look for signs of hormonal, nerve, and blood vessel disorders and examine the rectum.

The cause is sometimes clear from the history. For example, ED may occur soon after prostate surgery or beginning a new drug. One important clue is whether erections are present at night or on awakening. When erections are present, a physical cause is less likely than a psychologic cause because physical causes typically inhibit erections at all times. Other factors that suggest a psychologic cause are sudden development in a young healthy man, occurrence of symptoms only in certain situations, and resolution of ED without any treatment. Claudication or coolness or a blue color in the toes or feet may indicate a problem with the blood vessels such as peripheral vascular disease or vascular disease caused by diabetes.

TESTING

Testing is usually needed. Laboratory tests include the measurement of the level of testosterone in the blood. If the testosterone level is low, doctors measure additional hormones. Depending on the results of the history and physical examination, blood tests may also be done to check for previously unrecognized diabetes, thyroid disorders, and lipid disorders. Usually, these tests provide doctors with enough information to plan treatment.

Occasionally, doctors inject a drug into the penis that stimulates erection and then use ultrasonography to assess blood flow in the arteries and veins of the penis. Rarely, doctors may recommend the use of a home monitor that detects and records erections during sleep.

TREATMENT

Any underlying disorder is treated, and doctors often stop drugs that may be causing ED or switch the man to a different drug. However, men should talk with their doctor before they stop taking any drug.

Excess weight is a risk factor for many disorders that may cause ED, so weight loss may improve erectile function. Smoking is a risk factor for atherosclerosis, so stopping smoking may also improve erectile function. Stopping or decreasing alcohol use, if excessive, can also help.

Even ED caused by a physical disorder usually has a psychologic component, so doctors offer reassurance and education (including of the man's partner whenever possible). Couples counseling by a qualified sex therapist can help improve partner communication, reduce performance pressure, and resolve interpersonal conflicts that contribute to ED.

Supplemental testosterone can help restore erections in men with low testosterone levels. These testosterone preparations can be applied daily as a patch or a gel. Men with very low testosterone levels may need testosterone injections twice per month.

Noninvasive methods (mechanical devices and drugs) are tried first. Sometimes men must try the method a few times before doctors can determine whether it is effective. Although most men prefer drugs to other methods of treating ED, mechanical devices have the advantages of being highly effective and, because they are free of drug side effects, usually very safe. Penile implant surgery with an inflatable prosthesis is the last used, but most effective, way to achieve intercourse.

MECHANICAL DEVICES

Men who can develop but not sustain an erection may use a constriction ring. As soon as erection occurs, an elastic ring is placed around the base of the penis, helping prevent blood from flowing out and maintaining the firmness of the penis. If the man cannot develop an erection, a hand-held vacuum erection device can be applied over the penis. This device draws blood into the penis by exerting a gentle vacuum effect, after which the ring is placed on the base of the penis to retain the erection. Bruising of the penis, coldness of the tip of the penis, and lack of spontaneity are some drawbacks to this method. Sometimes a constriction ring and vacuum device are combined with drug therapy.

DRUGS

The primary drugs for ED are oral phosphodiesterase inhibitors. Other drugs include prostaglandins that are injected into the penis or inserted into the urethra. Oral phosphodiesterase inhibitors are used much more often than other drugs because they are simple to use and allow spontaneity in intercourse. Over-the-counter herbal remedies are sold for ED, but they are usually ineffective, contain hidden doses of a phosphodiesterase inhibitor, or both. The hidden phosphodiesterase inhibitor may expose the man to a drug with possible side effects.

Oral phosphodiesterase inhibitors (sildenafil, vardenafil, avanafil, and tadalafil) increase blood flow to the penis. These drugs work in the same way, but differ as to how long the effect lasts, their side effects, and their interactions with food. The effect of tadalafil lasts longer than those of the other drugs (up to 36 hours), which some men prefer.

Most phosphodiesterase inhibitors work best when taken on an empty stomach and at least 1 hour before sexual intercourse. Men who are taking nitrates (most often nitroglycerin for the treatment of angina but also recreational amyl nitrate ["poppers"]) should not take phosphodiesterase inhibitors because the combination can cause blood pressure to drop to unsafe levels. Other temporary side effects of phosphodiesterase inhibitors include flushing, vision abnormalities (including abnormal color perception), and headache. Priapism (prolonged erection) develops very rarely and may require emergency medical treatment (see page 111). In rare instances, men have reported blindness or hearing loss after taking phosphodiesterase inhibitors, but it is not clear whether the phosphodiesterase inhibitors have been the cause.

Alprostadil (the prostaglandin PGE_1) may be inserted into the urethra or injected into the penis using a very tiny needle, causing a suitable erection in most men. Alprostadil may cause priapism and penile pain. Usually, the doctor teaches the man to inject the drug himself during an office visit. After this, men may give themselves alprostadil. Alprostadil may be combined with a phosphodiesterase inhibitor for men in whom oral drugs are not effective. Sometimes other drugs are injected with alprostadil to cause an erection.

SURGERY

For some men, drug therapy is not effective or acceptable. In these men, surgery to implant a penile prosthesis may be done. Prostheses can take the form of rigid silicone rods or hydraulically operated devices that can be inflated and deflated. Both involve the risks of general anesthesia, infection, and prosthetic malfunction.

ESSENTIALS FOR OLDER PEOPLE

Although ED does increase with aging, it need not be accepted as a normal part of aging. Rather, because older men are more likely to have medical conditions that affect the blood vessels they are also more likely to have ED. Many older couples engage in satisfying sexual activity without erections or intercourse and may not choose to seek treatment.

O—π KEY POINTS

- ED commonly results from psychologic, nervous system, or blood vessel disorders, from injury, or from the side effects of some drugs or surgery.
- When considering the causes, doctors consider psychologic and interpersonal factors.
- Testosterone therapy may help restore erectile function in men with low serum testosterone levels and ED, but a low testosterone level is not a common cause of ED.
- Most men with ED may be successfully treated with an oral phosphodiesterase inhibitor such as sildenafil, vardenafil, avanafil, or tadalafil.
- Most men who do not respond to therapy with oral phosphodiesterase inhibitors can achieve erections with injections of alprostadil, either alone or combined with an oral phosphodiesterase inhibitor.
- Vacuum erection devices and penile prosthesis surgery are effective treatments for men with severe ED.

ERECTION, PERSISTENT (PRIAPISM)

Persistent erection (priapism) is a painful, persistent, abnormal erection unaccompanied by sexual desire or excitation. It is most common in boys aged 5 to 10 years and in men aged 20 to 50 years.

The penis is composed of three cylindrical spaces (sinuses) of tissue through which blood can flow (called erectile tissue). The larger two sinuses, the corpora cavernosa, occur side by side. The third sinus (the corpus spongiosum) surrounds the urethra and ends as the cone-shaped end of the penis (glans penis). When these sinuses fill with blood, the penis becomes larger and rigid (erect). Muscles then tighten around the veins of the groin, preventing blood from flowing out of the penis and keeping the penis erect.

ISCHEMIC PRIAPISM

Most cases of persistent erection involve failure of blood to flow out of the penis. Blood backs up, preventing new oxygen-rich blood from entering the penis. As a result, the penis can become starved of oxygen. This condition is known as ischemic priapism or low-flow priapism. Severe pain occurs if an erection lasts longer than 4 hours. The penis may be erect while the glans penis may be soft. Prolonged priapism can lead to erectile dysfunction or even the death of penile tissue.

Stuttering priapism is a recurring form of ischemic priapism in which episodes of erection alternate with periods when the penis is not erect.

NONISCHEMIC PRIAPISM

Less commonly, priapism is due to uncontrolled flow of blood into the penis. Such abnormal blood flow usually results from an injury to an artery in the groin area. Nonischemic priapism is also known as high-flow priapism. It is less painful than ischemic priapism and does not lead to tissue death. The penis is erect but not fully rigid. Subsequent erectile dysfunction is much less common than in ischemic priapism.

CAUSES

Priapism probably results from abnormalities of blood vessels, red blood cells, or nerves that cause blood to become trapped in the erectile tissue of the penis. Sometimes doctors are not able to determine the cause of priapism.

COMMON CAUSES

Causes differ somewhat based on age. In men, the most common cause is

- Drugs taken to treat erectile dysfunction

Drugs taken to cause an erection, including those taken by mouth (avanafil, sildenafil, tadalafil, and vardenafil) and those injected into the penis (for example, alprostadil), can cause priapism.

In boys, the most common causes are

- Blood disorders (for example, sickle cell disease and, less commonly, leukemia)

LESS COMMON CAUSES

Less common causes include

- Prostate cancer
- An injury to the penis or surrounding areas
- Spinal cord injury
- Use of drugs (other than those used to treat erectile dysfunction), such as certain antidepressants (for example, trazodone) or antihypertensive drugs, anticoagulants, corticosteroids, lithium, antipsychotic drugs, cocaine, and amphetamines

EVALUATION

The following information can help people know when to see a doctor and what to expect during the evaluation.

WARNING SIGNS

In boys and men with priapism, certain symptoms and characteristics are cause for concern. They include

- Severe pain
- Age less than 10 years

- Recent injury to the penis or groin area
- Fever and night sweats

necessary to determine whether the cause of priapism is something unusual or serious.

WHEN TO SEE A DOCTOR

All boys and men who have priapism should see a doctor immediately for treatment. If warning signs are present, further evaluation may be

WHAT THE DOCTOR DOES

Doctors first ask questions about symptoms and medical history and then do a physical examination. What they find during the history

SOME CAUSES AND FEATURES OF PRIAPISM

Cause	Common Features*	Tests
Drugs for erectile dysfunction (such as alprostadil, papaverine, phentolamine, avanafil, sildenafil, tadalafil, or vardenafil)	Painful priapism in men who took one of these drugs immediately before priapism started	Only a doctor's examination
Recreational drugs (such as amphetamines and cocaine)	Painful priapism If amphetamines or cocaine is the cause, agitation and anxiety	A doctor's examination Occasionally drug screening
Other drugs (such as anticoagulants, certain antidepressants, antihypertensive drugs, psychostimulants, antipsychotic drugs, corticosteroids, or lithium)	Painful priapism in boys or men being treated for a disorder	Only a doctor's examination
Blood disorders (such as leukemia, multiple myeloma, sickle cell disease or trait, or thalassemia)	In boys or young men, often of African or Mediterranean descent	A complete blood count Blood tests to check for abnormal hemoglobin (hemoglobin electrophoresis)
Prostate cancer that has spread to areas next to the prostate or any cancer that has spread to the genitals	In men over 50 who have worsening symptoms indicating that the opening from the bladder into the urethra (bladder outlet) is blocked (such as a weak urine stream, difficulty starting urination, and dribbling at the end of urination) Sometimes blood in the urine	Blood tests to measure the level of prostate-specific antigen CT or MRI
Spinal cord disorders, such as narrowing of the spinal canal (spinal cord stenosis) or compression of the spinal cord	Weakness or numbness in the legs Retention of urine or uncontrollable loss of urine or stool (urinary or fecal incontinence)	MRI or CT of the spine
Injury to an artery	Mildly painful and slightly rigid priapism In men who have had a recent injury to the penis or groin area	Duplex ultrasonography of the penis (ultrasonography that measures blood flow and shows structure of the blood vessels through which the blood is flowing) Angiography (x-rays of blood vessels) MRI

*Features include symptoms and the results of the doctor's examination. Features mentioned are typical but not always present.
CT = computed tomography; MRI = magnetic resonance imaging.

and physical examination often suggests a cause of priapism and the tests that may need to be done (see Table on page 110).

Doctors ask

- How long the erection has been present
- Whether there is pain
- Whether there has been an injury to the penis or the groin area
- Whether conditions (such as sickle cell disease) that may cause priapism are present
- What drugs have been taken, including drugs for erectile dysfunction and recreational drugs

Although doctors focus the physical examination on the genitals to detect signs of injury or cancer, they also examine the abdomen and do a digital rectal examination. Doctors may also do a neurologic examination to look for signs of a spinal cord disorder.

TESTING

The need for testing depends on what doctors find during the history and physical examination. Often, the type of priapism (ischemic or nonischemic) and cause are obvious, such as the use of a drug to treat erectile dysfunction. If it is not clear whether priapism is ischemic or nonischemic, doctors may take a sample of blood from the penis to test for the presence of oxygen and other gases (arterial blood gas measurement). They may also do duplex ultrasonography (ultrasonography that measures blood flow and shows structure of the blood vessels through which the blood is flowing). These tests help differentiate ischemic from nonischemic priapism. Ultrasonography may also show the blood flow patterns in priapism and the anatomic abnormalities contributing to priapism. If the cause is still not obvious, doctors test for blood disorders and urinary tract infections. Testing includes

- A complete blood count
- Urinalysis and urine culture
- Sometimes hemoglobin electrophoresis, particularly in boys and men of African or Mediterranean descent

Hemoglobin electrophoresis is a blood test to check for abnormal hemoglobin (the protein that carries oxygen in red blood cells).

Because some boys and men may be embarrassed to admit they have used recreational drugs, doctors sometimes do drug screening. Occasionally, magnetic resonance imaging (MRI) or computed tomography (CT) is also done.

TREATMENT

Simple measures that can be taken immediately include applying ice, climbing stairs, or both. However, priapism is an emergency. Treatment should begin as soon as possible, preferably by a urologist in an emergency department.

Doctors give boys and men who have significant pain a pain killer (analgesic). Other measures are usually needed if priapism is ischemic. After numbing the penis with a local anesthetic, doctors may inject the penis with a drug that causes the blood vessels carrying blood to the penis to narrow (for example, phenylephrine), decreasing blood flow to the penis and causing the swelling to subside. Doctors may also draw blood out of the penis using a needle and syringe (aspiration). Drawing out blood helps reduce pressure and swelling. Sometimes doctors also flush the veins of the penis with a salt water (saline) solution to help remove oxygen-depleted blood or blood clots.

These measures may be repeated. If they are still not effective, doctors may create a surgical shunt. A shunt is a passageway that is surgically inserted into the penis to divert excess blood flow and allow circulation in the penis to return to normal.

O—π KEY POINTS

- Priapism is an emergency that requires urgent evaluation and treatment.
- Drugs, including those used to treat erectile dysfunction, and sickle cell disease are the most common causes.
- Treatment usually involves injecting a drug into the penis and removing the excess blood from it.

EYE FLOATERS

Eye floaters are specks or strings that appear to move through a person's field of vision but do not correspond to external objects. Floaters are common.

CAUSES

Eye floaters result when something besides light from the environment stimulates the retina, which is the light-sensing structure at the back of the eye. This stimulation causes the retina to send a signal to the brain. The brain may interpret the signal as an apparent object floating in the field of vision (floater) or as a simple, sudden flash of light that can look like lightning, spots, or stars (photopsia). Photopsias can occur when the eyes are rubbed. The most common cause of eye floaters is

- Shrinking of the jellylike substance that fills the eyeball (vitreous humor)

Between about age 50 to 75 years, the vitreous humor shrinks and tugs on the retina from time to time. These tugs stimulate the retina, giving the illusion of light or objects, seen as floaters. Such floaters (idiopathic vitreous floaters) are not harmful. Less often, the vitreous humor pulls completely away from the retina (vitreous detachment).

Less common but more serious causes include

- Detachment of the retina
- Tear in the retina
- Detachment of the vitreous humor
- Bleeding in the vitreous humor
- Inflammation of the vitreous humor

Sometimes migraines cause vision symptoms. These vision symptoms may be white, jagged flashing lines that appear first in the middle of the field of vision and then spread across the entire field of vision (not single objects like floaters). They typically then resolve over about 20 minutes, disappearing first from the peripheral field of vision and last from the center of the field of vision. People may not have a headache with them. These symptoms are called ocular or retinal migraine. People can also have similar symptoms or lose vision in part of an eye for about 10 to 60 minutes, often before a migraine headache begins (called migraine aura). In these cases, symptoms are caused by a phenomenon in the brain, not in the retina.

Tumors (for example, lymphoma) of the eye are rare causes of floaters. Foreign objects in the eye can cause floaters but usually cause other symptoms, such as vision loss (see page 453), eye pain (see page 116), or eye redness (see page 122), that are more troublesome than floaters.

EVALUATION

Not every instance of eye floaters requires an immediate evaluation by a doctor. The following information can help people decide when a doctor's evaluation is needed and help them know what to expect during the evaluation.

WARNING SIGNS

In people with floaters, certain symptoms and characteristics are cause for concern. They include

- Sudden increase in floaters
- Repeated, often lightning-like flashes of light
- Complete or partial loss of vision (often feeling like part of the vision is covered by a shade or curtain)
- Recent eye surgery or eye injury
- Eye pain

WHEN TO SEE A DOCTOR

Although most often floaters are not serious, people who have warning signs should see an eye doctor right away. They may have a serious vitreous or retinal disorder, and waiting a few days, or sometimes even hours, may lead to a permanent loss of vision. People without warning signs who have begun to notice a few floaters should see a doctor when practical, although a delay of a few days or more is unlikely to be harmful. People who have had floaters for some time and have no other symptoms should have an eye examination at some point, but timing is not critical.

WHAT THE DOCTOR DOES

Doctors first ask questions about the person's symptoms and medical history. Doctors then do a physical examination. What they find during the history and physical examination often suggests a cause of the floaters and the tests that may need to be done (see Table, below).

Doctors ask the person to describe the floaters and then ask

- When the person noticed floaters
- What characteristics the floaters have (for example, shapes, movement, or whether they recur)
- Whether floaters occur in one or both eyes
- Whether the person sees flashing lights or whether any part of vision is missing or seems covered by a curtain
- Whether the person has had an eye injury or eye surgery
- Whether other symptoms (such as blurred vision, eye redness, eye pain, or headaches) are present
- Whether the person is nearsighted
- Whether the person has disorders that may affect vision, such as diabetes or immune system disorders (for example, AIDS)

The eye examination is the most important part of the physical examination. Doctors check sharpness of vision, eye movements, and the pupil's response to light. They also check the eyes for redness and the visual field for areas of vision loss.

Ophthalmoscopy is the most important part of the eye examination. Doctors first use drops to dilate the pupils. Then they use an ophthalmoscope (a light with magnifying lenses that shines into the back of the eye) to examine the inside of the person's eyes, including as much of the retina as possible. If one of the serious causes of floaters seems possible, ophthalmoscopy is repeated by an ophthalmologist. An ophthalmologist is a medical doctor who specializes in the evaluation and treatment (surgical and nonsurgical) of eye disorders.

Pressure in the eye (intraocular pressure) is measured after a drop of anesthetic is put into the eye.

Doctors put a drop of fluorescein stain in the eye and then use a slit lamp (an instrument that enables a doctor to examine the eye under high magnification) to examine the entire eye.

SOME CAUSES AND FEATURES OF EYE FLOATERS

Cause	Common Features*	Tests
Eye disorders that are not worrisome		
Vitreous contraction floaters (floaters due to shrinking of the jellylike substance that fills the back part of the eyeball, called the vitreous humor)	A few small, translucent clumps or strands that • Occasionally come into the field of vision • Move as the eye moves • May be more noticeable under certain lighting (such as bright sunlight) • May occur in both eyes, although not at the same time No recent change in the number or type of floaters No effect on vision	A doctor's examination
Eye disorders that are serious		
Detachment of the retina	Simple, sudden flashes of light that can look like lightning, spots, or stars (photopsias), that occur repeatedly or continuously Loss of vision that affects one area, usually what is seen out of the corners of the eye (peripheral vision) Loss of vision that spreads across the field of vision like a curtain Sometimes in people with risk factors for detachment of the retina (such as a recent eye injury, eye surgery, or severe nearsightedness)	Examination by an ophthalmologist

(continued)

SOME CAUSES AND FEATURES OF EYE FLOATERS *(continued)*

Cause	Common Features*	Tests
A tear in the retina	Photopsias Sometimes symptoms only in the peripheral field of vision	Examination by an ophthalmologist
Detachment of the vitreous humor from the retina	An increase in floaters over a period of 1 week–3 months, usually in older people Floaters that resemble cobwebs One large floater that moves in and out of the field of vision Photopsias that come and go	Examination by an ophthalmologist
Vitreous hemorrhage (bleeding into the vitreous humor)	In people who have risk factors for this disorder (such as diabetes, a tear in the retina, sickle cell disease, or an eye injury) Usually loss of the entire field of vision (not in just one or more spots)	Examination by an ophthalmologist Sometimes ultrasonography of the retina
Inflammation of the vitreous humor (as may occur when *Toxoplasma* parasites, fungi, or rarely cytomegalovirus infect the eye)	Pain Loss of vision affecting the entire field of vision Possibly affecting both eyes In people with risk factors for these infections (such as AIDS and other conditions that weaken the immune system)	Sometimes testing to detect microorganisms suspected of causing infection
Disorders not related to the eyes		
Ocular migraine (migraines that cause vision symptoms)	Jagged lines that appear first in the center of the field of vision, then spread outward, and disappear after about 20 minutes Sometimes blurring of central vision Sometimes a headache after the disturbances in vision Sometimes in people known to have migraines	A doctor's examination
Migraine aura	A blind spot, sometimes with shimmering spots and that lasts usually 10 to 60 minutes Usually a headache after the disturbances in vision Usually in people known to have migraines	A doctor's examination

*Features include symptoms and the results of the doctor's examination. Features mentioned are typical but not always present. Features occur in only one eye unless otherwise specified.

TESTING

Doctors can often identify less serious causes during an examination, but if a serious disorder seems possible, doctors refer people to an ophthalmologist to make a diagnosis. Ophthalmologists are medical doctors who specialize in the evaluation and treatment (surgical and nonsurgical) of eye disorders. The ophthalmologist does more detailed ophthalmoscopy and may order testing. For example, for vitreous inflammation due to infection, testing to identify organisms suspected of causing infection may be needed.

TREATMENT

Vitreous contraction floaters require no treatment.

Sometimes if a person has many floaters that interfere with vision, doctors may use a hollow needle to remove the vitreous humor from the eye and replace it with salt water. This surgical procedure is called vitrectomy. However, many doctors think vitrectomy should not be done for floaters because the procedure may cause detachment of the retina or cataracts and because sometimes floaters remain afterward.

Other disorders causing symptoms are treated. For example, surgery is done to repair a detached retina. Antimicrobial drugs are used for infections causing vitreous inflammation.

KEY POINTS

- People who have floaters but no warning signs rarely have a serious disorder.
- People with floaters and warning signs may need to be referred to an ophthalmologist.

EYE PAIN

Eye pain may be severe and seem sharp, aching, or throbbing, or people may feel only mild irritation of the eye surface or the sensation of a foreign object in the eye (foreign body sensation). Many causes of eye pain also cause the eye to look red (see page 122). Other symptoms may be present depending on the cause of eye pain. For example, people may have blurred vision (see page 445), a bulging eye (see page 131), or pain worsened by bright light.

The cornea (the clear layer in front of the iris and pupil) is highly sensitive to pain. Many disorders that affect the cornea also affect the anterior chamber (the fluid-filled space between the iris and the inner part of the cornea) and cause spasm of the muscle that controls the iris (the ciliary muscle). When such spasm is present, bright light causes muscle contraction, worsening pain.

CAUSES

Disorders that cause eye pain can be divided into disorders that affect primarily the cornea, disorders of other parts of the eye, and disorders of other areas of the body that cause pain to be felt in the eye.

COMMON CAUSES

Corneal disorders are the most common causes overall, particularly

- Corneal scratches (abrasions)
- Foreign objects

However, most corneal disorders can cause eye pain.

A feeling of scratchiness or a foreign body sensation may be caused by a disorder of the conjunctiva (the thin membrane that lines the eyelid and covers the front of the eye) or of the cornea.

EVALUATION

Mild eye irritation or a foreign body sensation is common and not usually serious. However, true pain in the eye can be a sign of a severe, vision-threatening disorder. The following information can help people decide when to see a doctor and help them know what to expect during the evaluation.

WARNING SIGNS

In people with eye pain, certain symptoms and characteristics are cause for concern. They include

- Vomiting
- Halos around lights
- Fever, chills, fatigue, or muscle aches
- Decreased sharpness of vision (visual acuity)
- Bulging of an eye (proptosis)
- Inability to move the eye in all directions (such as right, left, up, and down)

WHEN TO SEE A DOCTOR

People who have severe pain, eye redness, or warning signs should see a doctor right away. People with mild pain and no eye redness or warning signs can wait a day or two to see if the discomfort goes away on its own.

WHAT THE DOCTOR DOES

Doctors first ask questions about the person's symptoms and medical history. Doctors then do a physical examination. What they find during the history and physical examination often suggests a cause of the eye pain and the tests that may need to be done (see Table on pages 117 to 120).

Doctors ask the person to describe the pain, including when it started, how severe it is, and whether it hurts to look in different directions or blink. They ask about whether the person has ever had eye pain and whether the person is sensitive to light, has blurred vision, or feels as if the eye contains a foreign object.

During the physical examination, doctors check for the presence of fever or a runny nose. They check the face for tenderness.

Most important is the eye examination, including the entire eye, eyelids, and the region around the eye. Doctors check

- Whether the eyes are red or swollen
- How clearly a person can see using a standard eye chart (visual acuity)

- Whether the person can see in each part of the field of vision (visual field testing)
- How the pupils react to light
- Whether shining a light into the unaffected eye causes pain in the affected eye when the affected eye is closed (called true photophobia)

If doctors suspect a foreign object but do not see one, they turn the eyelids inside out to search for hidden foreign objects.

Doctors usually do a slit-lamp examination. A slit lamp is an instrument that enables a doctor to examine the eye under high magnification. Doctors place a drop of fluorescein stain on the cornea to show scratches or certain kinds of infection, including ulcers. Doctors use tonometry to measure the pressure inside the eye (intraocular pressure). They use an ophthalmoscope (a light with magnifying lenses that shines into the back of the eye) to examine the lens, vitreous humor (the jellylike substance that fills the eyeball), retina (the light-sensing structure at the back of the eye), optic nerve, and the retinal veins and arteries.

Sometimes findings are helpful in making a diagnosis. Particular findings or combinations may point to particular disorders.

Findings may also help suggest or eliminate certain types of disorders.

- Corneal disorders, among other disorders, tend to cause eye redness, tearing, and pain. If those symptoms are absent, a corneal disorder is very unlikely.
- Pain on the surface of the eye, a foreign body sensation, and pain with blinking suggest a foreign object.
- People who wear contact lenses may have a corneal scratch, a corneal ulcer, or contact lens keratitis.
- When measuring eye pressure, doctors put a drop of anesthetic into the eye. If pain then disappears, the cause of pain is probably a corneal disorder.
- Deep, aching, throbbing pain often indicates a possibly serious disorder such as acute closed-angle glaucoma, anterior uveitis, scleritis, endophthalmitis, orbital cellulitis, or orbital pseudotumor. If, in addition, there is eyelid swelling, bulging of the eye, or inability to move the eye to look in all directions, the most likely disorders are orbital pseudotumor, orbital cellulitis, or possibly severe endophthalmitis.

SOME CAUSES AND FEATURES OF EYE PAIN

Cause	Common Features*	Tests†
Disorders that affect the cornea primarily		
Contact lens keratitis (inflammation of the cornea—the clear layer in front of the iris and pupil—caused by wearing contact lenses for long periods of time)	Usually affecting both eyes Eye ache and a feeling of grittiness in the eye Eye redness, tearing, and sensitivity to light In people who wear contact lenses for long periods of time	A doctor's examination
Corneal scratch (abrasion) A foreign object (body)	Symptoms that begin after an eye injury, which may not be noticed in infants and young children Pain in the affected eye when blinking and a foreign body sensation Eye redness, tearing, and usually sensitivity to light	A doctor's examination
Corneal ulcer	Often a grayish patch on the cornea that later becomes an open, painful sore Eye ache and a foreign body sensation	A doctor's examination *(continued)*

SOME CAUSES AND FEATURES OF EYE PAIN *(continued)*

Cause	Common Features*	Tests†
Corneal ulcer *(continued)*	Eye redness, tearing, and sensitivity to light Sometimes in people who have had an eye injury or who have slept with their contact lenses in	Culture of a sample taken from the ulcer, done by an ophthalmologist
Epidemic keratoconjunctivitis (inflammation of the conjunctiva—the membrane that lines the eyelids and covers the front of the eye— and the cornea caused by an adenovirus)	Usually in both eyes Eye ache and a feeling of grittiness in the eye Eye redness, tearing, and usually sensitivity to light Often eyelid swelling and swollen, tender lymph nodes in front of the ears Rarely temporary, severe blurring of vision	A doctor's examination
Herpes simplex keratitis (infection of the cornea caused by the herpes simplex virus)	Usually affecting only one eye *Early*: Symptoms that begin after an episode of conjunctivitis Blisters on the eyelid, sometimes with crusting *Late or recurrent*: Eye redness and watering, eye pain, impaired vision, and sensitivity to light	Usually only a doctor's examination
Herpes zoster ophthalmicus (shingles that affects the face and eye, caused by the varicella-zoster virus)	Usually affecting only one eye *Early*: A rash with blisters and/or crusts on one side of the face, around the eye, on the forehead, and sometimes on the tip of the nose *Late*: Eye redness, tearing, usually sensitivity to light, and eyelid swelling	Usually only a doctor's examination
Welder's (ultraviolet) keratitis (inflammation of the cornea caused by exposure to excessive ultraviolet light)	Usually affects both eyes Symptoms that begin hours after exposure to excessive ultraviolet light (as is produced during arc welding, by a sunlamp, or by bright sun reflecting off snow, particularly at high altitudes) Eye ache and a feeling of grittiness in the eye Eye redness, tearing, and sensitivity to light	A doctor's examination
Other eye disorders		
Closed-angle glaucoma	Severe eye ache and redness Headache, nausea, vomiting, and pain with exposure to light Disturbances in vision such as halos seen around lights and/or decreased vision	Tonometry† Examination of the eye's drainage channels with a special lens (gonioscopy), done by an ophthalmologist *(continued)*

SOME CAUSES AND FEATURES OF EYE PAIN *(continued)*

Cause	Common Features*	Tests†
Anterior uveitis (inflammation of the anterior chamber—the fluid-filled space between the iris and cornea)	Eye ache and sensitivity to light Eye redness (particularly around the cornea) Blurring or loss of vision Often in people who have an autoimmune disorder or who recently had an eye injury	A doctor's examination
Endophthalmitis (infection inside the eye)‡	Affecting only one eye Eye ache, intense eye redness, sensitivity to light, and severely decreased vision Often in people who have had recent eye surgery or a serious eye injury	A doctor's examination Cultures of fluids inside of the eye, done by an ophthalmologist
Optic neuritis (inflammation of the optic nerve), which can be related to multiple sclerosis‡	Usually mild pain that may worsen when eyes are moved Partial or complete loss of vision Eyelids and corneas that appear normal	Often MRI with a radiopaque dye
Orbital cellulitis (infection of the tissue within the eye socket, or orbit)‡	Affecting only one eye Bulging of the eye, eye redness, pain deep within the eye, and aches in and around the eye Red and swollen eyelids Inability to fully move the eye in all directions Impaired vision or loss of vision Fever Sometimes preceded by symptoms of sinusitis (see Sinusitis on next page)	CT or MRI
Orbital pseudotumor (a noncancerous accumulation of inflammatory and fibrous tissue in the eye socket)‡	Aches in and around the eye, which may be very severe Often bulging of the eye Often inability to fully move the eye in all directions Swelling around the eye	CT or MRI Sometimes biopsy
Scleritis (inflammation of the white of the eye called the sclera)	Very severe pain, often described as boring, and sensitivity to light Watering of the eyes Red or violet patches on the white of the eye Often in people who have an autoimmune disorder	Usually only a doctor's examination

(continued)

SOME CAUSES AND FEATURES OF EYE PAIN *(continued)*

Cause	Common Features*	Tests†
Other disorders that cause eye pain		
Cluster or migraine headaches	In people who have had previous episodes of severe headaches	A doctor's examination
	Cluster headaches: Headaches that	
	■ Occur in clusters ■ Occur at the same time each day ■ Cause severe, piercing, knife-like pain, a runny nose, and watery eyes	
	Migraines: Headaches that	
	■ May be preceded by temporary disturbances in sensation, balance, coordination, speech, or vision (such as seeing flashing lights or having blind spots), called the aura ■ Typically cause a pulsating or throbbing pain ■ Are accompanied by nausea, vomiting, and sensitivity to sounds, light, and odors	
Sinusitis	Sometimes swelling around the eye but no other eye symptoms	Sometimes CT
	A yellow or green thick nasal discharge (sometimes with bleeding), headache, or eye or facial pain that varies with head position	
	Fever, tenderness of the face, sometimes a productive cough during the night, and bad breath	

*Features include symptoms and the results of the doctor's examination. Features mentioned are typical but not always present. Disorders usually affect only one eye unless otherwise specified.
†Doctors almost always do a slit-lamp examination with fluorescein staining and measure the pressure inside the eye (called tonometry).
‡These causes are uncommon.
CT = computed tomography; MRI = magnetic resonance imaging.

TESTING

The need for tests depends on what doctors find during the history and physical examination. Testing is usually not necessary. However, if doctors find increased intraocular pressure, they may refer the person to an ophthalmologist (a medical doctor who specializes in the evaluation and treatment—surgical and nonsurgical—of eye disorders) for gonioscopy. A gonioscope is a special lens that allows doctors to examine the drainage channels in the eye.

Bulging of the eye and inability of an eye to move in all directions without moving the head can indicate orbital cellulitis or orbital pseudotumor. Computed tomography (CT) or magnetic resonance imaging (MRI) is then done to check for these disorders. CT may also be done if sinusitis is suspected but the diagnosis is not otherwise clear or if complications are suspected. MRI with a radiopaque dye may be done if optic neuritis is suspected.

Doctors send a sample of fluids from inside the eye (vitreous or aqueous humor) to the laboratory if endophthalmitis seems likely. They may send a sample from the cornea or a blister if herpes simplex keratitis or herpes zoster ophthalmicus seems likely but the diagnosis is not certain. In the laboratory, technicians try to grow bacteria or viruses (culture) to confirm infections and determine the organism causing the infection.

dilating the pupil and thus reduces eye pain with light exposure. For example, homatropine may be used.

TREATMENT

The best way to treat eye pain is to treat the cause of the pain. People may also need to take pain relievers (analgesics) until the pain stops. If an over-the-counter analgesic such as acetaminophen or a nonsteroidal anti-inflammatory drug is ineffective, an opioid may be necessary. Sometimes people with pain caused by anterior uveitis or corneal disorders also need to use an eye drop that prevents ciliary muscle spasm by

O—π KEY POINTS

- Usually doctors can determine the cause of eye pain during an examination.
- People with severe pain, eye redness, or warning signs (vomiting, halos around lights, fever, decreased visual clarity, bulging eyes, and inability to move the eye in all directions) should see a doctor right away.

EYE REDNESS

Eye redness refers to a red appearance of the normally white part of the eye. The eye looks red or bloodshot because blood vessels on the surface of the eye widen (dilate), bringing excess blood into the eye. Pinkeye typically refers to eye redness caused by a specific viral infection called conjunctivitis.

Blood vessels can dilate as a result of

- Infection
- Allergy
- Inflammation caused by something other than an infection
- Elevated pressure inside the eye, typically caused by sudden, closed-angle glaucoma, in which fluid pressure increases in the front chamber of the eye

Several parts of the eye may be affected, most commonly the conjunctiva (the thin membrane that lines the eyelid and covers the front of the eye), but also the iris (the colored part of the eye), the sclera (the tough white fiber layer covering the eye), and the episclera (the connective tissue layer between the sclera and the conjunctiva).

Rarely is eye redness the only eye symptom. People may have tearing, itching, the feeling that a foreign object is in the eye (foreign body sensation), sensitivity to light, pain, or even changes in vision. Sometimes people have symptoms that affect other areas of the body, such as a runny nose or cough, or nausea and vomiting.

CAUSES

Many disorders can cause eye redness. Some are emergencies, but others are mild and go away without treatment. The degree of redness does not indicate the seriousness of the disorder. The presence of eye pain or vision problems is more likely to suggest a serious cause.

The most common causes of eye redness are

- Inflammation of the conjunctiva caused by an infection (infectious conjunctivitis, or pinkeye)
- Inflammation of the conjunctiva caused by an allergic reaction (allergic conjunctivitis)

Scratches of the cornea (the clear layer in front of the iris and pupil) and foreign objects in the eye are also common causes. In these cases, however, the person is more likely to consider the problem to be an eye injury, eye pain, or both. Corneal scratches may be caused by contact lenses or by foreign objects or tiny particles trapped under the eyelid. Occasionally, very dry air can cause some eye redness and irritation.

Serious causes of eye redness are much less common. They include corneal ulcers, herpes simplex keratitis (herpes infection in the cornea), herpes zoster ophthalmicus (shingles in or around the eye), acute closed-angle glaucoma, and scleritis (a deep, painful inflammation of the sclera).

EVALUATION

Not every case of eye redness requires evaluation by a doctor. The following information can help people decide when to see a doctor and to know what to expect during an evaluation. In most cases, people with eye redness can be evaluated by a general health care practitioner rather than an ophthalmologist (a medical doctor who specializes in the evaluation and treatment—surgical and nonsurgical—of eye disorders).

WARNING SIGNS

In people with eye redness, certain symptoms and characteristics are cause for concern. They include

- Sudden, severe pain and vomiting
- Rash on the face, particularly around the eyes or on the tip of the nose
- Decreased sharpness of vision (visual acuity)
- An open sore on the cornea

WHEN TO SEE A DOCTOR

Deep eye pain should be distinguished from irritation. People who have warning signs, particularly deep pain or a change in vision, should see a doctor right away. If no warning signs are present, it is safe to wait a couple of days or so, but people may want to see a doctor sooner so that they can start treatment quickly.

Doctors first ask questions about the person's symptoms and medical history and then do a physical examination. What they find during the history and physical examination often suggests a cause of eye redness and the tests that may need to be done (see Table, below).

Doctors ask

- How long redness has been present
- Whether redness has occurred before
- Whether there is pain or itching
- Whether there is discharge or the eyes are tearing
- Whether there is a change in vision
- Whether there has been an eye injury
- Whether the person wears contact lenses and whether they have been overused
- Whether the person has been exposed to substances (such as dust or eye drops) that could irritate the eyes
- Whether there are other symptoms (such as headache, halos around lights, runny nose, cough, or sore throat)
- Whether the person has allergies

Pain together with nausea or vomiting or halos around lights is a potentially serious combination of symptoms. These symptoms often occur in acute closed-angle glaucoma. Pain and sensitivity to light may indicate a disorder of the cornea, such as a scratch or a foreign object. An absence of pain and sensitivity to light may indicate a disorder of the conjunctiva.

During the physical examination, doctors examine the head and neck for signs of disorders that may cause eye redness, such as runny nose and cough that may indicate an upper respiratory infection or allergy or a rash that may indicate shingles (herpes zoster infection).

The eye examination is the most important part of the physical examination. Doctors check the person's eye and the area around the eye for injuries or swelling. They check the person's vision (with glasses or contacts if the person wears them), pupil size and response to a light, and eye movement.

Doctors use a slit lamp (an instrument that enables a doctor to examine the eye under high magnification) to examine the eye. Doctors put a drop of anesthetic and then a drop of fluorescein stain in the eye to diagnose corneal disorders. While the eye is anesthetized, pressure inside the eye (intraocular pressure) is often measured (called tonometry).

If pain develops in the affected eye (particularly if it is shut at this time) when a light is shined in the unaffected eye, the problem may be anterior uveitis or a corneal disorder. The use of an anesthetic makes the examination easier, and the person's response to the anesthetic may be a clue to the diagnosis. Anesthetic eye drops do not relieve pain that is caused by glaucoma, uveitis, or scleritis.

SOME CAUSES AND FEATURES OF EYE REDNESS

Cause	Common Features*	Tests
Conjunctival disorders and episcleritis†		
Allergic or seasonal conjunctivitis (inflammation of the conjunctiva—the membrane that lines the eyelid and covers the front of the eye)	Affecting both eyes An itching or scratching sensation and tearing In people with known allergies or other features of allergies (such as a runny nose that recurs during certain seasons) Sometimes in people who use eye drops (particularly neomycin)	A doctor's examination
Chemical (irritant) conjunctivitis	An itching or scratching sensation and tearing Exposure to potential irritants (such as dust, smoke, ammonia, or chlorine)	A doctor's examination *(continued)*

SOME CAUSES AND FEATURES OF EYE REDNESS *(continued)*

Cause	Common Features*	Tests
Episcleritis (inflammation of the tissue between the sclera—the white of the eye—and the overlying conjunctiva)	Affecting only one eye A spot of redness on the white of the eye Mild irritation of the eye	A doctor's examination
Infectious conjunctivitis (pinkeye)	An itching or scratching sensation, tearing, and sensitivity to light Sometimes a discharge from the eye and eyelid swelling Sometimes swollen lymph nodes in front of the ears	A doctor's examination
Subconjunctival hemorrhage (bleeding under the conjunctiva)	Affecting only one eye A red patch or large area of redness No tearing, irritation, itching, or discharge from the eye Sometimes in people who have had an eye injury, sneezed violently, or tried to exhale without letting air escape, as may occur during a bowel movement or while lifting a heavy weight (called the Valsalva maneuver) Often in people known to use drugs that help prevent blood from clotting (such as aspirin or warfarin)	A doctor's examination
Corneal disorders‡		
Contact lens keratitis (inflammation of the cornea—the clear layer in front of the iris and pupil)	Eye ache, redness, tearing, and sensitivity to light In people who have worn their contact lenses for too long	A doctor's examination
Corneal scratch (abrasion) or foreign object (body)	Symptoms that begin after an eye injury (which may not have been noticed in infants and young children) Pain when blinking and a foreign body sensation	A doctor's examination
Corneal ulcer	Sometimes a grayish patch on the cornea that later becomes an open, painful sore Sometimes in people who have had an eye injury or who slept with their contact lenses in	A doctor's examination Culture of a sample taken from the ulcer (done by an ophthalmologist)
Herpes simplex keratitis (infection of the cornea caused by the herpes simplex virus)	Affecting only one eye *Early*: Blisters on the eyelid and/or crusting *Late or recurrent*: Eye redness and tearing, eye pain, impaired vision, and sensitivity to light	Usually only a doctor's examination
Herpes zoster ophthalmicus (shingles that affects the face and eye, caused by the varicella-zoster virus)	Affecting only one eye *Early*: A rash with fluid-filled blisters and/or crusting on one side of the face,	Usually only a doctor's examination *(continued)*

SOME CAUSES AND FEATURES OF EYE REDNESS (continued)

Cause	Common Features*	Tests
Herpes zoster ophthalmicus (continued)	around the eye, on the forehead, and/or on the tip of the nose, and sometimes pain	
	Eye redness, tearing, and eyelid swelling	
	Late: Eye redness, usually sensitivity to light, and usually severe pain	
Other disorders		
Closed-angle glaucoma	Severe eye ache and redness	Measurement of pressure inside the eye (tonometry) and examination of the eye's drainage channels with a special lens (gonioscopy), done by an ophthalmologist
	Headache, nausea, vomiting, and pain with exposure to light	
	Disturbances in vision such as seeing halos around lights and/or decreased vision	
Anterior uveitis (inflammation of the anterior chamber—the fluid-filled space between the iris and cornea)	Eye ache and sensitivity to light	A doctor's examination
	Eye redness (particularly around the cornea)	
	Blurring or loss of vision	
	Often in people who have an autoimmune disorder or who recently had an eye injury	
Scleritis (inflammation of the white of the eye, called the sclera)	Pain, often described as boring, and severe enough to wake someone from a sound sleep	Usually only a doctor's examination
	Sensitivity to light	
	Tearing	
	Red or violet patches on the white of the eye	
	Often in people who have an autoimmune disorder	

*Features include symptoms and the results of the doctor's examination. Features mentioned are typical but not always present.
†Conjunctival disorders usually cause itching or a scratchy sensation, tearing, widespread eye redness, and often sensitivity to light. They usually do not cause pain or changes in vision.
‡Corneal disorders usually cause pain (particularly when the eyes are exposed to light), tearing, and sometimes impaired vision.

TESTING

Testing is usually unnecessary.

If doctors suspect a viral infection (herpes simplex virus or varicella-zoster virus), they may take samples of discharge or blister fluid to send to the laboratory. The sample is placed in a culture medium (a substance that allows bacteria or viruses to grow). Samples for culture may also be taken when the person has a corneal ulcer so doctors can give antibiotics that are most likely to be effective. Gonioscopy (use of a special lens to examine the drainage channels in the eye) is done in people with glaucoma. Sometimes people with uveitis are tested for autoimmune disorders, especially if there is no obvious cause (such as an injury) for the uveitis.

People with scleritis are usually referred to an ophthalmologist who often does additional tests.

TREATMENT

The cause is treated. Eye redness itself does not require treatment. It usually clears up on its own as the cause resolves (for example, a few days for infectious conjunctivitis or a couple of weeks for subconjunctival hemorrhage). Cool washcloths or artificial tears can be applied if any itching is particularly bothersome. Eye drops that aim to eliminate redness (available over-the-counter) are not recommended.

KEY POINTS

- Usually, eye redness is caused by conjunctivitis.
- Pain, a rash around the eye or nose, and changes in vision suggest a potentially serious cause.

EYELID SWELLING

A person may experience swelling in one or both eyelids. Swelling may be painless or accompanied by itching or pain. Eyelid swelling is distinct from bulging eyes (see page 131), although a few disorders can cause both.

CAUSES

Eyelid swelling has many causes (see Table on pages 128 to 129). It usually results from an eyelid disorder but may result from disorders in and around the eye socket (orbit) or from disorders elsewhere in the body that cause widespread swelling.

COMMON CAUSES

The most common causes are allergic, including

- Local allergy (contact sensitivity)
- More widespread allergic reaction (for example, angioedema or allergic rhinitis)

Swelling of one place in one eyelid is common and is most often caused by a blocked oil gland (chalazion) or a bacterial infection of a hair follicle (stye or hordeolum).

LESS COMMON CAUSES

Less common causes include disorders that cause generalized body swelling, particularly a type of kidney disease called nephrotic syndrome, bacterial infection of the skin of the eyelids and around the eyes (periorbital cellulitis), chronic inflammation of the eyelid margins (blepharitis), and underactive thyroid gland (hypothyroidism). An overactive thyroid gland can cause bulging eyeballs but does not cause swollen eyelids.

Rare but dangerous causes are infection within the orbit and around and behind the eye (orbital cellulitis) and blockage of a vein at the base of the brain by an infected blood clot (cavernous sinus thrombosis).

EVALUATION

The following information can help people decide whether a doctor's evaluation is needed and help them know what to expect during the evaluation.

WARNING SIGNS

In people with eyelid swelling, certain symptoms and characteristics are cause for concern. They include

- Fever
- Vision loss
- Double vision
- Abnormal bulging of one or both eyes (proptosis)

WHEN TO SEE A DOCTOR

People with warning signs should see a doctor right away. If pain occurs, people usually want to see a doctor within a day or two so that they can start to feel better.

WHAT THE DOCTOR DOES

Doctors first ask questions about the person's symptoms and medical history. Doctors then do a physical examination. What they find during the history and physical examination often suggests a cause of the swelling and the tests that may need to be done (see Table).

Doctors ask

- How long the swelling has been present
- Whether swelling affects the upper and/or lower eyelids in one or both eyes
- Whether any injury (including insect bites) or eye surgery has occurred
- Whether itching, pain, headache, changes in vision, fever, or eye discharge is present
- Whether symptoms affecting other areas of the body are also occurring
- Whether the person has disorders (for example, heart, kidney, or liver disease) or is taking drugs (for example, angiotensin-converting enzyme inhibitors) that are known to cause swelling or has changes in tolerance of cold or heat that might indicate a thyroid disorder
- Whether the person is using any drugs in or around the eye
- Whether there have been any changes in over-the-counter products used on the face or around the eye (for example, new makeup, face creams, or cleansers or new detergent to launder bed linens or towels)

SOME CAUSES AND FEATURES OF EYELID SWELLING

Cause	Common Features*	Tests
Eyelid disorders		
Allergic reaction affecting only the eyes	Itching but no pain	A doctor's examination
	Pale, puffy eyelid or eyelids and sometimes pale, puffy conjunctiva (the membrane that lines the eyelids and covers the front of the eye)	
	Sometimes in people who have had a previous episode, been exposed to an allergen, or both	
	Affecting one or both eyelids	
Blepharitis (inflammation of the edges of the eyelids)	Yellow crusts on lashes	A doctor's examination
	Eye itching, burning, redness, sores, or a combination	
	Sometimes accompanied by seborrheic dermatitis (inflammation of the skin characterized by greasy scales on the scalp and face)	
	Usually affecting both eyelids	
Blepharitis caused by herpes simplex virus	Clusters of fluid-filled blisters on reddened skin, open sores, and significant pain	A doctor's examination
	Usually affecting only one eye (may affect both eyes in children)	
Chalazion (enlargement of an oil gland deep in the eyelid)	An area of redness and pain on only one eyelid	A doctor's examination
	Eventually development of a round, painless swelling away from the edge of the eyelid	
Conjunctivitis, infectious (pinkeye, or inflammation of the conjunctiva, caused by bacteria or a virus) when severe	Redness of the white of the eyes, a discharge, and sometimes crusts on the lashes when the person wakes up	A doctor's examination
	Affecting one or both eyes	
Stye (hordeolum)	Redness and pain affecting one eyelid	A doctor's examination
	Eventually swelling at the edge of the eyelid, sometimes with small, raised, pus-filled bumps	
Insect bite	Itching, redness, and sometimes a small, raised bump	A doctor's examination
Disorders in and around the orbit		
Cavernous sinus thrombosis (blockage of a vein at the base of the brain by an infected blood clot)†	Headache, bulging eyes, weak eye muscles with double vision, a drooping eyelid, loss of vision, and fever	CT or MRI done immediately
	Usually affecting one eyelid first, then the other eyelid	
	Symptoms of sinusitis (pain behind the eyes or in the face that worsens when the head is moved and nasal discharge, sometimes with bleeding) or other infections of the face, such as orbital or preseptal cellulitis	

(continued)

SOME CAUSES AND FEATURES OF EYELID SWELLING *(continued)*

Cause	Common Features*	Tests
Orbital cellulitis (infection of tissue within and around the eye socket, or orbit)†	Bulging of the eye, eye redness, pain deep within the eye Red, swollen eyelids Sometimes double vision, inability to move the eye in certain directions, pain with eye movement, or loss of vision Usually affecting only one eye Fever Sometimes preceded by symptoms of sinusitis	CT or MRI
Preseptal (periorbital) cellulitis (infection of the eyelid and the skin and tissues around the front of the eye)	Swelling and redness around the eye but not bulging of the eye Sometimes pain (usually around the eye) and fever Usually affecting only one eye Normal vision and eye movement Sometimes preceded by a skin infection near the eye	Sometimes CT or MRI
Disorders that affect the entire body‡		
Allergic reactions	Itching Sometimes allergy symptoms that involve other areas (such as hives, wheezing, or a runny nose) Sometimes in people who have had a previous allergic episode, who have been exposed to an allergen, who tend to have many allergies, or a combination Usually affecting both eyes	A doctor's examination
Disorders that cause swelling throughout the body (such as chronic kidney disease, heart failure, liver failure, and, in pregnant women, preeclampsia)	Swelling of both eyelids and sometimes the forehead No itching, pain, redness, or other symptoms affecting the eyes Usually swelling of the feet	Testing for heart, liver, or kidney disorders, depending on which disorder is suspected
Hypothyroidism (an underactive thyroid gland)	A puffy face but no pain Dry, scaly skin and coarse hair Inability to tolerate cold	Blood tests to evaluate thyroid gland function

*Features include symptoms and the results of the doctor's examination. Features mentioned are typical but not always present.
†These disorders are rare.
‡These disorders cause swelling in both eyelids and do not cause redness.
CT = computed tomography; MRI = magnetic resonance imaging.

During the physical examination, doctors look for signs of disorders that may affect other parts of the body, but the focus is primarily on the eyes. They look for runny nose and other signs of allergies, toothache or headache, which may indicate a dental or sinus infection, fever, and changes in skin near the eye.

Any eyelid or eye sore is evaluated by using a slit lamp (an instrument that enables a doctor to examine the eye under high magnification). Doctors check the location and color of the swelling and whether the eyelid is tender or warm, whether vision is affected, whether eye muscles are functioning normally, and whether any discharge is present.

TESTING

In most cases, doctors can determine the cause of eyelid swelling based on the symptoms and the findings during the physical examination, and no testing is needed. However, if doctors suspect orbital cellulitis or cavernous sinus thrombosis, they immediately do computed tomography (CT) or magnetic resonance imaging (MRI). If a heart, liver, kidney, or thyroid disorder is suspected, doctors do laboratory tests and sometimes various imaging tests.

TREATMENT

The best way to treat eyelid swelling is to treat the disorder that is causing the swelling. There is no specific treatment for the swelling.

KEY POINTS

- Eyelid swelling may be caused by a disorder of the eye or eyelid or by a disorder elsewhere in the body.
- People with sudden double vision or loss of vision should see a doctor immediately.
- People with fever or a bulging eye should see a doctor within hours if possible.

EYES, BULGING

Bulging or protruding of one or both eyes is called proptosis or exophthalmos. Exophthalmos is usually used when describing bulging eyes caused by Graves disease, a disorder causing overactivity of the thyroid gland (hyperthyroidism). Bulging eyes are not the same as prominent eyes. Some disorders that may change the appearance of the face and eyes but that do not cause true eye bulging include Cushing disease and severe obesity.

Bulging sometimes causes other symptoms. The eyes may be dry and irritated (which causes watering) because the bulging may prevent the eyelids from closing properly. Also, people may blink less often or may appear to stare. Depending on the cause of bulging, people may have other symptoms such as double vision or difficulty focusing on objects. If bulging is prolonged, the optic nerve is stretched, which may impair vision. Vision may also be impaired if the disorder causing bulging also presses on the optic nerve.

CAUSES

The **most common cause** is Graves disease, which causes swelling of tissue behind and around the eye, pushing the eyeball forward.

Other causes are uncommon. They include tumors, bleeding, infections, and, rarely, inflammation of structures within the orbit without infection (called orbital pseudotumor). Glaucoma that is present from birth can cause the eyes to enlarge, which may seem to look similar to eyes that are pushed forward.

EVALUATION

The following information can help people decide when a doctor's evaluation is needed and help them know what to expect during the evaluation.

WARNING SIGNS

In people with bulging eyes, certain symptoms and characteristics are cause for concern. They include

- Loss or decrease of vision
- Double vision
- Eye pain or redness
- Headache

WHEN TO SEE A DOCTOR

People with warning signs should see a doctor as soon as possible, as should those with bulging that has developed over a few days or less. People with no warning signs should see a doctor when possible, but a delay of a week or so is unlikely to be harmful.

WHAT THE DOCTOR DOES

Doctors first ask questions about the person's symptoms and medical history. Doctors then do a physical examination. What they find during the history and physical examination often suggests a cause for eye bulging and the tests that may need to be done (see Table on page 132).

Doctors ask

- How long the bulging has been present
- Whether both eyes are bulging
- Whether bulging seems to be getting worse
- Whether the person has other eye symptoms, such as dryness, increased tear formation, double vision, loss of vision, irritation, or pain
- Whether the person has symptoms of hyperthyroidism, such as inability to tolerate heat, increased sweating, involuntary shaking movements (tremors), anxiety, increased appetite, diarrhea, palpitations, and weight loss

Bulging that has developed rapidly (over a few days) suggests different causes than bulging that has developed over years. Rapid bulging in only one eye suggests bleeding in the eye socket (orbit), which can occur after surgery or injury, or infection or inflammation of the eye socket. Bulging that develops slowly suggests Graves disease (when it affects both eyes) or a tumor in the eye socket (when it affects one eye).

The physical examination is focused on the eyes. Doctors examine the eyes for redness, sores, and irritation using a slit lamp (an instrument that enables a doctor to examine the eye under high magnification). They check whether the eyelids move as fast as the eyeball when the person looks down and check for staring. Slow eyelids and staring could indicate Graves disease.

Doctors may also check for other signs that could indicate hyperthyroidism, such as increased heart rate or blood pressure, tremors, and a swollen or tender thyroid gland in the neck.

TESTING

Doctors sometimes measure the degree of bulging with an instrument (exophthalmometry).

Magnetic resonance imaging (MRI) or computed tomography (CT) is often done when bulging affects only one eye. Blood tests to measure how well the thyroid is working are done when Graves disease is suspected.

TREATMENT

When bulging leads to severe dry eyes, lubrication with artificial tears is needed to protect the cornea (the clear layer in front of the iris and pupil). Sometimes if lubrication is not sufficient,

SOME CAUSES AND FEATURES OF BULGING EYES

Cause	Common Features*	Tests
Graves disease	*Eye symptoms*: Pain, watering, dryness, irritation, sensitivity to light, double vision, and loss of vision Usually affecting both eyes *General symptoms*: Palpitations, anxiety, increased appetite, weight loss, diarrhea, inability to tolerate heat, increased sweating, and insomnia	Blood tests to evaluate thyroid gland function
Orbital cellulitis (infection of the tissue within the eye socket, or orbit)	Affecting only one eye Eye redness, pain deep within the eye, pain when moving the eye, and aches in and around the eye Red and swollen eyelids Inability to fully move the eye in all directions Impaired vision or loss of vision Fever Sometimes preceded by symptoms of sinusitis	CT or MRI
A mass in the eye socket such as a tumor (cancerous or not) or blood vessel malformation	Loss of or a decrease in vision and pain in one eye Sometimes double vision or headache	MRI or CT
Retrobulbar hemorrhage (bleeding in the eye socket)	Usually affecting only one eye Symptoms that begin suddenly Loss of vision, double vision, and eye pain In people who have recently had eye surgery or an eye injury or who have a bleeding disorder	CT or treatment done immediately

*Features include symptoms and the results of the doctor's examination. Features mentioned are typical but not always present.
CT = computed tomography; MRI = magnetic resonance imaging.

surgery to provide better coverage of the eye surface or to reduce bulging may be needed.

Other treatments depend on the cause of bulging. For example, antibiotics are given for infections. Bulging due to Graves disease is not affected by treatment of the thyroid condition but may lessen over time. Corticosteroids (for example, prednisone) may help control swelling due to Graves disease or orbital pseudotumor. Tumors must be surgically removed.

KEY POINTS

- Graves disease is the most common cause of bulging eyes.
- People with headache, eye pain, or changes in vision should see a doctor quickly.
- Bulging of one eye is of greater concern than bulging of both eyes.

EYES, WATERY (EXCESS TEARING)

Excess tearing may cause a sensation of watery eyes or result in tears falling down the cheek. Other symptoms, such as eye irritation or pain, may be present depending on the cause.

Most tears are produced in the tear (lacrimal) glands located above the outer part of the upper eyelid. Tears run across the eye and drain through small openings at the inner corners of the eyelids near the nose (the upper and lower puncta) into a short channel (the canaliculus). They then run into the tear sac and through the nasolacrimal duct into the nose. Blockage anywhere along the tear drainage pathway can lead to a watery eye. Blockage also predisposes to infection of the tear sac (dacryocystitis). Such infection can sometimes spread to tissues around the eye (periorbital cellulitis).

CAUSES

Watery eyes can be caused by increased tear production or blockage of tear drainage (see Table on page 135).

Common causes of watery eyes are

- Upper respiratory infections
- Allergies that affect the nose (allergic rhinitis), eyes (allergic conjunctivitis), or both

Other causes include

- Dry eyes (the dry surface of the eye becomes irritated and thus, surprisingly, causes watery eyes)
- Inwardly turned eyelashes that rub against the eyeball (trichiasis)
- An outwardly turned eyelid (ectropion) that moves the punctum away from its normal position next to the eyeball so that it cannot drain away tears
- Age-related narrowing of the tear ducts
- Chronic infections in the tear sac

Any disorder that irritates the cornea (the clear layer in front of the iris and pupil) can increase tear production. However, most people with corneal disorders that cause watery eyes (such as a corneal scratch or sore, a foreign object in the eye, or inflammation of the cornea) have significant pain, redness, and/or sensitivity to light, which are the usual reasons they seek medical care.

EVALUATION

Not every case of watery eyes requires evaluation by a doctor. The following information can help people decide when a doctor's evaluation is needed and help them know what to expect during the evaluation.

WARNING SIGNS

In people with watery eyes, certain symptoms and characteristics are cause for concern. They include

- Repeated, unexplained episodes of red watery eyes
- A hard mass in or near the tear duct

WHEN TO SEE A DOCTOR

People with warning signs should see a doctor within a week or so. Other people who are bothered by watery eyes should see a doctor when it is convenient, but typically a delay of several weeks is not harmful.

WHERE TEARS COME FROM

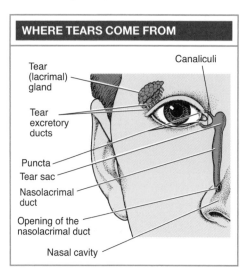

- Tear (lacrimal) gland
- Canaliculi
- Tear excretory ducts
- Puncta
- Tear sac
- Nasolacrimal duct
- Opening of the nasolacrimal duct
- Nasal cavity

WHAT THE DOCTOR DOES

Doctors first ask questions about the person's symptoms and medical history. Doctors then do a physical examination. What they find during the history and physical examination often suggests the cause of the watery eyes and the tests that may need to be done (see Table, below).

Doctors ask whether the person has

- Itching, a runny nose, or sneezing (especially after being exposed to a potential allergen)
- Eye irritation, redness, or pain
- Pain or discomfort with swelling or redness near the inner corner of the eye
- Other symptoms (for example, headache, shortness of breath, cough, fever, or rash)

- Had injuries, infections, burns, radiation therapy, or surgical procedures involving the eyes, nose, or sinuses
- Taken a drug that may cause watery eyes (such as chemotherapy drugs or eye drops containing echothiophate, epinephrine, or pilocarpine)

Doctors then do a physical examination. The physical examination focuses on the face, particularly the eyes and nose. Doctors look for tears running down the cheek. They examine the eyelids, the puncta, and the area at the inner corners of the eyes. They also examine the surface of the eye with a slit lamp to examine the eye under high magnification. The nose is examined for congestion, blockages, pus, discharge, and bleeding.

SOME CAUSES AND FEATURES OF WATERY EYES

Cause	Common Features*
Disorders that cause excess tear production	
Dry eyes	Watering that is worse when eyes are exposed to cold or windy weather, cigarette smoke, or dry heat
	A feeling of something in the eye (foreign object [body] sensation) that comes and goes, especially toward the end of the day
Irritation of the eye surface due to - Conjunctivitis (inflammation of the membrane that lines the back of the eyelid and covers the front of the eye) caused by allergies, chemicals, or infection - Blepharitis (inflammation of the edges of the eyelids) - An inwardly turned eyelid	Often a sensation of grittiness or something in the eye Eye redness In people with allergic conjunctivitis, itching
Nasal irritation caused by allergies or an upper respiratory infection	Runny nose, sneezing, and nasal congestion
Disorders that block tear drainage	
Blockage of a tear duct that is present at birth	Symptoms that begin weeks after birth
Age-related narrowing of tear ducts	Watery eyes that gradually become worse as people age
An inwardly turned eyelid	Usually seen during the examination
Dacryocystitis (infection of the tear sac)	Pain or discomfort near the corner of the eye and along the side of the nose Often swelling, redness, tenderness, and warmth in the same area
An outwardly turned eyelid	Usually seen during the examination
Tumors	Often in older people Sometimes a hard lump near the tear sac
Other causes (such as injuries or drugs)	Usually in people who know they have such causes

*Features include symptoms and the results of the doctor's examination. Features mentioned are typical but not always present.

Doctors can usually determine the cause based on the results of the history and physical examination. Testing is often unnecessary. If testing is needed, the person usually is referred to an ophthalmologist (a medical doctor who specializes in the evaluation and treatment—surgical and nonsurgical—of eye disorders).

Some tests are done in the ophthalmologist's office. Doctors may insert a small probe into the punctum and sometimes the canaliculus to try to detect blockage. They may also gently flush fluid through the canaliculus to see whether the fluid drains into the nose as it should.

Imaging tests and procedures (imaging of the tear ducts, computed tomography [CT], or examination of the inside of the nose with a flexible viewing tube [nasal endoscopy]) are sometimes done.

TREATMENT

Underlying disorders are treated. For example, doctors may give a nasal corticosteroid if allergic rhinitis is the cause.

Doctors sometimes recommend the use of artificial tears to decrease watery eyes when dry eyes or eye surface irritation is the cause.

In infants with blocked tear ducts, the blockage often resolves without treatment as the infant grows. Until the infant is about 1 year old, doctors often suggest that parents manually compress the tear sac 4 or 5 times per day to help relieve the obstruction. If the blockage is not relieved by the time the infant is about 1 year old, doctors may do a procedure to open the ducts. The infant is given a general anesthetic, and the doctor inserts a small probe into the tear duct to break through the blockage.

In children with blocked tear ducts, doctors may first try probing the tear duct. If blockage persists, doctors may need to insert a small plastic tube through the tear duct for a few months to keep a drainage pathway open.

In adults with blocked tear ducts, doctors first try different methods to treat the underlying disorder. If these methods do not work, doctors may have to do surgery to make a new drainage pathway for tears.

ESSENTIALS FOR OLDER PEOPLE

As people age, the tear ducts often narrow. Such narrowing is a common cause of unexplained watery eyes in older people. However, complete blockage of the tear duct is also possible. Rarely, a tumor of a tear sac is the cause.

O—ᴫ KEY POINTS

- Common causes of tearing include allergies, dry eyes, inward or outward turning of the eyelids, and infection, narrowing, or blockage of the tear drainage pathway.
- Testing, if necessary, can often be done in an ophthalmologist's office.
- Other testing, such as dacryoscintigraphy or dacryocystography (imaging tests of the tear ducts) or computed tomography is necessary when in-office tests do not reveal the cause or doctors suspect a tumor.

FAINTING AND LIGHT-HEADEDNESS

Light-headedness (near syncope) is a sense that one is about to faint. Fainting (syncope) is a sudden, brief loss of consciousness during which the person falls to the ground or slumps in a chair followed by a return to consciousness. The person is motionless and limp and usually has cool legs and arms, a weak pulse, and shallow breathing. Some people feel light-headed or dizzy before they faint. Others may have nausea, sweating, blurred or tunnel vision, tingling of lips or fingertips, chest pain, or palpitations. Less often, people faint suddenly, without any warning symptoms. Seizures, which are a disturbance of the brain's electrical activity, and cardiac arrest, in which the heart completely stops beating, can cause loss of consciousness but are not considered fainting.

Fainting can occur in people of any age, but dangerous causes of fainting are more common among older people.

CAUSES

A person cannot lose consciousness unless brain function is generally disturbed. This disturbance usually occurs because overall blood flow to the brain is reduced. Sometimes, however, blood flow is adequate but the blood does not contain sufficient oxygen or glucose (blood sugar), which the brain needs to function.

Blood flow to the brain can be reduced in several ways. Most often, the cause is something that interferes with the normal return of blood to the heart (and thus reduces blood flow out from the heart). Less often, the cause is a disorder that interferes with blood pumping (typically a heart disorder). Although strokes reduce blood flow to the brain, they only reduce flow to part of the brain. Thus, strokes rarely cause fainting except for the few strokes that involve the part of the brain that maintains consciousness.

The **most common causes** are

- Strong emotion (such as fear, pain, or sight of blood)
- Coughing or straining to pass stool or urine
- Prolonged standing
- Standing up suddenly

- Pregnancy
- Use of certain drugs
- Idiopathic (meaning that the cause cannot be determined)

These common causes nearly always cause fainting only when people are standing up. When they fall down, blood flow to the brain is increased, quickly restoring consciousness, although people may not feel completely normal for a few minutes. Some people feel tired or exhausted for several hours. These causes tend not to be serious unless people are injured when they fall.

Most of these causes involve decreased return of blood to the heart. Strong emotion (particularly that triggered by the sight of blood) or pain can activate the vagus nerve. Vagus nerve activation widens blood vessels, reducing the return of blood to the heart, and slows the heart rate. Both of these factors cause light-headedness and sometimes fainting (called vasovagal syncope).

Straining during bowel movements or urination or coughing increases chest pressure. Increased chest pressure can activate the vagus nerve and also reduce the return of blood to the heart—two factors that may cause fainting.

Healthy people may faint when standing still for a long time (most common in soldiers, a phenomenon called parade ground syncope), because the leg muscles have to be active to help return blood to the heart.

Sitting or standing up too quickly can cause fainting, because the change in position causes blood to pool in the legs, resulting in a fall in blood pressure. Normally, the body quickly increases the heart rate and constricts blood vessels to maintain blood pressure. If the body does not compensate in these ways, light-headedness is common and fainting may rarely occur. Certain brain and spinal cord disorders, prolonged bed rest, and certain drugs (particularly those used to treat high blood pressure) can interfere with this compensation and lead to fainting when standing up (see page 87).

Hormonal changes in early pregnancy sometimes lead to fainting.

Low blood sugar (hypoglycemia) initially causes confusion, light-headedness, shakiness, and other symptoms, but if hypoglycemia is severe or prolonged, people can lose consciousness. Because these other symptoms usually occur before fainting, people with hypoglycemia usually have some warning before they faint. Usually, the cause of hypoglycemia is use of drugs for diabetes, particularly insulin. Rarely, people have a tumor that secretes insulin.

Less common but more serious causes include

- Heart valve disorders (most commonly, the aortic valve)
- A heart rate that is too fast or too slow
- Blockage of an artery to the lungs by a blood clot (pulmonary embolism)
- Heart attack or other heart muscle disorders

Heart valve disorders can block blood from leaving the heart. A very fast heart rate may not allow the heart enough time to refill with blood, so less blood is pumped. A very slow heart rate may not pump enough blood. Blood clots in the lungs can keep the heart from pumping enough blood. People with a heart attack rarely have fainting when the heart attack occurs (more common in older people). Other uncommon heart muscle disorders called cardiomyopathies can cause fainting, particularly during exercise, typically because of an abnormal heart rhythm.

Although most strokes do not cause fainting, a stroke or transient ischemic attack (TIA) that involves certain blood vessels at the base of the brain (posterior circulation stroke) can cause fainting. Similarly, a migraine that involves these blood vessels sometimes causes fainting.

EVALUATION

If possible, someone who witnessed the faint should provide the doctor with a description of the event because the person who fainted may not remember.

WARNING SIGNS

In people who have fainted, certain symptoms and characteristics are cause for concern. They include

- Fainting during exercise
- Several episodes within a short time
- Sudden fainting without any warning symptoms or any apparent trigger

- Fainting preceded or followed by possible heart symptoms such as chest pain, palpitations, or shortness of breath
- Older age
- Significant injury as a result of fainting
- Family history of sudden unexpected death

WHEN TO SEE A DOCTOR

Although most causes of fainting are not serious, a doctor's evaluation is needed to distinguish serious causes from relatively harmless ones. People who fainted should see a doctor right away, especially if they have any warning signs.

WHAT THE DOCTOR DOES

Doctors first ask questions about the person's symptoms and medical history. Doctors then do a physical examination. What doctors find during the history and physical examination often suggests a cause of the fainting and the tests that may need to be done.

Doctors ask about the events leading up to the fainting episode. They ask whether the person was exercising, arguing, or in a potentially emotional situation. They ask whether the person was lying or standing, and, if standing, for how long. They also ask about symptoms that occurred immediately before or after the event, including whether the person felt light-headed or dizzy or experienced nausea, sweating, blurred or tunnel vision, tingling of lips or fingertips, chest pain, or palpitations. Doctors also ask any witnesses to describe the episode. A sudden, abrupt faint without any warning symptoms or apparent trigger suggests a heart disorder. If fainting is preceded by a brief period of symptoms such as light-headedness, nausea, yawning, blurred vision, or sweating and occurs during a painful or unpleasant situation, it is probably vasovagal syncope, which is not dangerous.

Doctors ask about previous episodes of dizziness or fainting and about other disorders, drugs, or symptoms that may be related to fainting. Doctors also check the person for injuries resulting from the fainting episode.

Then doctors measure the person's vital signs. Heart rate and blood pressure are measured with the person lying down and after 2 minutes of standing. Doctors listen to the heart for signs of an abnormal heart valve or abnormal blood flow. They do a neurologic examination for signs of a stroke.

SOME CAUSES AND FEATURES OF FAINTING

Cause	Common Features*	Tests†
Serious causes		
Heart valve disorders, such as aortic or mitral stenosis or failure of an artificial heart valve Cardiomyopathy (disorders affecting heart muscle), particularly hypertrophic cardiomyopathy	Fainting during or after exercise, followed by a prompt recovery In young or old people Often in people who are known to have had a heart murmur	Echocardiography (ultrasonography of the heart)
A very slow heart rate (typically less than 35 beats per minute), more common in older people A very rapid heart rate (typically over 150 beats per minute)	Fainting without warning, followed by recovery immediately after awakening Fainting that may occur in any position Sometimes in people taking certain drugs, especially drugs used to treat heart disorders such as abnormal heart rhythms (antiarrhythmic drugs)	ECG, sometimes continuous ambulatory ECG (using a Holter monitor worn for 24 hours or, rarely, a recording device implanted under the skin) Sometimes blood tests to measure electrolytes such as sodium and potassium
Pulmonary embolism (blockage of an artery to the lungs by a blood clot)	Often sharp pain when breathing in, shortness of breath, rapid breathing, and a rapid heart rate Sometimes mild fever, coughing up blood, or shock More likely in people with risk factors for pulmonary embolism (such as previous blood clots, recent surgery especially surgery on the legs, prolonged bed rest, a cast or splint on a leg, older age, smoking, or cancer)	CT or nuclear scanning of the lungs A blood test to detect blood clots (D-dimer test)
Heart attack (myocardial infarction)	Usually in older people Sometimes chest discomfort, feeling of indigestion, shortness of breath, or nausea	ECG Blood tests to measure substances that indicate heart damage (cardiac markers)
A severe allergic reaction (anaphylaxis) causing very low blood pressure	Fainting during or shortly after being exposed to a trigger for an allergic reaction, such as a drug or an insect bite Excessive sweating and pale skin color In people who may or may not have a history of allergies	Allergy testing
A low blood sugar level (hypoglycemia)	Fainting after a period of other symptoms, including confusion, shakiness, and sweating Unresponsiveness or confusion that remains until people are treated Almost always in people with diabetes	Fingerstick glucose measurement Immediate recovery following glucose infusion *(continued)*

SOME CAUSES AND FEATURES OF FAINTING *(continued)*

Cause	Common Features*	Tests†
Transient ischemic attack or stroke	Sudden fainting without warning	CT or MRI
	Fainting that may occur when people are upright or lying down	
	Sometimes loss of coordination or difficulty seeing, speaking, or swallowing	
	Usually in older people	
Less serious causes		
Increased pressure in the chest (for example, due to coughing or straining during urination or a bowel movement)	Fainting during an activity that increases pressure in the chest	Only a doctor's examination
	Warning symptoms (for example, dizziness, nausea, or sweating)	
	Recovery that is prompt but not immediate (within 5 to 15 minutes)	
Strong emotion (such as pain, fear, or distress at the sight of blood)	Fainting when experiencing strong emotion	Only a doctor's examination
	Warning symptoms (for example, dizziness, nausea, or sweating)	
	Recovery that is prompt but not immediate (within 5 to 15 minutes)	
	A cause that is usually apparent	
Migraine	Fainting sometimes preceded by disturbances in sensation, vision, or other functions (called the aura)	Only a doctor's examination
	Sensitivity to light	
Standing for a long time	A cause that is apparent based on the history	Only a doctor's examination
	No other symptoms	
Pregnancy	In healthy women of childbearing age	Urine pregnancy test
	No other symptoms	
	Usually in women with an early or unrecognized pregnancy	
Hyperventilation	Often tingling around the mouth or in the fingers before fainting	Only a doctor's examination
	Usually during or in response to an emotional situation	
	Rapid breathing, which may not be noticed by the person or by others	
	Typically in younger people	
Drugs such as most drugs used to lower the blood pressure (but rarely beta-blockers), antipsychotic drugs (mainly phenothiazines), loop diuretics, nitrates, quinidine, and tricyclic antidepressants	Light-headedness, followed by fainting within several minutes of sitting up or standing	A doctor's examination
	A drop in blood pressure when standing, detected during the examination	Sometimes tilt table testing

(continued)

SOME CAUSES AND FEATURES OF FAINTING *(continued)*

Cause	Common Features*	Tests†
Malfunction of the autonomic nervous system (which regulates internal body processes that require no conscious effort, such as blood pressure)	Light-headedness, followed by fainting within several minutes of sitting up or standing A drop in blood pressure when standing, detected during the examination	A doctor's examination Sometimes tilt table testing
Deconditioning caused by bed rest for many days	Light-headedness, followed by fainting within several minutes of sitting up or standing A drop in blood pressure when standing, detected during the examination	A doctor's examination Sometimes tilt table testing
Anemia	Light-headedness, followed by fainting within several minutes of sitting up or standing Chronic fatigue Sometimes dark stools or heavy menstrual periods	A complete blood count Stool tests to check for blood

*Features include symptoms and the results of the doctor's examination. Features mentioned are typical but not always present.

†In all people who have fainted, ECG is done, and oxygen levels in the blood are measured with a sensor placed on a finger (pulse oximetry).

CT = computed tomography; ECG = electrocardiography; MRI = magnetic resonance imaging.

TESTING

Testing typically is done unless people have an obvious, harmless emotional trigger and otherwise feel well. Doctors choose tests based on the suspected cause.

- Electrocardiography (ECG)
- Continuous ambulatory ECG (Holter monitor or event recorder)
- Measurement of oxygen in the blood (pulse oximetry)
- Fingerstick blood sugar measurement
- Sometimes ultrasonography of the heart (echocardiography)
- Sometimes tilt table testing
- Sometimes blood tests
- Rarely imaging of the central nervous system (brain and spinal cord)

In general, if fainting results in an injury or has happened several times (particularly within a brief period), more intensive evaluation is warranted.

People with suspected heart disorders, including heart attack, abnormal heart rhythm, or heart valve abnormality are usually admitted to the hospital for evaluation.

ECG is done. ECG may show a heart rhythm disturbance or other heart problem but sometimes is normal if the abnormal heart rhythm has resolved. Sometimes doctors admit the person to a hospital to monitor the heart's activity for 24 hours. Less often, doctors may have the person wear a small heart monitor while at home (called continuous ambulatory ECG).

Oxygen in the blood is measured. Pulse oximetry is done during or immediately after an episode to identify low levels of oxygen in the blood (which may indicate a blood clot). If the level of oxygen in the blood is low, doctors do computed tomography (CT) or a lung scan to check for a blood clot.

Laboratory tests are done if physical examination findings suggest they are needed. However, all women of childbearing age should have a pregnancy test.

Echocardiography may be done in people with exercise-induced fainting, heart murmurs, or fainting that occurs with sitting or standing.

Tilt table testing is sometimes done if people have fainting when they stand up. It is also used to evaluate fainting that is caused by exercise if echocardiography or exercise stress testing does not reveal a cause.

Stress testing is done when doctors suspect a heart rhythm disturbance brought on by exercise. It is often done for patients with exercise-induced symptoms.

Electrophysiologic testing (tests that record the electrical activity and electrical pathways of the heart by means of wires passed through blood vessels into the heart) is sometimes done if other testing does not identify a heart rhythm disturbance in a person with unexplained recurrent episodes of fainting.

Electroencephalography may be done when doctors suspect a seizure.

CT and magnetic resonance imaging of the head and brain may be done when doctors suspect a central nervous system disorder.

TREATMENT

Specific treatment depends on the cause. For example, people who have fainting caused by an abnormal heart rhythm may need to have a pacemaker and/or defibrillator implanted.

If people see someone faint, they should check whether the person is breathing. If the person is not breathing, bystanders should call for emergency medical assistance and begin cardiopulmonary resuscitation (CPR), including applying an automated external defibrillator (AED) if one is available. Once the person reaches the hospital, doctors will treat the cause of the fainting with drugs or appropriate measures, such as direct-current cardiac defibrillation to restart the heart or drugs or surgery to open blocked arteries.

A person who is breathing should remain lying down. If the person sits upright too rapidly, fainting may recur.

ESSENTIALS FOR OLDER PEOPLE

Older people are particularly susceptible to fainting because blood flow to the brain decreases as people age. The most common cause of fainting in older people is inability of blood pressure to rapidly adjust when the person stands. Blood flow decreases because arteries become more rigid and less able to adjust rapidly, physical inactivity reduces the muscle activity that pushes blood through the veins and back to the heart, and heart disease decreases the effectiveness of blood pumping.

In older people, fainting often has more than one cause. For example, the combination of taking several drugs to treat heart disorders or high blood pressure and standing in a hot church during a long or emotional service may lead to fainting even though no single factor might be enough to cause fainting.

O—π KEY POINTS

- Fainting usually results from insufficient blood flow to the brain.
- Most causes of fainting are not serious.
- Some less common causes are serious or potentially fatal.
- If fainting has an apparent trigger (such as strong emotion), is preceded by symptoms (such as light-headedness, nausea, or sweating), and requires a few minutes to recover, it is probably vasovagal syncope and is not serious.
- Fainting due to heart rhythm disturbances typically occurs abruptly and with a quick recovery.
- Doctors may ask a person who has fainted to restrict driving and operating machinery until the cause of fainting is determined and treated because if the cause is an unrecognized heart disorder, the next manifestation may be fatal.
- If fainting is caused by a slow heart rate, a pacemaker may be needed.

FATIGUE

Fatigue is when a person feels a strong need to rest and has so little energy that starting and sustaining activity is difficult. Fatigue is normal after physical exertion, prolonged stress, and sleep deprivation. However, fatigue that increases and develops after activities that previously did not cause it may be one of the symptoms or, occasionally, the first symptom of a disorder.

CAUSES

Most serious and many minor illnesses cause fatigue. However, most of these disorders have other more prominent symptoms (for example, pain, cough, fever, or jaundice) that are likely to bring the person to the doctor. This discussion focuses on disorders in which fatigue is the first or most severe symptom.

COMMON CAUSES

There is no firm dividing line between causes based on duration of fatigue. However, doctors find that certain causes tend to be more common depending on how long people have had fatigue before they seek medical care.

Recent fatigue (lasting less than 1 month) has many causes, but the most common are the following:

- Drug adverse effects
- Anemia
- Stress and/or depression

For prolonged fatigue (lasting 1 to 6 months), the most common causes are the following:

- Diabetes
- An underactive thyroid gland (hypothyroidism)
- Sleep disturbances (such as sleep apnea)
- Cancer

For chronic fatigue (lasting longer than 6 months), the most common causes are the following:

- Chronic fatigue syndrome
- Mental health disorder (such as depression)
- Drug adverse effects

Chronic fatigue syndrome is a disorder of unknown cause that results in fatigue and certain other symptoms. Not everyone who has fatigue for no apparent reason has chronic fatigue syndrome.

LESS COMMON CAUSES

Stopping cocaine can cause severe recent fatigue. Less common causes of prolonged or chronic fatigue include adrenal gland underactivity and pituitary gland underactivity.

EVALUATION

Fatigue can be highly subjective. People vary in what they consider to be fatigue and how they describe it. There are also few ways to objectively confirm fatigue or tell how severe it is. Doctors usually start an evaluation by trying to distinguish true fatigue from other symptoms that people may refer to as fatigue.

- Weakness: Weakness (see page 459) is lack of muscle strength that makes it difficult for people to move the affected muscles. Weakness is typically a symptom of a nervous system or muscle disorder. Disorders such as myasthenia gravis and Eaton-Lambert syndrome can cause weakness that worsens with activity, which may be confused with fatigue.
- Shortness of breath: People, such as those with certain heart and lung disorders, become short of breath with activity (see page 353) but do not feel fatigued at rest.
- Drowsiness: Excessive sleepiness (see page 212) is a symptom of sleep deprivation (for example, caused by lifestyle or by disorders such as allergic rhinitis, gastroesophageal reflux, painful musculoskeletal disorders, sleep apnea, and severe long-lasting disorders). Yawning and lapsing into sleep during daytime hours are common. However, many people with fatigue have disturbed sleep, so symptoms of sleep deprivation and fatigue can overlap.

In people with fatigue, certain symptoms and characteristics are cause for concern. They include

- Persistent, unintentional weight loss
- Chronic fever or night sweats
- Swollen lymph nodes throughout the body
- Muscle weakness and/or pain
- Serious accompanying symptoms (for example, coughing up or vomiting blood, bloody or black stools, shortness of breath, swelling in the abdomen, confusion, or suicidal thoughts)
- Involvement of more than one organ system (for example, rash plus joint pain and stiffness)
- Headache or loss of vision, particularly with muscle pains, in an older adult
- Older age (for example, older than about 65 years)

All people feel fatigue occasionally, and not every case of fatigue requires evaluation by a doctor, particularly those that accompany an acute illness (such as an acute infection) or that go away after a week or so. However, fatigue that seems to last longer or has no obvious explanation should be evaluated.

Older adults with a new or different headache or loss of vision and people who have serious accompanying symptoms should see a doctor immediately. Even if they have no other symptoms, older adults with fatigue should see their doctor as soon as possible. Other people who have other warning signs should see a doctor in a few days. People who have no warning signs should call their doctor. The doctor can decide how quickly they need to be seen. Typically a delay of a week or so is not harmful.

Doctors first ask questions about the person's symptoms and medical history. Doctors then do a physical examination. What they find during the history and physical examination often suggests a cause of the fatigue and the tests that may need to be done (see Table, below).

Doctors ask the person

- To describe what is meant by fatigue as precisely as possible
- How long fatigue has lasted
- When fatigue occurs in relation to rest and activity
- What other symptoms occur (such as fever, night sweats, or shortness of breath)
- What measures relieve or worsen fatigue
- How fatigue affects the person's work and social activities

Women are asked about their menstrual history. All people are asked about diet, anxiety, depression, and alcohol and drug use (including use of over-the-counter and recreational drugs).

Doctors then do a physical examination. Because many disorders can cause fatigue, the physical examination is very thorough, particularly in people with chronic fatigue. In particular, doctors also do a neurologic examination to evaluate the person's muscle strength and tone, reflexes, gait, mood, and mental status. The history and physical examination are more likely to reveal the cause of fatigue of more recent onset. A cause is also more likely to be found when fatigue is one of many symptoms than when fatigue is the only symptom. Fatigue that worsens with activity and lessens with rest suggests a physical disorder.

SOME COMMON CAUSES AND FEATURES OF PROLONGED OR CHRONIC FATIGUE		
Cause	Common Features*	Tests
Blood disorders or cancers		
Anemia	Decreased exercise tolerance with shortness of breath during activity greater than expected for the activity	CBC
	Sometimes paleness	
Cancers (such as digestive tract cancer, lung cancer, leukemia, lymphoma, multiple myeloma)	Widespread lymph node swelling, weight loss, and night sweats	CBC
	With multiple myeloma, low back or other bone pain, often severe at night	

(continued)

SOME COMMON CAUSES AND FEATURES OF PROLONGED OR CHRONIC FATIGUE *(continued)*

Cause	Common Features*	Tests
Infections		
Chronic hepatitis	Sometimes jaundice, loss of appetite, and fluid in the abdomen	Blood tests to determine how well the liver is functioning and to identify the hepatitis virus Sometimes liver biopsy
Cytomegalovirus infection	Enlarged spleen and lymph nodes, fever, and night sweats	Sometimes blood tests for antibodies to cytomegalovirus
Heart valve infection (endocarditis)	Fever and night sweats Sometimes joint pains Usually in people who have heart murmurs or inject drugs intravenously	Cultures of blood samples and echocardiography
HIV/AIDS	Fever, night sweats, and frequent infections Sometimes difficulty breathing, cough, diarrhea, and/or rash	HIV blood test
Mononucleosis	Recent sore throat and lymph node swelling	Mononucleosis blood test
Other infections (for example, fungal pneumonias such as histoplasmosis, parasitic infections, or tuberculosis)	Fever, night sweats, and weight loss Sometimes cough, difficulty breathing, and coughing up blood	Tests based on which type of infection seems likely
Other disorders and causes		
Chronic kidney disease	Shortness of breath, difficulty breathing when lying down that is relieved when upright (orthopnea), and/or swelling	Blood tests of kidney function
Connective tissue disorder (for example, rheumatoid arthritis or systemic lupus erythematosus [lupus])	Fever, night sweats, weight loss, joint pain, rash, and/or other organ involvement (for example, effects on the heart or lungs)	Blood tests for abnormal antibodies
Deconditioning	A history of lack of exercise or being bedbound or hospitalized	Only a doctor's examination
Diabetes (sometimes, other symptoms often more prominent)	Excessive thirst, excessive urination, increased appetite, and unexplained weight gain or loss	Measurement of sugar (glucose) level in the blood after the person fasts overnight and sometimes glucose tolerance testing
Drugs: Antidepressants, older antihistamines, antihypertensives, diuretics that cause low potassium levels in the blood, muscle relaxants, recreational drugs, and sedatives	History of taking a drug known to cause fatigue	Only a doctor's examination

(continued)

SOME COMMON CAUSES AND FEATURES OF PROLONGED OR CHRONIC FATIGUE *(continued)*

Cause	Common Features*	Tests
Giant cell (temporal) arteritis	Headache, pain in the jaw when chewing, pain when combing hair, loss of vision, and/or muscle pains in a person over 50	ESR and temporal artery biopsy
Mental health disorders: Anxiety, depression, drug addiction, panic disorder, or somatization disorder (physical symptoms caused mainly by anxiety)	Anxiety, sadness, loss of appetite, and unexplained sleep disturbance With somatization disorder, an excessive preoccupation with physical symptoms	Only a doctor's examination
Multiple sclerosis	Fatigue worse with exposure to heat Past symptoms of nervous system malfunction (such as numbness, loss of coordination, and weakness), particularly if people had more than one episode of symptoms	Brain and/or spinal cord MRI
Pregnancy	Cessation of menstrual periods, breast tenderness, morning sickness, and abdominal swelling	Pregnancy test
Sleep disorders	Excessive daytime sleepiness, frequent awakenings, breathing interruptions during sleep, difficulty falling asleep, unrefreshing sleep	Sleep laboratory testing (polysomnography)
Underactive thyroid gland (hypothyroidism)	Inability to tolerate cold, weight gain, constipation, and coarse skin	Blood tests of thyroid function
Undernutrition	Weight loss Sometimes loss of appetite, foul-smelling stool, abdominal pain, or a combination	A doctor's examination Sometimes other tests
Disorders of unknown cause		
Chronic fatigue syndrome	Sore throat, sleep that is not refreshing, difficulty with concentration or short-term memory, muscle aches, joint pain, headaches, and/or tender lymph nodes in the neck or under the arms	Only a doctor's examination
Fibromyalgia	Long-standing and widespread muscle and bone pain in areas outside the joints, trigger points, lower abdominal pain, gas, bloating, constipation or diarrhea, migraines, and anxiety	Only a doctor's examination

*Features include symptoms and the results of the doctor's examination. Features mentioned are typical but not always present.
CBC = complete blood count; ESR = erythrocyte sedimentation rate; HIV = human immunodeficiency virus; MRI = magnetic resonance imaging.

TESTING

The need for tests depends on what doctors find during the history and physical examination. For example, doctors test for human immunodeficiency virus infection and tuberculosis if people have risk factors. Testing for other infections or cancer is usually done only when people's findings suggest these causes. In general, people who have had fatigue for a long time and those who have warning signs are more likely to require testing.

If people do not have any other findings besides fatigue, many doctors do a few common blood tests. For example, they may do a complete blood count, blood tests to measure liver, thyroid gland, and kidney function, and a blood test called the erythrocyte sedimentation rate that suggests the presence of inflammation. However, such blood testing often does not reveal the cause.

TREATMENT

Treatment is directed at the cause. People with chronic fatigue syndrome or fatigue with no clear cause may be helped with physical therapy that includes increasing degrees of exercise and with psychologic support (for example, cognitive-behavioral therapy).

ESSENTIALS FOR OLDER PEOPLE

Although it is normal for people to slow down as they age, fatigue is not normal. Fatigue is more often the first symptom of a disorder in older people. For example, the first symptom of

a urinary tract infection in an older woman may be fatigue, rather than any urinary symptoms (such as burning during urination, frequent urination, or blood in the urine). Older people with pneumonia may have fatigue before they have a cough or fever. In older people, the first symptom of other disorders, such as giant cell arteritis, may also be fatigue. Because serious illness may become apparent soon after sudden fatigue in older people, it is important to determine the cause as quickly as possible.

KEY POINTS

- Fatigue is a common symptom.
- Fatigue caused primarily by a physical disorder increases with activity and lessens with rest.
- If a doctor uncovers no findings suggesting a cause of fatigue, tests are often not helpful in identifying the cause.
- Successful treatment of chronic fatigue may take work and persistence.
- Fatigue in older people is not a normal part of aging.

FEVER IN ADULTS

Fever is an elevated body temperature. Temperature is considered elevated when it is higher than 100° F (37.8° C) as measured by an oral thermometer or higher than 100.8° F (38.2° C) as measured by a rectal thermometer. Many people use the term "fever" loosely, often meaning that they feel too warm, too cold, or sweaty, but they have not actually measured their temperature.

Although 98.6° F (37° C) is considered normal temperature, body temperature varies throughout the day. It is lowest in the early morning and highest in the late afternoon—sometimes reaching 99.9° F (37.7° C). Similarly, a fever does not stay at a constant temperature. Sometimes temperature peaks every day and then returns to normal—a process called intermittent fever. Alternatively, temperature varies but does not return to normal—a process called remittent fever. Doctors no longer think that the pattern of the rise and fall of fever is very important in diagnosis of certain disorders.

CONSEQUENCES OF FEVER

The symptoms people have are due mainly to the condition causing the fever rather than the fever itself.

Although many people worry that fever can cause harm, the typical temporary elevations in body temperature to 100.4° to 104° F (38° to 40° C) caused by most short-lived (acute) illnesses are well-tolerated by healthy adults. However, a moderate fever may be slightly dangerous for adults with a heart or lung disorder because fever causes heart rate and breathing rate to increase. Fever can also worsen mental status in people with dementia.

Extreme temperature elevation (typically more than 105.8° F, or 41° C) may be damaging. A body temperature this high can cause malfunction and ultimately failure of most organs. Such extreme elevation sometimes results from very severe infection (such as sepsis, malaria, or meningitis) but is more typically caused by heatstroke or use of certain drugs. Drugs that can cause an extremely high temperature include certain illicit drugs (such as cocaine, amphetamines, or phencyclidine), anesthetics, and antipsychotic drugs.

CAUSES

Substances that cause fever are called pyrogens. Pyrogens can come from inside or outside the body. Microorganisms and the substances they produce (such as toxins) are examples of pyrogens formed outside the body. Pyrogens formed inside the body are usually produced by monocytes and macrophages (two types of white blood cells). Pyrogens from outside the body cause fever by stimulating the body to release its own pyrogens. However, infection is not the only cause of fever. Fever may also result from inflammation, a reaction to a drug, an allergic reaction, autoimmune disorders (when the body produces abnormal antibodies that attack its own tissues), and undetected cancer (especially leukemia or lymphoma).

Many disorders can cause fever. They are broadly categorized as

- Infectious (most common)
- Neoplastic (cancer)
- Inflammatory

An infectious cause is highly likely in adults with a fever that lasts 4 days or less. A noninfectious cause is more likely to cause fever that lasts a long time or recurs. Many cancers and inflammatory disorders cause fever. Inflammatory disorders include joint, connective tissue, and blood vessel disorders such as rheumatoid arthritis, systemic lupus erythematosus (lupus), and giant cell arteritis.

Drugs sometimes cause fever.

Also, an isolated, short-lived (acute) fever in people with cancer or a known inflammatory disorder is most likely to have an infectious cause. In healthy people, an acute fever is unlikely to be the first sign of a chronic illness.

MOST COMMON CAUSES

Virtually all infectious disorders can cause fever. But overall, the most likely causes are

- Upper and lower respiratory tract infections
- Gastrointestinal infections
- Urinary tract infections
- Skin infections

Most acute respiratory tract and gastrointestinal infections are viral.

Certain conditions (risk factors) make people more likely to have a fever. These factors include the person's health status, age, certain occupations, and use of certain medical procedures and drugs, as well as exposure to infections (for example, through travel or contact with infected people or insects).

EVALUATION

Usually, a doctor can determine that an infection is present based on a brief history, a physical examination, and occasionally a few simple tests, such as a chest x-ray and urine tests. However, sometimes the cause of fever is not readily identified.

When doctors initially evaluate people with an acute fever, they focus on two general issues:

- Identifying other symptoms such as headache or cough: These symptoms help narrow the range of possible causes.
- Determining whether the person is seriously or chronically ill: Many of the possible acute viral infections are difficult for doctors to diagnose specifically (that is, to determine exactly which virus is causing the infection). Limiting testing to people who are seriously or chronically ill can help avoid many expensive, unnecessary, and often fruitless searches.

In people with an acute fever, certain signs and characteristics are cause for concern. They include

- A change in mental function, such as confusion
- A headache, stiff neck, or both
- Flat, small, purplish red spots on the skin (petechiae), which indicate bleeding under the skin
- Low blood pressure
- Rapid heart rate or rapid breathing
- Shortness of breath (dyspnea)
- A temperature of > 104° F (40° C) or < 95° F (35° C)
- Recent travel to an area where malaria is common (endemic)
- Recent use of drugs that suppress the immune system (immunosuppressants)

People who have any warning sign should see a doctor right away. Such people typically need immediate testing and often admission to a hospital.

People without warning signs should call the doctor if the fever lasts more than 24 to 48 hours. Depending on the person's age, other symptoms, and known medical conditions, the doctor may ask the person to come for evaluation or recommend treatment at home. Typically, people should see a doctor if a fever lasts more than 3 or 4 days regardless of other symptoms.

Doctors first ask questions about the person's symptoms and medical history. Doctors then do a physical examination. What they find during the history and physical examination often suggests a cause of the fever and the tests that may need to be done.

A doctor begins by asking a person about present and previous symptoms and disorders, drugs currently being taken, exposure to infections, and recent travel. The pattern of the fever rarely helps the doctor make a diagnosis, except a fever that recurs every other day or every third day is typical of malaria. Doctors consider malaria as a possible cause only if people have traveled to an area where malaria is common.

Recent travel may give the doctor clues to the cause of a fever because some infections occur only in certain areas. For example, coccidioidomycosis (a fungal infection) occurs almost exclusively in the southwestern United States. Recent exposure to certain materials or animals is also important. For example, people who work in a meatpacking plant are more likely to develop brucellosis (a bacterial infection spread through contact with domestic animals).

Pain is an important clue to the possible source of fever, so the doctor asks about any pain in the ears, head, neck, teeth, throat, chest, abdomen, flank, rectum, muscles, and joints.

Other symptoms that help determine the cause of the fever include nasal congestion and/or discharge, cough, diarrhea, and urinary symptoms (frequency, urgency, and pain while urinating). Knowing whether the person has enlarged lymph nodes or a rash (including what it looks like, where it is, and when it appeared in relation to other symptoms) may help the doctor

SOME CAUSES OF FEVER

Risk Factor	Cause
None (healthy)	Upper or lower respiratory tract infection
	Gastrointestinal infection
	Urinary tract infection
	Skin infection
Hospitalization	Infection related to a catheter inserted in a vein (IV catheter infection)
	Urinary tract infection, particularly in people with a urinary catheter
	Pneumonia, particularly in people on a ventilator
	Atelectasis (collapse of part of a lung due to an airway blockage, rather than an infection)
	Infection or a pocket of blood (hematoma) at the site of surgery
	Deep vein thrombosis or pulmonary embolism
	Diarrhea (due to *Clostridium difficile*–induced colitis)
	Drugs
	Transfusion reaction
	Pressure sores
Travel to areas where an infection is common (endemic areas)	Malaria
	Viral hepatitis
	Disorders that cause diarrhea
	Typhoid fever
	Dengue fever (less common)
Exposure to insects or animals that carry disease-causing organisms, called vectors (in the United States)	Ticks: Rickettsiosis, ehrlichiosis, anaplasmosis, Lyme disease, babesiosis, or tularemia
	Mosquitoes: Arboviral encephalitis
	Wild animals: Tularemia, rabies, or hantavirus infection
	Fleas: Plague
	Domestic animals: Brucellosis, cat-scratch disease, Q fever, or toxoplasmosis
	Birds: Psittacosis
	Reptiles: *Salmonella* infection
	Bats: Rabies or histoplasmosis
A weakened immune system (immunocompromise)	Viruses: Varicella-zoster virus or cytomegalovirus infection
	Bacteria: Infection due to pneumococci, meningococci, *Staphylococcus aureus*, *Pseudomonas aeruginosa*, *Nocardia*, or mycobacteria
	Fungi: Infection due to *Candida*, *Aspergillus*, *Zygomycetes*, *Histoplasma*, *Coccidioides*, or *Pneumocystis jirovecii*
	Parasites: Infection due to *Toxoplasma gondii*, *Strongyloides stercoralis*, *Cryptosporidium*, microsporidia, or *Isospora belli*

(continued)

SOME CAUSES OF FEVER *(continued)*

Risk Factor	Cause
Drugs that can increase heat production	Amphetamines
	Cocaine
	Phencyclidine
	Methylenedioxymethamphetamine (MDMA, or Ecstasy)
	Antipsychotic drugs
	Anesthetics
Drugs that can trigger fever	Beta-lactam antibiotics
	Sulfa drugs
	Phenytoin
	Carbamazepine
	Procainamide
	Quinidine
	Amphotericin B
	Interferons (drugs that are based on substances produced by the immune system and that help block the reproduction of viruses)

pinpoint a cause. People with recurring fevers, night sweats, and weight loss may have a chronic infection such as tuberculosis or endocarditis (infection of the heart's lining and usually the heart valves).

The doctor may also ask about the following:

- Contact with anyone who has an infection
- Any known conditions that predispose to infection, such as HIV infection, diabetes, cancer, organ transplantation, sickle cell disease, or heart valve disorders, particularly if an artificial valve is present
- Any known disorders that predispose to fever without infection, such as lupus, gout, sarcoidosis, an overactive thyroid gland (hyperthyroidism), or cancer
- Use of any drugs that predispose to infection, such as cancer chemotherapy drugs, corticosteroids, or other drugs that suppress the immune system
- Use of illicit drugs that are injected

The physical examination begins with confirmation of fever. Fever is most accurately determined by measuring rectal temperature. Then the doctor does a thorough examination from head to toe to check for a source of infection or evidence of disease.

TESTING

The need for testing depends on what the doctor finds during the physical examination.

Otherwise healthy people who have an acute fever and only vague, general symptoms (for example, they feel generally ill or achy) probably have a viral illness that will go away without treatment. Therefore, they do not require testing. Exceptions are people who have been exposed to an animal or insect that carries and transmits a specific disease (called a vector), such as people with a tick bite, and people who have recently been in an area where a particular disorder (such as malaria) is common.

If otherwise healthy people have findings that suggest a particular disorder, testing may be needed. Doctors select tests based on those findings. For example, if people have a headache and stiff neck, a spinal tap (lumbar puncture) is done to look for meningitis. If people have a cough and lung congestion, a chest x-ray is done to look for pneumonia.

People who are at increased risk of infection and people who appear seriously ill often need testing even when findings do not suggest a particular disorder. For such people, doctors often do the following:

- A complete blood count (including the number and proportion of different types of white blood cells)
- A chest x-ray
- Urinalysis

An increase in the white blood cell count usually indicates infection. The proportion of different types of white blood cells (differential count) gives further clues. For example, an increase in neutrophils suggests a relatively new bacterial infection. An increase in eosinophils suggests the presence of parasites, such as tapeworms or roundworms. Also, blood and other body fluids may be sent to the laboratory to try to grow the microorganism in a culture. Other blood tests can be used to detect antibodies against specific microorganisms.

A fever of unknown origin may be diagnosed when people have a fever of at least 101° F (38.3° C) for several weeks and when extensive investigation does not detect a cause. In such cases, the cause may be an unusual chronic infection or something other than an infection, such as a connective tissue disorder or cancer. Ultrasonography, computed tomography (CT), or magnetic resonance imaging (MRI), particularly of areas that are causing discomfort, may help a doctor diagnose the cause. Radionuclide scanning, done after white blood cells labeled with a radioactive marker are injected into a vein, may be used to identify areas of infection or inflammation. If these test results are negative, doctors may need to take a sample of tissue from the liver, bone marrow, or another site of suspected infection for biopsy. The sample is then examined under a microscope and cultured.

TREATMENT

Because fever helps the body defend against infection and because fever itself is not dangerous (unless it is higher than about 106° F [41.1° C]), there is some debate as to whether fever should be routinely treated. However, people with a high fever generally feel much better when the fever is treated. Plus, people with a heart or lung disorder and those with dementia are considered to be at particular risk of dangerous complications, so when they have a fever, it should be treated.

Drugs used to lower body temperature are called antipyretics. The most effective and widely used antipyretics are acetaminophen and nonsteroidal anti-inflammatory drugs (NSAIDs), such as aspirin, ibuprofen, and naproxen. Typically, people may take 650 to 1000 milligrams of acetaminophen every 6 hours (not to exceed 4000 milligrams in 1 day). Alternatively, they may take 400 milligrams of ibuprofen every 6 hours. Because many over-the-counter cold or flu preparations contain acetaminophen, people must be careful not to take acetaminophen and one or more of these preparations at the same time.

Other cooling measures (such as cooling with a tepid water mist and using cooling blankets) are needed only if the temperature is about 106° F. Sponging with alcohol is avoided because alcohol can be absorbed through the skin and may have harmful effects.

ESSENTIALS FOR OLDER PEOPLE

Fever can be tricky in older people because the body may not respond the way it would in younger people. For example, in frail older people, infection is less likely to cause fever. Even when elevated by infection, the temperature may be lower than the standard definition of fever, and the degree of fever may not correspond to the severity of the illness. Similarly, other symptoms, such as pain, may be less noticeable. Frequently, a change in mental function or a decline in daily functioning is the only other initial sign of pneumonia or a urinary tract infection.

However, older people with a fever are significantly more likely to have a serious bacterial infection than are younger adults with a fever. As in younger adults, the cause is commonly a respiratory or urinary tract infection. Skin and soft-tissue infections are also common causes in older people.

Diagnosis is similar to that for younger adults, except that for older people, doctors usually recommend urine tests (including culture) and a chest x-ray. Samples of blood are cultured to rule out a blood infection. Older people with a blood infection or with abnormal vital signs (such as low blood pressure and a rapid pulse and breathing rate) are admitted to the hospital.

O—π KEY POINTS

- Most fevers in healthy people are caused by a respiratory or gastrointestinal infection due to a virus.
- If people with a fever have any warning signs (see page 149), they should see a doctor right away.
- Doctors can usually identify an infection based on a brief history, a physical examination, and occasionally a few simple tests, and then doctors use these results, particularly symptoms, to determine which other tests are needed.
- Doctors consider underlying chronic disorders, particularly those that impair the immune system, as a possible cause of fever that lasts a long time.
- Taking acetaminophen or an NSAID usually lowers fever and usually makes people feel better, although for most people, treatment is not crucial.
- In older people, infections are less likely to cause fever, and other symptoms may be less noticeable.

FEVER IN INFANTS AND CHILDREN

Normal body temperature varies from person to person and throughout the day (it is typically highest in the afternoon). Normal body temperature is higher in preschool-aged children and highest at about 18 to 24 months of age. However, despite these variations, most doctors define fever as a temperature of 100.4° F (about 38° C) or higher when measured with a rectal thermometer.

Although parents often worry about how high the temperature is, the height of the fever does not necessarily indicate how serious the cause is. Some minor illnesses cause a high fever, and some serious illnesses cause only a mild fever. Other symptoms (such as difficulty breathing, confusion, and not drinking) indicate the severity of illness much better than the temperature does. However, a temperature over 106° F (about 41° C), although quite rare, can itself be dangerous.

Fever can be useful in helping the body fight infection. Some experts think that reducing fever can prolong some disorders or possibly interfere with the immune system's response to infection. Thus, although a fever is uncomfortable, it does not always require treatment in otherwise healthy children. However, in children with a lung, heart, or brain disorder, fever may cause problems because it increases demands on the body (for example, by increasing the heart rate). So lowering the temperature in such children is important.

Infants with a fever are usually irritable and may not sleep or feed well. Older children lose their interest in play. Usually, the higher a fever gets, the more irritable and disinterested children become. However, sometimes children with a high fever look surprisingly well. Children may have seizures when their temperature rises or falls rapidly (febrile seizures). Rarely, a fever gets so high that children become listless, drowsy, and unresponsive.

HOW TO TAKE A CHILD'S TEMPERATURE

A child's temperature can be taken from the rectum, ear, mouth, forehead, or armpit. It can be taken with a glass or digital thermometer. Glass thermometers need to be shaken before use to make sure the temperature they show is below the normal body temperature (98.6° F, or about 37° C). Then they must be left in place for 2 to 3 minutes. Digital thermometers are easier to use and give much quicker readings (and usually give a signal when they are ready). Glass thermometers containing mercury are no longer recommended because they can break and expose people to mercury.

Rectal temperatures are most accurate. That is, they come closest to the child's true internal body temperature. For a rectal temperature, the bulb of the thermometer should be coated with a lubricant. Then the thermometer is gently inserted about 1/2 to 1 inch (about 1 1/4 to 2 1/2 centimeters) into the rectum while the child is lying face down. The child should be kept from moving.

Ear temperatures are taken with a digital device that measures infrared radiation from the eardrum. Ear thermometers are unreliable in infants under 3 months old. For an ear temperature, the thermometer probe is placed around the opening of the ear so that a seal is formed, then the start button is pressed. A digital readout provides the temperature.

Oral temperatures are taken by placing a glass or digital thermometer under the child's tongue. Oral temperatures provide reliable readings but are difficult to take in young children. Young children have difficulty keeping their mouth gently closed around the thermometer, which is necessary for an accurate reading. The age at which oral temperatures can be reliably taken varies from child to child but is typically after age 4.

Forehead (temporal artery) temperatures are taken with a digital device that measures infrared radiation from an artery in the forehead (the temporal artery). For a forehead temperature, the head of the thermometer is moved lightly across the forehead from hairline to hairline while pressing the scan button. A digital readout provides the temperature. Forehead temperatures are not as accurate as rectal temperatures, particularly in infants under 3 months old.

Armpit temperatures are taken by placing a glass or digital thermometer in the child's armpit, directly on the skin. Doctors rarely use this method because it is less accurate than others (readings are usually too low and vary greatly). However, if caretakers are uncomfortable taking a rectal temperature and do not have a device to measure ear or forehead temperature, measuring armpit temperature may be better than not measuring temperature at all.

CAUSES

Fever occurs in response to infection, injury, or inflammation and has many causes. Likely causes of fever depend on whether it has lasted 7 days or less (acute) or more than 7 days (chronic), as well as on the age of the child.

ACUTE FEVER

Acute fevers in infants and children are usually caused by an infection. Teething does not typically cause fever over 101° F.

The **most common causes** are

- Respiratory infections due to a virus, such as colds or flu
- Gastroenteritis (infection of the digestive tract) due to a virus
- Certain bacterial infections, particularly ear infections (otitis media), sinus infections, pneumonia, and urinary tract infections

Newborns and young infants are at higher risk of certain serious infections because their immune system is not fully developed. Such infections may be acquired before birth or during birth and include sepsis (a serious bodywide infection), pneumonia, and meningitis.

Children under 3 years old who develop a fever (particularly if their temperature is 102.2° F [39° C] or higher) sometimes have bacteria in their bloodstream (bacteremia). Unlike older children, they sometimes have bacteremia with no symptoms besides fever (called occult bacteremia). Vaccines against the bacteria that usually cause occult bacteremia (*Streptococcus pneumoniae and Haemophilus influenzae type B* [HiB]) are now widely used in the United States and Europe. As a result, occult bacteremia is less common. However, pneumococcal strains that are not a part of the current pneumococcal vaccine or other bacteria can sometimes cause it.

Less common causes of acute fevers include side effects of vaccinations and of certain drugs, bacterial infections of the skin (cellulitis) or joints (septic arthritis), and viral or bacterial infections of the brain (encephalitis), the tissues covering the brain (meningitis), or both. Heatstroke causes a very high body temperature.

Typically, a fever due to vaccination lasts a few hours to a day after the vaccine is given. However, some vaccinations can cause a fever even 1 or 2 weeks after the vaccine is given (as with measles vaccination). Children who have a fever when they are scheduled to receive a vaccine can still receive the vaccine.

CHRONIC FEVER

Chronic fever most commonly results from

- A prolonged viral illness
- Back-to-back viral illnesses, especially in young children

Chronic fever can also be caused by many other infectious and noninfectious disorders. Infectious causes include hepatitis, sinusitis, pneumonia, pockets of pus (abscesses) in the abdomen, infections of the digestive tract caused by bacteria or parasites, bone infections (osteomyelitis), heart infections (endocarditis), and tuberculosis. Noninfectious causes include Kawasaki disease, inflammatory bowel disease, juvenile idiopathic arthritis or other connective tissue disorders, and cancer (such as leukemia and lymphoma). Occasionally, children fake a fever, or caregivers fake a fever in the child they care for. Sometimes the cause is not identified.

EVALUATION

Detecting a fever is not difficult, but determining its cause can be.

WARNING SIGNS

Certain symptoms are cause for concern. They include

- Any fever in infants less than 2 months old
- Lethargy or listlessness
- Ill appearance
- Difficulty breathing
- Bleeding in the skin, appearing as tiny reddish purple dots (petechiae) or splotches (purpura)
- Continuous crying in an infant or toddler (inconsolability)
- Headache, neck stiffness, confusion, or a combination in an older child

WHEN TO SEE A DOCTOR

Children with fever should be evaluated by a doctor right away if they have any warning signs or are less than 2 months old.

Children without warning signs who are between 3 months and 36 months old should be seen by the doctor if the fever is 102.2° F

(39° C) or higher, if there is no obvious upper respiratory infection (that is, children are sneezing and have a runny nose and nasal congestion), or if the fever has continued more than 5 days. For children without warning signs who are over 36 months old, the need for and timing of a doctor's evaluation depend on the child's symptoms. Children who have upper respiratory symptoms but otherwise appear well may not need further evaluation. Children over 36 months of age with fever lasting more than 5 days should be seen by the doctor.

WHAT THE DOCTOR DOES

Doctors first ask questions about the child's symptoms and medical history. Doctors then do a physical examination. A description of the child's symptoms and a thorough examination usually enable doctors to identify the fever's cause (see Table on pages 157 to 159).

Doctors take the child's temperature. It is measured rectally in infants and young children for accuracy. The breathing rate is noted. If children appear ill, blood pressure is measured. If children have a cough or breathing problems, a sensor is clipped on a finger or an earlobe to measure the oxygen concentration in blood (pulse oximetry).

As doctors examine children, they look for warning signs (such as an ill appearance, lethargy, listlessness, and inconsolability), noting particularly how children respond to being examined—for example, whether children are listless and passive or extremely irritable.

Occasionally, the fever itself can cause children to have some of the warning signs including lethargy, listlessness, and ill appearance. Doctors may give children fever-reducing drugs (such as ibuprofen) and reevaluate them once the fever is reduced. It is reassuring when lethargic children become active and playful once the fever is reduced. On the other hand, it is worrisome when ill-appearing children remain ill-appearing despite a normal temperature.

TESTING

For acute fever, doctors can often make a diagnosis without testing. For example, if children do not appear very ill, the cause is usually a viral infection; a respiratory infection if they have a runny nose, wheezing, or a cough; or gastroenteritis if they have diarrhea and vomiting. In such children, the diagnosis is clear, and testing is not needed. Even if no specific symptoms suggest a diagnosis, the cause is still often a viral infection in children who otherwise do not appear very ill. Doctors try to limit testing to children who may have a more serious disorder. The chance of a serious disorder (and thus the need for tests) depends on the child's age, symptoms, and overall appearance, plus the particular disorders the doctor suspects (see Table).

If newborns (28 days old or younger) have a fever, they are hospitalized for testing because their risk of having a serious infection is high. Testing typically includes blood and urine tests, a spinal tap (lumbar puncture), and sometimes a chest x-ray.

In infants between 1 month and 3 months old, blood tests and urine tests (urinalysis) and cultures are done. The need for hospitalization, a chest x-ray, and a spinal tap depends on results of the examination and blood and urine tests, as well as how ill or well infants appear and whether a follow-up examination can be done. Testing in infants under 3 months old is done to look for occult bacteremia, urinary tract infections, and meningitis. Testing is necessary because the source of fever is difficult to determine in infants and because their immature immune system puts them a high risk of serious infection.

If children aged 3 to 36 months look well and can be watched closely, tests are not needed. If symptoms suggest a specific infection, doctors do the appropriate tests. If children have no symptoms suggesting a specific disorder but look ill or have a temperature of 102.2° F (39° C) or higher, blood and urine tests are usually done. The need for hospitalization depends on how well or ill children look and whether a follow-up examination can be done.

In children over 36 months old, tests are typically not done unless children have specific symptoms suggesting a serious disorder.

For chronic fever, tests are often done. If doctors suspect a particular disorder, tests for that disorder are done. If the cause is unclear, screening tests are done. Screening tests include a complete blood cell count, urinalysis and culture, and blood tests to check for inflammation. Tests for inflammation include the erythrocyte sedimentation rate (ESR) and measurement of C-reactive protein (CRP) levels. Other tests doctors sometimes do when there is no clear cause include stool tests, tuberculosis tests, chest x-rays, and computed tomography (CT) of the sinuses.

SOME COMMON CAUSES AND FEATURES OF FEVER IN CHILDREN

Cause	Common Features*	Tests
Acute (lasting 7 days or less)		
Respiratory infections due to a virus	A runny or congested nose	A doctor's examination
	Usually a sore throat and cough	
	Sometimes swollen lymph nodes in the neck, without redness and tenderness	
Other infections due to a virus	In some infants or children, no symptoms except fever	A doctor's examination
Gastroenteritis	Diarrhea	A doctor's examination
	Often vomiting	Sometimes examination and testing of stool
	Possibly recent contact with infected people or certain animals or consumption of contaminated food or water	
Ear infection (otitis media)	Pain in one ear (difficult to detect in infants and young children who do not talk)	A doctor's examination
	Sometimes rubbing or pulling at the ear	
Throat infections (pharyngitis)	A red, swollen throat	A doctor's examination
	Pain when swallowing	Sometimes a throat culture or rapid strep test (both done on a sample taken from the back of the throat with a swab)
Occult bacteremia	In children under 3 years old	Blood tests
	No other symptoms	
Pneumonia	Cough and rapid breathing	A doctor's examination
	Often chest pain, shortness of breath, or both	Usually a chest x-ray
Skin infections (cellulitis)	A red, painful, slightly swollen area of skin	A doctor's examination
Urinary tract infection	Pain during urination	Urine tests
	Sometimes blood in urine	
	Sometimes back pain	
	In infants, vomiting and poor feeding	
Encephalitis (a rare infection of the brain)	**Infants:** Sometimes bulging of the soft spots (fontanelles) between the skull bones, sluggishness (lethargy) or inconsolability	A spinal tap (lumbar puncture)
	Older children: Headache, confusion, or lethargy	
Meningitis (uncommon)	**Newborns:** Bulging of the soft spots (fontanelles) between the skull bones, inconsolability, poor feeding, and/or lethargy	A spinal tap
	Infants: Fussiness and irritability especially when held, inconsolability, poor feeding, and/or lethargy	
	Older children: Headache, sensitivity to light, lethargy, vomiting, and/or a stiff neck that makes lowering the chin to the chest difficult	

(continued)

SOME COMMON CAUSES AND FEATURES OF FEVER IN CHILDREN (continued)

Cause	Common Features*	Tests
Vaccines	Recent vaccination	A doctor's examination
Kawasaki disease	Fever for more than 5 days	A doctor's examination
	Red eyes, lips, and tongue	Blood tests
	Painful swelling of hands and feet	ECG and echocardiography
	Often a rash	Sometimes urine tests, ultrasonography of the abdomen, or an eye examination
	Sometimes swollen lymph nodes in the neck	
Acute rheumatic fever	Swollen, painful joints	Blood tests
	New heart murmur detected during a doctor's examination	A throat culture
		ECG and echocardiography
	Sometimes a rash or bumps under the skin	
	Sometimes jerky, uncontrollable movements or changes in behavior	
	Often a history of strep throat	

Chronic (lasting more than 7 days)

Cause	Common Features*	Tests
Infections due to a virus, such as ■ Epstein-Barr virus ■ Cytomegalovirus ■ Hepatitis viruses ■ Arboviruses	Long-lasting weakness and tiredness Sometimes swollen lymph nodes in the neck, a sore throat, or both Sometimes yellow discoloration of the whites of the eyes (jaundice)	Blood tests
Sinusitis	Intermittent headaches, a runny nose, and congestion	CT of the sinuses
Abdominal abscess (a pocket of pus inside the abdomen)	Abdominal pain and often tenderness to the touch	CT of the abdomen
Joint infection (septic arthritis)	Swollen, red, painful joint	Testing of a sample of fluid taken from the joint with a needle
Bone infection (osteomyelitis)	Pain in affected bone Sometimes a skin infection near the affected bone	Bone scan, MRI of bone, or both Sometimes biopsy of bone to check for bacteria (culture)
Endocarditis	Sometimes a heart murmur	Blood tests for bacteria (blood culture) Echocardiography
Tuberculosis (uncommon)	Poor weight gain or weight loss Night sweats Cough	Chest x-ray Skin tests Possibly culture of a sputum sample, and/or blood tests
Malaria (varies by geographic location)	A shaking chill followed by a fever that can exceed 104° F (40° C) Fatigue and vague discomfort (malaise), headache, body aches, and nausea	Blood tests

(continued)

SOME COMMON CAUSES AND FEATURES OF FEVER IN CHILDREN *(continued)*

Cause	Common Features*	Tests
Lyme disease	Sometimes headache and neck pain	A doctor's examination
	Sometimes a swollen, painful joint (such as the knee)	Sometimes blood tests
	Sometimes a bull's-eye rash in one or more locations	
	Occasionally a known history of a tick bite	
Cat-scratch disease	Often a swollen, painful lymph node	Blood tests
	Sometimes a bump on the skin where scratched by a cat	
Inflammatory bowel disease ■ Crohn disease ■ Ulcerative colitis	Blood in stool, crampy abdominal pain, weight loss, and loss of appetite Sometimes arthritis, rashes, sores in the mouth, and tears in the rectum	Colonoscopy Sometimes CT or x-rays after barium is inserted in the rectum (barium enema)
Joint and connective tissue disorders, such as ■ Juvenile idiopathic arthritis ■ Systemic lupus erythematosus (lupus)	Swollen, red, tender joints Often a rash Sometimes fatigue	Blood tests
Cancer, such as ■ Leukemia ■ Lymphoma ■ Neuroblastoma ■ Bone tumors	Poor weight gain or weight loss and loss of appetite Night sweats Possibly bone pain	A complete blood cell count Removal (aspiration) of a sample of bone marrow for examination Sometimes a bone scan, and/or MRI of bone Sometimes CT of the chest or abdomen
Periodic fever syndromes, such as ■ Periodic fever with aphthous stomatitis, pharyngitis, and adenitis (PFAPA) ■ Familial Mediterranean fever ■ Cyclic neutropenia	Fever that recurs in often predictable cycles with periods of wellness in between Sometimes mouth sores, sore throat, and swollen lymph nodes Sometimes chest or abdominal pain Sometimes family members who have had similar symptoms or have been diagnosed with one of the familial periodic fever syndromes	A doctor's examination during episodes of fever Blood tests during and between fever episodes Sometimes genetic testing
Pseudo fever of unknown origin	Usually a misinterpretation of normal fluctuations in body temperature or overinterpretation of frequent, minor viral illnesses Usually no other symptoms of concern Normal examination findings	A doctor's examination Thorough and accurate recording of illnesses and temperatures as well as a description of the overall function of the child and family Occasionally blood tests to rule out other causes and reassure parents

*Features include symptoms and results of the doctor's examination. Features mentioned are typical but not always present. Disorders that cause chronic fever also cause fever during the first 7 to 10 days.

CT = computed tomography; ECG = electrocardiogram; MRI = magnetic resonance imaging.

Rarely, fevers persist, and doctors cannot identify the cause even after extensive testing. This type of fever is called fever of unknown origin. Children with a fever of unknown origin are much less likely to have a serious disorder than are adults.

TREATMENT

If the fever results from a disorder, that disorder is treated. Other treatment focuses on making children feel better.

GENERAL MEASURES

Ways to help children with a fever feel better without using drugs include

- Giving children plenty of fluids to prevent dehydration
- Putting cool, wet cloths (compresses) on their forehead, wrists, and calves
- Placing children in a warm bath (only slightly cooler than the temperature of the child)

Because shivering may actually raise the child's temperature, methods that may cause shivering, such as undressing and cool baths, should be used only for dangerously high temperatures of 106° F (about 41° C) and above.

Rubbing the child down with alcohol or witch hazel must not be done because alcohol can be absorbed through the skin and cause harm. There are many other unhelpful folk remedies, ranging from the harmless (for example, putting onions or potatoes in the child's socks) to the uncomfortable (for example, coining or cupping).

DRUGS TO LOWER FEVER

Fever in an otherwise healthy child does not necessarily require treatment. However, drugs called antipyretic drugs may make children feel better by lowering the temperature. These drugs do not have any effect on an infection or other disorder causing the fever. However, if children have a heart, lung, brain, or nerve disorder or a history of seizures triggered by fever, using these drugs is important because they reduce the extra stress put on the body by fever.

Typically, the following drugs are used:

- Acetaminophen, given by mouth or by suppository
- Ibuprofen, given by mouth

Acetaminophen tends to be preferred. However, some doctors are concerned that acetaminophen use has contributed to the recent increase in asthma in children and thus do not recommend its use in children with asthma or who have a family history of asthma. Ibuprofen, if used for a long time, can irritate the stomach's lining. These drugs are available over the counter without a prescription. The recommended dosage is listed on the package or may be specified by the doctor. It is important to give the correct dose at the correct interval. The drugs do not work if too little drug is given or it is not given often enough. And although these drugs are relatively safe, giving too much of the drug or giving it too often can cause an overdose.

Rarely, acetaminophen or ibuprofen is given to prevent a fever, as when infants have been vaccinated.

Aspirin is no longer used for lowering fever in children because it can interact with certain viral infections (such as influenza or chickenpox) and cause a serious disorder called Reye syndrome.

KEY POINTS

- Usually, fever is caused by a viral infection.
- The likely causes of fever and need for testing depend on the age of the child.
- Infants under 2 months of age with a temperature of 100.4° F or higher need to be evaluated by a doctor.
- Children aged 3 to 36 months with fever who have no symptoms suggesting a specific disorder but look ill or have a temperature of 102.2° F (39° C) or higher need to be evaluated by a doctor.
- Teething does not cause significant fever.
- Drugs that lower fever may make children feel better but do not affect the disorder causing the fever.

GAS

Gas is normally present in the digestive system and may be expelled through the mouth (belching) or through the anus (flatus).

There are three main gas-related complaints:

- Excessive belching (eructation)
- Abdominal bloating (distention)
- Excessive flatus (known colloquially as farting)

Belching is more likely to occur shortly after eating or during periods of stress. Some people feel a tightness in their chest or stomach just before belching that is relieved as the gas is expelled.

People who complain of flatulence often have a misconception of how much flatus people normally produce. There is great variability in the quantity and frequency of flatus. People typically have flatus about 13 to 21 times a day, and some people pass flatus more or less often. Such gas may or may not have an odor.

Although flatus is flammable (due to the hydrogen and methane gas that it contains), this does not pose a routine problem. For example, working near open flames is not hazardous. However, there are rare reports of gas explosion during intestinal surgery and colonoscopy when electrical cautery was used in people whose bowels were incompletely cleaned out before the procedure.

In the past, colic in infants 2 to 4 months of age was attributed to excessive abdominal gas. Today, however, most doctors do not think colic is related to gas, because tests do not show excess gas in the abdomen of these infants. The actual cause of colic remains unclear.

CAUSES

Causes vary depending on the gas-related symptom.

BELCHING

Belching is caused by

- Swallowed air
- Gas generated by carbonated beverages

People normally swallow small amounts of air while eating and drinking. However, some people unconsciously swallow larger amounts of air (aerophagia) repeatedly while eating or smoking and sometimes when they feel anxious or nervous. Excessive salivation, which may occur with gastroesophageal reflux, ill-fitting dentures, certain drugs, gum chewing, or nausea of any cause, also increases air swallowing.

Most swallowed air is later belched up, and very little passes from the stomach into the rest of the digestive system. The small amount of air that does pass into the intestines is mostly absorbed into the bloodstream and very little is passed as flatus.

FLATUS

Flatus results from hydrogen, methane, and carbon dioxide gases that are produced by the bacteria normally present in the large intestine. These bacteria always produce some gas, but excessive gas can be produced

- When people consume certain foods
- When the digestive tract is unable to absorb food properly (malabsorption syndromes)

Foods that increase gas production include any with poorly digestible carbohydrates (for example, dietary fiber such as in baked beans and cabbage), certain sugars (such as fructose) or sugar alcohols (such as sorbitol), and fats. Almost anyone who eats large amounts of vegetables or fruits develops some degree of flatulence.

Malabsorption syndromes can increase gas production. People who have carbohydrate deficiencies (deficiencies of the enzymes that break down certain sugars), such as those with lactase deficiency, tend to produce large amounts of gas when they eat foods containing these sugars. Other malabsorption syndromes, such as tropical sprue, celiac disease, and pancreatic insufficiency, also may lead to the production of large amounts of gas.

However, some people may simply have more or different bacteria naturally living in their digestive tract, or they may have a motility (movement) disorder of the muscles in their digestive tract. These variations may account for differences in flatus production. People can record their flatus frequency in a diary before being evaluated by a doctor.

BLOATING

A sensation of bloating or abdominal swelling (distention) can be present in people who have digestive disorders such as poor stomach emptying (gastroparesis) or irritable bowel syndrome or other physical disorders such as ovarian or colon cancer. Sometimes, the sensation is caused by disorders that do not involve the abdomen. For example, in some people, the only symptom of a heart attack is a feeling of bloating or a strong urge to belch. However, many people who feel bloated do not have any physical disorder.

Doctors are not sure what role intestinal gas plays in the sensation of bloating. Aside from people who drink carbonated beverages or swallow excessive air, most people who have a sensation of bloating actually do not have excessive gas in their digestive system. However, studies do show that some people, such as those who have irritable bowel syndrome, are particularly sensitive to normal amounts of gas. Similarly, people with eating disorders (such as anorexia nervosa or bulimia) often misperceive and are particularly stressed by symptoms such as bloating. Thus, the basic abnormality in people with gas-related symptoms may be an intestine that is extremely sensitive (hypersensitive intestine). A motility disorder may contribute to symptoms as well.

EVALUATION

Most gas-related symptoms do not require immediate evaluation by a doctor. The following information can help people decide whether a doctor's evaluation is needed and help them know what to expect during the evaluation.

WARNING SIGNS

In people with gas, certain symptoms and characteristics are cause for concern. They include

- Weight loss (unintentional)
- Blood in stool
- Chest pain

WHEN TO SEE A DOCTOR

People with a bloating sensation in their chest, especially if the bloating sensation is accompanied by chest pain, should see a doctor promptly because this may be a sign of heart disease. People with any gas-related symptoms who have other warning signs, abdominal discomfort, or diarrhea should see a doctor within a week or so. People who have none of these symptoms or signs should see a doctor at some point, but it is not urgent.

WHAT THE DOCTOR DOES

Doctors first ask questions about the person's symptoms and medical history. Doctors then do a physical examination. What they find during the history and physical examination often suggests a cause of the symptoms and the tests that may need to be done (see Table on pages 163 to 164).

For excessive belching, the history is focused on finding the cause of air swallowing, especially dietary causes. For excessive flatus, doctors seek dietary causes and also symptoms of malabsorption (such as diarrhea and/or fatty, foul-smelling stool).

In people with any gas-related complaint, doctors need to understand the relationship between symptoms and meals (both timing and type and amount of food) and bowel movements. Doctors ask people about changes in frequency and color and consistency of stool. Doctors also need to know whether people have lost any weight.

In people with bloating or flatus, the physical examination is focused on finding signs of an underlying physical disorder (such as ovarian cancer). Doctors do abdominal, rectal, and (for women) pelvic examinations.

TESTING

Doctors do not usually do any testing on people with gas-related complaints unless they have other symptoms that suggest a specific disorder (see Table). For example, people who also have diarrhea may need testing for a malabsorption syndrome. An exception is middle age or older people who develop persistent bloating or distention, particularly those who have not had digestive system symptoms in the past. For such people, doctors may do tests for cancer of the ovary and/or colon.

TREATMENT

Doctors reassure people who have chronic bloating or flatus that their condition is not

SOME CAUSES AND FEATURES OF GAS-RELATED COMPLAINTS

Cause	Common Features*	Tests†
Belching		
Air swallowing	People with or without awareness of swallowing air	A doctor's examination
	Sometimes in people who smoke or chew gum excessively	
	Sometimes in people who have esophageal reflux or ill-fitting dentures	
Gas from carbonated beverages	Beverage consumption usually obvious based on person's history	A doctor's examination
Distention or bloating		
Air swallowing	See Belching, above	A doctor's examination
Irritable bowel syndrome	Chronic, recurrent bloating or distention associated with a change in the frequency of bowel movements or consistency of stool	A doctor's examination
		Examination of stool
	No warning signs	Blood tests
	Typically begins during the teens and 20s	
Poor emptying of the stomach (gastroparesis), usually due to other disorders such as diabetes, connective tissue disorders, or neurologic disorders	Nausea, abdominal pain, and sometimes vomiting	Upper endoscopy‡ and/or nuclear scanning that evaluates stomach emptying
	Early fullness (satiety)	
	Sometimes in people known to have a disorder that causes it	
Eating disorders	Long-standing symptoms, particularly in young women	A doctor's examination
	In people who are thin but still very concerned about excess body weight	
Chronic constipation	A long history of hard, infrequent bowel movements	A doctor's examination
Cancer (rarely) of the ovary or large intestine	New, persistent bloating in middle-aged or older people	If ovarian cancer is suspected, ultrasonography of the pelvis
	For colon cancer, sometimes blood in stool (blood may be visible or detected during a doctor's examination)	If colon cancer is suspected, colonoscopy
Passing of gas (flatulence)		
Foods, including beans, dairy products, vegetables (such as onions, celery, carrots, Brussels sprouts), fruits (such as raisins, bananas, apricots, or prune juice), and foods containing complex carbohydrates (such as pretzels, bagels, or wheat germ)	Symptoms that develop mainly when food that can cause gas is consumed	A doctor's examination
		Elimination of the suspected food from diet to see whether symptoms go away
Lactose intolerance	Bloating, cramps, and diarrhea after consuming milk products	A breath test to detect hydrogen, indicating undigested food

(continued)

SOME CAUSES AND FEATURES OF GAS-RELATED COMPLAINTS *(continued)*

Cause	Common Features*	Tests†
Celiac disease	Light-colored, soft, bulky, and unusually foul-smelling stools that may appear oily	Blood tests to measure antibodies produced when people with celiac disease eat foods containing gluten and biopsy of the upper small intestine
	Weakness, loss of appetite, and diarrhea	
	Often begins in childhood	
Tropical sprue	Light-colored, soft, bulky, and unusually foul-smelling stools that may appear oily	Blood tests and biopsy of the small intestine
	Nausea, loss of appetite, diarrhea, abdominal cramps, and weight loss	

*Features include symptoms and the results of the doctor's examination. Features mentioned are typical but not always present.
†Doctors usually do a urine pregnancy test for all girls and women of childbearing age.
‡Upper endoscopy is examination of the esophagus, stomach, and the first segment of the small intestine (duodenum) using a flexible viewing tube called an endoscope.

caused by another disorder and that these gas-related symptoms are not harmful to their health.

Bloating and belching are difficult to relieve because they are usually caused by unconscious air swallowing or an increased sensitivity to normal amounts of gas. If belching is the main problem, reducing the amount of air being swallowed can help, which is difficult because people usually are not aware of swallowing air. Avoiding chewing gum and eating more slowly in a relaxed atmosphere may help. Avoiding carbonated beverages helps some people. Doctors may also recommend that people try to minimize air swallowing by practicing open-mouth breathing from the diaphragm and fully control any associated upper digestive tract diseases (such as peptic ulcers).

People who pass flatus excessively should avoid foods that are likely to cause flatus. Typically, people should eliminate one food or group of foods at a time. Thus, people can start by eliminating foods containing hard-to-digest carbohydrates (such as beans and cabbage), then milk and dairy products, then fresh fruits, and then certain vegetables and other foods. Roughage (such as bran and psyllium seeds) may be added to the diet to try to increase movement through the large intestine. However, additional roughage may make symptoms worse for some people.

DRUG TREATMENT

Drugs do not provide much relief. Some doctors try anticholinergic drugs (such as bethanechol) and simethicone, which is present in some antacids and is also available by itself. However, there is little scientific evidence that these are of benefit.

Activated charcoal tablets can sometimes help reduce flatus and its unpleasant odor. However, charcoal stains the mouth and clothing. Charcoal-lined undergarments are available. Probiotics (such as VSL#3), which are bacteria found naturally in the body that promote the growth of good bacteria, may reduce bloating and flatulence by promoting growth of normal intestinal bacteria.

Some people with indigestion (dyspepsia) and upper abdominal fullness after a meal may be helped by antacids, a low dose of antidepressants (such as nortriptyline), or both to reduce a hypersensitive intestine.

O—π KEY POINTS

- Testing is done mainly when other symptoms suggest a certain disorder.
- Doctors should be aware of new and persistent symptoms of bloating in older people.

GASTROINTESTINAL BLEEDING

Bleeding may occur anywhere along the digestive (gastrointestinal [GI]) tract, from the mouth to the anus. Blood may be easily seen by the naked eye (overt) or may be present in amounts too small to be visible (occult). Occult bleeding is detected only by chemical testing of a stool specimen.

Blood may be visible in vomit (hematemesis), which indicates the bleeding is coming from the upper GI tract, usually from the stomach or the first part of the small intestine. When blood is vomited, it may be bright red if bleeding is brisk and ongoing. Alternatively, vomited blood may have the appearance of coffee grounds if bleeding has slowed or stopped, due to the partial digestion of the blood by acid in the stomach.

Blood may also be passed from the rectum, either as black, tarry stools (melena), as bright red blood (hematochezia), or in apparently normal stool if bleeding is less than a few teaspoons per day. Melena is more likely when bleeding comes from the esophagus, stomach, or small intestine. The black color of melena is caused by blood that has been exposed for several hours to stomach acid and enzymes and to bacteria that normally reside in the large intestine. Melena may continue for several days after bleeding has stopped. Hematochezia is more likely when bleeding comes from the large intestine, although it can be caused by very rapid bleeding from the upper portions of the digestive tract as well.

People who have lost only a small amount of blood may feel well otherwise. However, serious and sudden blood loss may be accompanied by a rapid pulse, low blood pressure, and reduced urine flow. A person may also have cold, clammy hands and feet. Severe bleeding may reduce the flow of blood to the brain, causing confusion, disorientation, sleepiness, and even extremely low blood pressure (shock). Slow, chronic blood loss may cause symptoms and signs of anemia (such as weakness, easy fatigue, paleness [pallor], chest pain, and dizziness). People with underlying ischemic heart disease may develop chest pain (angina) or a have a heart attack (myocardial infarction) because of decreased blood flow through the heart.

CAUSES

The causes are divided into three areas: upper GI tract, lower GI tract, and small intestine (see Table on pages 167 to 168).

The most common causes are difficult to specify because causes vary by the area that is bleeding and the person's age.

However, in general, the most common causes of **upper GI bleeding** are

- Ulcers or erosions of the esophagus, stomach, or duodenum
- Varicose veins of the esophagus (esophageal varices)
- A tear in the lining of the esophagus after vomiting (Mallory-Weiss syndrome)

The most common causes of **lower GI bleeding** are

- Polyps of the large intestine
- Diverticular disease
- Hemorrhoids
- Inflammatory bowel disease
- Colon cancer

Other causes of lower GI bleeding include abnormal blood vessels in the colon, a split in the skin of the anus (anal fissure), ischemic colitis, and large bowel inflammation resulting from radiation or poor blood supply.

Bleeding from the small intestine is rare but can result from blood vessel abnormalities, tumors, or a Meckel diverticulum.

Bleeding from any cause is more likely, and potentially more severe, in people who have chronic liver disease (caused by alcohol abuse or chronic hepatitis), who have hereditary disorders of blood clotting, or who are taking certain drugs. Drugs that can cause or worsen bleeding include anticoagulants (such as heparin and warfarin), those that affect platelet function (such as aspirin and certain other nonsteroidal anti-inflammatory drugs [NSAIDs] and clopidogrel), and those that affect the stomach's protective barrier against acid (such as NSAIDs).

EVALUATION

GI bleeding typically requires evaluation by a doctor. The following information can help people decide when a doctor's evaluation is needed and help them know what to expect during the evaluation.

WARNING SIGNS

In people with GI bleeding, certain symptoms and characteristics are cause for concern. They include

- Fainting (syncope)
- Sweating (diaphoresis)
- Rapid heart rate (over 100 beats per minute)
- Passing more than 1 cup (250 milliliters) of blood

WHEN TO SEE A DOCTOR

People who have GI bleeding should see a doctor right away unless the only sign of bleeding is black stool or blood on the toilet paper after a bowel movement. If people with such findings have no warning signs and feel otherwise well, a delay of a day or two is not harmful.

WHAT THE DOCTOR DOES

Doctors first ask questions about the person's symptoms and medical history. Doctors then do a physical examination. What they find during the history and physical examination often suggests a cause of the GI bleeding and the tests that may need to be done (see Table on pages 167 to 168).

The history is focused on finding out exactly where the bleeding is coming from, how rapid it is, and what is causing it. Doctors need to know how much blood (for instance, a few teaspoons or several clots) is being passed and how often blood is being passed. Doctors ask people with hematemesis whether blood was passed the first time they vomited or only after they vomited a few times with no blood.

Doctors ask people with rectal bleeding whether pure blood was passed; whether it was mixed with stool, pus, or mucus; or whether blood simply coated the stool. People with bloody diarrhea are asked about recent travel or other possible forms of exposure to other agents that can cause digestive tract illness (for instance, food poisoning).

Doctors then ask about symptoms of abdominal discomfort, weight loss, and easy bleeding or bruising and symptoms of anemia (such as weakness, easy exhaustion [fatigability], and dizziness).

Doctors need to know about any current or past digestive tract bleeding and the results of any previous colonoscopy (examination of the entire large intestine, the rectum, and the anus using a flexible viewing tube). People should tell doctors whether they have inflammatory bowel disease, bleeding tendencies, and liver disease and whether they use any drugs that increase the likelihood of bleeding or chronic liver disease (such as alcohol).

The physical examination is focused on the person's vital signs (such as pulse, breathing rate, blood pressure, and temperature) and other indicators of shock or a decrease in the volume of circulating blood (hypovolemia—rapid heart rate, rapid breathing, pallor, sweating, little urine production, and confusion) and anemia.

Doctors also look for small purplish red (petechiae) and bruise-like (ecchymoses) spots on the skin, which are signs of bleeding disorders. Doctors also look for signs of chronic liver disease (such as spider angiomas, fluid in the abdominal cavity [ascites], and red palms) and portal hypertension (such as an enlarged spleen [splenomegaly] and dilated abdominal wall veins).

Doctors do a rectal examination to search for stool color, masses, and fissures and to check the stool for blood. Doctors also examine the anus to look for hemorrhoids.

TESTING

The need for tests depends on what doctors find during the history and physical examination, particularly whether warning signs are present.

There are four main testing approaches to GI bleeding:

- Blood tests and other laboratory studies
- Upper endoscopy for suspected upper GI tract bleeding
- Colonoscopy for lower GI tract bleeding (unless clearly caused by hemorrhoids)
- Sometimes insertion of a nasogastric tube

The person's blood count helps indicate how much blood has been lost. A low platelet count is a risk factor for bleeding. Other blood tests include prothrombin time (PT), partial

SOME CAUSES AND FEATURES OF GASTROINTESTINAL BLEEDING

Cause*	Common Features†	Tests
Upper digestive tract (indicated by vomiting blood or dark brown material)		
Ulcers or erosions of the esophagus, stomach, or first part of the small intestine (duodenum)	Pain that <ul><li>Is steady and mild or moderately severe</li><li>Is usually located just below the breastbone</li><li>May awaken the person during the night and/or be relieved by eating</li></ul>	Upper GI endoscopy (examination of esophagus, stomach, and duodenum using a flexible viewing tube called an endoscope) Sometimes angiography (x-rays taken after injecting a dye that can be seen on x-rays into an artery through a catheter)
Esophageal varices (varicose veins of the esophagus)	Usually very heavy bleeding Often in people known to have chronic liver disease such as cirrhosis Sometimes signs of chronic liver disease such as a swollen abdomen and yellowish discoloration of the skin and whites of the eyes (jaundice)	Upper GI endoscopy
Mallory-Weiss tear (a tear in the esophagus caused by vomiting)	In people who vomited one or more times before they started vomiting blood Sometimes pain in the lower chest during vomiting	Upper GI endoscopy
Abnormal growths in blood vessels (such as angiomas)	Sometimes pink, red, purple, or reddish brown patches on the skin around or inside the mouth	Upper GI endoscopy
Abnormal connections between the arteries and veins (arteriovenous malformations) in the intestine	Usually no other symptoms	Upper GI endoscopy
Lower digestive tract (indicated by passing blood in the stool)		
Anal fissures	Pain during bowel movements Bright red blood only on toilet paper or on the surface of formed stools Fissure seen during the doctor's examination	A doctor's examination
Abnormal blood vessels (angiodysplasia) in the intestine	Painless, bright red blood from the rectum (hematochezia)	Colonoscopy (examination of the entire large intestine, rectum, and anus using an endoscope)
Inflammation of the large intestine due to radiation therapy, infection, or disruption of the blood supply (as occurs in ischemic colitis)	Bloody diarrhea, fever, and abdominal pain	Colonoscopy
Colon cancer	Sometimes fatigue, weakness, and/or a bloating sensation Usually in middle-aged or older people	Colonoscopy and biopsy (examination of tissue samples taken from the lining of the intestine) *(continued)*

SOME CAUSES AND FEATURES OF GASTROINTESTINAL BLEEDING *(continued)*

Cause*	Common Features†	Tests
Colon polyps	Often no other symptoms	Colonoscopy
Diverticular disease (such as diverticulosis)	Painless hematochezia Sometimes in people already known to have diverticular disease	Colonoscopy
Inflammatory bowel disease (such as ulcerative proctitis, ulcerative colitis, or Crohn disease)	Bloody diarrhea, fever, and abdominal pain and cramps Sometimes in people who have had several episodes of bleeding from the rectum	Colonoscopy and biopsy
Internal hemorrhoids	Bright red blood only on toilet paper or on the surface of formed stools	Anoscopy (examination of the anus and rectum with a short, rigid tube) or sigmoidoscopy

*Causes are listed in order from the most common to the least.
†Features include symptoms and the results of the doctor's examination. Features mentioned are typical but not always present.
GI = gastrointestinal.

thromboplastin time (PTT), and tests of liver function, all of which help detect problems with blood clotting. Doctors often do not do blood tests on people who have minor bleeding caused by hemorrhoids.

If the person has vomited blood or dark material (which may represent partially digested blood), the doctor passes a small, hollow plastic tube through the person's nose down into the stomach (nasogastric tube) and suctions out the stomach contents. Bloody or pink contents indicate active upper GI bleeding, and dark or coffee-ground material indicates that bleeding is slow or has stopped. Sometimes, there is no sign of blood even though the person was bleeding very recently. A nasogastric tube may be inserted in anyone who has not vomited but has passed a large amount of blood from the rectum (if not from an obvious hemorrhoid) because this blood may have originated in the upper digestive tract. The nasogastric tube is usually left in place until it is clear that all bleeding has stopped.

If the nasogastric tube reveals signs of active bleeding, or the person's symptoms strongly suggest the bleeding is originating in the upper digestive tract, the doctor usually does upper endoscopy. Upper endoscopy is a visual examination of the esophagus, stomach, and the first segment of the small intestine (duodenum) using a flexible tube called an endoscope. An upper endoscopy allows the doctor to see the bleeding source and often treat it.

People with symptoms typical of hemorrhoids may need only sigmoidoscopy (examination of the lower part of the large intestine, the rectum, and anus using an endoscope). All other people with hematochezia should have colonoscopy (examination of the entire large intestine, the rectum, and the anus using an endoscope).

Rarely, endoscopy (both upper and lower) and colonoscopy do not show the cause of bleeding. There are still other options for finding the source of the bleeding. Doctors may do a small-bowel follow-through, which is a series of detailed x-rays of the small intestine. Doctors may do endoscopy of the small bowel (enteroscopy). If bleeding is rapid or severe, doctors sometimes do angiography. During angiography, doctors use a catheter to inject an artery with a dye that can be seen on x-rays. Angiography helps doctors diagnose upper digestive tract bleeding and allows them to do certain treatments (such as embolization and vasoconstrictor infusion). Doctors may also inject the person with red blood cells labeled with a radioactive marker (radionuclide scanning). With the use of a special scanning camera, the radioactive marker can sometimes show the approximate location of the bleeding.

Another option is capsule endoscopy, in which people swallow a tiny camera that takes pictures as it passes through the intestines. Capsule endoscopy is especially useful in the small intestine but it is not very useful in either the colon or stomach, because these organs are too big to get good pictures of their inner lining.

TREATMENT

There are two goals to treating people with GI bleeding:

- Replace lost blood with fluid given by vein (intravenously) and sometimes with a blood transfusion
- Stop any ongoing bleeding

Hematemesis, hematochezia, or melena should be considered an emergency. People with severe GI bleeding should be admitted to an intensive care unit and should be seen by a gastroenterologist and a surgeon.

FLUID REPLACEMENT

People with sudden, severe blood loss require intravenous fluids and sometimes an emergency blood transfusion to stabilize their condition. People with blood clotting abnormalities may require transfusion of platelets or fresh frozen plasma or injections of vitamin K.

STOPPING THE BLEEDING

Most GI bleeding stops without treatment. Sometimes, however, it does not. The type and location of bleeding tells the doctors what treatment to use. For example, doctors can often stop peptic ulcer bleeding during endoscopy by using a device that uses an electrical current to produce heat (electrocautery), heater probes, laser, or injections of certain drugs (injection sclerotherapy). If endoscopy does not stop the bleeding, surgery is required.

Doctors stop bleeding of varicose veins with endoscopic banding, injection sclerotherapy, or a transjugular intrahepatic portosystemic shunting (TIPS) procedure.

Doctors can sometimes control severe, ongoing lower GI bleeding caused by diverticula or angiomas during colonoscopy by using an electrocautery device, coagulation with a heater probe, or injection with epinephrine. Polyps can be removed by a wire snare or electrocautery. If these methods do not work or are impossible, doctors do angiography during which they may pass a catheter into the bleeding vessel and then inject a chemical, fragments of a gelatin sponge, or a wire coil to block the blood vessel and thereby stop the bleeding (embolization) or inject vasopressin to reduce blood flow to the bleeding vessel. People with continued bleeding may need surgery, so it is important for doctors to know the location of the bleeding site.

Internal hemorrhoid bleeding stops spontaneously in most cases. For people whose bleeding does not stop without treatment, doctors do anoscopy and may place rubber bands around the hemorrhoids or inject them with substances that stop bleeding or do electrocautery or surgery.

ESSENTIALS FOR OLDER PEOPLE

In older people, hemorrhoids and colorectal cancer are the most common causes of minor bleeding. Peptic ulcers, diverticular disease (such as diverticulitis), and abnormal blood vessels (angiodysplasia) are the most common causes of major bleeding. Bleeding from varicose veins of the esophagus is less common than in younger people.

Older people poorly tolerate massive GI bleeding. Doctors must diagnose older people quickly, and treatment must be started sooner than in younger people, who can better tolerate repeated episodes of bleeding.

⚬━π KEY POINTS

- Rectal bleeding may result from upper or lower GI bleeding.
- Most people stop bleeding spontaneously.
- Endoscopy is usually the first choice for people whose bleeding will not stop without treatment.

HAIR LOSS
(ALOPECIA; BALDNESS)

Hair loss, also called alopecia, can occur on any part of the body. Hair loss that occurs on the scalp is generally called baldness. Hair loss is often of great concern to people for cosmetic reasons, but it can also be a sign of a bodywide (systemic) disorder.

Hair grows in cycles. Each cycle consists of a long growing phase (anagen), a brief transitional phase (catagen), and a short resting phase (telogen). At the end of the resting phase, the hair falls out, and the cycle begins again as a new hair starts growing in the follicle. Normally, about 50 to 100 scalp hairs reach the end of resting phase each day and fall out. When many more than 100 hairs/day go into resting phase, hair loss (telogen effluvium) may occur. A disruption of the growing phase causing loss of hairs is called anagen effluvium.

Doctors sometimes classify hair loss as focal (confined to one part of the scalp) or diffuse (widespread).

CAUSES

The **most common cause** of hair loss is

- Male-pattern and female-pattern hair loss (androgenetic alopecia)

Other common causes of hair loss are

- Alopecia areata
- Certain systemic disorders, such as those that cause high fever, systemic lupus erythematosus (lupus), hormonal disorders, and nutritional deficiencies
- Drugs, particularly chemotherapy
- Fungal infections, such as ringworm of the scalp (tinea capitis)
- Physical stresses, such as a high fever, surgery, a major illness, sudden weight loss, or pregnancy (which can lead to a telogen effluvium)
- Psychologic stresses, including habitual pulling out of normal hair (trichotillomania)
- Traction alopecia (hair loss caused by continuous traction such as from braids, rollers, or ponytails)

Less common causes are primary hair shaft abnormalities (that is, the abnormality originates in the hair shaft), sarcoidosis, heavy metal poisoning, radiation therapy, and rare skin conditions.

ANDROGENETIC ALOPECIA

This form of alopecia eventually affects up to 80% of white men by the age of 70 (male-pattern hair loss) and about half of all women (female-pattern hair loss). The hormone dihydrotestosterone plays a major role, along with heredity. The hair loss can begin at any age during or after puberty, even during the teenage years.

In men, hair loss usually begins at the forehead or on the top of the head toward the back. Some men lose only some hair and have only a receding hairline or a small bald spot in the back. Others, especially when hair loss begins at a young age, lose all of the hair on the top of the head but retain hair on the sides and back of the scalp. This pattern is called male-pattern hair loss.

In women, hair loss occurs on the top of the head and is usually a thinning of the hair rather than a complete loss of hair. The hairline typically stays intact. This pattern is called female-pattern hair loss.

ALOPECIA AREATA

In alopecia areata, round, irregular patches of hair are suddenly lost. The cause is believed to be an autoimmune reaction.

CUTANEOUS LUPUS

Systemic lupus erythematosus (lupus), an autoimmune disorder, affects various organs throughout the body. When the skin is affected, the disorder is called cutaneous lupus. If skin lesions affect the scalp or hair follicles, areas of hair may be lost. Hair loss may be permanent if the hair follicle is completely destroyed.

HORMONE IMBALANCE

If women have excessive amounts of male hormones, they can develop masculine characteristics (called virilization), such as a deepened voice, acne, and hair in locations more typical of

LOSING HAIR

In men, hair is usually first lost at the forehead or on the top of the head toward the back. This pattern is called male-pattern hair loss.

In women, hair is usually first lost on the top of the head. Typically, the hair thins rather than is completely lost, and the hairline stays intact. This pattern is called female-pattern hair loss.

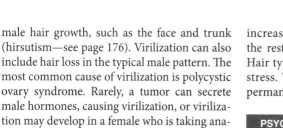

male hair growth, such as the face and trunk (hirsutism—see page 176). Virilization can also include hair loss in the typical male pattern. The most common cause of virilization is polycystic ovary syndrome. Rarely, a tumor can secrete male hormones, causing virilization, or virilization may develop in a female who is taking anabolic steroids to enhance athletic performance.

Hair loss can also occur after childbirth or during menopause.

DRUGS

Male or female-pattern baldness can occur when anabolic steroids are used. It can also occur frequently with the use of chemotherapy drugs.

NUTRITIONAL DISORDERS

Nutritional disorders are a less common cause of hair loss. Symptoms vary according to the specific nutritional disorder:

- Excess vitamin A: Rash, scaly chapped lips, painful swelling of the limbs, sluggishness, loss of appetite, and weight loss
- Iron deficiency: Anemia, with easy fatigability and a decreased ability to exercise
- Zinc deficiency: Rash, diarrhea, underdeveloped genitals, frequent infections, loss of appetite, and poor wound healing

PHYSICAL STRESSES

Stresses such as a high fever, surgery, a major illness, weight loss, or pregnancy can increase the number of hairs that go into the resting phase (causing telogen effluvium). Hair typically falls out a few months after the stress. This type of hair loss tends not to be permanent.

PSYCHOLOGIC STRESSES

These stresses include the habitual pulling out of normal hair (trichotillomania). The habit is most common among children but may occur in adults. The hair pulling may not be noticed for a long time, confusing doctors and parents, who may mistakenly think that a disorder such as alopecia areata or a fungal infection is causing the hair loss.

RINGWORM OF THE SCALP (TINEA CAPITIS)

This fungal infection is a common cause of patchy hair loss in children. The infection begins as a red patch with scaling that gradually enlarges. Hairs may eventually break off, usually flush with the scalp, looking like black dots. Sometimes parts of the hair remain above the scalp. Hair loss may be permanent, especially if the infection is left untreated.

TRACTION ALOPECIA

This disorder is hair loss caused by tight braids, rollers, or ponytails that pull constantly on hair. Hair loss most often occurs at the hairline of the forehead and temples.

EVALUATION

The following information can help people decide whether a doctor's evaluation is needed and help them know what to expect during the evaluation.

WARNING SIGNS

The following are of particular concern:

- Signs of a bodywide disorder or poisoning
- In women, development of masculine characteristics (virilization), such as a deepened voice, hair in locations more typical of male hair growth (hirsutism), irregular menstrual periods, and acne

WHEN TO SEE THE DOCTOR

People who have hair loss and signs of a bodywide disorder or poisoning should see a doctor within a day or two. Women who have developed masculine characteristics should see a doctor within a week or so. Other people should see a doctor when possible, but an appointment is not urgent unless other symptoms develop.

WHAT THE DOCTOR DOES

Doctors first ask questions about the person's symptoms and medical history and then do a physical examination. What doctors find during the history and physical examination often suggests a cause and the tests that may need to be done.

Doctors ask about the hair loss:

- Whether hair loss began gradually or suddenly
- How long it has been present
- Whether hair loss is increasing
- Whether hair is being lost over the entire head or in one specific area

They note other symptoms such as itching and scaling. They ask about hair care, including whether braids, rollers, and hair dryers are used and whether the hair is routinely pulled or twisted.

Doctors ask whether the person has been recently exposed to drugs, toxins, or radiation or has experienced significant stress (such as that from surgery, chronic illness, or fever or psychologic stress). The person is asked about other characteristics that may suggest a cause, including dramatic weight loss, dietary practices (including vegetarianism), and obsessive-compulsive behavior. Current and recent drug use is reviewed. The person is asked whether any family member has had hair loss.

During the physical examination, doctors focus on the scalp, noting the distribution of hair loss, the presence and characteristics of any skin abnormalities, and the presence of any scarring. They measure the width of the part and check for abnormalities of hair shafts.

Doctors evaluate hair loss elsewhere on the body (such as the eyebrows, eyelashes, arms, and legs). They look for rashes that may be associated with certain types of alopecia and for signs of virilization in women, such as a deepened voice, hirsutism, an enlarged clitoris (the smaller female organ that corresponds to the penis), and acne. They also examine the thyroid gland.

TESTING

Testing is usually unnecessary if a cause is identified based on the doctor's examination. For example, male-pattern and female-pattern hair loss generally requires no testing. However, if hair loss occurs in a young man with no family history of hair loss, the doctor may question him about anabolic steroid use and other drugs. If women have significant hair loss and have developed masculine characteristics, blood tests are done to measure levels of the hormones testosterone and dehydroepiandrosterone sulfate (DHEAS). If the doctor's examination detects signs of other hormonal abnormalities or other serious illness, blood tests to identify those disorders may be needed.

The **pull test** helps doctors evaluate hair loss. Doctors gently pull on a bunch of hairs (about 40) on at least 3 different areas of the scalp. Doctors then count the number of hairs that come out with each pull and examine them under a microscope to determine their phase of growth. If more than 4 to 6 hairs in the telogen phase come out with each pull, the pull test is positive, and the person most likely has telogen effluvium.

During the **pluck test,** doctors abruptly pull out about 50 individual hairs ("by the roots"). Doctors examine the roots and shafts of the plucked hairs under a microscope to assess the hair shaft and determine the phase of growth. These results help doctors tell whether the

SOME CAUSES AND FEATURES OF HAIR LOSS

Cause	Common Features*	Tests
Hair loss over the entire scalp		
Male-pattern hair loss (androgenetic alopecia)	Often a family history Sometimes a history of using anabolic steroids	A doctor's examination
Female-pattern hair loss (androgenetic alopecia)	Often a family history Sometimes occurring during menopause Sometimes in women with masculine characteristics (virilization), a history of using anabolic steroids such as dihydrotestosterone, polycystic ovary syndrome, or a tumor that produces male hormones	A doctor's examination Sometimes measurement of blood levels of the male hormones testosterone and dehydroepiandrosterone sulfate (DHEAS)
Drugs and toxins	A history of using a specific drug such as certain chemotherapy drugs, anticoagulants, retinoids, oral contraceptives, ACE inhibitors, beta-blockers, lithium, antithyroid drugs, anticonvulsants, or high doses of vitamin A or of being exposed to heavy metals	A doctor's examination
Stress (psychologic or physical) causing telogen effluvium	Psychologic symptoms Recent weight loss, surgery, severe illness with a fever, or delivery of a baby	A doctor's examination Sometimes blood tests to check for anemia and iron deficiency and to evaluate thyroid function
Thyroid disorders	With hyperthyroidism (an overactive thyroid gland), difficulty tolerating heat, sweating, weight loss, bulging eyes, shakiness (tremor), restlessness, and an enlarged thyroid gland (goiter) With hypothyroidism (an underactive thyroid gland), difficulty tolerating cold, weight gain, coarse and thick skin, and sluggishness	A doctor's examination Blood tests that evaluate thyroid function
Nutritional disorders, such as vitamin A excess or a deficiency of iron or zinc	Symptoms of the specific nutritional disorder	A doctor's examination Sometimes blood tests to check for nutritional disorders
Hair loss only in a specific area of the scalp		
Alopecia areata	Round patches of hair loss with short broken hairs (resembling exclamation points) around the edges of the patches Sometimes loss of all body hair Sometimes a burning sensation or itching	A doctor's examination

(continued)

SOME CAUSES AND FEATURES OF HAIR LOSS *(continued)*

Cause	Common Features*	Tests
Cutaneous lupus (systemic lupus erythematosus—called lupus—of the skin)	Scattered patches of hair loss Sometimes a rash on the scalp that tends to be red, raised, and scaly Sometimes areas of scarring Sometimes itching	A doctor's examination Blood tests to check for lupus[†]
Lichen planopilaris (lichen planus of the scalp)	Shiny, reddish-purplish, flat-topped bumps Scattered patches of hair loss Often areas of scarring	A doctor's examination Biopsy of the scalp
Burns, injuries, or radiation (for example, from radiation therapy)	A history of burns, radiation therapy, or injury Often scarring	A doctor's examination Sometimes other tests to check for the cause doctors suspect
Tinea capitis (ringworm of the scalp)	Bald areas with small black dots (due to hair that has broken off at the scalp surface) or hairs broken just above the scalp surface Round, scaly areas of skin, which can be red or inflamed	A doctor's examination[†] Examination of plucked hairs under a microscope and/or culture of plucked hairs Sometimes a Wood's light examination
Traction alopecia	Braids, rollers, or ponytails that are left in too long or pulled too tight	A doctor's examination[†]
Trichotillomania (compulsive hair pulling)	Typically an asymmetric, bizarre, irregular hair loss pattern Sometimes obsessive-compulsive behavior Affects women 4 times more often than men	A doctor's examination[†]

*Features include symptoms and results of the doctor's examination. Features mentioned are typical but not always present.
[†]Rarely, biopsy of the scalp is done.

person has a telogen effluvium, a primary hair shaft abnormality, or some other problem.

Daily hair counts can be done to quantify hair loss when it is not clear whether hair loss is actually excessive. Hairs lost in the first morning combing or during washing are collected in clear plastic bags daily for 14 days. The number of hairs in each bag is then recorded. Loss of more than 100 hairs/day is abnormal except after shampooing, when up to 250 hairs may be lost. Hairs may be brought in by the person for examination under a microscope.

A biopsy of the scalp skin is done if the diagnosis is not clear after a doctor's examination and other tests. A biopsy helps determine whether hair follicles are normal and can help differentiate alopecia that causes scarring (by destroying the hair follicle) from alopecia that does not. If the hair follicles are abnormal, the biopsy may indicate possible causes.

TREATMENT

Specific causes of hair loss are treated when possible. For example, antifungal drugs are used to treat scalp ringworm. Drugs that are causing hair loss are switched or stopped. Hormonal disorders can be treated with drugs or surgery, depending on the cause. Iron or zinc supplements can be given if these minerals are deficient. Cutaneous lupus and lichen planopilaris can usually be treated with corticosteroids or other drugs applied to the scalp or taken by mouth.

Traction alopecia is treated by eliminating physical traction or stress to the scalp.

Scalp ringworm is treated with antifungal drugs taken by mouth.

Trichotillomania is difficult to treat, but behavioral modification, clomipramine, or a selective serotonin reuptake inhibitor (such as fluoxetine, fluvoxamine, paroxetine, sertraline, escitalopram, or citalopram) may be useful.

Hair loss due to physical stresses such as recent weight loss, surgery, a severe illness with a fever, or delivery of a baby (telogen effluvium) is not typically treated because it tends to resolve on its own. Applying minoxidil to the scalp may be helpful for some people.

If hair does not regrow on its own, hair replacement methods can be tried, including

- Drugs
- Hair transplantation
- Wigs

DRUGS

Male-pattern and female-pattern hair loss can sometimes be treated effectively with drugs.

Minoxidil may prevent further hair loss and increase hair growth when applied directly to the scalp twice a day. Hair regrowth can take 8 to 12 months and is noticeable in only about 30 to 40% of people. The most common side effect is skin irritation, such as itching and rash.

Finasteride works by blocking the effects of male hormones on the hair follicles and is taken by mouth daily. Finasteride is not used in women who have hair loss. In men, its effectiveness at stopping hair loss and stimulating hair growth is usually evident within 6 to 8 months of treatment and increases over time. After 2 years of treatment, about 66% of men have noticeable hair regrowth. Finasteride can decrease libido, increase breast size, and

contribute to erectile dysfunction. Finasteride can also decrease prostate-specific antigen levels. Men should discuss how finasteride can affect prostate cancer screening with their doctor before they begin treatment.

The most important effect of minoxidil or finasteride may be to prevent further hair loss. The effects last only as long as the drugs are taken.

Hormonal modulators, such as birth control pills (oral contraceptives) or spironolactone, may be useful in some women, especially those who have developed masculine characteristics.

HAIR TRANSPLANTATION

Transplantation is a more permanent solution. In this procedure, hair follicles are removed from one part of the scalp and transplanted to the bald area. In a newer hair transplantation technique, only one or two hairs are transplanted at a time. Although this technique is more time-consuming, it does not require removal of large plugs of skin and allows the implants to be oriented in the same direction as the natural hair.

Another surgical option involves removing some bald parts of the scalp skin and stretching the parts that have hair over a wider area.

WIGS

Wigs often offer the best treatment for temporary hair loss (for example, that caused by chemotherapy). People undergoing chemotherapy should consult a wig maker even before therapy begins so that an appropriate wig can be ready when needed.

KEY POINTS

- Male-pattern and female-pattern hair loss is the most common type of hair loss.
- Doctors look for an underlying disorder in women with signs of virilization.
- Microscopic hair examination or scalp biopsy may be required to determine the reason for the hair loss.

In men, the amount of body hair varies greatly, but very few men are concerned enough about excess hair to see a doctor. In women, the amount of hair that is considered excessive varies depending on ethnic background and culture. Usually, excess body hair is only a cosmetic and psychologic concern. However, the cause sometimes is a serious hormonal disorder, particularly in women who develop masculine characteristics.

Hairiness can be categorized as

- Hirsutism
- Hypertrichosis

Hirsutism is excessive growth of thick or dark body hair in women in locations that are more typical of male hair growth. Such locations include the face (on the upper lip, chin, or sideburn area), torso (around the nipples or on the chest, lower abdomen, or back), and limbs (on the inner thigh). Hirsutism usually results from high levels of male hormones (androgens, such as testosterone) or from increased sensitivity to normal levels of male hormones in the body. Sometimes other masculine characteristics develop—a condition called virilization. For example, the voice deepens, muscle size increases, hair is lost from the head, the clitoris (the smaller female organ that corresponds to the penis) becomes larger, and menstruation becomes irregular or stops completely. Acne may also develop.

Hypertrichosis is an increase in the amount of hair anywhere on the body in either sex. The excess hair may grow all over the body or only in specific locations. The hair may be fine, light-colored, and downlike or thick, dark, and long. This disorder may be present at birth or develop later. Hypertrichosis that develops later can usually be treated.

CAUSES

Hair growth depends on the balance between male and female hormones. Male hormones stimulate the growth of thick, dark hair. Female hormones (such as estrogen) slow hair growth or make the hair finer and lighter-colored. Women normally produce small amounts of male hormones, and men produce small amounts of female hormones.

HIRSUTISM

Conditions that tip the hormonal balance in favor of male hormones can cause hirsutism. The balance may be tipped by excess production of male hormones. However, in hirsutism that runs in families (familial hirsutism), women's hair follicles simply appear to be more sensitive to normal levels of male hormones.

The most common cause of hirsutism is

- Polycystic ovary syndrome

There are many uncommon causes of hirsutism (see Table on pages 177 to 178):

- Pituitary, ovarian, or adrenal gland disorders that result in overproduction of male hormones
- Tumors that produce male hormones (including certain tumors of the ovaries, adrenal glands, lungs, or digestive tract)
- Use of certain drugs, such as anabolic steroids, danazol, or birth control pills (oral contraceptives) that have a high dose of progesterone
- A familial trait, most often occurring in people of Mediterranean, Middle Eastern, or South Asian descent

HYPERTRICHOSIS

Most commonly, hypertrichosis is caused by

- Certain complications of cancer (paraneoplastic syndromes)
- A drug, most commonly minoxidil, phenytoin, or cyclosporine
- A serious bodywide disorder, such as AIDS, brain disorders or injuries, undernutrition (as occurs in carbohydrate deficiencies and eating disorders including anorexia nervosa), dermatomyositis, and porphyria
- Repeated injury to and/or friction or inflammation of areas of skin (for example, an increase in hair growth that is noticed after a cast has been removed from a previously broken arm or leg)

Rarely, hypertrichosis is caused by a gene mutation. In such cases, it is usually present at birth.

EVALUATION

Doctors must determine whether the excess hair results from a disorder or is simply a cosmetic concern.

WARNING SIGNS

In women with excess body hair, certain symptoms are cause for concern:

- Development of masculine characteristics (virilization), such as a deepened voice, increased muscle size, baldness, decreased or absent menstrual periods, and acne
- Sudden appearance and rapid growth of excess hair (over weeks to months)

The sudden appearance of excess hair may suggest cancer.

WHEN TO SEE A DOCTOR

If warning signs are present, people should see a doctor promptly, within a week or so. If excess hair appears gradually without warning signs, people should see a doctor, but the visit need not be scheduled as quickly.

Typically, women without warning signs do not need to see a doctor if they have always had excess hair, they otherwise feel well, they have regular menstrual periods and no other masculine characteristics, and have family members who also have excess hair. Such women have excess body hair because it runs in their family.

WHAT THE DOCTOR DOES

Doctors first ask questions about the person's symptoms and medical history. Doctors then do a physical examination. What they find during the history and physical examination often suggests a cause and the tests that may need to be done (see Table).

Women are asked when hair began to grow excessively and where it is located, whether they have menstrual periods, and, if so, whether periods are regular. Doctors also ask whether women have had problems conceiving a child and whether any family members also have excess hair.

SOME CAUSES AND FEATURES OF HIRSUTISM

Cause	Common Features*	Tests
Adrenal gland disorders		
Development of masculine characteristics (virilization) caused by adrenal hyperplasia (enlarged adrenal glands that produce abnormally large amounts of male hormones)	The presence of masculine characteristics, such as a deepened voice, baldness, an enlarged clitoris, increased muscle size, irregular or absent menstrual periods, and acne When adrenal hyperplasia is present at birth, external genital organs that are not clearly male or female (ambiguous)	Blood and sometimes urine tests to measure hormone levels A dexamethasone suppression test (dexamethasone, taken by mouth, followed several hours later by a blood test to measure hormone levels)
Adrenal tumors (usually cancerous)	Development of masculine characteristics or Cushing syndrome, which can occur suddenly In girls who have not gone through puberty, an unusually fast increase in height or an early end of growth, resulting in a short adult height	MRI or CT
Cushing syndrome	Excess fat throughout the torso, a pad of fat between the shoulders (buffalo hump), thin arms and legs, purple streaks on the abdomen, and a large, round face (moon face)	Urine tests to measure the level of cortisol (which may be high in Cushing syndrome) Sometimes a dexamethasone suppression test Sometimes blood tests to measure the level of cortisol *(continued)*

SOME CAUSES AND FEATURES OF HIRSUTISM *(continued)*

Cause	Common Features*	Tests
No disorder present		
Familial hirsutism	Hirsutism in family members	A doctor's examination
	No other symptoms (normal menstrual cycles and no other masculine characteristics)	Blood tests to measure hormone levels (which are normal)
Ovarian disorders		
Polycystic ovary syndrome	Hirsutism that begins after puberty Development of masculine characteristics, obesity, infertility, menstrual irregularities, acne, decreased sensitivity to insulin, and darkened and thickened skin in the underarms, on the nape of the neck, and in skinfolds (acanthosis nigricans)	A doctor's examination Blood tests to measure levels of hormones, such as testosterone, luteinizing hormone, and follicle-stimulating hormone Usually ultrasonography
Tumors	Sometimes one or more of the following symptoms, which often begin suddenly: ■ Pelvic pain ■ Abdominal swelling or bloating ■ Weight loss ■ Development of other masculine characteristics	Ultrasonography Sometimes CT or MRI
Pituitary disorders		
A pituitary adenoma (a noncancerous tumor) that secretes prolactin	Production of breast milk in women who are not breastfeeding (galactorrhea) No menstrual periods Sometimes vision problems	Blood tests to measure the level of prolactin MRI of the brain
A pituitary disorder that causes Cushing disease (such as a pituitary tumor)	See Cushing syndrome, above	Blood and sometimes urine tests to measure the level of cortisol (which may be high in Cushing disease) A dexamethasone suppression test MRI of the brain
Drugs		
Androgenic drugs: ■ Anabolic steroids, including those taken to enhance athletic performance, such as testosterone products and danazol ■ Birth control pills that have a high dose of progesterone	Development of male characteristics Use of anabolic steroids (sometimes not admitted by the user)	A doctor's examination

*Features include symptoms and results of the doctor's examination. Features mentioned are typical but not always present.
CT = computed tomography; MRI = magnetic resonance imaging.

Doctors ask people about all the drugs they are taking, particularly anabolic steroids and other drugs known to cause hair growth.

During the physical examination, doctors note the pattern of hair growth and look for other masculine characteristics and for other features that suggest a cause. For example, a lump felt during the pelvic examination suggests a tumor in an ovary.

TESTING

Unless doctors confirm that the cause is use of a drug, blood tests are done to measure levels of various hormones and thus identify the cause.

Ultrasonography or computed tomography (CT) of the pelvis or both are usually done to rule out cancer, particularly if a lump is found in the pelvis or if male hormone levels are high.

If Cushing syndrome is suspected or an adrenal tumor is detected, urine tests are also done.

TREATMENT

The underlying condition is treated or corrected. For example, drugs that may cause hirsutism are stopped or changed.

Treatment for the excess hair is unnecessary unless women wish to minimize or remove it for cosmetic reasons. If excess hair growth is not related to increased levels of male hormones, physical methods are used to remove the hair. If increased levels of male hormones are the cause, hormone therapy is needed in addition to physical methods.

PHYSICAL METHODS

Several methods are available.

Depilation removes the part of the hair above the surface of the skin. Methods include shaving and over-the-counter (OTC) creams, which may contain barium sulfate and/or calcium thioglycolate.

Epilation involves removing intact hairs with their roots. Methods to temporarily remove hairs include tweezing, plucking, waxing, and epilating devices used at home. Some methods have longer-lasting, sometimes permanent effects, but the treatments often must be repeated. These methods include electrolysis, thermolysis, and laser treatments.

HORMONAL THERAPY

Usually, hormones used to treat hirsutism must be taken a long time because most of the disorders that cause high male hormone levels cannot be cured. These hormones include birth control pills and drugs that block the effects of male hormones, such as finasteride, flutamide, or spironolactone. Women who are pregnant should not take a drug that blocks male hormones because it can cause feminine characteristics to develop in a male fetus.

Metformin, a drug used to treat diabetes, can reduce levels of testosterone, but it is less effective than other drugs. Gonadotropin-releasing hormone agonists (such as leuprolide) can be used if the ovaries are producing extremely high levels of male hormones, but use of these drugs requires close supervision by a gynecologist or an endocrinologist. Corticosteroids can be used to reduce levels of male hormones produced by adrenal gland tumors.

OTHER METHODS

Bleaching is an alternative to hair removal. It is inexpensive and works well when women have only a small amount of excess hair. Bleaches lighten the color of the hair, making it less noticeable. Several types of hair-bleaching products are available. Most contain hydrogen peroxide.

Eflornithine cream, applied twice a day, slows the rate of hair growth and, with long-term use, may increase the amount of time between hair removal treatments.

O—π KEY POINTS

- Excess body hair may run in families, and what is considered excessive may vary with ethnic background and culture.
- Hirsutism, which occurs only in women, causes excess hair to grow in a male pattern and differs from hypertrichosis, which is excess hair anywhere on the body and can occur in men or women.
- Polycystic ovary syndrome is the most common cause of hirsutism.
- If women also develop male characteristics (such as a deepened voice, increased muscle mass, scalp hair loss, or irregular or absent menstrual periods), they may have a disorder that requires prompt evaluation by a doctor.
- If excess body hair appears suddenly and grows rapidly, the cause may be cancer.
- Treatment may include hair removal and/or hormonal therapy.

HEADACHE

A headache is pain in any part of the head, including the scalp, upper neck, face, and interior of the head. Headaches are one of the most common reasons people visit a doctor. Headaches interfere with the ability to work and do daily tasks. Some people have frequent headaches. Other people hardly ever have them.

CAUSES

Although headaches can be painful and distressing, they are rarely due to a serious condition. Headaches can be divided into two types:

- Primary headaches: Not caused by another disorder
- Secondary headaches: Caused by another disorder

Primary headache disorders include migraine, cluster headache, and tension-type headache.

Secondary headaches may result from disorders of the brain, eyes, nose, throat, sinuses, teeth, jaws, ears, or neck or from a bodywide (systemic) disorder.

COMMON CAUSES

The two most common causes of headache are primary headaches:

- Tension-type (most common overall)
- Migraine

LESS COMMON CAUSES

Less often, headaches are due to a less common primary headache disorder called cluster headache or to one of the many secondary headache disorders (see Table on pages 182 to 185). Some secondary headache disorders are serious, particularly those that involve the brain, such as meningitis, a brain tumor, or bleeding within the brain (intracerebral hemorrhage).

Fever can cause headaches, as can many infections that do not specifically involve the brain. Such infections include Lyme disease, Rocky Mountain spotted fever, and influenza. Headaches also commonly occur when people stop consuming caffeine or stop taking pain relievers (analgesics) after using them for a long time (called medication overuse headache).

Contrary to what most people think, eye strain and high blood pressure (except for extremely high blood pressure) do not typically cause headaches.

EVALUATION

The following information can help people decide when a doctor's evaluation is needed and help them know what to except during the evaluation.

WARNING SIGNS

In people with headaches, certain characteristics are cause for concern:

- Changes in sensation or vision, sudden weakness, loss of coordination, seizures, difficulty speaking or understanding speech, or changes in levels of consciousness such as drowsiness or confusion (suggesting a brain disorder)
- A fever and a stiff neck that makes lowering the chin to the chest painful and sometimes impossible
- A very sudden, severe headache (thunderclap headache)
- Tenderness at the temple (as when combing hair) or jaw pain when chewing
- The presence of cancer or a disorder that weakens the immune system
- Use of a drug that suppresses the immune system
- Red eyes and halos seen around lights

WHEN TO SEE A DOCTOR

People who have any warning sign should see a doctor immediately. If a warning sign is present, headaches may be caused by a serious disorder. For example, a severe headache with a fever and a stiff neck suggests meningitis—a life-threatening infection of the fluid-filled space between the tissues covering the brain and spinal cord (meninges). A thunderclap headache may suggest a subarachnoid hemorrhage—bleeding within the meninges, which is often due to a ruptured aneurysm. Tenderness at the temple, particularly in older people who have lost weight and have muscle aches, may indicate giant cell arteritis. Headaches in people who have cancer or who have a weakened immune system (due to a disorder or drug) may be caused by meningitis or spread of cancer to the brain. Having red eyes and seeing halos around lights suggests glaucoma, which, if untreated, leads to irreversible loss of vision.

People without warning signs but with certain other symptoms require prompt evaluation within a few days to a week. These symptoms include

- Headaches that increase in frequency or severity
- Headaches that begin after age 50
- Worsening vision
- Weight loss
- A new headache that is worse when the person awakens in the morning or that awakens the person from sleep (sometimes indicating a brain tumor)

If people with none of the above symptoms or characteristics start having headaches that are different from any they have had before or if their usual headaches become unusually severe, they should call their doctor. Depending on their other symptoms, the doctor may advise taking an analgesic or ask them to come for an evaluation.

WHAT THE DOCTOR DOES

Doctors first ask questions about the person's symptoms and medical history. Doctors then do a physical examination. What they find during the history and physical examination often suggests a cause of the pain and tests that may need to be done (see Table on pages 182 to 185).

Doctors ask about the characteristics of the headache: how often it occurs, how long it lasts, where the pain is, how severe is it, whether any symptoms accompany it, and how long a sudden headache takes to reach its maximum intensity. Doctors also ask what triggers the headache, what makes it worse, and what relieves it.

Risk factors for headache are identified. They include whether people take or have stopped taking certain drugs, whether they have had a spinal tap recently, and whether they have a disorder that may account for the headache. A general physical examination is done. It focuses on the head and neck and on the brain, spinal cord, and nerves (neurologic examination).

A free website at http://promyhealth.org provides a questionnaire that can help people with headaches communicate with their doctor. The questionnaire asks many of the questions that headache specialists use to help diagnose the cause of headaches. People can fill out the questionnaire, print the results, and take them to their doctor. This approach can save people and their doctor time and help guide the evaluation.

TESTING

Most people do not need testing. However, if doctors suspect a serious disorder, tests are usually done. For some suspected disorders, tests are done as soon as possible. In other cases, testing can be done within one or more days.

Magnetic resonance imaging (MRI) or computed tomography (CT) is done immediately if people have

- A thunderclap headache
- Changes in levels of consciousness, such as drowsiness or confusion
- Swelling of the optic nerve, detected by eye examination with an ophthalmoscope
- Symptoms that suggest a brain disorder, such as changes in sensation or vision, sudden weakness, loss of coordination, seizures, or difficulty speaking or understanding speech
- Extremely high blood pressure

MRI (usually) or CT is done within a day or so if people have cancer or a weakened immune system (due to a disorder or a drug). MRI or CT is done within a few days if people have certain other characteristics—for example, headaches that begin after age 50, weight loss, double vision, a new headache that is worse when the person awakens in the morning or that awakens the person from sleep, and sometimes an increase in the frequency, duration, or intensity of chronic headaches.

A spinal tap (lumbar puncture) is done immediately if acute meningitis or encephalitis (a brain infection) is suspected. Sometimes doctors do CT or MRI before the spinal tap if they think that a mass (such as a tumor, an abscess, or a hematoma) may be present. A spinal tap can be dangerous if people have such a mass. Doctors

SOME CAUSES AND FEATURES OF HEADACHES

Type or Cause	Common Features*	Tests
Primary headache (*not* due to another disorder)		
Cluster	A severe, piercing headache that ■ Affects one side of the head and is focused around the eye ■ Lasts 30 to 180 minutes ■ Occurs at the same time of day ■ Occurs in clusters, separated by periods of time when no headaches occur ■ Is usually not worsened by light, sounds, or odors ■ Is not accompanied by vomiting Inability to lie down and restlessness (sometimes expressed by pacing) On the same side as the pain: A runny nose, tearing, drooping of the eyelid, and sometimes swelling of the area below the eye	Occasionally CT or MRI of the head to rule out other disorders, particularly if the headaches have developed recently or if the pattern of symptoms has changed
Migraine	A moderate to severe headache that ■ Is typically pulsating or throbbing, usually on one side but sometimes on both sides of the head ■ Lasts several hours to days ■ Can occur frequently for a long time, then disappear for weeks, months, or years ■ May be triggered by exertion, lack of sleep, a head injury, hunger, or certain wines and foods ■ Is lessened with sleep ■ May be accompanied by nausea, vomiting, and sensitivity to loud sounds, bright light, and/or odors Often a sensation that a migraine is beginning (called a prodrome), which may include mood changes, loss of appetite, and nausea Sometimes preceded by temporary disturbances in sensation, balance, muscle coordination, speech, or vision, such as seeing flashing lights and having blind spots (these symptoms are called the aura)	Same as those for cluster headaches
Tension-type	Usually a mild to moderate headache that ■ Feels like tightening of a band around the head ■ Affects the whole head ■ Lasts 30 minutes to several days ■ May be worse at the end of the day ■ Is not worsened by physical activity, light, sounds, or odors ■ Is not accompanied by nausea, vomiting, or any other symptoms	Same as those for cluster headaches *(continued)*

SOME CAUSES AND FEATURES OF HEADACHES *(continued)*

Type or Cause	Common Features*	Tests
Secondary headache (due to another disorder)		
Altitude illness	Light-headedness, loss of appetite, nausea and vomiting, fatigue, weakness, irritability, or difficulty sleeping In people who have recently gone to a high altitude (including flying 6 hours or more in an airplane)	A doctor's examination
Brain tumor, abscess, or another mass in the brain, such as a hematoma (an accumulation of blood)	A mild to severe headache that ■ May become progressively worse ■ Worsens when a person lies down and may awaken a person from sleep ■ Usually recurs more and more often and eventually becomes constant without relief ■ May result in blurred vision when a person suddenly changes position ■ May be accompanied by clumsiness, weakness, confusion, nausea, vomiting, seizures, or impaired vision	MRI or CT
Carbon monoxide exposure (during winter, people may breathe this gas if heating equipment is not adequately vented)	Possibly no awareness of the exposure because carbon monoxide is colorless and odorless	A blood test
Dental infections (in upper teeth)	Pain that is ■ Usually felt over the face and mostly on one side ■ Worse when chewing Toothache	Dental examination
Encephalitis (infection of the brain)	Headaches with varying characteristics Often accompanied by fever, worsening drowsiness, confusion, agitation, weakness, and/or clumsiness Seizures and coma	MRI or CT and a spinal tap
Giant cell (temporal) arteritis	A throbbing pain felt on one side of the head at the temple Pain when combing the hair or while chewing Sometimes enlarged arteries in the temples (temporal arteries) and aches and pains, particularly in the shoulders, thighs, and hips Possibly impaired vision or loss of vision More common among people over 60	A blood test to measure the erythrocyte sedimentation rate (ESR), which can detect inflammation Biopsy of the temporal artery

(continued)

SOME CAUSES AND FEATURES OF HEADACHES *(continued)*

Type or Cause	Common Features*	Tests
Glaucoma—a type called closed-angle glaucoma—that starts abruptly (acute)	Moderate or severe pain that ■ Occurs at the front of the head or in or over an eye ■ May begin when the person is in a dark room Red eyes, halos seen around lights, nausea, and loss of vision	An eye examination as soon as possible
Head injury (postconcussion syndrome)	Headache that begins immediately or shortly after a head injury (with or without loss of consciousness) Sometimes a faulty memory, personality changes, or both	CT or MRI with normal results
Idiopathic intracranial hypertension (increased pressure within the skull without any evidence of a cause)	Headaches that ■ Occur daily or almost daily, with fluctuating intensity ■ Affect both sides of the head Sometimes nausea or ringing in the ears that occurs in time with the pulse	MRI and magnetic resonance venography, followed by a spinal tap
Intracerebral hemorrhage	Mild or severe pain that ■ Begins suddenly ■ Occurs on one or both sides of the head ■ Is accompanied often by nausea and sometimes by vomiting Possibly severe drowsiness, clumsiness, weakness, difficulty speaking or understanding speech, loss of vision, loss of sensation, or confusion Occasionally seizures or coma	CT or MRI
Medication overuse headache	Chronic and often daily headaches Often in people who have migraine or tension-type headaches Overuse of pain relievers (analgesics such as NSAIDs or opioids), barbiturates, caffeine, or sometimes triptans or other drugs to treat headaches	A doctor's examination
Meningitis	A severe, constant headache Fever Neck stiffness that makes lowering the chin to the chest painful and sometimes impossible A feeling of illness, drowsiness, nausea, or vomiting	A spinal tap (often preceded by CT)
Obstructive sleep apnea	Headaches that occur in the morning Snoring with episodes of gasping or choking, typically after pauses in breathing during sleep Daytime sleepiness	A doctor's examination Sleep laboratory evaluation with polysomnography *(continued)*

SOME CAUSES AND FEATURES OF HEADACHES (continued)

Type or Cause	Common Features*	Tests
Sinusitis	Pain that ■ Is sometimes felt in the face, at the front of the head, or as tooth pain ■ May begin suddenly and last only days or hours or begin gradually and be persistent ■ Is worse when facing the floor A runny nose, sometimes with pus or blood A feeling of illness, possibly a cough at night, and often a fever	Possibly CT of the sinuses or endoscopy of the nose
Subarachnoid hemorrhage (bleeding between the inner and middle layers of tissues covering the brain)	Severe, constant pain that ■ Begins suddenly and peaks within a few seconds (thunderclap headache) ■ Is often described as the worst headache ever experienced Possibly brief loss of consciousness as the headache begins Possibly drowsiness, confusion, difficulty being aroused, or coma A stiff neck, nausea and vomiting, dizziness, and low back pain	MRI or CT If MRI or CT results are negative or inconclusive, a spinal tap
Subdural hematoma (a pocket of blood between the outer and middle layers of tissues covering the brain)	Headaches with varying characteristics Possibly sleepiness, confusion, forgetfulness, and/or weakness or paralysis on one side of the body	MRI or CT
Temporomandibular disorders	Pain when chewing hard foods Sometimes pain in or around the jaw or in the neck Sometimes clicking or popping when the mouth is opened, locking of the jaw, or difficulty opening the mouth wide	Physical examination Occasionally MRI, x-rays, or CT

*Features include symptoms and results of the doctor's examination. Features mentioned are typical but not always present.
CT = computed tomography; MRI = magnetic resonance imaging; NSAIDs = nonsteroidal anti-inflammatory drugs.

also do a spinal tap if people have a thunderclap headache (suggesting subarachnoid hemorrhage) and the results of CT or MRI are normal.

Other tests are done within hours or days, depending on the examination results and the causes that are suspected (see Table).

TREATMENT

Treatment depends on the cause. If the headache is a tension headache or if it accompanies a minor viral infection, people can take acetaminophen or a nonsteroidal anti-inflammatory drug (NSAID).

ESSENTIALS FOR OLDER PEOPLE

If headaches begin after age 50, doctors usually assume they result from another disorder until proved otherwise. Disorders that cause headaches, such as giant cell arteritis, brain tumors, and subdural hematomas (which may result from falls), are more common among older people.

Treatment of headaches may be limited in older people. They are more likely to have disorders that prevent them from taking some of the drugs used to treat migraines and cluster headaches (triptans and dihydroergotamine). These disorders include angina, coronary artery disease, and uncontrolled high blood pressure. If older people need to take drugs to treat headaches that can have sedating effects, they must be monitored closely.

O—π KEY POINTS

- Most headaches do not have a serious cause, particularly if the headaches began at a young age, if they have not changed over time, and if results of the examination are normal.
- If warning signs are present, people should see a doctor.
- Most headaches do not require testing.
- Doctors can usually determine the type or cause of headaches based on the medical history, symptoms, and results of a physical examination.
- If doctors suspect that the cause is a serious disorder (such as a hemorrhage or an infection), CT or MRI is done, often immediately.
- If doctors suspect meningitis or encephalitis, a spinal tap is done.

HEARING LOSS

Overall, about 10% of people in the United States have some degree of hearing loss. The incidence increases with age. Although less than 2% of children under 18 have a permanent hearing loss, hearing loss during infancy and early childhood can be detrimental to language and social development. Over one third of people over 65 years and over half of people over age 75 are affected.

Most hearing loss develops slowly over time. However, sudden deafness (see page 194) occurs in about 1 in 5,000 people each year in the United States.

CAUSES

Hearing loss has many causes (see Table on pages 189 to 190). Different parts of the hearing pathway can be affected, and loss is classified as conductive, sensorineural, or mixed, depending on the part of the pathway that is affected.

Conductive hearing loss occurs when something blocks sound from reaching the sensory structures in the inner ear. The problem may involve the external ear canal, the eardrum (tympanic membrane—TM), or the middle ear.

Sensorineural hearing loss occurs when sound reaches the inner ear, but either sound cannot be translated into nerve impulses (sensory loss) or nerve impulses are not carried to the brain (neural loss). The distinction between sensory and neural loss is important because sensory hearing loss is sometimes reversible and is seldom life threatening. A neural hearing loss rarely goes away and may be due to a potentially life-threatening brain tumor—commonly a cerebellopontine angle tumor.

Mixed loss involves both conductive and sensorineural loss. It may be caused by severe head injury, chronic infection, or one of many rare genetic disorders.

COMMON CAUSES

The **most common causes** overall are

- Earwax (cerumen) accumulation
- Noise
- Aging
- Ear infections (particularly among children and young adults)

Earwax accumulation is the most common cause of treatable hearing loss, especially among older people.

Noise can cause sudden or gradual sensorineural hearing loss. Exposure to a single, extreme noise (such as a nearby gunshot or explosion) can cause a sudden hearing loss referred to as acoustic trauma. Some people with acoustic trauma also have ringing or buzzing in the ears (tinnitus). Hearing loss from acoustic trauma usually goes away within a day (unless there is also blast damage to the eardrum or middle ear). However, long-term exposure to noise causes most noise-induced hearing loss. Noise louder than about 85 decibels (dB) can cause hearing loss if exposure continues long enough. Although people vary somewhat in susceptibility to noise-induced hearing loss, nearly everyone loses some hearing if they are exposed to sufficiently intense noise for a long enough time.

Ear infections are a common cause of temporary mild to moderate hearing loss (mainly in children). Most children regain normal hearing in 3 to 4 weeks after an ear infection resolves, but a few have persistent hearing loss. Hearing loss is more likely in children who have recurring ear infections.

LESS COMMON CAUSES

Less common causes include the following:

- Autoimmune disorders
- Congenital disorders
- Drugs that damage the ear (ototoxic drugs)
- Injuries
- Tumors

EVALUATION

The following information can help people decide when to see a doctor and know what to expect during the evaluation.

WARNING SIGNS

In people with hearing loss, certain symptoms and characteristics are cause for concern. They include

MEASUREMENT OF LOUDNESS

Loudness is measured on a logarithmic scale. This means that an increase of 10 decibels (dB) represents a 10-fold increase in sound intensity and a doubling of the perceived loudness. Thus, 20 dB is 100 times the intensity of 0 dB and seems 4 times as loud; 30 dB is 1,000 times the intensity of 0 dB and seems 8 times as loud.

Decibels	Example
0	Faintest sound heard by human ear
30	Whisper, quiet library
60	Normal conversation, sewing machine, or typewriter
90	Lawnmower, shop tools, or truck traffic (8 hours per day is the maximum exposure without protection*)
100	Chainsaw, pneumatic drill, or snowmobile (2 hours per day is the maximum exposure without protection)
115	Sandblasting, loud rock concert, or automobile horn (15 minutes per day is the maximum exposure without protection)
140	Gun muzzle blast or jet engine (noise causes pain, and even brief exposure injures unprotected ears, and injury may occur even with hearing protectors)
180	Rocket launching pad

*This level is the mandatory federal standard, but protection is recommended for anything more than very brief exposure to sound levels above 85 dB.

- Hearing loss in only one ear
- Any neurologic abnormalities (such as difficulty chewing or speaking, numbness of the face, dizziness, or loss of balance)

WHEN TO SEE A DOCTOR

People with warning signs should see a doctor right away. People with hearing loss and no warning signs should see their doctor at some point, but a delay of a week or so is not harmful.

Because people may not notice gradual hearing loss, doctors recommend routine screening hearing tests for children and older people. Childhood screening should begin at birth so that hearing deficits can be found and treated before they interfere with language development. Screening of older people should be done routinely by asking questions that seek evidence of impaired communication. Such screening is important because some older people who might benefit from treatment do not realize or even deny they have a hearing problem.

WHAT THE DOCTOR DOES

Doctors first ask questions about the person's symptoms and medical history. Doctors then do a physical examination. What they find during the history and physical examination may suggest a cause of the hearing loss and the tests that may need to be done (see Table on pages 189 to 190).

Doctors ask how long people have noticed hearing loss, whether the loss is in one or both ears, and whether the loss followed any sudden event (for example, a head injury, sudden change in pressure, or starting of a drug). It is also important for them to note

- Ear symptoms such as pain or fullness, tinnitus, or discharge
- Balance symptoms such as disorientation in the dark or a false sensation of spinning or moving (vertigo)
- Neurologic symptoms such as headache, weakness of the face, or an abnormal sense of taste

In children, important associated symptoms include delays in speech or language development and delayed motor development.

Doctors explore people's medical history for disorders that might cause hearing loss, including repeated ear infections, chronic exposure to loud noise, head injury, and autoimmune disorders such as rheumatoid arthritis and systemic lupus erythematosus. Doctors note whether people have a family history of hearing loss. Doctors also ask people whether they are taking drugs that can damage the ear (ototoxic drugs—see Table on page 189).

The physical examination focuses on the ears and hearing and the neurologic examination.

SOME CAUSES AND FEATURES OF HEARING LOSS

Cause*	Common Features†	Tests‡
External ear (conductive loss)		
Obstruction (as caused by wax, a foreign object [body], an outer ear infection, or, rarely, a tumor)	Visible during a doctor's examination	A doctor's examination
Middle ear (conductive loss)		
Middle ear infection (acute or chronic)	Sometimes dizziness, pain or fullness in the ear, or a discharge from the ear Usually an eardrum that looks abnormal (seen during a doctor's examination) Often many previous ear infections	A doctor's examination
Ear trauma§	Often visible perforation of the eardrum, blood behind the eardrum, or both In a person with an obvious recent injury	A doctor's examination
Tumors (cancerous or not)	Often visible tumor during a doctor's examination Hearing loss in only one ear	CT or MRI
Inner ear (sensory loss)		
Genetic disorders	Often family members with similar hearing loss Sometimes a white forelock of hair or different colored eyes (as occurs in Waardenburg syndrome)	A doctor's examination Genetic testing CT of the inner ear
Noise exposure	Usually apparent by history Possibly temporary hearing loss	A doctor's examination
Presbycusis	Older age (over 55 in men and over 65 in women) Progressive loss of hearing in both ears Normal neurologic examination	A doctor's examination
Drugs that can damage the ear (ototoxic drugs), such as ■ Aspirin ■ Aminoglycosides ■ Vancomycin ■ Cisplatin ■ Furosemide ■ Ethacrynic acid ■ Quinine	In a person who recently used a causative drug Hearing loss in both ears Sometimes dizziness and loss of balance	A doctor's examination
Infections, such as ■ Meningitis ■ An inner ear infection that produces pus	Obvious history of infection Hearing loss during or shortly after an infection	A doctor's examination
Autoimmune disorders such as ■ Rheumatoid arthritis ■ Systemic lupus erythematosus (lupus)	Joint pains and a rash Sometimes a sudden change in vision or eye irritation Often in a person known to have the disorder	Blood tests

(continued)

SOME CAUSES AND FEATURES OF HEARING LOSS *(continued)*

Cause*	Common Features†	Tests‡
Meniere disease	Episodes of hearing loss (typically in only one ear) Sometimes ringing or buzzing in the ear (tinnitus) and/or a false sensation of spinning or moving (vertigo)	MRI using a contrast agent (gadolinium)
Pressure changes (as may occur during diving)§	Occurring during an activity that causes abrupt changes in pressure or after a blow to the ear Sometimes severe ear pain or vertigo	Tympanometry and balance testing If vertigo persists, surgery to look for the cause
Head injury (often with fracture of the base of the skull)§	In a person with an obvious recent severe injury Possibly dizziness or drooping facial muscles Sometimes fluid (bloody, blood-tinged, or clear) coming from the affected ear or blood behind the eardrum	CT or MRI
Nervous system (neural loss)		
Tumors, such as ■ Acoustic neuroma (an auditory nerve tumor) ■ Meningioma (a spinal cord tumor)	Hearing loss in only one ear, often with tinnitus Often dizziness or vertigo, trouble with balance Sometimes drooping facial muscles and/or numbness of the face and taste abnormalities	MRI using a contrast agent
Demyelinating disorders, such as multiple sclerosis	Hearing loss in only one ear Sometimes weakness or numbness that comes and goes and that occurs in different parts of the body	MRI using a contrast agent Sometimes a spinal tap (lumbar puncture)

*Each group is listed in approximate order of frequency.
†Features include symptoms and the results of the doctor's examination. Features mentioned are typical but not always present.
‡All patients should have audiologic testing.
§Mixed conductive and sensorineural loss may be present.
CT = computed tomography; MRI = magnetic resonance imaging.

Doctors inspect the external ear for obstruction, infection, malformations that are present at birth (congenital), and other visible abnormalities. The eardrum is examined for tears (perforations), drainage, and signs of acute or chronic infection. Doctors often do several tests using a tuning fork to differentiate conductive from sensorineural hearing loss.

TESTING

Testing includes

■ Audiologic tests
■ Sometimes MRI or CT

Doctors perform audiologic tests on all people who have hearing loss. Audiologic tests help doctors understand the type of hearing loss and determine what other testing may be needed.

Audiometry is the first step in hearing testing. In this test, a person wears headphones that play tones of different frequency (pitch) and loudness into one ear or the other. The person signals when a tone is heard, usually by raising the corresponding hand. For each pitch, the test identifies the quietest tone the person can hear in each ear. The results are presented in comparison to what is considered normal hearing. Because loud tones presented to one ear may also be heard by the other ear, a sound other than the test tone (usually white noise) is presented to the ear not being tested.

Speech threshold audiometry measures how loudly words have to be spoken to be understood. A person listens to a series of two-syllable, equally accented words (spondees), such as "railroad," "stairway," and "baseball," presented at different volumes. The volume at which the person can correctly repeat half of the words (spondee threshold) is recorded.

Discrimination, the ability to hear differences between words that sound similar, is tested by presenting pairs of similar one-syllable words. The percentage of words correctly repeated is the discrimination score. People with a conductive hearing loss usually have a normal discrimination score, although at a higher volume. People with sensorineural hearing loss may have abnormal discrimination at all volumes. Doctors sometimes test people's ability to recognize words within full sentences. This test helps decide which people who do not have acceptable results with a hearing aid might benefit from an implanted device.

Tympanometry tests how well sound can pass through the eardrum and middle ear. This test does not require the active participation of the person being tested and is commonly used in children. A device containing a microphone and a sound source is placed snugly in the ear canal, and sound waves are bounced off the eardrum as the device varies the pressure in the ear canal. Abnormal tympanometry results suggest a conductive type of hearing loss.

Tuning fork tests can help distinguish between conductive and sensorineural hearing loss. The **Rinne test** compares how well a person hears sounds conducted by air with how well the person hears sounds conducted by the skull bones. To test hearing by air conduction, the tuning fork is placed near the ear. To test hearing by bone conduction, the base of a vibrating tuning fork is placed against the head so the sound bypasses the middle ear and goes directly to the nerve cells of the inner ear. If hearing by air conduction is reduced but hearing by bone conduction is normal, the hearing loss is conductive. If both air and bone conduction hearing are reduced, the hearing loss is sensorineural or mixed. People

with sensorineural hearing loss may need further evaluation to look for other conditions, such as Meniere disease or brain tumors. In the **Weber test,** the stem of a vibrating tuning fork is placed on the top of the head in the middle. The person indicates in which ear the tone is louder. In one-sided conductive hearing loss, the tone is louder in the ear with hearing loss. In one-sided sensorineural hearing loss, the tone is louder in the normal ear because the tuning fork stimulates both inner ears equally and the person hears the stimulus with the unaffected ear.

Auditory brain stem response is a test that measures nerve impulses in the brain stem resulting from sound signals in the ears. The information helps determine what kind of signals the brain is receiving from the ears. Test results are abnormal in people with some sensorineural types of hearing loss and in people with many types of brain tumors. Auditory brain stem response is used to test infants and also can be used to monitor certain brain functions in people who are comatose or undergoing brain surgery.

Electrocochleography measures the activity of the cochlea and the auditory nerve by means of an electrode placed on, or through, the eardrum. This test and the auditory brain stem response can be used to measure hearing in people who cannot or will not respond voluntarily to sound. For example, these tests are used to find out whether infants and very young children have profound hearing loss (deafness) and whether a person is faking or exaggerating hearing loss (psychogenic hypacusis).

Otoacoustic emissions testing uses sound to stimulate the inner ear (cochlea). The ear itself then generates a very low-intensity sound that matches the stimulus. These cochlear emissions are recorded using sophisticated electronics and are used routinely in many nurseries to screen newborns for congenital hearing loss and to monitor the hearing of people who are using ototoxic drugs. This test is also used in adults to help determine the reason for a hearing loss.

Other tests can measure the ability to interpret and understand distorted speech, understand a message presented to one ear when a competing message is presented to the other ear, fuse incomplete messages to each ear into a meaningful message, and determine where a sound is coming from when it is presented to both ears at the same time. People who have an abnormal neurologic examination or who have certain findings on audiologic tests also need a gadolinium-enhanced MRI of the head. This type of MRI can help doctors detect certain disorders of the inner ear, brain tumors near the ear, or tumors in the nerves coming from the ear.

PREVENTION

Limiting exposure to loud noise can help prevent hearing loss. Both the duration and intensity of noise should be limited. People regularly exposed to loud noise must wear ear protectors (such as plastic plugs in the ear canals or glycerin-filled muffs over the ears). The Occupational Safety and Health Administration (OSHA) of the U.S. Department of Labor and similar agencies in many other countries have standards regarding the length of time that people can be exposed to noise. The louder the noise, the shorter is the permissible time of exposure.

TREATMENT

Any cause of hearing loss is treated. For example, doctors remove benign or cancerous growths. When possible, they stop giving ototoxic drugs (unless the need for the drug outweighs the risk of additional hearing loss).

Many causes of hearing loss have no cure, and treatment involves compensating for the hearing loss with hearing aids and various coping mechanisms.

COPING MECHANISMS

Alerting systems that use light let people with hearing loss know when the doorbell is ringing, a smoke detector is sounding, or a baby is crying. Special sound systems transmitting infrared or FM radio signals help people hear in theaters, churches, or other places where competing noise exists. Many television programs carry closed captioning. Telephone communication devices are also available.

People with profound hearing loss often communicate by using sign language. American Sign Language (ASL) is the most common version in the United States. Other forms include Signed English, Signing Exact English, and Cued Speech.

TREATMENT IN CHILDREN

In addition to having any cause treated and hearing aids provided, children with hearing loss require support of language development with appropriate therapy. Because children must be able to hear language to learn it spontaneously, most deaf children develop language only with special training. Ideally, this training begins as soon as the hearing loss is identified. An exception would be a deaf child growing up with deaf parents who are fluent sign language users. Deaf infants also need a way to communicate before they learn to speak. For example, a sign language that is tailored to infants can provide a foundation for later development of spoken language if a cochlear implant is not available. However, for children, there is no substitute for access to the sounds of speech (phonemes) to enable a refined and nuanced understanding of speech and language.

A cochlear implant may be helpful for infants as young as 1 month of age who have profound hearing loss in both ears and who cannot hear sounds with a hearing aid. Although cochlear implants help many children with either congenital or acquired deafness hear, they are more effective in children who already have developed language. Sometimes the inner ear hardens into bone (ossifies) in children who become deaf after having meningitis. In such cases, cochlear implants should be used early to maximize effectiveness. Children whose acoustic nerves have been destroyed by tumors may be helped by having electrodes implanted in the base of the brain (brain stem) as well. Children with cochlear implants may have a slightly greater risk of meningitis than children without cochlear implants or adults with cochlear implants.

Children who are deaf in only one ear should be allowed to use a special system in the classroom, such as an FM auditory trainer. With these systems, the teacher speaks into a microphone that sends signals to a hearing aid in the child's normal ear. This process improves the child's greatly impaired ability to hear speech against a noisy background.

ESSENTIALS FOR OLDER PEOPLE

Older people typically have a progressive decrease in hearing, called presbycusis. Hearing impairment is present in over one third of people over 65 and in over half of those over 75. Even so, doctors should evaluate older people with hearing loss because the cause may not be aging. Some people may have a tumor, a neurologic or autoimmune disorder, or an easily correctable cause of hearing loss.

Even mild hearing loss makes understanding speech difficult and causes older people with hearing loss to exhibit certain common behaviors. An older person with mild hearing loss may avoid conversations. Understanding speech may be particularly difficult if there is background noise or more than one person is talking, such as in a restaurant or at a family gathering. Constantly asking others to talk louder can frustrate both the listener and the speaker. People with hearing loss may misunderstand a question and give an apparently bizarre answer, leading others to believe they are confused. They may misjudge the loudness of their own speech and thus shout, discouraging others from conversing with them. Thus, hearing loss can lead to social isolation, inactivity, loss of social support, and depression. In a person with dementia, hearing loss can make communicating even more difficult. For people affected by dementia, correcting a hearing loss makes dementia easier to cope with. Correcting hearing loss has clear physical and psychosocial health benefits.

PRESBYCUSIS

Presbycusis is age-related hearing loss. It probably results from a combination of age-related deterioration and the effects of a lifetime of noise exposure.

Hearing loss usually affects the highest sound frequencies first, usually beginning at about age 55 to 65 (sometimes sooner). The loss of high-frequency hearing makes speech particularly hard to understand, even when the overall loudness of speech seems normal. That is because certain consonants (such as C, D, K, P, S, T) are high-frequency sounds. These consonant sounds are the most important for speech recognition. For example, when the words "shoe," "blue," "true," "too," or "new" are spoken, many people with presbycusis can hear the "oo" sound, but they cannot recognize which word has been spoken because they cannot distinguish the consonants. Affected people typically think the speaker is mumbling. A speaker attempting to speak louder usually accentuates vowel sounds (which are low frequency), doing little to improve speech recognition. Excessive background noise makes speech comprehension particularly difficult.

SCREENING

Screening older people for hearing loss is important because many do not notice it themselves. Family members or doctors can ask the person a series of questions:

- Does a hearing problem cause you to feel embarrassed when you meet people?
- Does a hearing problem cause you to feel frustrated when talking to a family member?
- Do you have difficulty hearing when someone whispers?
- Do you feel handicapped by a hearing problem?
- Does a hearing problem cause you difficulty when visiting friends, relatives, or neighbors?
- Does a hearing problem cause you to attend religious services less often than you would like?
- Does a hearing problem cause you to have arguments with family members?
- Does a hearing problem cause you difficulty when listening to the television or radio?
- Do you feel that any difficulty with your hearing hampers your personal or social life?
- Does a hearing problem cause you difficulty when in a restaurant with relatives or friends?

For each question, a "no" answer = 0 points, "sometimes" = 2 points, and "yes" = 4 points. A score over 10 suggests significant hearing loss, and follow up with a hearing specialist is recommended.

⚬—π KEY POINTS

- Earwax, infections, aging, and noise exposure are the most common causes of hearing loss.
- All people with hearing loss should have audiologic testing.
- People with neurologic symptoms (such as dizziness or vertigo) usually should undergo imaging tests.

HEARING LOSS: SUDDEN DEAFNESS

Sudden deafness is severe or complete hearing loss that develops over a few hours or is noticed on awakening. Such hearing loss typically affects only one ear (unless the cause is a drug). Depending on the cause of sudden deafness, people may have other symptoms such as ringing in the ears (tinnitus), dizziness, or a false sensation of spinning or moving (vertigo). About 1 in 5,000 people each year develop sudden deafness. For hearing loss that develops gradually, see page 187.

CAUSES

Causes of sudden deafness fall into three general categories:

- An unknown cause
- An obvious explanatory event (such as a brain infection or head injury)
- An underlying disorder that has caused few or no other symptoms

UNKNOWN CAUSE

In most people, no cause can be found for their sudden deafness. However, doctors have several theories. Possible causes include viral infections (particularly infections with herpes simplex virus), an attack on the inner ear or its nerves by the body's immune system (autoimmune reaction), and blockage of the small blood vessels of the inner ear or the blood vessels of its nerves. Perhaps different causes affect different people.

OBVIOUS EVENT

In many other people, a cause for the sudden deafness is obvious. Such causes include

- Head injury
- Severe pressure change
- Drugs that damage the inner ear (ototoxic drugs)
- Infections

Head injury (such as a fracture of the temporal bone in the skull or sometimes a severe concussion without a fracture) can damage the inner ear and cause sudden hearing loss.

Severe pressure changes (such as those that can occur with diving or less often by bearing down during weightlifting) can cause a hole (fistula) to form between the middle and inner ear. Sometimes, such a fistula is present from birth and can spontaneously cause sudden hearing loss or make the person more susceptible to hearing loss after a head injury or pressure changes.

Ototoxic drugs (see Table on page 195) are drugs that have damaging side effects to the ears. Some drugs can rapidly cause hearing loss, sometimes within a day (especially with an overdose). A few people have a rare genetic disorder that makes them more susceptible to hearing loss from the class of antibiotics called aminoglycosides.

A number of infections cause sudden deafness during or immediately after acute illness. Common infections include bacterial meningitis, Lyme disease, and many viral infections. The most common viral causes in the developed world are mumps and herpes simplex brain infection. Measles is a very rare cause because most people are immunized against the infection.

UNDERLYING DISORDERS

Sudden deafness rarely can be the first symptom of some disorders that usually have other initial symptoms. Such disorders include a tumor of the auditory nerve called acoustic neuroma, multiple sclerosis, Meniere disease, or a small stroke of the balance center of the brain (the cerebellum). Sometimes a syphilis infection reactivates in people who have HIV infection. This reactivation can cause sudden deafness.

Rarer disorders include Cogan syndrome, in which an autoimmune reaction attacks the inner ear (and also the surface of the eye); certain disorders involving blood vessel inflammation (vasculitis); and blood disorders such as Waldenström macroglobulinemia, sickle cell disease, and some forms of leukemia.

EVALUATION

The following information can help people decide when a doctor's evaluation is needed and help them know what to expect during the evaluation.

In people with sudden deafness, certain symptoms and characteristics are cause for concern. They include

- Any abnormalities of the nervous system (other than hearing loss)

Anyone with sudden deafness should see a doctor right away because some causes must be treated quickly.

Doctors first ask questions about the person's symptoms and medical history. Doctors then do a physical examination. What they find during the history and physical examination may suggest a cause of the sudden deafness and the tests that may need to be done (see Table, below).

Doctors note whether hearing loss affects one or both ears and whether a specific event such as head injury, diving injury, or infectious illness occurred. They ask about accompanying symptoms that involve the ear (such as ringing

SOME CAUSES AND FEATURES OF SUDDEN DEAFNESS

Cause	Common Features*	Tests†
Unknown		
—	Deafness in only one ear No other symptoms	MRI using a contrast agent (gadolinium)
Obvious causes		
Acute infection (such as bacterial meningitis, Lyme disease, mumps, or herpes simplex)	Deafness in one or both ears In people with a serious, acute illness Often headache and confusion With Lyme disease, deafness preceded by a typical rash and flu-like symptoms With mumps, pain in cheeks with swallowing	A doctor's examination If not already done, blood tests and a spinal tap (lumbar puncture)
Head injury	Deafness in only one ear Sometimes fluid (bloody, blood-tinged, or clear) coming from the affected ear	CT or MRI
Pressure changes (as may occur during diving)	Deafness in only one ear Sudden onset during causative activity Sometimes accompanied by an explosive sound, dizziness, or ringing in the ear	Tympanometry (placement of a device in the ear to measure how well sound passes through the ear) Electronystagmography (a test to record involuntary movements of the eye caused by a condition known as nystagmus) CT
Drugs that can damage the ear (ototoxic drugs) including - Aminoglycosides (such as gentamicin or tobramycin) - Cisplatin - Ethacrynic acid - Furosemide - Vancomycin	Deafness in both ears Sometimes dizziness and loss of balance In people who recently started taking an ototoxic drug	A doctor's examination

(continued)

SOME CAUSES AND FEATURES OF SUDDEN DEAFNESS *(continued)*

Cause	Common Features*	Tests†
Hidden disorders‡		
Acoustic neuroma (a tumor of the auditory nerve)	Deafness in only one ear	MRI using a contrast agent (gadolinium)
	Often dizziness or a false sensation of spinning or moving (vertigo) and loss of balance	
	Sometimes drooping facial muscles and/or numbness of the face and taste abnormalities	
Autoimmune disorders, such as Cogan syndrome, some blood disorders, and disorders that cause vasculitis	Deafness in one or both ears	Blood tests
	Sometimes joint pains or a rash	
Meniere disease	Deafness in only one ear in about three fourths of people	A doctor's examination
	Sometimes dizziness and/or ringing in the ear	MRI using a contrast agent (gadolinium)
Multiple sclerosis	Deafness in only one ear	MRI using a contrast agent
	Sometimes weakness or numbness that comes and goes and that occurs in different parts of the body	Sometimes a spinal tap
Stroke (affecting the cerebellum)	Deafness in only one ear	MRI using a contrast agent
	Sometimes difficulty with balance or coordination	
Reactivation of syphilis in people with HIV infection	Deafness in one or both ears	Blood tests
	Sometimes risk factors for sexually transmitted diseases (such as unprotected sex, multiple partners)	

*Features include symptoms and the results of the doctor's examination. Features mentioned are typical but not always present. Features overlap between causes.
†All people should have an audiogram.
‡Rarely, sudden deafness is the first symptom of a disorder that usually has other symptoms first. Symptoms typical of these disorders may not be present at all. However, some people disregard mild symptoms that may be discovered by the doctor through careful questioning and examination.
CT = computed tomography; MRI = magnetic resonance imaging.

in the ears or ear discharge), balance center (such as disorientation in the dark or vertigo), and other parts of the brain and nervous system (such as headache, weakness, or an abnormal sense of taste). They try to identify whether people are currently taking (or recently took) any ototoxic drugs.

The physical examination focuses on the ears and hearing and on examination of the nervous system.

TESTING

Typically, people should have an audiogram (a hearing test). Unless doctors think the problem is clearly an acute infection or drug toxicity, they usually also do gadolinium-enhanced magnetic resonance imaging (MRI), particularly when the hearing loss is greater in one ear. Other tests are done based on the likely cause (see Table). For example, people who had a head injury should have MRI. People at risk of sexually transmitted diseases should have blood tests for HIV infection and syphilis.

TREATMENT

Treatment is directed at any known cause of the sudden deafness. When the cause is unknown, many doctors try giving corticosteroids along with antiviral drugs effective against herpes simplex (such as valacyclovir or famciclovir).

When the cause is a viral infection or is unknown, about half of people regain normal hearing and the other half recover partial hearing. Improvement, if it can be achieved, usually occurs within 10 to 14 days. Recovery from an ototoxic drug varies greatly depending on the drug and the dosage. With some drugs (such as aspirin and diuretics), hearing returns within 24 hours. However, antibiotic and chemotherapy drugs often cause permanent hearing loss if safe dosages have been exceeded.

KEY POINTS

- Why sudden deafness occurs is usually unknown.
- A few people have an obvious cause (such as severe head injury or infection or use of drugs that can damage hearing).
- In a very few people, sudden deafness is the first sign of an underlying disorder.

Indigestion (dyspepsia) is pain or discomfort in the upper abdomen. People may also describe the sensation as gassiness, a sense of fullness, or gnawing or burning. The sense of fullness may occur after a small meal (early satiety), be a feeling of excessive fullness after a normal meal (postprandial fullness), or be unrelated to meals. For more about severe abdominal discomfort, see page 1.

Because dyspepsia is usually a vague, mild discomfort, many people do not seek medical care until it has been present (or coming and going) for a long time. Sometimes, dyspepsia is a more sudden, noticeable (acute) sensation.

Depending on the cause of the dyspepsia, people may have other symptoms such as a poor appetite, nausea, constipation, diarrhea, flatulence, and belching. For some people, eating makes symptoms worse. For others, eating relieves symptoms.

CAUSES

Dyspepsia has many causes, which, despite common use of the term indigestion, do not involve a problem digesting food.

Acute dyspepsia may occur briefly after ingestion of

- A large meal
- Alcohol
- Certain irritating drugs (such as bisphosphonates, erythromycin, iron, or nonsteroidal anti-inflammatory drugs [NSAIDs])

Also, some people having a heart attack or unstable angina (coronary artery ischemia) may feel only a sensation of dyspepsia, rather than chest pain (see page 31).

For recurrent dyspepsia, common causes include

- Achalasia
- Cancer (of the stomach or esophagus)
- Delayed gastric (stomach) emptying
- Drugs
- Gastroesophageal reflux disease (GERD)
- Gastritis or peptic ulcer disease
- Unknown (nonulcer dyspepsia)

Achalasia is a disorder in which the rhythmic contractions of the esophagus greatly decrease and the lower esophageal muscle does not relax normally.

Delayed gastric emptying is a situation in which food remains in the stomach for an abnormally long period of time. Delayed emptying is usually caused by a disorder (such as diabetes, a connective tissue disorder, or a neurologic disorder) that affects the nerves to the digestive tract.

Anxiety by itself does not cause dyspepsia. However, anxiety can sometimes worsen dyspepsia by increasing the person's concern about unusual or unpleasant sensations, so that minor discomfort becomes very distressing.

In many people, doctors find no abnormality during a physical examination or after looking in the esophagus and stomach with a flexible viewing tube (upper endoscopy). In such cases, called nonulcer (functional) dyspepsia, the person's symptoms may be due to an increased sensitivity to sensations in the stomach or to intestinal contractions.

EVALUATION

Not every episode of dyspepsia requires immediate evaluation by a doctor. The following information can help people decide when a doctor's evaluation is needed and help them know what to expect during the evaluation.

WARNING SIGNS

In people with dyspepsia, certain symptoms and characteristics are cause for concern. They include

- Shortness of breath, sweating, or fast heart rate accompanying an episode of dyspepsia
- Loss of appetite (anorexia)
- Nausea or vomiting
- Weight loss
- Blood in the stool
- Difficulty swallowing (dysphagia) or pain with swallowing (odynophagia)

People who have a single, sudden episode of dyspepsia should see a doctor right away, especially if their symptoms are accompanied by shortness of breath, sweating, or a fast heart rate. Such people may have acute coronary ischemia. People with chronic dyspepsia that occurs when they exert themselves but that goes away when they rest may have angina and should see a doctor within a few days.

People with dyspepsia and one or more of the other warning signs should see a doctor within a few days to a week. Those with recurrent dyspepsia and no warning signs should see a doctor at some point, but a delay of a week or so is not harmful.

Doctors first ask questions about the person's symptoms and medical history. Doctors then do a physical examination. What they find during the history and physical examination often suggests a cause of the dyspepsia and the tests that may need to be done (see Table on page 200).

The history is focused on obtaining a clear description of the symptoms, including whether they are sudden or chronic. Doctors need to know the timing and frequency of recurrence, any difficulty swallowing, and whether the symptoms occur only after eating, drinking alcohol, or taking certain drugs. Doctors also need to know what factors make the symptoms worse (particularly exertion, certain foods, or alcohol) or relieve them (particularly eating or taking antacids).

Doctors also ask the person about gastrointestinal symptoms such as anorexia, nausea, vomiting, vomiting of blood (hematemesis), weight loss, and bloody or black stools. Other symptoms include shortness of breath and sweating.

Doctors need to know whether the person has been diagnosed with a gastrointestinal and/or heart disorder, has any heart risk factors (such as high blood pressure [hypertension] or an excessive amount of cholesterol in the blood [hypercholesterolemia]), and the results of previous tests that have been done and treatments that have been tried.

The physical examination usually does not give doctors clues to a specific diagnosis. However, doctors look for signs of chronic disease, such as very pale skin, wasting away of muscle or fat tissue (cachexia), or yellowing of the eyes and skin (jaundice). They also do a rectal examination to detect any blood. Doctors are more likely to recommend testing for people with such abnormal findings.

Possible tests include

- Upper endoscopy
- Blood tests

Because of the risk of cancer, doctors typically look in the esophagus and stomach with a flexible tube (upper endoscopy) in people who are over age 45 and in younger people with warning signs. Those who are younger and have no symptoms other than dyspepsia are often treated with acid-blocking drugs. If this treatment is unsuccessful, doctors usually do an endoscopy.

People with symptoms of acute coronary ischemia, particularly those with risk factors, should go to the emergency department for an immediate evaluation, including electrocardiography (ECG) and blood tests for damage to heart muscle cells.

People with chronic, nonspecific symptoms should undergo blood tests. If results of the blood tests are abnormal, doctors consider additional tests (such as imaging studies or endoscopy). Some doctors recommend screening for *Helicobacter pylori* infection with a breath test or a test of a stool sample.

Doctors do esophageal manometry and pH (acidity) studies for people who still have reflux symptoms after they have undergone an upper endoscopy and have been taking a proton pump inhibitor (PPI) for 2 to 4 weeks.

Sometimes an abnormality found during testing (such as gastritis or gastroesophageal reflux) is not the cause of the person's dyspepsia. Doctors know this only when the disorder clears up but symptoms of dyspepsia do not.

The best way to treat dyspepsia is to treat any underlying disorders. People with no identifiable disorders are observed over time and reassured.

SOME CAUSES AND FEATURES OF INDIGESTION

Cause	Common Features*	Tests
Achalasia (rhythmic contractions of the esophagus are greatly decreased, and the lower esophageal muscle does not relax normally)	Difficulty swallowing (dysphagia) that worsens over months to years Sometimes spitting up (regurgitation) of undigested food while sleeping Discomfort in the chest Fullness after a small meal (early satiety), nausea, vomiting, bloating, and symptoms that are worsened by food	X-rays of the upper digestive tract after barium is given by mouth (barium swallow) Measurements of pressure produced during contractions of the esophagus (esophageal manometry)
Cancer (such as cancer of the esophagus or stomach)	Chronic, vague discomfort Later, dysphagia with esophageal cancer or early satiety with stomach cancer Weight loss	Upper digestive tract endoscopy (examination of the esophagus, stomach, and duodenum using a flexible viewing tube called an endoscope)
Coronary ischemia (inadequate blood flow to the coronary arteries)	Sometimes in people who have symptoms when exerting themselves Risk factors for heart disorders (such as high blood pressure, diabetes, and/or high cholesterol levels)	Electrocardiography (ECG) Blood tests Sometimes stress testing
Drugs (such as bisphosphonates, erythromycin and other macrolide antibiotics, estrogens, iron, nonsteroidal anti-inflammatory drugs [NSAIDs], and potassium)	In people who are taking a drug that can cause indigestion Symptoms occur shortly after taking the drug	A doctor's examination
Esophageal spasm	Sometimes difficulty swallowing liquids and solids	Barium swallow Esophageal manometry
Gastroesophageal reflux disease (GERD)	Heartburn and/or sometimes reflux of acid or stomach contents into mouth Symptoms sometimes triggered by lying down Relief with antacids	A doctor's examination Sometimes trying treatment with drugs to suppress acid production Sometimes endoscopy of the upper digestive tract
Peptic ulcer disease	Burning or gnawing pain occurring before meals and partially relieved by eating food or taking antacids or histamine-2 (H_2) blockers May awaken people at night	Endoscopy of the upper digestive tract
Poor stomach emptying (gastroparesis)—usually due to other disorders such as diabetes, connective tissue disorders, and/or neurologic disorders	Nausea, abdominal pain, and sometimes vomiting Early satiety Sometimes in people who are known to have a causative disorder	Endoscopy of the upper digestive tract and/or nuclear scanning to evaluate stomach emptying

*Features include symptoms and the results of the doctor's examination. Features mentioned are typical but not always present. Features overlap between causes.

CT = computed tomography; MRI = magnetic resonance imaging.

For people who do not appear to have a specific disorder, doctors often try treatment with acid-blocking drugs (such as proton pump inhibitors or histamine-2 [H$_2$] blockers) or drugs that combat ulcers by increasing the amount of mucus in the stomach (cytoprotective agents). Alternatively, doctors may give a drug that helps stimulate movement of the digestive tract muscles (prokinetic drugs—such as metoclopramide and erythromycin). Doctors may prescribe an antidepressant for some people.

KEY POINTS

- People with severe "gas" discomfort in the upper abdomen or chest may have acute coronary ischemia.
- People who have warning signs and who are over age 45 require an endoscopy.
- People who have no warning signs and who are under age 45 are treated with an acid-blocking drug.
- People whose symptoms do not lessen in 2 to 4 weeks require further evaluation.

HICCUPS

Hiccups are repeated involuntary spasms of the diaphragm, followed by quick, noisy closings of the glottis. The diaphragm is the muscle that separates the chest from the abdomen and that is responsible for each breath. The glottis is the opening between the vocal cords, which closes to stop the flow of air to the lungs. Hiccups are more common among men.

Brief episodes of hiccups (lasting a few minutes) are very common. Occasionally, hiccups persist for some time, even in healthy people. Sometimes hiccups can last more than 2 days or even more than 1 month. These longer episodes are called persistent or intractable (difficult to treat or cure). These longer episodes are uncommon but can be quite distressing.

CAUSES

Doctors are not clear why hiccups happen but they think it may involve irritation of the nerves or the parts of the brain that control muscles of respiration (including the diaphragm).

Brief episodes of hiccups often have no obvious cause but sometimes are triggered by

- A bloated stomach
- Alcohol consumption
- Swallowing hot or irritating substances

In such cases, hiccups usually start in a social situation, perhaps triggered by some combination of laughing, talking, eating, and drinking (particularly alcohol). Sometimes hot or irritating food or liquids are the cause. Hiccups are more likely to occur when carbon dioxide levels in the blood decrease. Such a decrease can occur when people hyperventilate.

Persistent or intractable episodes of hiccups sometimes have more serious causes (see Table on pages 203 to 204). For example, the diaphragm may become irritated because of pneumonia, chest or stomach surgery, or waste products that accumulate in the blood when the kidneys malfunction (uremia). Rarely, hiccups develop when a brain tumor or stroke interferes with the breathing center in the brain.

When the cause is serious, hiccups tend to persist until the cause is corrected. Hiccups due to a brain tumor or stroke may be very hard to stop and may become exhausting.

EVALUATION

Brief episodes of hiccups do not require evaluation by a doctor. For persistent hiccups, the following information can help people decide whether a doctor's evaluation is needed and help them know what to expect during the evaluation.

WARNING SIGNS

In people with hiccups, certain symptoms and characteristics are cause for concern. They include

- Neurologic symptoms (such as headache, weakness, numbness, and loss of balance)

WHEN TO SEE A DOCTOR

People who have hiccups and warning signs should see a doctor right away. People without warning signs should see a doctor if hiccups last more than 2 or 3 days.

WHAT THE DOCTOR DOES

Doctors first ask questions about the person's symptoms and medical history. Doctors then do a physical examination. What doctors find during the history and physical examination often suggests a cause of the hiccups and the tests that may need to be done (see Table).

The history is focused on how long the hiccups have lasted, what remedies the person has tried, and whether the person has recently been ill or had surgery. Doctors also ask people whether they have any

- Symptoms of gastroesophageal reflux
- Swallowing difficulties
- Cough, fever, or chest pain
- Neurologic symptoms (such as headaches and/or difficulty walking, talking, speaking, or seeing)

Doctors also ask people about their use of alcohol.

SOME CAUSES AND FEATURES OF PERSISTENT OR INTRACTABLE HICCUPS

Cause	Common Features*	Tests
Esophagus		
Gastroesophageal reflux disease	Heartburn (burning pain that begins in the upper abdomen and travels up to the throat, sometimes with an acid taste in the mouth)	A doctor's examination
		Sometimes trying treatment with drugs to suppress acid production
	Chest pain	Sometimes endoscopy of the upper digestive tract (examination of the esophagus and stomach using a flexible viewing tube)
	Sometimes a cough, hoarseness, or both	
	Symptoms sometimes triggered by lying down	
	Relief with antacids	
Abdomen		
Abdominal surgery (recent)	Obvious history of recent surgery	A doctor's examination
Gallbladder disease	Pain in the upper right part of the abdomen, under the rib cage	Ultrasonography
	Sometimes nausea and vomiting	
Hepatitis	A general feeling of illness (malaise)	Blood tests
	Poor appetite	
	Nausea and sometimes vomiting	
	Sometimes yellowing of the skin and whites of the eyes (jaundice)	
	Mild discomfort in the upper right part of the abdomen	
Liver cancers (including cancers that metastasized to the liver)	Long-standing discomfort in the upper part of the abdomen	Ultrasonography, CT, or MRI of the abdomen
	Weight loss	
	Fatigue	
Pancreatitis	Severe, constant pain in the upper part of the abdomen	Blood tests
	Usually vomiting	
Pregnancy	Usually a missed menstrual period	A pregnancy test
	Sometimes morning sickness and/or breast swelling	
Chest		
Chest surgery (recent)	Obvious history of recent surgery	A doctor's examination
Inflammation of the membrane around the heart (pericarditis)	Sharp chest pain that worsens with breathing and coughing	Electrocardiography (ECG)

(continued)

SOME CAUSES AND FEATURES OF PERSISTENT OR INTRACTABLE HICCUPS *(continued)*

Cause	Common Features*	Tests
Inflammation of the part of the membrane around the lung (pleura) near the diaphragm (diaphragmatic pleurisy)	Sharp chest pain that worsens with breathing and coughing	A chest x-ray
Pneumonia	Cough, fever, chills, and chest pain Sometimes shortness of breath	A chest x-ray
Other		
Alcoholism	History of excessive consumption of alcohol	A doctor's examination
Certain brain tumors or strokes	Sometimes in people who are known to have had a stroke or who have a tumor Sometimes recurring headaches and/or difficulty walking, talking, speaking, or seeing	MRI and/or CT of the brain
Kidney failure	Usually in people who are known to have kidney failure	Blood tests

*Features include symptoms and the results of the doctor's examination. Features mentioned are typical but not always present.
CT = computed tomography; MRI = magnetic resonance imaging.

The physical examination is focused on a full neurologic examination. A general examination usually does not reveal much, but doctors look for signs of chronic disease such as severe wasting away of muscle and fat tissue (cachexia).

TESTING

Doctors generally do not do any testing for people who have brief hiccups.

People who have warning signs or whose hiccups are persistent and have no obvious cause should have testing. Doctors typically begin with blood tests, chest x-rays, and electrocardiography (ECG). Other tests are done based on the other symptoms people have (see Table). If these tests do not reveal a cause, doctors may do magnetic resonance imaging (MRI) of the brain and computed tomography (CT) of the chest even if people do not have other symptoms specifically related to these areas.

TREATMENT

The best way to treat hiccups is to treat the underlying disorder. For example, doctors give people antibiotics for pneumonia and proton pump inhibitors for gastroesophageal reflux disease.

BRIEF HICCUPS

Nearly all hiccups go away with or without treatment. Many home remedies have been used to treat brief hiccups. Most do not work or are only slightly effective. However, because these remedies typically are safe and simple to do, there is no harm in trying them. Many methods involve ways to raise the level of carbon dioxide in the blood, such as the following:

- Holding the breath
- Breathing deeply into a paper (not plastic) bag

Other methods are done to try to stimulate the vagus nerve, which runs from the brain to the stomach. The following can stimulate this nerve:

- Drinking water quickly
- Swallowing dry bread, granulated sugar, or crushed ice
- Gently pulling on the tongue
- Stimulating gagging (such as by sticking a finger down the throat)
- Gently rubbing the eyeballs

PERSISTENT AND INTRACTABLE HICCUPS

For persistent hiccups, treatment is needed, particularly when the cause cannot be easily corrected. Several drugs have been used with varying success. They include but are not limited to chlorpromazine, baclofen, metoclopramide, and gabapentin.

If drugs do not work, doctors may block one of the phrenic nerves, which control the contractions of the diaphragm. Doctors block the nerve by injecting it with small amounts of a local anesthetic called procaine. If blocking the nerve works but hiccups return, doctors may surgically cut the nerve (phrenicotomy), but even this procedure does not cure all cases.

KEY POINTS

- The cause is usually unknown.
- Although rare, a serious disorder is sometimes present.
- A doctor's evaluation typically does not reveal a cause but should be done for hiccups that are persistent or intractable.
- Numerous remedies exist, but none is superior to or more effective than the other ones.

HIVES

Hives (urticaria) are red, itchy, slightly elevated swellings. Itching may be severe. Hives have clearly defined borders and may have a clear center. Typically, crops of hives come and go. One hive may remain for several hours, then disappear, and later, another may appear elsewhere. After the hive disappears, the skin usually looks completely normal. The swelling is caused by the release of chemicals (such as histamine) from mast cells in the skin, which cause fluid to leak out of small blood vessels temporarily.

Hives may occur with angioedema, which, likes hives, involves swelling. However, the swelling caused by angioedema is under the skin rather than on its surface. Sometimes angioedema affects the face, lips, throat, tongue, and airways. It can be life threatening if the swelling interferes with breathing.

Hives and angioedema are often allergic reactions.

CAUSES

Hives may occur when certain chemicals are inhaled, consumed, injected, or touched. These chemicals can be in the environment, foods, drugs, insects, plants, or other sources. They are harmless in most people. But if people are sensitive to them, these chemicals (called triggers or allergens) can cause an allergic reaction. That is, the immune system overreacts to the chemicals.

However, hives are not always part of an allergic reaction. For example, they may result from autoimmune disorders. In these disorders, the immune system malfunctions, misinterpreting the body's own tissues as foreign and attacking them. Also, some drugs cause hives directly without triggering an allergic reaction. Emotional stress and some physical conditions (such as heat or light) may cause hives for reasons that are not well understood.

Hives usually last less than 6 weeks and are classified as acute. If hives last more than 6 weeks, they are classified as chronic.

Acute hives are most commonly caused by

- Allergic reactions
- Nonallergic reactions

Allergic reactions are often triggered by foods, particularly eggs, fish, shellfish, nuts, and fruits, or by insect stings. Eating even a tiny amount of some foods can suddenly cause hives. But with other foods (such as strawberries), an allergic reaction occurs only after a large amount is eaten. Many drugs, particularly antibiotics, may cause hives. Immediate allergic reactions may also occur when a substance comes into direct contact with the skin (such as latex), after an insect bite, or as a reaction to a substance that is inhaled into the lungs or through the nose.

Nonallergic causes of hives include infections, some drugs, some physical stimuli (such as pressure or cold), and some food additives.

Even though acute hives usually have a specific cause, the cause cannot be identified in about half of cases.

Chronic hives are most commonly caused by

- Unidentified (idiopathic) conditions
- Autoimmune disorders

Sometimes the cause is easily overlooked, as when people repeatedly consume a food not known to be a trigger, such as a preservative or dye in foods or penicillin in milk. Sometimes, despite the best efforts, the cause remains unidentified.

Chronic hives can last for months or years, then sometimes go away for no apparent reason.

EVALUATION

Not every episode of hives requires immediate evaluation by a doctor. The following information can help people decide whether a doctor's evaluation is needed and help them know what to expect during the evaluation.

WARNING SIGNS

Certain symptoms and characteristics are cause for concern:

- Swelling of the face, lips, throat, tongue, or airways (angioedema)

- Difficulty breathing, including wheezing
- Hives that are deeply colored, that become open sores, or that persist more than 48 hours
- Fever, swollen lymph nodes, jaundice, weight loss, and other symptoms of a bodywide (systemic) disorder

WHEN TO SEE A DOCTOR

People should call an ambulance if

- They have difficulty breathing or are wheezing.
- Their throat feels as if it is closing up.

People should go to an emergency department or a doctor's office as soon as possible if

- Their symptoms are severe.
- They feel progressively weak or light-headed or have severe fever or chills.
- They are vomiting or have abdominal pain or diarrhea.

People should see a doctor if

- A bee sting triggers hives (to obtain advice about treatment if another bee sting occurs).
- They have other symptoms, such as fever, joint pains, weight loss, swollen lymph nodes, or night sweats.
- Hives recur without exposure to a trigger.
- Symptoms last for more than 2 days.

If children have hives that appear suddenly, disappear quickly, and do not recur, an examination by a doctor is usually unnecessary. The cause is usually a viral infection.

WHAT THE DOCTOR DOES

Doctors first ask questions about the symptoms and medical history. Doctors then do a physical examination. What they find during the history and physical examination often suggests a cause and the tests that may need to be done (see Table on pages 208 to 210).

Doctors ask the person to describe each episode of hives in detail and any other symptoms that occurred (such as itching, difficulty breathing, or swelling of the face and tongue). They ask about the person's activities before and during the episode and about possible exposure to substances that can trigger allergic reactions, including drugs being taken. The person is also asked about specific symptoms that could suggest a cause, past allergic reactions, and recent travel.

The trigger is not always clear from the history, often because the trigger is something that may have been tolerated previously.

During the physical examination, doctors first check to see whether the lips, tongue, throat, or airways are swollen. If there is swelling, they begin treatment right away. Then doctors note how the hives look, determine which parts of the body are affected, and check for other symptoms that may help confirm the diagnosis. Doctors may use various physical stimuli to see whether they can trigger the hives. For example, they may apply light pressure, heat, or cold to the skin or stroke the skin.

TESTING

Usually, testing is not needed for a single episode of hives unless symptoms suggest a specific disorder that requires treatment (such as some infections). But if hives have unusual characteristics, recur, or persist, tests are usually done.

Typically, tests include a complete blood cell count and blood tests to measure levels of electrolytes, sugar (glucose), and thyroid-stimulating hormone and to determine how well the kidneys and liver are functioning. Skin tests, such as a skin prick test, are done by an allergist (a doctor who specializes in allergic disorders) to identify specific allergens. Imaging and other blood tests are done based on results of the history and physical examination. If results suggest that the cause is a bodywide disorder, a thorough evaluation is needed to identify the cause.

A skin biopsy is done if the diagnosis is unclear or if hives last more than 48 hours.

TREATMENT

Hives often go away on their own after a day or two. If the cause is obvious or if the doctor identifies a cause, people should avoid it if possible. If the cause is not obvious, people should stop taking all nonessential drugs until the hives subside.

Bathing and showering with only cool water, refraining from scratching, and wearing loose clothing may help relieve symptoms.

SOME CAUSES AND FEATURES OF HIVES

Cause	Common Features*	Tests
Acute hives (lasting less than 6 weeks)		
Drugs such as ■ Aspirin and other nonsteroidal anti-inflammatory drugs (NSAIDs) ■ Some opioids ■ Vancomycin ■ Succinylcholine (sometimes given before surgery) ■ Contrast agents (used with imaging tests such as computed tomography) ■ Possibly any drug, whether prescription, over-the-counter, or herbal, if people are allergic to it	Hives that start within 48 hours after the drug was used	A doctor's examination
Emotional or physical stimuli ■ Stress or anxiety ■ Cold ■ Exercise ■ Pressure on the skin (dermatographism) ■ Heat ■ Sunlight ■ Sweating as occurs during a warm bath, exercise, or fever	For most stimuli, hives that typically start within seconds or minutes of exposure to the stimulus For pressure on the skin, hives that start within 4–6 hours and affect only the area of the skin pressed For sunlight, hives that affect only the area of the skin exposed to sunlight	A doctor's examination Exposure to the suspected physical stimulus to see whether it triggers symptoms
Foods that trigger an allergic reaction (food allergens), such as peanuts, nuts, fish, shellfish, wheat, eggs, milk, and soybeans	Hives that start within minutes or hours after consumption	A doctor's examination, particularly the medical history Sometimes allergy skin prick testing
Infections (rare causes) ■ Bacterial, such as some urinary tract, streptococcal, and *Helicobacter pylori* infections ■ Parasitic, such as *Toxocara canis, Giardia intestinalis (lamblia), Schistosoma mansoni, Strongyloides stercoralis, Trichuris trichiura,* and *Blastocystis hominis* infections ■ Viral, such as hepatitis (A, B, or C) and HIV, cytomegalovirus, Epstein-Barr virus, and enterovirus infections	Fever, chills, and fatigue Symptoms of the particular infection Particularly for parasitic infections, recent travel to a developing country	Tests depending on the suspected infection (suggested by results of the medical history and examination) Diagnosis confirmed if hives disappear after the infection is eliminated
Insect bites or stings	Hives that start within seconds or minutes after an insect bite or sting	A doctor's examination, particularly the medical history *(continued)*

SOME CAUSES AND FEATURES OF HIVES *(continued)*

Cause	Common Features*	Tests
Serum sickness	Hives that start within 7–10 days after injection of ■ A blood product (as in a transfusion) ■ A drug derived from animal blood such as horse serum (which is used to treat poisonous snake and spider bites) ■ Possibly another drug May be accompanied by fever, joint pain, swollen lymph nodes, and abdominal pain	A doctor's examination
Substances that trigger an allergic reaction through contact (contact allergens), such as latex, animal saliva or dander, dust, pollen, or molds	Hives that start within minutes or hours after contact	A doctor's examination, particularly the medical history Sometimes allergy testing
Transfusion reactions	Hives that usually start within a few minutes after transfusion of a blood product	A doctor's examination, particularly the medical history

Chronic hives (lasting more than 6 weeks)

Cause	Common Features*	Tests
Autoimmune disorders ■ Systemic lupus erythematosus (lupus) ■ Sjögren syndrome ■ Urticarial vasculitis	Various symptoms depending on the autoimmune disorder For systemic lupus erythematosus, symptoms may include fever, fatigue, headache, joint pain and swelling, painful breathing, and mouth sores For Sjögren syndrome, dry eyes and dry mouth For urticarial vasculitis, hives that ■ May be painful rather than itchy ■ Usually last more than 24 hours ■ Do not whiten (blanch) when pressure is applied ■ Can be accompanied by small blisters and reddish purple blotches (purpura)	For all autoimmune disorders, blood tests to check for abnormal antibodies Sometimes skin biopsy For Sjögren syndrome, a test that estimates the amount of tears people are producing For urticarial vasculitis, skin biopsy
Cancer, typically of the digestive organs or lungs, or lymphoma	Weight loss, night sweats, abdominal pain, cough (sometimes bringing up blood), jaundice, swollen lymph nodes, or a combination	Various tests depending on the cancer suspected
Chronic idiopathic hives (diagnosed when no specific cause is identified)	Hives that occur daily (or almost daily) and itching that lasts for at least 6 weeks, with no obvious cause	A doctor's examination Blood and sometimes other tests, such as skin prick tests and exposure to various triggers, to rule out other causes

(continued)

SOME CAUSES AND FEATURES OF HIVES *(continued)*

Cause	Common Features*	Tests
Drugs (same as those for acute hives)	Hives that occur in a person who has been taking a prescription, an over-the-counter, or an herbal drug for a long time when there is no other explanation for them	A doctor's examination Sometimes allergy testing Trial of avoidance to see whether hives disappear after the drug is stopped
Emotional or physical stimuli (same as those for acute hives)	For most stimuli, hives that typically occur within seconds or minutes of exposure to the stimulus For pressure on the skin, hives that start within 4–6 hours and affect only the area of the skin pressed For sunlight, hives that affect only the area of the skin exposed to sunlight	A doctor's examination Exposure to the suspected stimulus to see whether it triggers symptoms
Endocrine abnormalities such as a thyroid disorder or an elevated level of progesterone (a female hormone)	For thyroid disorders, difficulty tolerating heat or cold, a slow or fast heart rate, and shaking (tremor) or sluggishness Occurring in women who take birth control pills (oral contraceptives) or hormone therapy containing progesterone or who have hives appearing just before their menstrual periods start and disappearing when periods stop	A doctor's examination If a thyroid disorder is suspected, a blood test to measure thyroid-stimulating hormone
Mastocytosis	Small red bumps that turn into hives when touched Sometimes abdominal pain, easy flushing, and recurring headaches	Skin and sometimes bone marrow biopsy Sometimes blood tests to measure levels of substances released when certain immune cells (called mast cells) are activated

*Features include symptoms and results of the doctor's examination. Features mentioned are typical but not always present.
HIV = human immunodeficiency virus.

DRUGS

For hives, antihistamines are used. These drugs partially relieve the itching and reduce the swelling. To be effective, they must be taken regularly, rather than as needed. Several antihistamines, including cetirizine, diphenhydramine, and loratadine, are available without a prescription. Diphenhydramine is an older drug that is more likely to cause drowsiness than the other two. Other antihistamines include desloratadine, fexofenadine, hydroxyzine, and levocetirizine.

If symptoms are severe and other treatments are ineffective, corticosteroids, such as prednisone, taken by mouth, are used. They are given for as short a time as possible. When taken by mouth for more than 3 to 4 weeks, corticosteroids have many, sometimes serious, side effects. Corticosteroid or antihistamine creams do not help.

People who have severe reactions should carry a self-injecting epinephrine pen and, if a reaction occurs, use it immediately.

In about half the people with chronic hives, the hives disappear without treatment within 2 years. In some adults, the antidepressant doxepin, which is also a potent antihistamine, helps relieve chronic hives.

ESSENTIALS FOR OLDER PEOPLE

Older people are more likely to have side effects when they take the older antihistamines (such as hydroxyzine and diphenhydramine). In addition to drowsiness, these drugs can cause confusion and delirium and can make starting and continuing to urinate difficult. Usually, older people should not take these drugs for hives.

⊶ KEY POINTS

- Hives may or may not be an allergic reaction.
- If hives have lasted less than 6 weeks, the cause is usually an allergic reaction to a specific substance, an acute infection, or a nonallergic reaction to a specific substance.
- If hives have lasted 6 weeks or more, the cause usually cannot be identified (is idiopathic) or is an autoimmune disorder.
- People should call an ambulance if they have difficulty breathing or if their throat feels as if it is closing up.
- People with mild symptoms should avoid any known or suspected triggers and can take antihistamines to relieve symptoms.
- People who have severe reactions should carry a self-injecting epinephrine pen and, if a reaction occurs, use it immediately.

INSOMNIA AND EXCESSIVE DAYTIME SLEEPINESS

The most commonly reported sleep-related problems are insomnia and excessive daytime sleepiness (EDS).

- Insomnia is difficulty falling asleep or staying asleep or a disturbance in sleep quality that makes sleep seem inadequate or unrefreshing.
- EDS refers to being unusually sleepy or falling asleep during the day in people who are not sleep-deprived.

Difficulty falling and staying asleep and waking up earlier than desired are common among young and old. About 10% of adults have long-standing (chronic) insomnia, and about 50% sometimes have insomnia.

People with insomnia or EDS are sleepy, tired, and irritable during the day and have trouble concentrating and functioning. People with EDS may fall asleep when working or driving.

There are several types of insomnia:

- **Difficulty falling asleep (sleep onset insomnia):** Commonly, people have difficulty falling asleep when they cannot let their mind relax and they continue to think and worry. Sometimes the body is not ready for sleep at what is considered a usual time for sleep. That is, the body's internal clock is out of sync with the earth's cycle of light and dark—a type of circadian rhythm sleep disorder. This problem is common among adolescents and young adults.
- **Difficulty staying asleep (sleep maintenance insomnia):** Older people are more likely to have difficulty staying asleep than are younger people. People with this type of insomnia fall asleep normally but wake up several hours later and cannot fall asleep again easily. Sometimes they drift in and out of a restless, unsatisfactory sleep.
- **Early morning awakening:** This type may be a sign of depression in people of any age.

CAUSES

Insomnia and EDS may be caused by conditions inside or outside the body. Some conditions cause insomnia and EDS, and some cause one or the other. Some people have chronic insomnia that has little or no apparent relationship to any particular cause.

COMMON CAUSES

Insomnia is most often caused by

- Poor sleep habits, such as drinking a caffeinated beverage in the afternoon or evening, exercising late at night, or having an irregular sleep-wake schedule
- Mental health disorders, particularly mood and anxiety disorders
- Other disorders such as heart and lung disorders, disorders that affect muscles or bones, or chronic pain
- Stress, such as that due to hospitalization or loss of a job (called adjustment insomnia)
- Excessive worrying about sleeplessness and another day of fatigue (called psychophysiologic insomnia)

Sleeping late or napping to make up for lost sleep may make sleeping during the night even harder.

EDS is most often caused by

- Insufficient sleep despite having ample opportunity to sleep (called insufficient sleep syndrome)
- Obstructive sleep apnea (a serious disorder in which breathing frequently stops during sleep)
- Various disorders, particularly mental health disorders, brain or nerve (neurologic) disorders (such as encephalitis, meningitis, or a brain tumor), and disorders that affect muscles or bones
- Disorders that disrupt people's internal sleep-wake schedule (circadian rhythm disorders), such as jet lag and shift work disorder

Most major mental health disorders are accompanied by insomnia and EDS. About 80% of people with major depression have EDS and insomnia, and about 40% of people with insomnia have a mental health disorder, usually a mood disorder.

Any disorder that causes pain or discomfort, particularly if worsened by movement, can cause brief awakenings and interfere with sleep.

LESS COMMON CAUSES

Drugs, when used for a long time or when stopped (withdrawal), can cause insomnia and EDS (see Table, below).

Many mind-altering (psychoactive) drugs can cause abnormal movements during sleep and may disturb sleep. Sedatives that are commonly prescribed to treat insomnia can cause irritability and apathy and reduce mental alertness. Also, if a sedative is taken for more than a few days, stopping the sedative can make the original sleep problem suddenly worse.

Sometimes the cause is a sleep disorder.

Central sleep apnea is often first identified when people report insomnia or disturbed or unrefreshing sleep. This disorder causes breathing to become shallow or to stop repeatedly throughout the night.

Narcolepsy is a sleep disorder characterized by EDS with uncontrollable episodes of falling asleep during normal waking hours and sudden, temporary episodes of muscle weakness.

Periodic limb movement disorder interrupts sleep because it causes repeated twitching or kicking of the legs during sleep. As a result, people are sleepy during the day.

Restless legs syndrome makes falling and staying asleep difficult because people feel as if they have to move their legs and, less often, their arms when they sit still or lie down. People usually also have creepy, crawly sensations in the limbs.

SOME DRUGS THAT INTERFERE WITH SLEEP	
Type	**Examples**
When the drug is used	
Anticonvulsants	Phenytoin
Chemotherapy drugs	All
Drugs that stimulate the brain	Amphetamines
	Caffeine
Birth control pills (oral contraceptives)	All
Propranolol	—
Steroids	Anabolic steroids
	Corticosteroids
Thyroid hormone preparations	—
When the drug is stopped	
Illegal drugs	Cocaine
	Heroin
	Marijuana
	Phencyclidine
Drugs that slow the brain	Barbiturates
	Opioids
	Sedatives
When the drug is used or stopped	
Alcohol	—
Antidepressants	Some

EVALUATION

Usually, the cause can be identified based on the person's description of the current problem and results of a physical examination. Many people have obvious problems, such as poor sleep habits, stress, or coping with shift work.

WARNING SIGNS

Certain symptoms are cause for concern:

- Falling asleep while driving or during other potentially dangerous situations
- Frequently falling asleep without warning
- Stopping breathing during sleep or waking up with gasping or choking (reported by a bed partner)
- Moving violently or injuring self or others during sleep
- Sleepwalking
- A heart or lung disorder that is constantly changing (is unstable)

WHEN TO SEE A DOCTOR

People should see a doctor if they have warning signs or if their sleep-related symptoms interfere with their daily activities. If healthy people have sleep-related symptoms for a short time (less than 1 or 2 weeks) but do not have warning signs, they can try changes in behavior that can help improve sleep (see Table on page 216). If these changes do not help after a week or so, people should see a doctor.

WHAT THE DOCTOR DOES

The doctor asks people about their sleep patterns, habits around bedtime, use of drugs (including illegal drugs), use of other substances (such as alcohol, caffeine, and tobacco), degree of stress, medical history, and level of physical activity. People may be asked to keep a sleep log. In it, they record a detailed description of their sleep habits, with sleep and wake times (including awakening during the night), use of naps, and any problems with sleeping. When considering the diagnosis of insomnia, the doctor considers that some people need less sleep than others.

If people have EDS, the doctor may ask them to fill out a questionnaire indicating how likely they are to fall asleep in various situations. The doctor may ask their sleep partner to describe any abnormalities that occur during sleep, such as snoring or pauses in breathing.

A physical examination is done to check for disorders that can cause insomnia or EDS.

TESTING

Doctors sometimes refer people to a sleep disorders specialist for evaluation in a sleep laboratory. Reasons for such a referral include

- An uncertain diagnosis
- Suspicion of certain disorders (such as sleep apnea, a seizure disorder, narcolepsy, and periodic limb movement disorder)
- Insomnia or EDS persisting despite basic measures to correct it (changing behavior to improve sleep and taking sleep aids for a short time)
- Presence of warning signs or other symptoms such as nightmares and twitching of the legs or arms during sleep
- Dependence on sleep aids
- An irresistible urge to move the legs or arms just before or during sleep

Tests are not needed if symptoms suggest a cause such as restless legs syndrome, poor sleep habits, stress, or shift work disorder.

The evaluation consists of polysomnography and observation (and sometimes video recording) of unusual movements during an entire night's sleep. Other tests are sometimes also done.

Polysomnography is usually done overnight in a sleep laboratory. Electrodes are pasted to the scalp and face to record the brain's electrical activity (electroencephalography, or EEG) as well as eye movements. These recordings help provide doctors with information about sleep stages. Electrodes are also attached to other areas of the body to record heart rate (electrocardiography, or ECG), muscle activity (electromyography), and breathing. A painless clip is attached to a finger or an ear to record oxygen levels in the blood. Polysomnography can detect breathing disorders (such as obstructive sleep apnea), seizure disorders, narcolepsy, periodic limb movement disorder, and unusual movements and behaviors during sleep (parasomnias).

A multiple sleep latency test is done to distinguish between physical fatigue and EDS and to check for narcolepsy. People spend the day in a sleep laboratory, taking four or five naps at 2-hour intervals. Polysomnography is used as part of this test to assess how quickly people fall asleep. It detects when people fall asleep and is used to monitor the stages of sleep during the naps.

The **maintenance of wakefulness test** is used to determine how well people can remain awake while sitting in a quiet room.

Tests to evaluate the heart, lungs, and liver may be done in people with EDS if symptoms or results from the physical examination suggest that another disorder is the cause.

TREATMENT

Treatment of insomnia depends on its cause and severity. If insomnia results from another disorder, that disorder is treated. Such treatment may improve sleep.

If insomnia is mild, general measures may be all that is needed. They include

- Changes in behavior (such as following a regular sleep schedule and avoiding caffeine after lunch time)
- Prescription sleep aids
- Nonprescription sleep aids

If stress is the cause, reducing stress, if possible, typically eliminates the symptoms. If symptoms persist, talk therapy (cognitive-behavioral therapy), done by trained specialists, may be the most effective and safest treatment. It helps people understand the problem, unlearn bad sleeping habits, and eliminate unhelpful thoughts, such as worrying about losing sleep or the next day's activities. This therapy also includes relaxation training. But if daytime sleepiness and fatigue develop, especially if they interfere with daytime functioning, treatment with sleep aids is warranted for a short time. A combination of cognitive-behavioral therapy and sleep aids is often best.

If people have insomnia and depression, the depression should be treated, which often relieves the insomnia. Some antidepressant drugs also have sedative effects that help with sleep when the drugs are given before bed. However, these drugs may also cause daytime sleepiness, particularly in older people.

PRESCRIPTION SLEEP AIDS

When a sleep disorder interferes with normal activities and a sense of well-being, taking prescription sleep aids (also called hypnotics or sleeping pills) occasionally for up to a few weeks may help.

NONPRESCRIPTION SLEEP AIDS

Some sleep aids are available without a prescription (over-the-counter, or OTC), but an OTC sleep aid may be no safer than a prescription sleep aid, especially for older people. OTC sleep aids contain diphenhydramine or doxylamine, both antihistamines, which may have side effects, such as daytime drowsiness or sometimes nervousness, agitation, falls, and confusion, especially in older people.

OTC sleep aids should not be taken for more than 7 to 10 days. They are intended to manage an occasional sleepless night, not chronic insomnia, which could signal a serious underlying problem. If these drugs are used a long time or stopped abruptly, they may cause problems.

Melatonin is sometimes used to treat insomnia, especially in older people, who may have a low level of melatonin. It may be effective when sleep problems are caused by consistently going to sleep and waking up late (for example, going to sleep at 3 AM and waking up at 10 AM or later) —called delayed sleep phase syndrome. To be effective, melatonin must be taken when the body normally produces melatonin (the early evening for most people). Otherwise, melatonin can worsen sleep problems. Use of melatonin is controversial. It appears to be safe for short-term use (up to a few weeks), but the effects of using it for a long time are unknown. Also, melatonin products are unregulated, and thus purity and content cannot be confirmed.

Many other medicinal herbs and dietary supplements, such as skullcap and valerian, are available in health food stores, but their effects on sleep and their side effects are not well understood.

ESSENTIALS FOR OLDER PEOPLE

Because sleep patterns deteriorate as people age, older people are more likely to report insomnia than younger people. As people age, they tend to sleep less and to awaken more often during the night and to feel sleepier and to nap during the day. The periods of the deep sleep

CHANGES IN BEHAVIOR TO IMPROVE SLEEP

What to Do	How to Do It
Follow a regular sleep-wake schedule	People should go to bed at the same time each night and, more importantly, get up at the same time each morning, even on weekends and vacations.
Follow a regular routine before bedtime	A regular pattern of activities—such as listening to soft music, brushing the teeth, washing the face, and setting the alarm clock—can set the mood for sleep. This routine should be followed every night, at home or away. As part of this routine, people should avoid bright lights before bedtime.
Make the environment conducive to sleep	The bedroom should be kept dark, quiet, and not too warm or too cold. Loud noises can disturb sleep even when people are not awakened by them. Wearing ear plugs, using a white-noise machine or a fan, or installing heavy curtains in the bedroom (to block out outside noises and light) can help. Wearing a mask over the eyes can help people who must sleep during daylight in a room that cannot be completely darkened. If people wake up during the night, they should avoid bright lights.
Use pillows	Pillows between the knees or under the waist can make some people more comfortable. For people with back problems, lying on the side with a large pillow between the knees may help.
Use the bed primarily for sleeping	The bed should be used for sleep and sex. It should not be used for eating, reading, watching television, paying bills, or other activities associated with being awake.
Get up	When unable to fall asleep within 20 minutes, getting up and doing something else in another room and coming back to bed when sleepy may be more effective than lying in bed and trying harder and harder to fall asleep.
Exercise regularly	Exercise can help people fall asleep naturally. However, exercise within 5 hours of bedtime can stimulate the heart and brain and keep people awake.
Relax	Stress and worry interfere with sleep. People who are not sleepy at bedtime can relax by reading or taking a warm bath. Relaxation techniques, such as visual imagery, progressive muscle relaxation, and breathing exercises, can be used. People can aim to leave their problems at the bedroom door. Scheduling a worry time during the day to think about concerns can diminish the need to worry at bedtime.
Avoid stimulating activity before bedtime	Watching exciting television shows, playing thrilling computer games, or dealing with complicated work-related matters during the hour or so before bedtime can make sleeping difficult.
Avoid substances that interfere with sleep	Food and beverages that contain alcohol or caffeine (such as coffee, tea, cola drinks, and chocolate) can interfere with sleep, as can appetite suppressants, diuretics, and nicotine (in cigarettes and nicotine patches). Caffeinated substances should not be consumed within 12 hours of bedtime. Drinking a large amount of alcohol in the evening causes early morning awakenings. Quitting smoking may help.
Eat a light snack	Hunger can interfere with going to sleep. A light snack, especially if warm, can help, unless a person has gastroesophageal reflux. However, heavy meals near bedtime should be avoided. They may cause heartburn, which can interfere with sleep.
Eliminate behaviors that provoke anxiety	People can turn the clock away so that time is not a focus. They should not watch the clock while they are in bed.
Spend time in bright light during the day	Exposure to light during the day can help people readjust their sleep-wake schedule to be in sync with the earth's cycle of light and dark.

PRESCRIPTION SLEEP AIDS: NOT TO BE TAKEN LIGHTLY

Among the most commonly used sleep aids are sedatives, minor tranquilizers, and antianxiety drugs. Most are safe as long as a doctor supervises their use.

Most sleep aids require a doctor's prescription because they may cause problems. Many of these problems are less common with newer sleep aids.

- **Loss of effectiveness:** Once people become accustomed to a sleep aid, it may become ineffective. This effect is called tolerance.
- **Withdrawal symptoms:** If a sleep aid is taken for more than a few days, stopping it can make the original sleep problem suddenly worse (causing rebound insomnia) and can increase anxiety. Thus, doctors recommend reducing the dose slowly over a period of several weeks until the drug is stopped.
- **Habit-forming or addiction potential:** If people use sleep aids for more than a few days, they may feel that they cannot sleep without them. Stopping the drug makes them anxious, nervous, and irritable or causes disturbing dreams.
- **Potential for overdose:** If taken in higher than recommended doses, some of the older sleep aids can cause confusion, delirium, dangerously slow breathing, a weak pulse, blue fingernails and lips, and even death.
- **Serious side effects:** Most sleep aids, even when taken at recommended doses, are particularly risky for older people and for people with breathing problems because sleep aids tend to suppress areas of the brain that control breathing. Some can reduce daytime alertness, making driving or operating machinery hazardous. Sleep aids are especially dangerous when taken with other drugs that can cause daytime drowsiness and suppress breathing, such as alcohol, opioids (narcotics), antihistamines, or antidepressants. The combined effects are more dangerous. Rarely, especially if taken at higher than recommended doses or with alcohol, sleep aids have been known to cause people to walk or even drive during sleep and to cause severe allergic reactions.

Newer sleep aids can be used for longer periods of time without losing effect, becoming habit-forming, or causing withdrawal. They are also less dangerous if an overdose is taken.

Benzodiazepines are the most commonly used sleep aids. Some benzodiazepines (such as chlordiazepoxide, diazepam, flurazepam, and nitrazepam) are longer acting than others (such as temazepam and triazolam). Doctors try to avoid prescribing long-acting benzodiazepines for older people. Older people cannot metabolize and excrete drugs as well as younger people. Thus for them, taking these drugs may be more likely to cause daytime drowsiness, slurred speech, and falls.

Other useful sleep aids are not benzodiazepines but affect the same areas of the brain as benzodiazepines. These drugs (eszopiclone, zaleplon, and zolpidem) are shorter acting than most benzodiazepines and are less likely to lead to daytime drowsiness. Older people appear to tolerate these drugs well. Zolpidem also comes in a longer-acting (extended-release, or ER) form and a very short acting (low-dose) form. Ramelteon, a newer sleep aid, has the same advantages as these shorter-acting drugs. In addition, it can be used longer than benzodiazepines without losing its effectiveness or causing withdrawal symptoms. It is not habit-forming and does not appear to have overdose potential. Ramelteon affects the same area of the brain as melatonin (a hormone that helps promote sleep) and is thus called a melatonin receptor agonist. Doxepin, used as an antidepressant when given in high doses, is an effective sleep aid when given in very low doses.

Some **antidepressants** (such as paroxetine, trazodone, and trimipramine) can relieve insomnia and prevent early morning awakening when they are given in lower doses than those used to treat depression. These drugs may be used in the rare instances when people who are not depressed cannot tolerate other sleep aids. However, side effects, such as daytime sleepiness, can be a problem, especially for older people.

---

that is most refreshing become shorter and eventually disappear. Usually, these changes alone do not indicate a sleep disorder in older people.

Older people who have interrupted sleep can benefit from regular bedtimes, lots of exposure to light during the day, regular exercise, and less napping during the day (because napping may make getting a good night's sleep even harder).

Many older people with insomnia do not need to take sleep aids. But if they do, they should keep in mind that these drugs can cause problems Thus, caution is required.

O—ᴛᴛ KEY POINTS

- Poor sleep habits, stress, and conditions that disrupt people's internal sleep-wake schedule (such as shift work) cause many cases of insomnia and excessive daytime sleepiness.
- However, sometimes the cause is a disorder, such as obstructive sleep apnea or a mental disorder.
- Evaluation in a sleep laboratory, including polysomnography, is usually recommended when doctors suspect the cause is obstructive sleep apnea or another sleep disorder, when the diagnosis is uncertain, or when general measures do not help.
- If insomnia is mild, general measures, such as following a regular sleep schedule, may be all that is needed.
- If insomnia interferes with daily activities and general measures are ineffective, taking a sleep aid for up to a few weeks may help.
- Sleep aids are more likely to cause problems in older people.

ITCHING

Itching can be very uncomfortable. It is one of the most common reasons people see dermatologists. Itching can be triggered by wool fibers or irritants, such as solvents or cosmetics.

Itching can result from disorders that affect the skin, the nervous system (which senses itching), or other parts of the body (such as bile ducts or kidneys) or from drugs. Causes that affect more of the body than just the skin are called systemic causes.

Itching makes people want to scratch. Scratching temporarily relieves itching but can damage the skin, sometimes resulting in more itching or infection. Over time, the skin can become thick and scaly.

CAUSES

The **most common causes** of itching are related to skin disorders:

- Dry skin
- Eczema (also called atopic dermatitis)
- Contact dermatitis (an allergic rash resulting from direct contact with a particular substance)
- Fungal skin infections

Systemic causes are less common but are more likely if there is no visible skin problem. Some of the more common systemic causes are

- Allergic reactions that have internal effects—for example, to foods, drugs, bites, or stings (internal allergic reactions)
- Disorders of the gallbladder or liver, such as gallstones
- Chronic kidney disease

Less common systemic causes include an overactive thyroid gland (hyperthyroidism), an underactive thyroid gland (hypothyroidism), diabetes, iron deficiency, and polycythemia vera (a cancerous overproduction of red blood cells). Drugs can cause itching by causing allergic reactions. Drugs can also cause itching without causing an allergic reaction. For example, morphine and some radiopaque dyes given by vein (intravenously) may cause itching.

EVALUATION

Not every episode of itching requires immediate evaluation by a doctor. The following information can help people decide whether a

---

WHEN THE SKIN IS DRY

Normal skin owes its soft, pliable texture to its water content. To help protect against water loss, the outer layer of skin contains oil, which slows evaporation and holds moisture in the deeper layers of skin. If the oil is depleted, the skin becomes dry.

Dry skin (xerosis) is common, especially among people past middle age. Common causes are cold weather and frequent bathing. Bathing washes away surface oils, allowing the skin to dry out. Dry skin may become irritated and often itches—sometimes it sloughs off in small flakes and scales. Scaling most often affects the lower legs. Rubbing or scratching dry skin can lead to infection and scarring.

A form of severe dry skin is called ichthyosis. Ichthyosis can be an inherited disorder or can result from a number of other disorders, such as an underactive thyroid gland (hypothyroidism), lymphoma, and AIDS.

The key to treating simple dry skin is keeping the skin moist. Taking fewer baths allows protective oils to remain on the skin. Moisturizing ointments or creams containing petroleum jelly, mineral oil, or glycerin can also hold water in the skin. Harsh soaps, detergents, and the perfumes in some moisturizers irritate the skin and may further dry it.

When scaling is a problem, solutions or creams containing salicylic or lactic acid or urea may help remove the scales. For some forms of severe ichthyosis, creams containing substances related to vitamin A, such as tretinoin, help the skin shed excessive scales.

SOME CAUSES AND FEATURES OF ITCHING

Cause	Common Features*	Tests
Skin causes		
Contact dermatitis	Redness and sometimes blisters in a shape or location corresponding to the substance causing the reaction (such as along the hairline when caused by hair dyes, on the wrist when caused by a watch, or on exposed skin when caused by poison ivy)	A doctor's examination
Dry skin	Dry, scaly skin, usually on the legs, that develops or becomes worse in winter, after a hot bath, or after prolonged exposure to water	A doctor's examination
Eczema (atopic dermatitis)	Dryness, redness, and sometimes thickening and scaling, often in the folds of the elbows or behind the knees Usually a family history of allergies or rashes	A doctor's examination
Fungal skin infections, such as ringworm, jock itch, or athlete's foot	A circular rash with raised borders, scaling, and often hair loss In adults, usually on the feet or genital area In children, usually on the scalp or body	Sometimes examination of skin scales under a microscope
Hives (urticaria)	Red, raised swellings that have sharp borders and are often clear in the center Each hive resolving within hours, but new hives continuing to appear, sometimes repeatedly	Usually only a doctor's examination
Insect bite	Sudden appearance of one or a few bumps that are usually small, red, and raised	A doctor's examination
Lice infestation (pediculosis)	Areas of scratched, irritated skin and sometimes tiny, pinpoint bites Usually in the scalp, armpits, or pubic area or on the waist or eyelashes	Sometimes examination of skin scales or debris under a microscope
Lichen simplex chronicus	Areas where repeatedly scratched skin has thickened Areas are red, scaly, raised, rough, and separated from surrounding skin	A doctor's examination
Psoriasis	Raised red patches with silver scales Usually on the outer exposed surface of the elbows or knees or on the scalp or trunk	A doctor's examination
Scabies	Burrows, which are small red or dark bumps, next to a fine, wavy, slightly scaly short line Usually in the web spaces between the fingers or toes, along the belt (waist) line, on the inner surfaces of the elbows, behind the knees, around the nipples (in women), or near the genitals (in men)	Sometimes examination of skin scales or debris under a microscope
Systemic causes (conditions that affect more of the body than just the skin)		
Allergic reactions that have internal effects	Widespread itching Often a raised red rash and sometimes hives	Avoiding things one at a time to see what the cause is Sometimes skin testing

(continued)

SOME CAUSES AND FEATURES OF ITCHING *(continued)*

Cause	Common Features*	Tests
Cancer, such as Hodgkin lymphoma, certain other lymphomas such as mycosis fungoides, and polycythemia vera	Itching sometimes as the first symptom of cancer With Hodgkin lymphoma, burning with itching, particularly in the legs With mycosis fungoides, various raised or flat skin patches or reddening of the skin With polycythemia vera, itching without a rash	A complete blood count A chest x-ray A biopsy of lymph nodes for Hodgkin lymphoma, of skin for mycosis fungoides, or of bone marrow for polycythemia vera
Chronic kidney disease	Widespread itching and no rash Sometimes worse during dialysis and sometimes worse on the back	Tests to exclude other causes of itching, based on the person's symptoms
Diabetes	Frequent urination, thirst, and weight loss Itching usually occurring only after other symptoms have developed	Blood tests for level of sugar (glucose) and glycosylated hemoglobin (which indicates the level of blood sugar over time)
Drugs, such as aspirin, barbiturates, cocaine, morphine, penicillin, and some antifungal and chemotherapy drugs	Sometimes no rash	A doctor's examination
Gallbladder or liver disorders	Other symptoms of gallbladder or liver disorders, such as jaundice, fatigue, oily stools, and abdominal pain	Usually blood tests to measure liver enzymes and ultrasonography
Iron deficiency anemia	Tendency to tire easily Sometimes paleness, weakness, or difficulty breathing	Blood tests for anemia and iron deficiency
Multiple sclerosis	Intense itching that comes and goes Other symptoms of multiple sclerosis, such as numbness and tingling, weakness, loss of vision, vertigo, and clumsiness	Magnetic resonance imaging (MRI) of the brain, spinal cord, or both Sometimes a spinal tap Sometimes electroencephalography or electromyography
Pregnancy	Usually widespread itching without rash, developing sometimes in late pregnancy Sometimes resulting from mild liver problems	Sometimes blood tests to check for a liver disorder
Psychologic factors	Linear skin scratches and/or scabs in different stages of healing, and psychologic symptoms	Tests to exclude other causes of itching, based on the person's symptoms
Thyroid disorders	With hyperthyroidism (an overactive thyroid gland): Difficulty tolerating heat, sweating, weight loss, bulging eyes, shakiness (tremor), restlessness, and sometimes an enlarged thyroid gland (goiter) With hypothyroidism (an underactive thyroid gland): Difficulty tolerating cold, weight gain, coarse and thick skin, and sluggishness	Blood tests to evaluate thyroid function

*Features include symptoms and results of the doctor's examination. Features mentioned are typical but not always present.

doctor's evaluation is needed and help them know what to expect during the evaluation. Most conditions causing itching are not serious.

WARNING SIGNS

The following may indicate that the cause could be serious:

- Weight loss, fatigue, or night sweats—symptoms that may indicate a serious infection or a tumor
- Weakness, numbness, or tingling—symptoms that may indicate a nervous system disorder
- Abdominal pain or a yellowish discoloration of the skin and eyes (jaundice)—symptoms that may indicate a gallbladder or liver disorder
- Excessive thirst, abnormally frequent urination, and weight loss—symptoms that may indicate diabetes

WHEN TO SEE A DOCTOR

People who have weight loss, fatigue, or night sweats should see a doctor as soon as convenient, probably within a week or so. People with any of the other warning signs or with severe itching should probably see a doctor immediately or as soon as possible.

WHAT THE DOCTOR DOES

Doctors ask many questions and look at the skin. Often, a person needs to undress so that the entire skin surface can be checked. If no clear cause is found after checking the skin, doctors may do a complete physical examination to check for systemic causes. Testing may be necessary to diagnose certain systemic causes and sometimes skin disorders.

If itching is widespread and begins shortly after use of a drug, that drug is a likely cause. If itching (usually with a rash) is confined to an area in contact with a substance, particularly if the substance is known to cause contact dermatitis, that substance is a likely cause. However, allergic causes of widespread itching can be difficult to identify because affected people have usually eaten several different foods and have been exposed to many substances that could cause an allergic reaction before itching develops. Similarly, identifying a drug that is causing the reaction in a person taking several drugs

may be difficult. Sometimes the person has been taking the drug causing the reaction for months or even years before a reaction occurs.

TESTING

Most causes of itching can be diagnosed without testing. If the diagnosis of a skin abnormality is not clear from its appearance and the person's history, removal (biopsy) of a skin sample may be necessary so that it can be analyzed. If the cause of itching seems to be an allergic reaction but the substance causing the allergic reaction is not evident, skin testing may be necessary. In skin testing, substances that can cause allergic reactions on contact are applied to the skin, either in a patch (called patch testing) or with a small needle (called prick testing).

If the cause seems not be an allergic reaction or skin disorder, testing is done based on the person's other symptoms. For example, tests may be done for gallbladder or liver disorders, chronic kidney disease, thyroid disorders, diabetes, or cancer.

TREATMENT

Disorders that cause itching are treated. Sometimes other measures can also help relieve itching.

SKIN CARE

Skin care measures can help relieve itching regardless of cause. Baths or showers should be short, no more frequent than necessary, and taken with cool or lukewarm (not hot) water. Using moisturizing soap and skin lubricants can also help, as can humidifying dry air (for example, in winter) and not wearing tight or wool clothing.

TOPICAL TREATMENTS

Topical treatments can be applied to the skin if only a specific area is affected. To be effective, capsaicin cream should be used for at least 2 weeks. It tends to burn, but the burning decreases over time. Menthol and camphor creams have strong odors but can be used, as can tacrolimus or pimecrolimus creams.

Corticosteroid creams can help relieve itching and often clear up the rash and other skin abnormalities in disorders such as eczema, contact dermatitis, psoriasis, and lichen simplex chronicus. Corticosteroids should usually not be used when the skin is infected, when an infestation is present, when no rash or skin abnormalities are present, and when the cause is systemic.

Type B ultraviolet light can relieve itching but can cause sunburn-like effects and increases the risk of skin cancers.

SYSTEMIC TREATMENTS

Systemic treatments are drugs that are taken internally, usually by mouth. They are used if itching is widespread or if topical treatments are ineffective.

Antihistamines, particularly hydroxyzine, are used most often. Some antihistamines, such as cyproheptadine, diphenhydramine, and hydroxyzine, cause drowsiness. They help relieve itching and, when used before bedtime, aid in sleep. However, these drugs are usually not given during the day to older people, who are at higher risk of falling because of drowsiness. Cetirizine and loratadine cause less drowsiness but rarely can have this effect in older people. Fexofenadine causes less drowsiness but sometimes causes a headache. Doxepin makes people very drowsy and is effective, so it can be taken at bedtime if itching is severe.

Cholestyramine is used to treat itching caused by gallbladder or liver disorders, chronic kidney disease, or polycythemia vera. However, cholestyramine has an unpleasant taste, causes constipation, and can decrease absorption of other drugs. Naltrexone can be used to treat itching caused by gallbladder or liver disorders but may increase pain if pain is present. Gabapentin can help relieve itching caused by chronic kidney disease but can cause drowsiness.

O──ᴛᴛ KEY POINTS

- Itching usually results from dry skin, a skin disorder, or an allergic reaction.
- If the person has no rash or skin abnormalities, the cause may be a drug, an allergic reaction that has internal effects, or a systemic disorder.
- Skin care measures (such as limiting bathing, moisturizing the skin, and humidifying the air) can usually help relieve itching.
- Itching can usually be relieved by topical or systemic treatments.

ITCHING, ANAL

Itching of the anus and the skin around the anus (perianal skin) is called anal itching or pruritus ani.

CAUSES

The **most common** causes of anal itching are

- Unknown (the majority)
- Related to hygiene

Most often, doctors do not identify a specific disorder as the cause of anal itching, and the itching goes away without treatment after a period of time. Many of the other cases of anal itching are due to hygiene issues. Only a very few cases are caused by a specific disorder (see Table on pages 225 to 226), such as pinworms or a fungal infection. Of the specific causes, only inflammatory bowel disease and anal cancer (rare causes) are considered serious.

Extremes in hygiene can lead to anal itching. For instance, inadequate cleansing leaves irritating stool and sweat residue on the anal skin. More commonly, overly vigorous cleansing, often with sanitary wipes and strong soaps, can dry or irritate the skin or occasionally cause an allergic reaction. Hemorrhoids can make it difficult for people to thoroughly clean themselves after a bowel movement. Some hemorrhoids produce mucus or cause stool leakage, both of which can cause itching.

Once anal itching starts, an itch-scratch-itch cycle can begin, in which scratching causes more itching. Often, people scratch and rub the itchy area so much that they scrape the skin open. The scrapes sometimes become infected, which causes yet more itching. Also, people sometimes become allergic to the ointments or other treatments they use for the itching.

EVALUATION

Not every episode of anal itching requires immediate evaluation by a doctor. The following information can help people decide whether a doctor's evaluation is needed and help them know what to expect during the evaluation.

WARNING SIGNS

In people with anal itching, certain symptoms and characteristics are cause for concern. They include

- Pus draining from the anus or around it (draining fistula)
- Bloody diarrhea
- Bulging or protruding hemorrhoids
- Perianal skin soiled with fecal material
- Dull or thickened perianal skin

WHEN TO SEE A DOCTOR

People who have anal itching plus bloody diarrhea or draining pus should see a doctor in a day or two. Other people should see a doctor if the itching has lasted for more than a few days, but the visit is not urgent.

WHAT THE DOCTOR DOES

Doctors first ask questions about the person's symptoms and medical history. Doctors then do a physical examination. What they find during the history and physical examination often suggests a cause of the itching and the tests that may need to be done (see Table).

The history is focused on when the itching started and how long it has lasted. Doctors ask about the following:

- Ingestion of irritating foods, particularly acidic or spicy foods
- Bowel habits, including use of wipes, ointments (even those used to treat itching), sprays, and soaps applied to the anus
- Hygiene habits, particularly frequency of showers and baths
- Known infections or disorders (such as diabetes, hemorrhoids, or psoriasis)
- Recent use of antibiotics

The physical examination is focused on the appearance of the anus and the perianal skin. Doctors examine this area for

- Dullness and thickness
- Signs of infection due to scratching
- Hemorrhoids, lesions, fistulas, and scrapes (caused by scratching and rubbing)
- Scabies or pinworms

CAUSES AND FEATURES OF ANAL ITCHING

Cause	Common Features*	Tests
Anal or rectal disorders		
Inflammatory bowel disease (such as Crohn disease)	Discharge of pus Pain in the rectum (sometimes) and/or abdomen (often) Sometimes diarrhea	Examination of the lower portion of the large intestine, the rectum, and the anus with an endoscope (sigmoidoscopy) or of the entire large intestine (colonoscopy)
Hemorrhoids (internal or external)	With internal hemorrhoids, bleeding (a small amount of blood on toilet paper or in the toilet bowl) With external hemorrhoids, a painful, swollen lump on the anus	A doctor's examination Usually examination of the rectum with an endoscope (anoscopy) or sigmoidoscopy
Infections		
Bacterial infection (caused by scratching)	Inflamed, red area, sometimes visible scratching	A doctor's examination
Yeast infection (*Candida*)	A rash around the anus	A doctor's examination Sometimes examination of a sample of skin scrapings under a microscope (to identify the fungus)
Pinworms	Usually in children Sometimes present in several family members	Microscopic examination of transparent tape that was applied to the anal area to check for pinworm eggs
Scabies	Intense itching, usually worse at night Possibly itching of other body areas Possibly pink, thin, slightly raised lines or bumps (burrows) on the affected areas	A doctor's examination Examination of skin scrapings
Skin disorders		
Atopic dermatitis	An itchy, red, oozing, and crusty rash	A doctor's examination
Psoriasis	Sometimes itchy or painful patches on the skin	A doctor's examination
Drugs		
Antibiotics	Current or recent use of an antibiotic	Elimination of the drug to see whether symptoms are relieved
Foods and dietary supplements		
Beer, caffeine, chocolate, hot peppers, milk products, nuts, tomato products, citrus fruits, spices, or vitamin C tablets	Symptoms that occur after a substance is ingested	Elimination of the substance from the diet to see whether symptoms are relieved
Hygiene-related problems		
Excessive sweating	Excessive sweating described by the person, particularly with wearing of tight and/or synthetic clothing	Measures to limit sweating (such as wearing loose cotton underwear and changing underwear frequently) to see whether symptoms are relieved

(continued)

CAUSES AND FEATURES OF ANAL ITCHING (continued)

Cause	Common Features*	Tests
Overly meticulous or aggressive cleansing of the anal area	Inappropriate cleansing practices described by the person	A change in cleansing practices to see whether symptoms are relieved
Poor cleansing		
Skin irritants		
Anesthetic preparations, ointments, soaps, and sanitary wipes	Use of a possibly irritating substance described by the person	Avoidance of the substance to see whether symptoms are relieved

*Features include symptoms and the results of the doctor's examination. Features mentioned are typical but not always present.

TESTING

If doctors do not see any abnormalities on or around the anus, they usually do not do tests and simply treat the person's symptoms. If there are any visible skin abnormalities, doctors may examine a scraping of the perianal skin to rule out a fungal infection. Sometimes they give the person a local anesthetic and remove a small piece of tissue to examine under a microscope (skin biopsy). If pinworms are suspected, eggs can be collected from the anal region using sticky transparent tape to confirm the diagnosis.

Doctors may also examine the rectum with a short, rigid tube (a procedure called anoscopy) to check for internal hemorrhoids.

TREATMENT

The best way to treat anal itching is to treat the underlying disorder. For example, drugs can be taken for parasitic infections, and creams can be applied for fungal infections. Irritating foods can be eliminated from the diet or avoided for a while to see whether the itching lessens. If possible, antibiotics can be stopped or switched.

Proper hygiene is important. After bowel movements, the anal area should be cleaned with absorbent cotton or plain soft tissue moistened with warm water or a commercial cleanser made specifically for hemorrhoids. People should avoid using soaps and premoistened wipes. Frequent dusting with nonmedicated cornstarch or talcum powder helps combat excess moisture. Corticosteroid ointments (such as 1% hydrocortisone) often help relieve symptoms. Clothing should be loose, and bed clothing should be lightweight.

KEY POINTS

- Pinworms in children and hygiene-related issues in adults are common causes.
- Foods and detergents or soaps can cause anal itching.
- Appropriate hygiene practices (careful but gentle cleansing, avoiding strong soaps and chemicals, and decreasing skin moisture) can help relieve symptoms.

JAUNDICE IN ADULTS

In jaundice, the skin and whites of the eyes look yellow. Jaundice occurs when there is too much bilirubin (a yellow pigment) in the blood—a condition called hyperbilirubinemia.

Bilirubin is formed when hemoglobin (the part of red blood cells that carries oxygen) is broken down as part of the normal process of recycling old or damaged red blood cells. Bilirubin is carried in the bloodstream to the liver, where it binds with bile. Bilirubin is then moved through the bile ducts into the digestive tract, so that it can be eliminated from the body. Most bilirubin is eliminated in stool, but a small amount is eliminated in urine. If bilirubin cannot be moved through the liver and bile ducts quickly enough, it builds up in the blood and is deposited in the skin. The result is jaundice.

Many people with jaundice also have dark urine and light-colored stool. These changes occur when a blockage or other problem prevents bilirubin from being eliminated in stool, causing more bilirubin to be eliminated in urine.

High bilirubin levels may cause people to itch all over, but jaundice itself causes few other symptoms in adults. However in newborns, high bilirubin levels (see page 233) can cause a form of brain damage called kernicterus. Also, many disorders that cause jaundice cause other symptoms or serious problems. These symptoms may include nausea, vomiting and abdominal pain, and small spiderlike blood vessels that are visible in the skin (spider angiomas). Men may have enlarged breasts, shrunken testes, and pubic hair that grows as it does in women.

Serious problems can include

- Ascites: Accumulation of fluid within the abdomen
- Coagulopathy: A tendency to bleed or bruise
- Hepatic encephalopathy: Deterioration of brain function because the liver malfunctions, allowing toxic substances to build up in the blood, reach the brain, and cause changes in mental function (such as confusion and drowsiness)
- Portal hypertension: High blood pressure in the veins that bring blood to the liver, which can lead to bleeding in the esophagus and sometimes stomach

If people eat large amounts of food rich in beta-carotene (such as carrots, squash, and some melons), their skin may look slightly yellow, but their eyes do not turn yellow. This condition is not jaundice and is unrelated to liver disease.

CAUSES

Jaundice has many causes. Most causes involve disorders and drugs that

- Damage the liver
- Interfere with the flow of bile
- Trigger the destruction of red blood cells (hemolysis), thus producing more bilirubin than the liver can handle

The **most common causes** are

- Hepatitis
- Alcoholic liver disease
- A blockage of a bile duct by a gallstone (usually) or tumor
- A toxic reaction to a drug or medicinal herb

Hepatitis damages the liver, making it less able to move bilirubin into the bile ducts. Hepatitis may be acute (short-lived) or chronic (lasting at least 6 months). It is usually caused by a virus. Acute viral hepatitis is a common cause of jaundice, particularly jaundice that occurs in young and otherwise healthy people. Sometimes hepatitis is caused by an autoimmune disorder or use of certain drugs. When hepatitis is caused by an autoimmune disorder or a drug, it cannot be spread from person to person.

Drinking large amounts of alcohol over a long period of time damages the liver. The amount of alcohol and time required to cause damage varies, but typically, people must drink heavily for at least 8 to 10 years. Other drugs, toxins, and some herbal products can also damage the liver (see Table on page 231).

If the bile ducts are blocked, bilirubin can build up in the blood. Most blockages are caused by a gallstone, but some are caused by cancer (such as cancer in the pancreas or bile ducts) or rare liver disorders (such as primary biliary cirrhosis or primary sclerosing cholangitis).

Less common causes of jaundice include hereditary disorders that interfere with how the body processes bilirubin. They include Gilbert syndrome and other, less common disorders such as Dubin-Johnson syndrome. In Gilbert syndrome, bilirubin levels are slightly increased but usually not enough to cause jaundice. This disorder is most often detected during routine screening tests in young adults. It causes no other symptoms and no problems.

EVALUATION

Jaundice is obvious, but identifying its cause requires a doctor's examination, blood tests, and sometimes other tests.

WARNING SIGNS

In people with jaundice, the following symptoms are cause for concern:

- Severe abdominal pain and tenderness
- Changes in mental function, such as drowsiness, agitation, or confusion
- Blood in stool or tarry black stool
- Blood in vomit
- Fever
- A tendency to bruise or to bleed easily, sometimes resulting in a reddish purple rash of tiny dots or larger splotches (which indicate bleeding in the skin)

WHEN TO SEE A DOCTOR

If people have any warning signs, they should see a doctor as soon as possible. People with no warning signs should see a doctor within a few days.

WHAT THE DOCTOR DOES

Doctors first ask questions about the person's symptoms and medical history. Doctors then do a physical examination. What they find during the history and physical examination often suggests a cause and the tests that may need to be done (see Table on pages 229 to 231).

Doctors ask when the jaundice started and how long it has been present. They also ask when urine started to look dark (which usually occurs before jaundice develops). People are asked about other symptoms, such as itching, fatigue, changes in stool, and abdominal pain. Doctors are particularly interested in symptoms that suggest a serious cause. For example,

sudden loss of appetite, nausea, vomiting, pain in the abdomen, and fever suggest hepatitis, particularly in young people and people with risk factors for hepatitis. Fever and severe, constant pain in the upper right part of the abdomen suggest acute cholangitis (infection of the bile ducts), usually in people with a blockage in a bile duct. Acute cholangitis is considered a medical emergency.

Doctors ask people whether they have had liver disorders, whether they have had surgery that involved the bile ducts, and whether they take any drugs that can cause jaundice (including alcohol, over-the-counter drugs, medicinal herbs, and other herbal products such as teas). Knowing whether family members have also had jaundice or other liver disorders can help doctors identify hereditary liver disorders.

Because hepatitis is a common cause, doctors ask particularly about conditions that increase the risk of hepatitis, such as

- Working at a day care center
- Living in or working at an institution with long-term residents, such as a mental health care facility, prison, or long-term care facility
- Living in or traveling to an area where hepatitis is widespread
- Participating in anal sex
- Eating raw shellfish
- Injecting illegal or recreational drugs
- Having hemodialysis
- Sharing razor blades or toothbrushes
- Getting a tattoo or body piercing
- Working in a health care facility without being vaccinated against hepatitis
- Having had a blood transfusion before 1992
- Having sex with someone who has hepatitis

During the physical examination, doctors look for signs of serious disorders (such as fever, very low blood pressure, and a rapid heart rate) and for signs that liver function is greatly impaired (such as easy bruising, a rash of tiny dots or splotches, or changes in mental function). They gently press on the abdomen to check for lumps, tenderness, swelling, and other abnormalities, such as an enlarged liver or spleen.

TESTING

Tests include the following:

- Blood tests to evaluate how well the liver is functioning and whether it is damaged (liver function tests)

SOME CAUSES AND FEATURES OF JAUNDICE

Cause	Common Features*	Tests†
Liver and gallbladder disorders		
Alcoholic liver disease	Jaundice that develops slowly	A doctor's examination
	A history of heavy alcohol consumption	Blood tests
	In men, development of feminine characteristics, including loss of muscle tissue, smooth skin, enlarged breasts, shrunken testes, and growth of pubic hair in a female pattern	Sometimes liver biopsy
	Sometimes swelling of the abdomen due to accumulation of fluid (ascites)	
Blockage of a bile duct by a gallstone or, less commonly, by a tumor of the pancreas or bile ducts	Dark urine and light-colored, soft, bulky, oily-looking, and unusually foul-smelling stool	Imaging such as
	Usually pain in the upper right part or middle of the abdomen	■ Ultrasonography (done by putting the ultrasound probe on the abdomen)
	If the cause is a tumor, weight loss and sometimes chronic abdominal pain	■ Endoscopic ultrasonography (done with a probe inserted via a flexible viewing tube into the small intestine)
		■ CT cholangiography (CT of the bile ducts done after a radiopaque dye is injected into a vein)
		■ MRCP (MRI of the bile and pancreatic ducts using specialized techniques)
		■ ERCP (x-rays of the bile and pancreatic ducts taken after a radiopaque dye is injected into these ducts through a flexible viewing tube inserted through the mouth and into the small intestine)
		Biopsy if imaging results suggest cancer
Cholestasis of pregnancy	Severe itching	Blood tests
	Later, jaundice and dark urine	Usually ultrasonography
	Usually develops during late pregnancy	
Hepatitis (viral)	Symptoms that occur before jaundice develops:	Blood tests for hepatitis viruses
	■ Nausea or vomiting ■ Loss of appetite ■ Fatigue ■ Constant pain in the upper right part of the abdomen ■ Fever ■ Sometimes joint pain	Usually liver biopsy if hepatitis is chronic
	Often in people with risk factors, such as recreational use of injected drugs or participation in anal sex	

(continued)

SOME CAUSES AND FEATURES OF JAUNDICE *(continued)*

Cause	Common Features*	Tests†
Primary biliary cirrhosis (an autoimmune disorder causing destruction of the small bile ducts in the liver)	Symptoms that often occur before jaundice develops: ■ Fatigue ■ Itching ■ Dry mouth and eyes Sometimes discomfort in the upper right part of the abdomen, darkening of the skin, and small yellow deposits of fat in the skin (xanthomas) or eyelids (xanthelasmas)	Blood tests to check for the antibodies that occur in most people with this disorder Ultrasonography and often MRI of the abdomen Liver biopsy
Primary sclerosing cholangitis (scarring and destruction of small and large bile ducts)	Symptoms that occur before jaundice develops: ■ Worsening fatigue ■ Itching Pain in the upper right part of the abdomen Sometimes light-colored, soft, bulky, oily-looking, and unusually foul-smelling stool Often in people with inflammatory bowel disease	MRI of the abdomen ERCP
Other disorders		
Breakdown of red blood cells (hemolysis), which may be caused by ■ Drugs ■ Toxins (including some snake venoms) ■ Hereditary red blood cell disorders ■ Enzyme deficiencies (such as G6PD deficiency) ■ Infections (such as malaria)	Symptoms of anemia (paleness, weakness, and fatigue) Sometimes use of a drug that causes hemolysis or presence of a red blood cell disorder in a family member	Blood tests
Wilson disease (which causes copper to accumulate in the liver)	Tremors, difficulty speaking and swallowing, involuntary movements, loss of coordination, and personality changes Gold or greenish gold rings in the cornea of the eyes (Kayser-Fleischer rings)	Slit-lamp examination of the eyes to check for Kayser-Fleischer rings Blood tests to measure levels of copper and copper proteins Urine tests to measure the level of copper eliminated in the urine If the diagnosis is still unclear, liver biopsy
Surgical complications such as ■ Scarring of the bile ducts due to surgery on or near these ducts ■ Reduced blood flow to the liver due to blood loss or other complications of major surgery	Develops soon after surgery, particularly major surgery	A doctor's examination Sometimes other tests, depending on the likely causes

(continued)

SOME CAUSES AND FEATURES OF JAUNDICE *(continued)*

Cause	Common Features*	Tests†
Drugs and toxins		
Acetaminophen (in high doses or as an overdose)	Use of a substance that can cause jaundice	A doctor's examination
Certain medicinal herbs such as germander, kava, or pyrrolizidine		
Isoniazid		
Iron when taken in large amounts		
Amanita phalloides mushroom toxin		

*Features include symptoms and results of the doctor's examination. Features mentioned are typical but not always present.
†Doctors typically measure bilirubin levels in the blood and do blood tests to determine how well the liver is functioning and whether it is damaged (liver function tests) and to assess the blood's ability to clot.
CT = computed tomography; ERCP = endoscopic retrograde cholangiopancreatography; G6PD = glucose-6-phosphate dehydrogenase; MRCP = magnetic resonance cholangiopancreatography; MRI = magnetic resonance imaging.

- Usually imaging tests such as ultrasonography
- Sometimes biopsy or laparoscopy

Liver function tests help doctors determine whether the cause is liver malfunction or a blocked bile duct. If a bile duct is blocked, imaging tests, such as ultrasonography, are usually required.

Other blood tests are done based on the disorder doctors suspect and the results of the examination and the initial tests. They may include

- Tests to assess the blood's ability to clot (prothrombin time and partial thromboplastin time)
- Tests to check for hepatitis viruses or abnormal antibodies (due to autoimmune disorders)
- A complete blood count
- Blood cultures to check for infection of the bloodstream
- Examination of a blood sample under a microscope to check for excessive destruction of red blood cells

If imaging is needed, ultrasonography of the abdomen is often done first. It can usually detect blockages in the bile ducts. Alternatively, computed tomography (CT) or magnetic resonance imaging (MRI) may be done.

If ultrasonography shows a blockage in a bile duct, other tests may be needed to determine the cause. Typically, magnetic resonance cholangiopancreatography (MRCP) or endoscopic retrograde cholangiopancreatography (ERCP) is used. MRCP is MRI of the bile and pancreatic ducts, done with specialized techniques that make the fluid in the ducts appear bright and the surrounding tissues appear dark. Thus, MRCP provides better images of the ducts than conventional MRI. For ERCP, a flexible viewing tube (endoscope) is inserted through the mouth and into the small intestine, and a radiopaque dye is injected through the tube into the bile and pancreatic ducts. Then x-rays are taken. When available, MRCP is usually preferred because it is just as accurate and is safer. But ERCP may be used because it enables doctors to take a biopsy sample, remove a gallstone, or do other procedures.

Occasionally, liver biopsy is needed. It may be done when certain causes (such as viral hepatitis, use of a drug, or exposure to a toxin) are suspected or when the diagnosis is unclear after doctors have the results of other tests.

Laparoscopy may be done when other tests have not identified why bile flow is blocked. For this procedure, doctors make a small incision just below the navel and insert a viewing tube (laparoscope) to examine the liver and gallbladder directly. Rarely, a larger incision is needed (a procedure called laparotomy).

TREATMENT

The underlying disorder and any problems it causes are treated as needed. If jaundice is due to acute viral hepatitis, it may disappear gradually, without treatment, as the condition of the liver improves. However, hepatitis may become chronic, even if the jaundice disappears. Jaundice itself requires no treatment in adults (unlike in newborns—see page 235).

Usually, itching gradually disappears as the liver's condition improves. If itching is bothersome, taking cholestyramine by mouth may help. However, cholestyramine is ineffective when a bile duct is completely blocked.

If the cause is a blocked bile duct, a procedure may be done to open the bile duct. This procedure can usually be done during ERCP, using instruments threaded through the endoscope.

ESSENTIALS FOR OLDER PEOPLE

In older people, the disorder causing jaundice may not cause the same symptoms as it typically does in younger people, or the symptoms may be milder or harder to recognize. For example, if older people have acute viral hepatitis, they often have much less abdominal pain than younger people. When older people become confused, doctors may mistakenly diagnose dementia and not realize that the cause is hepatic encephalopathy. That is, doctors may not realize that brain function is deteriorating because the liver is unable to remove toxic substances from the blood (as it usually does) and, thus, the toxic substances can reach the brain.

In older people, jaundice usually results from a blockage in the bile ducts, and the blockage is more likely to be cancer. Doctors suspect that the blockage is cancer when older people have lost weight, have only mild itching, have no abdominal pain, and have a lump in the abdomen.

⊶ KEY POINTS

- If damage to the liver is severe, jaundice may be accompanied by serious problems, such as deterioration of brain function and a tendency to bleed or bruise.
- Acute viral hepatitis is a common cause of jaundice, particularly in young and otherwise healthy people.
- People should see a doctor promptly if they have jaundice so that the doctor can check for serious causes.
- Cholestyramine may help relieve itching.

JAUNDICE IN NEWBORNS

In jaundice, the skin and whites of the eyes look yellow. Jaundice is common in newborns. It occurs when the level of bilirubin (a yellow pigment produced during the normal breakdown of red blood cells) in the blood rises. When the bilirubin level gets too high, bilirubin can be deposited in the skin, the whites of the eyes, and other tissues. As bilirubin levels increase, the whites of the eyes turn yellow first, followed by the skin. Slightly more than half of all full-term newborns develop jaundice during the first week of life. Jaundice is even more common among premature infants.

Newborns normally have a high red blood cell count at birth, and their red blood cells have a shorter life span than adult red blood cells. The high red blood cell count and shorter life span mean that more of the newborn's red blood cells undergo the normal daily breakdown of aging red blood cells (a process called hemolysis). Aging red blood cells are normally removed by the spleen. Hemoglobin (the substance in red blood cells that carries oxygen) is broken down and recycled. One portion of the hemoglobin molecule is converted into bilirubin, which is carried by the blood to the liver. The liver chemically changes the bilirubin by binding it to another substance, creating conjugated bilirubin. The conjugated bilirubin passes into the bile, which is then excreted into the digestive tract. In adults, bilirubin is further broken down by the bacteria that normally reside in the digestive tract. This form of bilirubin is excreted in the stool and gives stool its typical brown color. However, newborns do not yet have these bacteria or other digestive enzymes needed to process bilirubin. Thus, because newborns produce more bilirubin than older children and adults and eliminate bilirubin at a slower rate than older children and adults, high levels of bilirubin can build up in their blood relatively quickly. This disorder is called hyperbilirubinemia.

COMPLICATIONS

Whether jaundice is dangerous depends on what is causing it, how high the bilirubin level is, and how quickly the bilirubin level rises. Some disorders that cause jaundice are dangerous regardless of what the bilirubin level is. However, an extremely high bilirubin level, regardless of cause, is dangerous.

The most serious consequence of a high bilirubin level is kernicterus—a disorder in which bilirubin is deposited in the brain and causes brain damage. Kernicterus occurs only when the level of bilirubin is high. The risk of this disorder is higher for newborns who are premature, who are seriously ill, or who are given certain drugs. If untreated, kernicterus may lead to unresponsiveness (stupor) or lethargy, loss of muscle tone, a high-pitched cry, poor feeding, and seizures. Later, children can have cerebral palsy, hearing loss, a permanent upward gaze, or other signs of brain damage. Kernicterus is now rare because of increased screening for hyperbilirubinemia and early treatment.

CAUSES

COMMON CAUSES

The most common causes of jaundice in the newborn are

- Physiologic jaundice (most common)
- Breastfeeding jaundice
- Breast milk jaundice
- Excessive breakdown of red blood cells (hemolysis)

Physiologic jaundice occurs in most newborns. It develops because the red blood cells in newborns normally break down at a slightly increased rate and because the digestive tract and liver function in newborns are immature. As the digestive tract and liver mature, bilirubin is processed faster, and jaundice quickly disappears. Physiologic jaundice typically appears 2 to 4 days after birth (jaundice that appears in the first 24 to 48 hours after birth is usually due to a disorder). Physiologic jaundice usually causes no other symptoms and resolves within 1 to 2 weeks.

Breastfeeding jaundice is common. It develops in 1 of 6 breastfed infants a few days after birth. It occurs in newborns who do not consume enough breast milk (often because the mother's milk has not yet come in well). Newborns who consume less breast milk have fewer bowel movements and thus eliminate less bilirubin. As newborns continue to breastfeed and consume more milk, the jaundice usually disappears on its own.

Breast milk jaundice is less common. It develops in only 1 to 2% of breastfed newborns. It occurs when breast milk contains a high level of a substance that slows bilirubin excretion and thus causes the bilirubin level to increase. Breast milk jaundice appears when newborns are 5 to 7 days old, peaks at about 2 weeks, and can last for 3 to 12 weeks.

Excessive breakdown of red blood cells can overwhelm the liver with more bilirubin than it can process. There are several causes of excessive breakdown of red blood cells. In hemolytic disease of the newborn, the newborn's blood type is incompatible with the mother's (as occurs in Rh incompatibility). Because their blood types are different, antibodies from the mother can cross the placenta and attack the newborn's red blood cells, rapidly breaking them down. This causes a sudden rise in bilirubin level. Less common causes of excessive red blood cell breakdown include hereditary deficiency of the red blood cell enzyme glucose-6-phosphate dehydrogenase (G6PD) and hereditary red blood cell disorders such as severe alpha-thalassemia. Events during delivery sometimes lead to excessive breakdown of red blood cells. Newborns who were injured during birth sometimes have a collection of blood (hematoma) under their skin. The breakdown of blood in a large hematoma may cause jaundice. If the umbilical cord was not clamped quickly, newborns may get excess blood from the placenta. The breakdown or this blood can also cause jaundice.

LESS COMMON CAUSES

Less common disorders that cause jaundice include

- Severe infections
- An underactive thyroid gland (hypothyroidism)
- Certain hereditary liver disorders
- Obstruction of bile flow from the liver

Overwhelming bacterial infection (sepsis) acquired during or shortly after birth can cause jaundice. Infections acquired by the fetus in the womb are sometimes the cause. Such infections include toxoplasmosis and infections with cytomegalovirus or the herpes simplex virus or rubella virus.

Hypothyroidism may be present at birth or shortly thereafter, and up to 10% of affected newborns have jaundice for weeks to months.

Hereditary liver disorders that can cause jaundice include Dubin-Johnson syndrome, Rotor syndrome, Crigler-Najjar syndrome, and Gilbert syndrome.

Bile flow may be reduced or blocked because of a birth defect of the bile ducts (such as biliary atresia), pyloric stenosis, or because a disorder such as cystic fibrosis has damaged the liver.

RISK FACTORS

Major risk factors for jaundice include prematurity (35 to 36 weeks' gestation), blood type incompatibility with the mother, jaundice that begins soon after birth (high levels occur in the first 24 hours), birth-related bruising, and family history of jaundice. Also at major risk of jaundice are newborns who are exclusively breastfed and who have lost a significant amount of weight and have a high-risk bilirubin level before discharge from the hospital.

Newborns who have a low-risk level of bilirubin before discharge from the hospital, who are postmature (over 41 weeks' gestation), and who are exclusively bottle-fed are at low risk of jaundice.

EVALUATION

While newborns are in the hospital, doctors periodically check them for jaundice. Jaundice is sometimes obvious in the color of the whites of the newborn's eyes or skin. But most doctors also measure the newborn's bilirubin level before discharge from the hospital. If the newborn has jaundice, doctors focus on determining whether it is physiologic and, if not, identifying its cause.

WARNING SIGNS

In newborns with jaundice, the following symptoms are cause for concern:

- Jaundice that appears in the first 24 hours of life
- Jaundice in newborns over 3 weeks old
- Lethargy, poor feeding, irritability, or difficulty breathing

- Jaundice that rapidly worsens
- A fever

Doctors are also concerned when the bilirubin level is very high or is increasing rapidly and when blood tests suggest that the flow of bile is reduced or blocked.

WHEN TO SEE A DOCTOR

Newborns with warning signs should be evaluated by a doctor right away. If the newborn is discharged from the hospital on the first day after birth, a bilirubin level should be done before discharge. A follow-up visit to measure the bilirubin level should be scheduled within 2 days of discharge. Newborns with risk factors for a high jaundice level or who had a high level before discharge may need to be seen at least twice after discharge from the hospital.

Once at home, if the newborn had not been jaundiced before but parents now notice that their newborn's skin or eyes look yellow, they should contact their doctor immediately. The doctor can decide how urgently to evaluate the newborn based on whether the newborn has any symptoms or risk factors (such as prematurity).

WHAT THE DOCTOR DOES

Doctors first ask questions about the newborn's symptoms and medical history. Doctors then do a physical examination. What they find during the history and physical examination often suggests a cause and the tests that may need to be done.

Doctors ask when the jaundice started, how long has it been present, and whether the newborn has other symptoms such as lethargy and poor feeding. Doctors ask what, how much, and how often the newborn is being fed. They ask how well the newborn is latching onto the breast or taking the nipple of the bottle, whether the mother feels that her milk has come in, and whether the newborn is swallowing during feedings and seems satisfied after feedings. Information about how much urine and stool the newborn produces can help doctors evaluate whether the newborn is being fed enough.

Doctors ask the mother whether she has had infections or disorders that can cause jaundice, what her blood type is, and what drugs she is taking. They also ask whether family members have had any of the hereditary disorders that can cause jaundice.

During the physical examination, doctors check the newborn's skin to see how far jaundice has spread. They also look for other clues suggesting a cause, particularly signs of infection, injury, and thyroid disease.

TESTING

The bilirubin level is measured to confirm the diagnosis of jaundice and determine its severity. The level may be measured in a sample of blood or by using a sensor placed on the skin.

If the bilirubin level is high, other blood tests are done. They include

- Hematocrit (the percentage of red blood cells in blood)
- Examination of a blood sample under a microscope
- Reticulocyte count (the number of newly formed red blood cells)
- Direct Coombs test (which checks for certain antibodies attached to red blood cells)
- Measurement of different types of bilirubin
- Blood type and Rh status (positive or negative) of the newborn and mother
- Albumin (a protein that binds bilirubin, keeping it from being able to enter the brain) level

Other tests may be done depending on results of the history and physical examination and on the newborn's bilirubin level. They may include culturing samples of blood, urine, or cerebrospinal fluid to check for infection and measuring levels of red blood cell enzymes to check for unusual causes of red blood cell breakdown.

TREATMENT

When a disorder is identified, it is treated if possible (for example, doctors may give immune globulin to infants with hemolytic disease of the newborn). A high bilirubin level itself may also require treatment.

Physiologic jaundice usually does not require treatment. More frequent feedings (for breastfed newborns, nursing at least 8 to 12 times per day and similar or slightly fewer feedings for formula-fed newborns) can help prevent jaundice or reduce its severity. Frequent feedings increase the frequency of bowel movements and thus eliminate more bilirubin in stool. The type of formula does not seem to matter. Newborns should not be fed water or sugar water because these liquids do not prevent the bilirubin level from rising, do not provide nutrition, and will decrease the amount of milk or formula the newborn drinks.

Breastfeeding jaundice may also be prevented or reduced by increasing the frequency of feedings to at least 8 to 12 times per day. If the bilirubin level continues to increase, temporarily supplementing breast milk feedings with formula or expressed breast milk may help.

Breast milk jaundice is not relieved by more frequent nursing because the breast milk contains a substance that worsens jaundice. In some cases, mothers may be advised to stop breastfeeding for 1 or 2 days and to express breast milk regularly during this break from breastfeeding. They can resume breastfeeding as soon as the newborn's bilirubin level starts to decrease. In most cases, mothers are advised to breastfeed as usual because the benefits of breastfeeding are greater than the risk of developing kernicterus with breast milk jaundice.

A high bilirubin level may be treated with

- Exposure to light (phototherapy)
- Exchange transfusion

PHOTOTHERAPY

This treatment is most commonly used. It uses bright light to change unconjugated bilirubin into forms that can be eliminated rapidly through the urine. Blue light is the most effective light, and most doctors use special commercial phototherapy units. Newborns are undressed to expose as much skin as possible. They are turned frequently and left under the lights until the bilirubin level comes down and stays low. The lights may be needed for as few as 2 days to a week. Intensive phototherapy can prevent kernicterus if started early when the bilirubin level is rising. However, it is useful only for a high level of bilirubin that has not been changed (conjugated) by the liver. To determine how well the treatment is working, doctors periodically measure the bilirubin level in the blood. Skin color is not a reliable guide. Light therapy is relatively safe for newborns. However, newborns need eye shields to protect their eyes from the bright light.

EXCHANGE TRANSFUSION

This treatment is used when the bilirubin level is very high and continues to rise despite use of intensive phototherapy. It can rapidly remove bilirubin from the bloodstream. A small amount of the newborn's blood is gradually removed (one syringe at a time) and replaced with an equal amount of donor blood. The procedure usually takes 2 to 4 hours. Typically, the total amount of blood that is removed and replaced is equal to twice the newborn's total blood volume.

Exchange transfusions may need to be repeated if the bilirubin level continues to rise. The procedure has risks and complications, such as heart and breathing problems, blood clots, and electrolyte imbalances in the blood.

The need for exchange transfusion has decreased since early bilirubin screening has become the normal practice and because phototherapy (and immune globulin treatment for hemolytic disease of the newborn) has become increasingly effective.

O—π KEY POINTS

- In many newborns, jaundice develops 2 or 3 days after birth and disappears on its own within a week.
- Whether jaundice is of concern depends on what is causing it, how high the bilirubin level is, and how quickly the bilirubin level rises.
- Doctors check newborns for risk factors, do bilirubin tests before newborns leave the hospital, and follow up within 2 to 3 days after discharge from the hospital to identify newborns who may need treatment.
- Jaundice may result from serious disorders, such as incompatibility of the newborn's and mother's blood type, excessive breakdown of red blood cells, or a severe infection.
- If jaundice develops in a newborn, parents should call their doctor right away.
- If jaundice is caused by a disorder, that disorder is treated.
- If a high bilirubin level requires treatment, it is typically treated with phototherapy and sometimes with exchange transfusions.

Pains that seem to be coming from joints can sometimes be coming from structures outside the joints, such as ligaments, tendons, or muscles. Examples of such disorders are bursitis and tendinitis.

True joint pain (arthralgia) may or not be accompanied by joint inflammation (arthritis). The most common symptom of joint inflammation is pain. Inflamed joints may also be warm and swollen, and less often the overlying skin may be red. Arthritis may involve only joints of the limbs or also joints of the central part of the skeleton, such as the spine or pelvis. Pain may occur only when a joint is moved or also be present at rest. Other symptoms, such as rash, fever, eye pain, or mouth sores, may be present depending on the cause of the joint pain.

Different disorders tend to affect different numbers of joints. Because of this, doctors consider different causes of pain when the pain affects only one joint (see page 243) than when it affects more than one joint. When multiple joints are involved, some disorders are more likely to affect the same joint on both sides of the body (for example, both knees or both hands) than other disorders. This is termed symmetric arthritis. Also, in some disorders, an attack of arthritis remains in the same joints throughout the attack. In other disorders, the arthritis moves from joint to joint (migratory arthritis).

CAUSES

In most cases, the cause of pain originating inside multiple joints is arthritis. Disorders that cause arthritis may differ from each other in certain tendencies, such as the following:

- How many and which joints they usually involve
- Whether the central part of the skeleton, such as the spine or pelvis, is typically involved
- Whether arthritis is sudden (acute) or longstanding (chronic)

Acute arthritis affecting multiple joints is most often due to

- Viral infection

- The beginning of a joint disorder or a flare up of an existing chronic joint disorder (such as rheumatoid arthritis or psoriatic arthritis)

Less common causes of acute arthritis in multiple joints include Lyme disease (which also may affect only one joint), gonorrhea and streptococcal bacterial infections, reactive arthritis (arthritis that develops after an infection of the digestive or urinary tract), and gout.

Chronic arthritis affecting multiple joints is most often due to

- Inflammatory disorders such as rheumatoid arthritis, psoriatic arthritis, or systemic lupus erythematosus (in adults)
- The noninflammatory disorder osteoarthritis (in adults)
- Juvenile idiopathic arthritis (in children)

Other causes of chronic arthritis in multiple joints include autoimmune disorders that affect the joints, for example, systemic lupus erythematosus, psoriatic arthritis, ankylosing spondylitis, and vasculitis.

Some chronic inflammatory disorders can affect the spine as well as the limb joints (called the peripheral joints). Some affect certain parts of the spine more frequently. For example, ankylosing spondylitis more commonly affects the lower (lumbar) part of the spine, whereas rheumatoid arthritis more typically affects the upper (cervical) part of the spine in the neck.

The most common disorders **outside the joints** that cause pain around the joints are

- Fibromyalgia
- Polymyalgia rheumatica
- Bursitis or tendinitis

Bursitis and tendinitis often result from injury, usually affecting only one joint. However, certain disorders cause bursitis or tendinitis in many joints.

EVALUATION

In evaluating joint pain, doctors first try to decide whether joint pain is caused by a disorder of the joints or a serious bodywide (systemic) illness. Serious bodywide disorders may need specific immediate treatment. The following information can help people decide when to see a doctor and know what to expect during the evaluation.

WARNING SIGNS

In people with pain in more than one joint, symptoms that should prompt rapid evaluation include

- Joint swelling, warmth, and redness
- New skin rashes, spots, or purple blotches
- Sores in the mouth or nose or on the genitals
- Chest pain, shortness of breath, or new or severe cough
- Abdominal pain
- Fever, sweats, or chills
- Eye redness or pain

WHEN TO SEE A DOCTOR

People with warning signs should see a doctor right away. People without warning signs should call a doctor. The doctor decides how quickly they need to be seen based on the severity and location of pain, whether joints are swollen, whether the cause has been diagnosed previously, and other factors. Typically, a delay of several days or so is not harmful.

WHAT THE DOCTOR DOES

Doctors first ask questions about the person's symptoms and medical history. Then they do a physical examination. What doctors find during the history and physical examination often suggests a cause for joint pain and guides the tests that may need to be done (see Table on pages 239 to 241).

Doctors ask about pain severity, onset (sudden or gradual), how symptoms vary over time, and what increases or decreases pain (for example, rest or movement or time of day when the symptoms worsen or abate). They ask about joint stiffness and swelling, previously diagnosed joint disorders, and risk of exposure to sexually transmitted diseases and Lyme disease.

Doctors then do a complete physical examination. They check all joints (including those of the spine) for swelling, redness, warmth, tenderness, and noises that are made when the joints are moved (called crepitus). The joints are moved through their full range of motion, first by the person without assistance (called active range of motion) and then by the doctor (called passive range of motion). This examination helps determine which structure is causing the pain and if inflammation is present. They also check the eyes, mouth, nose, and genital area for sores or other signs of inflammation. The skin is examined for rashes. Lymph nodes are felt and the lungs and heart examined. Doctors usually test function of the nervous system so that they can detect disorders of the muscles or nerves.

Some findings give helpful clues as to the cause. For example, if the tenderness is around the joint but not over the joint, bursitis or tendinitis is the likely cause. If tenderness is present all over, fibromyalgia is possible. If the spine is tender as well as the joints, possible causes include osteoarthritis, reactive arthritis, ankylosing spondylitis, and psoriatic arthritis. Findings in the hand can help doctors differentiate between rheumatoid arthritis and osteoarthritis, two particularly common types of arthritis. For example, rheumatoid arthritis is more likely to involve the large knuckle joints (those that join the fingers with the hand) and wrist. Osteoarthritis is more likely to involve the finger joint near the fingernail. The wrist is unlikely to be affected in osteoarthritis, except at the base of the thumb.

TESTING

The following tests are the most important overall:

- Tests of joint fluid
- Blood tests for autoantibodies
- Erythrocyte sedimentation rate (ESR) and C-reactive protein

If joints are swollen, doctors usually insert a needle into the joint to take a sample of the fluid in the joint for testing (a procedure called joint aspiration or arthrocentesis). Doctors numb the area before taking a sample, so people experience little or no pain during the procedure. Doctors generally do a culture on the fluid to see whether infection is present. They look under a microscope for crystals in the fluid, which indicate gout or related disorders. The numbers of white blood cells in the fluid indicate whether the joint is inflamed.

Doctors also often do blood tests for autoantibodies. Examples of such tests are antinuclear antibodies, anti–double-stranded DNA, anticyclic citrullinated peptide, and rheumatoid factor. Autoantibodies in the blood may indicate an autoimmune disorder such as rheumatoid arthritis or systemic lupus erythematosus.

SOME CAUSES AND FEATURES OF PAIN IN MORE THAN ONE JOINT

Cause	Common Features*	Tests†
Disorders usually causing symmetric joint pain		
Fibromyalgia	Joints not inflamed	Sometimes testing unnecessary
	Chronic widespread pain and tenderness of muscles (that may involve joints and/or the back)	
	Fatigue	
	Sometimes irritable bowel syndrome or sleep disturbances	
	Usually chronic, often affecting women	
	Often depression or other mood disorders	
Infectious arthritis caused by viruses	Joint pain with or without inflammation, typically developing over hours or days	Analysis of joint fluid
		Blood tests to identify the virus (most often hepatitis C or B or parvovirus)
	Other symptoms of viral infection (for example, hepatitis B may cause jaundice, hepatitis C may cause purple blotches on legs, and HIV causes swollen lymph nodes)	
Juvenile idiopathic arthritis	Chronic,‡ symmetric joint inflammation during childhood	Blood tests for autoantibodies§
	Lower back pain	
	Swollen glands throughout the body or episodes of fever	
	An enlarged liver and spleen	
	Excess fluid around the heart or lungs	
	Rash or eye pain and redness	
Other diseases that cause joint inflammation (such as Sjögren syndrome and systemic sclerosis)	Pain in many joints with or without mild swelling	Blood tests for autoantibodies§
Rheumatoid arthritis	Chronic,‡ symmetric inflammation of small and large joints	X-rays
	Fatigue and morning stiffness	Blood tests for autoantibodies§
	Eventually, deformity of joints (particularly the knuckles and wrist joints)	
	Sometimes hard swellings under the skin and carpal tunnel syndrome	
	More common among young adults but can affect people aged 60 or older	
Serum sickness (a reaction by the immune system against large amounts of foreign proteins in the bloodstream)	Pain and inflammation in several joints	Sometimes blood tests
	Fever, rash, and swollen glands	
	In people known to have been exposed to foreign proteins (for example, from a blood transfusion) up to 21 days before the start of symptoms	

(continued)

SOME CAUSES AND FEATURES OF PAIN IN MORE THAN ONE JOINT *(continued)*

Cause	Common Features*	Tests†
Syndromes that cause unusual joint flexibility (such as Ehlers-Danlos syndrome)	Usually pain in many joints Joint inflammation very uncommon Increased looseness (laxity) of skin In people known to have a history of recurring joint dislocations or misalignment In people known to have affected family members	Sometimes genetic testing
Systemic lupus erythematosus and other, less common, autoimmune diseases (for example, polymyositis, dermatomyositis, Sjögren syndrome, and vasculitis such as immunoglobulin A–associated vasculitis)	Joint pain‡ with or without inflammation that can occur when the disorder flares up Other symptoms depending on specific autoimmune disease, such as skin changes; abdominal pain; muscle soreness; kidney disease; fluid around the lungs, heart, or other organs (serositis); or dry eyes and dry mouth	Blood tests for various autoantibodies§ Sometimes biopsy of skin, kidney, or other involved organs Analysis of urine
Disorders usually causing asymmetric joint pain		
Ankylosing spondylitis	Involvement of the large joints Lower back pain in most people Eye redness and pain (iritis) Achilles tendinitis Leakage of blood back through the aortic valve (aortic insufficiency)	X-rays Sometimes CT or MRI
Behçet syndrome	Chronic‡ or recurrent mouth and genital ulcers Sometimes eye pain and redness Often begins in the 20s Usually in parts of Asia and the middle east (relatively rare in the United States)	Sometimes testing unnecessary
Gout and related disorders (for example, pseudogout)	Sudden and severe pain, warmth, and swelling (particularly in the big toe or knee, but can be almost any joint) Sometimes fever Often only one joint affected, but sometimes many	Tests of joint fluid
Infective endocarditis (infection of the lining of the heart and usually also of the heart valves)	Joint pain and swelling Fever, night sweats, rash, weight loss, and heart murmur are common	Blood tests Echocardiography
Osteoarthritis	Chronic pain, most often in the knees and hips and small joints in the fingers, which may also be enlarged and slightly deformed No redness Often back and neck pain	X-rays

(continued)

SOME CAUSES AND FEATURES OF PAIN IN MORE THAN ONE JOINT (continued)

Cause	Common Features*	Tests†
Psoriatic arthritis	Psoriasis (sometimes with few or no skin lesions)	X-rays
	Sometimes chronic,‡ symmetric inflammation of joints	
	Chronic deformities of fingers, toes, and nails	
	Tendinitis	
	Eye redness and pain	
Reactive arthritis and enteropathic arthritis	Sudden pain, usually involving the large joints of the legs or feet, often 1 to 3 weeks after an infection of the gastrointestinal tract (such as gastroenteritis) or genitourinary tract (such as urethritis)	Tests for sexually transmitted diseases
	Sometimes involvement of the spine	

*Features include symptoms and the results of the doctor's examination. Features mentioned are typical but not always present.
†X-rays are often unnecessary. If fluid is in the joint, the fluid often needs to be removed for testing.
‡Symptoms may begin suddenly, but the disorder is typically chronic or recurs.
§Autoantibodies are antibodies directed against a person's own tissues. Examples include antinuclear antibodies, anti–double-stranded DNA, anticyclic citrullinated peptide, and rheumatoid factor.
CT = computed tomography; MRI = magnetic resonance imaging.

The ESR is a test that measures the rate at which red blood cells settle to the bottom of a test tube containing a blood sample. Blood that settles quickly typically means that bodywide (systemic) inflammation is likely, but many factors can affect the ESR test including age and anemia, so the test is sometimes inaccurate. To help determine whether bodywide inflammation is present, doctors sometimes do another blood test called C-reactive protein (a protein that circulates in the blood and dramatically increases in level when there is inflammation) in addition to the ESR test.

If a particular disorder is suspected, other tests may be required (see Table).

Imaging tests are sometimes necessary, especially if there is a possibility of bone or joint tumors. X-rays are done first, but sometimes computed tomography (CT) or magnetic resonance imaging (MRI) is needed.

TREATMENT

The underlying disorder is treated. For example, people with an autoimmune disorder (such as systemic lupus erythematosus) may need a drug that suppresses the immune system. People with a gonorrhea infection in the joint need antibiotics.

Symptoms can usually be relieved before the diagnosis is known. Inflammation can usually be relieved with nonsteroidal anti-inflammatory drugs (NSAIDs). Pain without inflammation is usually treated more safely with acetaminophen. Immobilizing the joint with a splint or sling can sometimes relieve pain. Applying heat (for example, with a heating pad) may decrease pain by relieving spasm in the muscles around joints (for example, after an injury). Applying cold (for example, with ice) may help relieve pain caused by joint inflammation. Heat or cold should be applied for at least 15 minutes at a time to allow deep penetration. The skin must be protected from extremes of heat and cold. For example, ice should be put in a plastic bag and wrapped in a towel.

After the acute pain and inflammation have lessened, physical therapy may be useful to regain or maintain range of motion and strengthen surrounding muscles. In people with chronic arthritis, continued physical activity is important to prevent permanent joint stiffness (contractures) and muscle loss (atrophy).

ESSENTIALS FOR OLDER PEOPLE

Osteoarthritis is the most common cause of multiple joint pains in the elderly. Although more common among younger adults (those aged 30 to 40), rheumatoid arthritis can also begin later in life (after age 60). Older adults who may have rheumatoid arthritis may also have cancer. People over age 55 who have hip and shoulder stiffness and pain that is usually worse in the morning may have polymyalgia rheumatica. Recognizing polymyalgia rheumatica is important because treating it can help prevent other problems.

KEY POINTS

- Acute pain in multiple joints is most often due to inflammation or the beginning or flare up of a chronic joint disorder.
- Chronic pain in multiple joints is usually due to osteoarthritis or an inflammatory disorder (such as rheumatoid arthritis) or, in children, juvenile idiopathic arthritis.
- When significant fluid accumulates inside of a joint, a fluid sample usually must be withdrawn and tested.
- Lifelong physical activity helps maintain range of motion in people with chronic arthritis.

JOINT PAIN: SINGLE JOINT

Pain that is isolated to just one joint is called monoarticular joint pain. A joint may simply be painful (arthralgia) or may also be inflamed (arthritis). Arthritis usually causes warmth, swelling, and rarely redness of the overlying skin. Pain may occur only when the joint is moved or also be present at rest. Fluid may collect within the joint (called an effusion).

Pain that seems to be coming from a joint sometimes originates in a structure outside of the joint, such as a ligament, tendon, or muscle. Examples of such disorders are bursitis, tendinitis, sprains, and strains. Pains caused by these disorders are usually not considered true joint pains.

CAUSES

Common causes of arthritis in a single joint include infectious arthritis, gout and related disorders, and osteoarthritis. Joint pain may be the first symptom of a disorder that affects other organs in the body, such as an autoimmune disorder or a bodywide infection. Symptoms of some autoimmune disorders can include fever, mouth sores, and rash. Pain that develops in one joint may also be the first symptom of a disorder that eventually affects many joints (see page 237).

COMMON CAUSES

At all ages, injury is the most common cause of sudden pain in a single joint.

Among **young adults** who have not been injured, the most common cause is

- Infectious arthritis (often caused by gonorrhea that has spread throughout the body or bloodstream [disseminated gonococcal infection], particularly if the joint is warm and swollen)

Among **older adults** who have not been injured, the most common causes are

- Osteoarthritis
- Gout or pseudogout (caused by crystals in the joint, and thus often called crystal-induced arthritis)

The most dangerous cause at any age is acute infectious arthritis. Infectious arthritis can damage structures inside the joint within hours, which can lead to permanent arthritis. Rapid treatment can minimize permanent damage and prevent sepsis and death.

Common causes of pain in a single joint are listed in the Table on page 245.

LESS COMMON CAUSES

Less common causes include destruction of part of the nearby bone caused by poor blood supply (osteonecrosis), joint tumors (such as pigmented villonodular synovitis), and blood in the joint (hemarthrosis).

EVALUATION

The following information can help people decide when a doctor's evaluation is needed and help them know what to expect during the evaluation.

WARNING SIGNS

In people with pain in a single joint, certain symptoms and characteristics are cause for concern and are more likely to require immediate treatment. They include

- Sudden or severe pain
- Joint redness, warmth, swelling, or limitation of motion
- Fever
- Broken, red, warm, or tender skin near the joint
- Presence of a bleeding disorder, use of blood thinners (for example, warfarin), or abnormal blood hemoglobin (for example, sickle cell disease)
- Signs of sudden illness other than joint pain
- Possibility of a sexually transmitted disease (for instance, due to unprotected sex with a new partner)

WHEN TO SEE A DOCTOR

People with warning signs should see a doctor right away. Doctors are better able to treat symptoms more rapidly and completely if treatment occurs early in certain disorders, including crystal-induced arthritis, hemarthrosis, and infectious arthritis. People without warning signs, particularly if the cause of pain is known (for example, if typical pain recurs in a joint affected by osteoarthritis or if pain occurs after a minor injury) and symptoms are mild, the person can wait a few days and see whether symptoms resolve before seeing a doctor.

WHAT THE DOCTOR DOES

Doctors first ask questions about the person's symptoms and medical history. Doctors then do a physical examination. What they find during the history and physical examination often suggests a cause of the pain and the tests that may need to be done (see Table on page 245).

During the history, doctors ask about the following:

- When the pain started, how it has progressed, where it is located, and its severity
- What makes the pain better or worse (for example, movement, weight-bearing exercise, or rest)
- Previous injuries or previous joint pain
- Symptoms in other joints (such as swelling)
- Risk factors for sexually transmitted diseases and Lyme disease
- Known disorders, particularly those that could cause or contribute to joint pain (such as osteoarthritis, gout, or sickle cell disease)

The physical examination focuses on the joints for signs of inflammation (including swelling, warmth, and rarely redness), tenderness, limitation of motion, and noises made when the joint moves (called crepitus). Doctors compare the affected joint with the coordinating unaffected joint on the opposite side of the body to look for any subtle changes. Doctors also look for signs of infection elsewhere on the body, particularly on the skin and genitals.

Several findings from the history and examination give clues to the cause of joint pain:

- Based on the examination, doctors can usually tell whether the source of the pain is the joint or nearby structures. For example, if only one side of a joint seems abnormal, the source of the pain is probably outside of the joint.
- Based on the examination, doctors can usually tell whether fluid is in the joint.

- Inflammation that develops over hours is usually caused by crystal-induced arthritis, particularly if similar symptoms have occurred previously. Infectious arthritis is another major cause of acute arthritis.
- Fever is most often caused by infectious arthritis or crystal-induced arthritis.

TESTING

The need for tests depends on what doctors find during the history and physical examination, particularly whether warning signs are present.

Possible tests include

- Testing of joint fluid
- X-rays and other imaging tests

Doctors usually test the fluid in the joint if the joint is swollen. Doctors extract the fluid from the joint by first sterilizing the area with an antiseptic solution and then numbing the skin with an anesthetic. Then a needle is inserted into the joint and joint fluid is withdrawn (a procedure called joint aspiration or arthrocentesis). This procedure causes little or no pain. The fluid is usually tested for, among other things, bacteria that can cause infection and is examined under a microscope for crystals that cause gout and related disorders. Sometimes doctors do not test the fluid if the cause of the joint pain is obvious, for example, the pain occurs after an injury or fluid accumulates repeatedly in a joint with a chronic joint disorder such as osteoarthritis.

X-rays may be taken, but they are usually unnecessary in people with acute arthritis. X-rays do not show abnormalities of soft tissues or cartilage. X-rays are most helpful in diagnosing fractures and sometimes bone tumors or osteonecrosis. Magnetic resonance imaging (MRI) or computed tomography (CT) can show abnormalities of bones, joints, tendons, and muscles in more detail than x-rays. Thus, MRI or CT is used to diagnose bone and joint abnormalities that may not be evident or clear on x-rays (for example, hip fractures that are too small to be seen on x-rays). MRI is used to diagnose certain soft-tissue abnormalities, such as rotator cuff abnormalities in the shoulder and ligament and meniscus cartilage abnormalities in the knee.

Blood tests are occasionally necessary, for example, to help diagnose or rule out Lyme disease.

SOME CAUSES AND FEATURES OF PAIN IN A SINGLE JOINT

Cause	Common Features*	Tests
Crystal-induced arthritis (gout and related disorders such as pseudogout)	Sudden and severe pain, swelling, warmth, and decreased range of motion, particularly in the great toe, ankle, wrist, or knee Sometimes with redness of the skin Often prior similar episodes of pain that resolved with or without treatment	Withdrawal and testing of joint fluid
Hemarthrosis (blood in the joint)†	Symptoms may be spontaneous or begin soon after an injury Usually in a person with a recent injury or a bleeding disorder	Withdrawal and testing of joint fluid Sometimes CT or MRI
Infectious arthritis (for example, a bacterial, fungal, or viral infection or tuberculosis)‡	Sudden and severe pain, swelling, warmth, and decreased range of motion Sometimes gradual pain and swelling	Withdrawal and testing of joint fluid
Injury, such as a fracture or abnormality inside the joint that interferes with joint motion (for example, abnormal joint cartilage due to a torn knee meniscus)	Symptoms begin immediately after injury Often swelling	X-rays Frequently MRI Sometimes insertion of a viewing scope into the joint (arthroscopy)
Lyme disease	Sudden start of pain in one joint that may move from one joint to another Usually body aches, fever, and severe fatigue Usually begins several days to weeks after person had a rash with one or more red blotches with a clear center Often after a tick bite (tick bite may not be noticed)	Blood test for antibodies against *Borrelia burgdorferi,* the bacterium that causes Lyme disease
Osteoarthritis	Slowly progressive pain in older people or young people who frequently stress the affected joint (for example, doing manual labor or high-impact sports)	X-rays
Osteonecrosis†	Joint pain in people who have taken or currently take corticosteroids or who have sickle cell disease	X-rays plus MRI
Psoriatic arthritis	Pain in a single joint, usually with swelling Usually in people known to have psoriasis	Withdrawal and testing of joint fluid the first time the disorder develops Sometimes x-rays
Tumor	Slowly progressive joint pain usually with swelling Often pain at night	X-rays and MRI

*Features include symptoms and the results of the doctor's examination. Features mentioned are typical but not always present.

†These causes are rare.

‡Infectious arthritis occurs more frequently in people with a weakened immune system (caused by a disorder or drugs), intravenous drug users, people with diabetes, and people at risk of sexually transmitted diseases.

CT = computed tomography; MRI = magnetic resonance imaging.

TREATMENT

The most effective way to relieve joint pain is to treat the disorder causing the pain. For example, antibiotics can be given to treat infectious arthritis. Bones with fractures may need to be immobilized (for example, set in a cast).

Drugs can also be used to relieve joint inflammation regardless of the cause. Such drugs include nonsteroidal anti-inflammatory drugs (NSAIDs) or, for very severe inflammation, sometimes corticosteroids. Joint pain without inflammation, regardless of the cause, can be relieved with NSAIDs, although acetaminophen tends to be as effective and safer for most people.

Immobilizing a joint with a splint or sling is sometimes a useful temporary way to relieve pain. Applying cold (for example, with ice) is the best treatment immediately after an injury has occurred and can be used for relieving pain caused by joint inflammation. Applying heat (for example, with a heating pad) may decrease pain by relieving spasms in the muscles around joints. However, people should protect their skin from extremes of heat and cold. For example, ice should be put in a rubber ice bag or a plastic bag wrapped in a towel and not applied to the skin directly. Also, hot and cold materials should be applied for at least 15 minutes at a time to penetrate deeply enough to affect the most painful or inflamed tissues.

After the severe pain has lessened, doctors may recommend people have physical therapy to regain or maintain range of motion and strengthen surrounding muscles.

O—π KEY POINTS

- Single-joint pain in older adults is most often caused by osteoarthritis or gout.
- Single-joint pain in young adults or adolescents may be caused by a sexually transmitted disease such as gonorrhea.
- People who have sudden joint pain with swelling should be evaluated by a doctor as soon as possible so that infectious arthritis, if present, can be promptly treated.
- Fluid from swollen joints is usually withdrawn and tested for infection and the presence of crystals.

LIMB PAIN

Pain may affect all or part of a leg or arm. Most disorders that cause limb pain affect the legs more commonly. Pain in the joints is discussed elsewhere (see pages 237 and 243).

Limb pain may be constant or occur irregularly. Pain may be precipitated by motion or have no relation to movement. Other symptoms, such as warmth, redness, numbness, or tingling, may also be present depending on the cause of the limb pain.

CAUSES

Injuries and overuse are the most common causes of pain in a limb, but people usually know the cause of these injuries. This discussion covers limb pain unrelated to injury or strain. There are many causes.

The most common causes are the following:

- Blood clot in a deep-lying vein (deep vein thrombosis)
- Bacterial infection of the skin (cellulitis)
- Pressure on a spinal nerve root

Uncommon but serious causes that require immediate evaluation and treatment include

- Sudden blockage of an artery in the limb (acute arterial occlusion)
- Deep soft-tissue infection
- Heart attack (arm pain only)

Other less common causes include bone tumors, bone infections (osteomyelitis), and nerve problems such as pressure on nerves or degeneration of nerves (such as caused by diabetes or long-term alcohol abuse).

EVALUATION

It is particularly important to make sure the person does not have a sudden blockage of an artery because the limb can develop gangrene if there is no blood flow for more than a few hours. The following information can help people decide when a doctor's evaluation is needed and help them know what to expect during the evaluation.

WARNING SIGNS

In people with limb pain, certain symptoms and characteristics are cause for concern. They include

- Sudden, severe pain
- Limb that is cold to the touch or pale
- Chest pain, sweating, shortness of breath, or palpitations
- Signs of severe illness (for example, confusion, fever, or collapse)
- Limb swollen, blistered, or has black spots
- Risk factors for deep vein thrombosis, such as recent surgery, bed rest, or a cast on a leg
- New nerve deficits, such as weakness or numbness of the affected limb

WHEN TO SEE A DOCTOR

People who have warning signs should see a doctor right away. People without warning signs should call a doctor. The doctor will decide how quickly the person needs to be seen based on the symptoms, age, and presence of other medical disorders. Typically, a delay of several days is not harmful.

WHAT THE DOCTOR DOES

Doctors first ask questions about the person's symptoms and medical history. Doctors then do a physical examination. What they find during the history and physical examination often suggests a cause of the limb pain and the tests that may need to be done.

Doctors ask

- How long limb pain has been present
- Whether pain occurs at certain times or during specific activities
- How intense the pain is
- Whether the pain is sharp or throbbing
- Where the pain is located
- What activities trigger or worsen pain
- What the person does to relieve pain
- What other symptoms (such as numbness or tingling) occur along with the pain

Doctors look for symptoms that may indicate a cause of the pain. Some obvious findings may be very helpful in diagnosing the cause of limb pain. For example, back or neck pain suggests that a nerve root may be affected and fever suggests that the person has an infection. Shortness of breath and a rapid heart rate suggest blockage of an artery by a blood clot that has traveled from a leg to the lungs (pulmonary embolism). An irregular pulse suggests that the person may have a certain abnormal heart rhythm (atrial fibrillation) that has caused a blood clot to travel from the heart to block an artery in the leg.

The painful limb is inspected for color, swelling, and any skin or hair changes. The doctor also checks for pulses, temperature, tenderness, and crepitation (a subtle crackling sensation indicating gas in the soft tissue caused by a serious infection). Strength, sensation, and reflexes are compared between affected and unaffected sides. Blood pressure is measured in the ankle or wrist of the affected limb and compared with the blood pressure in an unaffected arm or leg. If blood pressure is much lower in the painful limb, it is likely that the arteries in the limb are blocked.

SOME CAUSES AND FEATURES OF LIMB PAIN

Cause*	Common Features†	Tests
Sudden, severe pain that develops within a few minutes		
Blockage of an artery in a limb, usually a leg, by a blood clot	Coolness and paleness of the limb After several hours, signs of nerve malfunction, such as weakness, numbness, tingling, or cramping Weak or no pulse felt in the limb	Arteriography done immediately
Sudden herniation of a disk in the spine	Pain and sometimes numbness that occurs in a line down the limb Pain that is often worsened by movement Often neck or back pain Usually weakness in part of the affected limb	Usually MRI
Heart attack (myocardial infarction)	Pain in an arm, not a leg Sometimes pain or pressure in the chest or jaw Sometimes nausea, sweating, and shortness of breath Sometimes in people known to have heart disease	ECG Blood tests for substances that indicate heart damage (cardiac markers) Sometimes angiography of the arteries of the heart
Fatty deposits in artery walls (atherosclerosis), which reduce blood flow, almost always in a leg	Intermittent episodes of leg pain that occur only when walking and are relieved by a few minutes of rest (intermittent claudication)	Ultrasonography Sometimes arteriography
Pain that develops gradually (over hours to days)		
Bacterial infection of the skin (cellulitis)	An irregular area of redness, warmth, and tenderness Sometimes fever	A doctor's examination Sometimes blood cultures *(continued)*

SOME CAUSES AND FEATURES OF LIMB PAIN *(continued)*

Cause*	Common Features†	Tests
Deep vein thrombosis (a blood clot in a deep-lying vein in a leg [typically] or an arm)	Swelling of an entire part of a limb (for example, whole calf or calf and upper leg) Usually pain, redness, warmth, and/or tenderness in the affected area Sometimes in people with risk factors for blood clots, such as recent surgery, an injury, bed rest, a cast on a leg, use of hormone therapy, or cancer	Ultrasonography Sometimes a blood test to detect blood clots (D-dimer)
Bacterial infection deep under the skin and/or in the muscle (myonecrosis)	Deep, constant pain Redness, warmth, tenderness, and swelling that feels tight Signs of severe illness (such as fever, confusion, and a rapid heart rate) Sometimes a foul discharge, blisters, or areas of blackened, dead skin	Blood and tissue cultures X-rays Sometimes MRI
Bone infection (osteomyelitis)	Deep, constant pain that often occurs at night Bone tenderness and fever Often in people with risk factors (such as a weakened immune system, use of injection drugs, or a known source for the infection)	X-rays and MRI and/or CT Sometimes bone culture
Chronic pain (present for a week or more)		
A bone tumor (originating in the bone or spread to the bone from cancer elsewhere in the body)	Deep, constant pain that is often worse at night Bone tenderness Often in people known to have cancer	X-rays and MRI and/or CT
Pressure on certain nerves, as occurs in ■ A disorder of the brachial plexus (a network of nerves in the shoulder and back) ■ Thoracic outlet syndrome (which involves nerves that pass between the neck and chest)	Usually weakness and sometimes numbness or tingling along part of the limb	Usually electromyography and nerve conduction studies Sometimes MRI
Pressure on a spinal nerve root (the part of a spinal nerve next to the spinal cord), which may be caused by a herniated disk or bone spurs	Pain and sometimes numbness that occurs in a line down the limb Pain that is often worsened by movement Often neck or back pain Usually weakness in part of the affected limb	Usually MRI

(continued)

SOME CAUSES AND FEATURES OF LIMB PAIN (continued)

Cause*	Common Features†	Tests
Degeneration or inflammation of many nerves throughout the body (polyneuropathy)	Chronic numbness and burning pain, typically in both hands and/or both feet	Only a doctor's examination
	Often in people with a disorder that causes nerve damage, such as diabetes or alcohol abuse	
Complex regional pain syndrome	Severe burning or aching pain	Only a doctor's examination
	Sometimes increased sensation and pain caused by a stimulus that would not ordinarily be considered painful	
	Often skin that appears red, mottled, or ashen and increased or decreased sweating in the affected limb	
	Typically in people who have had an injury (sometimes many years before)	
Chronic venous insufficiency (causing blood to pool in the legs)	Swelling of the ankles or legs	Only a doctor's examination
	Chronic mild discomfort, aching, or cramps in the legs but no pain	
	Sometimes reddish brown, leathery areas on the skin and shallow sores on the lower legs	
	Often varicose veins	

*Arm or leg pain that is caused by injury is not included.
†Features include symptoms and the results of the doctor's examination. Features mentioned are typical but not always present.
CT = computed tomography; ECG = electrocardiography; MRI = magnetic resonance imaging.

TESTING

Testing is not needed for all people with limb pain. Doctors can often diagnose some causes of limb pain, including cellulitis, myofascial pain, and painful polyneuropathy, based on the people's symptoms and the physical examination findings. Testing is usually needed for other possible causes of pain.

TREATMENT

The best way to treat limb pain is to treat the underlying disorder. Analgesics such as acetaminophen and nonsteroidal anti-inflammatory drugs can help relieve pain. Sometimes opioids are needed.

KEY POINTS

- In people with sudden, severe pain, blood flow to the limb has often been stopped or reduced, and testing must be done quickly.
- Symptoms and characteristics found during the doctor's examination usually provide clues to the cause of limb pain.

LUMP IN THROAT (GLOBUS SENSATION)

Some people feel as if they have a lump or mass in their throat when no mass is actually there. If this sensation is unrelated to swallowing, it is termed globus sensation, or globus hystericus (which does not mean the person is hysterical). Some people have the sensation but also notice difficulty swallowing (see page 371). Some people can actually feel a lump on the side of their neck (see page 302).

- Neck or throat pain
- Weight loss
- Abrupt appearance after age 50
- Pain, choking, or difficulty with swallowing (dysphagia)
- Spitting up (regurgitation) of food
- Muscle weakness
- A mass that is visible or that can be felt
- Progressive worsening of symptoms

CAUSES

Doctors are not sure what causes globus sensation. It may involve increased muscle tension in muscles of the throat or just below the throat, or it may also be due to gastroesophageal reflux. The sensation sometimes comes when people experience certain emotions, such as grief or pride, but is often independent of such feelings.

Globus sensation is not dangerous and does not cause complications. However, certain more serious disorders that affect the esophagus can sometimes be confused with globus sensation. Such disorders include upper esophageal webs; esophageal spasm; gastroesophageal reflux disease (GERD); muscle disorders such as myasthenia gravis, myotonic dystrophy, or polymyositis; and tumors in the neck or upper chest. Such disorders typically affect swallowing and/or cause other symptoms besides the sensation of a lump.

EVALUATION

People with globus sensation rarely require immediate evaluation by a doctor. The following information can help people decide whether a doctor's evaluation is needed and help them know what to expect during the evaluation.

WARNING SIGNS

In people with globus sensation, certain symptoms and characteristics suggest another disorder is present and are cause for concern. They include

WHEN TO SEE A DOCTOR

People who have warning signs should see a doctor within a few days to a week. People who have no warning signs should call their doctor. Depending on the severity and nature of the sensation, doctors may suggest people wait to see how symptoms develop or suggest a mutually convenient time.

WHAT THE DOCTOR DOES

Doctors ask questions about the person's symptoms and medical history and do a physical examination. What doctors find during the history and physical examination helps decide what, if any, tests need to be done.

The history is focused on distinguishing globus sensation from difficulty swallowing, which suggests a structural or motility (movement) disorder of the throat or esophagus. Doctors ask people to clearly describe their symptoms, particularly their relationship to swallowing (such as a sensation of food sticking) and emotional events. They also seek any other warning signs.

The physical examination is focused on the mouth and neck. Doctors inspect and feel the floor of the mouth and the neck for masses. Doctors look down the throat with a thin, flexible viewing scope to inspect the back of the throat and the voice box. Doctors also observe the person swallowing water and a solid food such as crackers.

Warning signs or abnormal findings found during the examination suggest a mechanical or motility disorder of swallowing. People who have chronic symptoms that occur during episodes of grief that may be relieved by crying suggest globus sensation.

TESTING

People who have symptoms that are not related to swallowing, have no warning signs (particularly no pain or difficulty with swallowing), and a normal examination (including swallowing observed by the doctor) most likely have globus sensation. Such people rarely need tests.

If the diagnosis is unclear, warning signs are present, or the doctor cannot adequately see the throat, swallowing tests (as for difficulty swallowing—see page 372) are done. Typical tests include plain or video esophagography, measurement of swallowing time, chest x-ray, and manometry of the esophagus.

TREATMENT

Globus sensation does not require any treatment besides reassurance and sympathetic concern. Sometimes, simply understanding that globus sensation comes with certain moods is all the help people need. No drugs are helpful. However, if any underlying depression, anxiety, or other behavioral disorder seems to be making symptoms more disturbing to people, doctors may try giving an antidepressant drug or referring people to a psychiatrist.

KEY POINTS

- Globus symptoms are not related to swallowing.
- People do not need tests unless their symptoms are related to swallowing, their physical examination is abnormal, or they have warning signs.

MEMORY LOSS

Memory loss is one of the most common reasons that people, particularly older people, visit a doctor. Sometimes family members notice and report the memory loss. The biggest concern for the person, family members, and doctors is usually whether the memory loss is the first sign of Alzheimer disease, a progressive and incurable form of dementia (a type of brain disorder). People with dementia have lost the ability to think clearly. Usually, if people are aware enough of their memory loss to be concerned about it, they do not have early dementia.

Memories may be stored in short-term or long-term memory, depending on what they are and how important they are to the person. Short-term memory holds a small amount of information that a person needs temporarily, such as a list of things to buy at the grocery store. Long-term memory, as the name suggests, stores memories (such as the name of the person's high school) for a long time. Short-term memory and long-term memory are stored in a different parts of the brain. Long-term memory is stored in many areas of the brain. One part of the brain (the hippocampus) helps sort new information and associate it with similar information already stored in the brain. This process turns short-term memories into long-term memories. The more often short-term memories are recalled or rehearsed, the more likely they are to become long-term memories.

CAUSES

COMMON CAUSES

The most common causes of memory loss are

- Age-related changes in memory (most common)
- Mild cognitive impairment
- Dementia
- Depression

Age-related changes in memory refer to the normal slight decline in brain function that occurs as people age. Most older people have some memory problems. Retrieving memories of new things, such as what is a new neighbor's name or how to use a new computer program, takes longer. Older people also have to rehearse new memories more often for the memories to be stored. People with this type of memory loss occasionally forget things, such as where they left their car keys. But for them, unlike people with dementia, the ability to do daily activities or to think is not impaired. Given enough time, these people usually remember, although sometimes later than is convenient. This type of memory loss is not a sign of dementia or early Alzheimer disease.

Mild cognitive impairment is an imprecise term used to describe impairments in mental function that are more severe than normal age-related changes but less severe than those caused by dementia. Memory loss is often the most obvious symptom. People with mild cognitive impairment have trouble remembering recent conversations and may forget important appointments or social events, but they typically remember past events. Attention and the ability to do daily activities are not affected. However, about half of people with mild cognitive impairment develop dementia within 3 years.

Dementia is a much more serious decline in mental function. Memory loss, particularly for recently acquired information, is often the first symptom, and it becomes worse with time. People who have dementia may forget entire events, not just the details. They have difficulty remembering how to do things they have done many times before and how to get to places they have often been to. They can no longer do things that require many steps, such as following a recipe. People may forget to pay bills or keep appointments. They may forget to turn off a stove, lock the house when they leave, or take care of a child left in their care. They are unaware of their memory loss and often deny that they have such loss. Finding the right word, naming objects, understanding language, and doing, planning, and organizing daily activities become more and more difficult. People with dementia eventually become disoriented, not knowing what time or even what year it is or where they are.

Their personality may change. They may become more irritable, anxious, paranoid, inflexible, or disruptive.

There are many forms of dementia. Alzheimer disease is the most common. Most forms of dementia progressively worsen until the person's death.

Some conditions that increase the risk of heart and blood vessel disorders (such as high blood pressure, high levels of cholesterol, and diabetes) seem to increase the risk of dementia.

Depression can cause a type of memory loss (called pseudodementia) that resembles memory loss due to dementia. Also, dementia commonly causes depression. Thus, determining whether dementia or depression is the cause of memory loss can be difficult. However, people with memory loss due to depression, unlike those with dementia, are aware of their memory loss and complain about it. Also, they rarely forget important current events or personal matters, and usually have other symptoms, such as intense sadness, sleeping problems (too little or too much), sluggishness, or loss of appetite.

Stress can interfere with forming a memory and with recalling a memory, partly by preoccupying people and thus preventing them from paying attention to other things. However in certain circumstances, particularly when stress is mild to moderate and does not last long, it can enhance memory.

LESS COMMON CAUSES

Many disorders can cause a deterioration of mental function that resembles dementia. Some of these disorders can be reversed with treatment. They include normal-pressure hydrocephalus (due to excess fluid around the brain), subdural hematomas (pockets of blood under the outer layer of the membranes covering the brain), hypothyroidism (an underactive thyroid gland), and vitamin B_{12} deficiency.

Other disorders are only partially reversible. They include those that interfere with the supply of blood or nutrients to the brain, such as a cardiac arrest, certain types of stroke, unusually long seizures, head injuries, a brain infection, HIV infection, brain tumors, and overuse of certain drugs (including alcohol). In people with these disorders, treatment can sometimes improve memory and mental function. If damage is more extensive, treatment may not improve mental function but can often prevent further deterioration.

In delirium, memory is affected, but memory loss is not the most noticeable symptom. Rather, people with delirium are very confused, disoriented, and incoherent. Severe alcohol withdrawal (delirium tremens), a severe bloodstream infection (sepsis), lack of oxygen (as may result from pneumonia), and many other disorders can cause delirium, as can use of illegal drugs.

EVALUATION

Doctors focus on determining whether the cause is normal age-related changes in the brain, mild cognitive impairment, depression, or early dementia.

WARNING SIGNS

In people with memory loss, certain symptoms are cause for concern:

- Difficulty doing usual daily activities
- Difficulty paying attention and fluctuations in level of consciousness—symptoms that suggest delirium
- Depression

WHEN TO SEE A DOCTOR

People with warning signs should see a doctor. They should see a doctor immediately if they

- Cannot pay attention and seem very confused, unfocused, and disoriented—symptoms that suggest delirium
- Feel depressed and are thinking of hurting themselves
- Have other symptoms that suggest a problem with the nervous system, such as headaches, difficulty using or understanding language, sluggishness, vision problems, or dizziness

People who have difficulty doing daily activities should see a doctor within a week or so.

People who do not have warning signs but are concerned about their memory should call their doctor. The doctor can determine how quickly they need to be seen based on other symptoms they have and the severity of the symptoms.

Doctors ask about the person's symptoms and medical history. Doctors then do a physical examination. Having a family member present is helpful because people with memory difficulties may not be able to describe their symptoms accurately. What doctors find during the history and physical examination often suggests a cause and the tests that may need to be done (see Table on page 256).

Doctors often talk to the person and the person's family members separately because family members may not feel free to describe the symptoms candidly with the person listening.

Doctors ask specific questions about the memory loss:

- What types of things the person forgets (for example, whether the person forgets words or names or gets lost)
- When the memory problems started
- Whether memory loss is getting worse
- How the memory loss is affecting the person's ability to function at work and at home

Doctors also ask whether the person has other symptoms, such as difficulty using or understanding language and changes in their eating and sleeping habits or mood. They ask about all disorders the person has had and all the drugs the person is taking, including recreational or illegal drugs, to check for possible causes. Information about the person's education, jobs, and social activities can help doctors better assess the person's previous mental function and gauge the severity of the problem. Doctors ask whether any family members have had dementia or early mild cognitive impairment.

During the physical examination, doctors evaluate all body systems but focus on the nervous system (neurologic examination), including evaluation of mental function (mental status testing).

In mental status testing, doctors ask people to answer questions or do specific tasks to evaluate various aspects of mental function, such as

- Orientation to time, place, and person: State the current date and place and who they are.
- Attention: Repeat a short list of words.
- Concentration: Spell "world" backwards or repeat their phone number forward, then backward.

- Short-term memory: Recall the short list of words after several minutes.
- Long-term memory: Describe events from the distant past.
- Use of language: Name common objects and body parts, and read, write, and repeat certain phrases.

This testing also assesses abstract thinking, comprehension, the ability to follow commands and solve math problems, awareness of the illness, and mood.

Doctors can usually determine whether the cause is age-related changes, mild cognitive impairment, or early dementia based on the type of memory loss and the symptoms that accompany it. However, when the diagnosis is unclear, neuropsychologic testing can provide more information. This testing is similar to mental status testing except it is much more detailed. Complete testing may take a full day. These tests must be given by a trained, licensed psychologist or psychiatrist with expertise in memory loss. These tests may not be as useful in people over 65.

If doctors suspect dementia or find any abnormalities during the neurologic examination, they usually do magnetic resonance imaging (MRI) or computed tomography (CT) to check for abnormalities such as a brain tumor, normal-pressure hydrocephalus, damage due to a head injury, and stroke. They may also do blood tests to measure levels of vitamin B_{12} and thyroid hormones to determine whether vitamin B_{12} deficiency or a thyroid disorder could be causing memory loss. If a brain infection is suspected, doctors usually do a spinal tap (lumbar puncture) to obtain samples of the fluid around the brain (cerebrospinal fluid) for analysis.

TREATMENT

Treating any disorders contributing to memory loss may help restore memory. For example, vitamin B_{12} deficiency is treated with vitamin B_{12} supplements, and an underactive thyroid gland is treated with thyroid hormone supplements. For depression, treatment involves drugs, psychotherapy, or both. Doctors choose antidepressants that do not worsen memory loss, such as

SOME CAUSES AND FEATURES OF MEMORY LOSS

Cause	Common Features*	Tests
Age-related memory changes	Occasional forgetfulness of such things as names or the location of car keys No effect on thinking, other mental functions, or the ability to do daily activities	A doctor's examination (particularly a neurologic examination and mental status testing to assess functions such as attention, orientation, and memory)
Mild cognitive impairment	Memory loss that is more severe than expected for a person's age, particularly difficulty remembering recent events and conversations (short-term memory loss) No effect on the ability to do daily activities An increased risk of developing dementia	A doctor's examination Sometimes formal neuropsychologic testing, which resembles mental status testing but evaluates function in more detail
Dementia	Memory loss that becomes worse as time passes, eventually with no awareness of the loss Difficulty using and understanding language, doing usual manual tasks, thinking, and planning (for example, planning and shopping for meals), resulting in not being able to function normally Disorientation (for example, not knowing the time or location) Changes in personality or behavior (for example, becoming irritable, agitated, paranoid, inflexible, or disruptive)	A doctor's examination Usually MRI or CT of the brain Sometimes formal neuropsychologic testing Possibly a spinal tap (lumbar puncture) to measure levels of two abnormal proteins (amyloid and tau) that occur in Alzheimer disease Sometimes blood tests to check for certain causes, such as an underactive thyroid gland (hypothyroidism) or a vitamin deficiency
Depression	Memory loss and awareness of the loss, usually accompanied by intense sadness, and lack of interest in usual pleasures Sometimes sleep problems (too little or too much), loss of appetite, and slowing of thinking, speech, and general activity Common among people with dementia, mild cognitive impairment, or age-related changes in memory	A doctor's examination Sometimes use of standardized questionnaires to identify depression
Drugs, such as ■ Drugs with anticholinergic effects, including some antidepressants and many antihistamines (used in OTC sleep aids, cold remedies, and allergy drugs) ■ Opioids ■ Drugs that help people sleep (sedatives)	Use of a drug that can cause memory loss Often recent use of a new drug, an increase in a drug's dose, or a change in health that prevents the drug from being processed and eliminated from the body normally, as can occur in kidney or liver disorders	Typically stopping the drug to see whether memory improves

*Features include symptoms and results of the doctor's examination. Features mentioned are typical but not always present.
CT = computed tomography; MRI = magnetic resonance imaging; OTC = over-the-counter.

selective serotonin reuptake inhibitors (SSRIs). For normal-pressure hydrocephalus, a shunt can be surgically placed to drain the excess fluid around the brain. If a person is taking drugs that affect brain function, doctors may stop the drug, decrease the dose, or try substituting another drug.

If the only cause is age-related changes in memory, doctors reassure people that the problem is not serious, that these changes do not mean that mental function will decline substantially, and that there are ways to compensate for losses and possibly to improve mental function.

Some generally healthful measures are often recommended:

- Exercising regularly
- Eating a healthy diet with lots of fruits and vegetables
- Getting enough sleep
- Not smoking
- Using alcohol only in moderation
- Participating in social and intellectually stimulating activities
- Getting regular check-ups
- Avoiding high levels of stress
- Protecting the head from injury

These measures, along with controlling blood pressure, cholesterol levels, and blood sugar levels, also tend to reduce the risk of heart and blood vessel disorders. Some evidence suggests that they may reduce the risk of dementia, but this effect has not been proved.

Some experts recommend learning new things (such as a new language or a new musical instrument), doing mental exercises (such as memorizing lists, doing word puzzles, or playing chess, bridge, or other games that use strategy), reading, working on the computer, or doing crafts (such as knitting and quilting). These activities may help maintain or improve mental function, possibly because they strengthen connections between nerves. Having stronger nerve connections helps people postpone the decline in mental function that results from changes in the brain and then helps them compensate for that decline.

Mild cognitive impairment may be treated with donepezil, a drug used to treat Alzheimer disease. This drug may temporarily improve memory, but the benefit appears to be slight. No other drug has been shown to help.

Dementia may be treated with donepezil or certain other cholinesterase inhibitors, such as galantamine and rivastigmine. These drugs may temporarily and slightly improve mental function, including memory, in some people. A different type of drug, memantine, may also help and can be used with a cholinesterase inhibitor. However, no treatment can restore mental function or completely stop the progression of dementia. Thus, treatment focuses on keeping the person safe and providing support as the person declines.

If memory loss is relatively severe or family members are concerned about the person's safety, the person's home can be evaluated by occupational or physical therapists. They can recommend ways to prevent falls and other accidents and may suggest protective measures, such as hiding knives, unplugging the stove, and taking the car keys away. Eventually, the person may need a housekeeper or home health aide or may need to move to a one-story home, an assisted-living facility, or a skilled nursing facility.

ESSENTIALS FOR OLDER PEOPLE

As people age, most start having some memory problems. Usually, memory loss is caused by normal age-related changes in the brain and does not lead to dementia. Understanding such changes can reduce anxiety and thus help older people adjust and compensate. However, about 14 to 18% of people over 70 have mild cognitive impairment. Dementia occurs in about 1% of people aged 60 to 64 but becomes more likely with increasing age. About 30 to 50% of those over 85 have Alzheimer disease (a type of dementia).

COPING

Strategies that can help people cope with a declining memory include

- Making lists
- Keeping a detailed calendar
- Establishing routines
- Making associations or relating new information to information already known, such as associating a new person's name with the name of a movie star

- Repeating information, such as repeating a new person's name several times
- Focusing on (paying attention to) one thing at a time
- Improving organizational skills, such as keeping frequently used items such as car keys in the same place

Making sure that they can hear and see well can help people stay engaged with others and participate in social activities. Such participation helps people maintain confidence in themselves and often improves mental function.

O━ᴨ KEY POINTS

- Memory loss and fear of dementia are common sources of worry among older people.
- Usually, memory loss results from normal age-related changes in the brain, which slow mental functions slightly but do not significantly impair them.
- Memory loss due to dementia usually interferes with the ability to do daily activities and becomes progressively worse.
- Most people who are aware of memory loss do not have dementia.
- Doctors can usually identify the cause based on results of the examination, imaging tests (such as MRI or CT), and other tests, including formal tests of mental function.
- Having a healthy lifestyle, staying mentally active, and participating in social activities may help maintain mental function or postpone its decline.
- Using lists and other memory aids, focusing on one thing at a time, and getting organized can help older people compensate for age-related changes in memory.

Having no menstrual periods is called amenorrhea. Amenorrhea is normal before puberty, during pregnancy, while breastfeeding, and after menopause. At other times, it may be the first symptom of a serious disorder.

Amenorrhea may be accompanied by other symptoms, depending on the cause. For example, women may develop masculine characteristics (virilization), such as excess body hair (hirsutism), a deepened voice, and increased muscle size. They may have headaches, vision problems, or a decreased sex drive. They may have difficulty becoming pregnant. In most women with amenorrhea, the ovaries do not release an egg. Such women cannot become pregnant.

If amenorrhea lasts a long time, problems similar to those associated with menopause may develop. They include hot flashes, vaginal dryness, decreased bone density (osteoporosis), and an increased risk of heart and blood vessel disorders. Such problems occur because in women who have amenorrhea, the estrogen level is low.

TYPES OF AMENORRHEA

There are two main types of amenorrhea:

- **Primary:** Menstrual periods never start.
- **Secondary:** Periods start, then stop.

Usually if periods never start, girls do not go through puberty, and thus secondary sexual characteristics, such as breasts and pubic hair, do not develop normally.

If women have been having menstrual periods, which then stop, they may have secondary amenorrhea. Secondary amenorrhea is much more common than primary.

HORMONES AND MENSTRUATION

Menstrual periods are regulated by a complex hormonal system. Each month, this system produces hormones in a certain sequence to prepare the body, particularly the uterus, for pregnancy. When this system works normally and there is no pregnancy, the sequence ends with the uterus shedding its lining, producing a menstrual period. The hormones are produced by the hypothalamus (part of the brain that helps control the pituitary gland), the pituitary gland (which produces luteinizing hormone and follicle-stimulating hormone), and the ovaries (which produce estrogen and progesterone). Other hormones, such as thyroid hormones and prolactin (produced by the pituitary gland), can affect the menstrual cycle.

The most common reason for no menstrual periods is malfunction of any part of this hormonal system. Less commonly, the hormonal system is functioning normally, but another problem prevents periods from occurring. For example, menstrual bleeding may not occur because the uterus is scarred or because a birth defect, fibroid, or polyp blocks the flow of menstrual blood out of the vagina.

High levels of prolactin, which stimulates the breasts to produce milk, can result in no periods.

CAUSES

Amenorrhea can result from conditions that affect the hypothalamus, pituitary gland, ovaries, uterus, cervix, or vagina. These conditions include hormonal disorders, birth defects, genetic disorders, and drugs.

Which causes are most common depends on whether amenorrhea is primary or secondary.

PRIMARY AMENORRHEA

The disorders that cause primary amenorrhea are relatively uncommon, but the most common are

- A genetic disorder
- A birth defect of the reproductive organs that blocks the flow of menstrual blood

Genetic disorders include Turner syndrome, Kallman syndrome, overproduction of male hormones by the adrenal glands (congenital adrenal hyperplasia), and disorders that result in ambiguous—neither male nor female—genitals (pseudohermaphroditism or true hermaphroditism). Genetic disorders and birth defects that cause primary amenorrhea may not be noticed until puberty. These disorders cause only primary amenorrhea, not secondary.

All disorders that cause secondary amenorrhea can cause primary amenorrhea.

Sometimes puberty is delayed in girls who do not have a disorder, and normal periods simply begin at a later age. Such delayed puberty may run in families.

SECONDARY AMENORRHEA

The most common causes are

- Pregnancy
- Breastfeeding
- Malfunction of the hypothalamus
- Polycystic ovary syndrome
- Premature menopause (premature ovarian failure)
- Malfunction of the pituitary gland
- Use of certain drugs, such as birth control pills (oral contraceptives), antidepressants, or antipsychotic drugs

Pregnancy is the most common cause of amenorrhea among women of childbearing age.

The hypothalamus may malfunction for several reasons. Stress or excessive exercise (as done by competitive athletes, particularly women who participate in sports that involve maintaining a low body weight) may affect the hypothalamus, causing periods to stop. Poor nutrition (as occurs in women with eating disorders) and mental disorders (such as depression or obsessive-compulsive disorder) may cause the hypothalamus to malfunction. Radiation therapy or an injury may also damage the hypothalamus or cause it to malfunction.

The pituitary gland may malfunction because it is damaged or because levels of prolactin are high. Antidepressants, antipsychotic drugs, or certain other drugs can cause prolactin levels to increase, as can pituitary tumors and some other disorders.

Less common causes of secondary amenorrhea include chronic disorders (particularly of the lungs, digestive tract, blood, kidneys, or liver), some autoimmune disorders, thyroid disorders, cancer, HIV infection, radiation therapy, head injuries, a hydatidiform mole (overgrowth of tissue from the placenta), Cushing syndrome, and malfunction of the adrenal glands. Scarring of the uterus (usually due to an infection or surgery), polyps, and fibroids can also cause secondary amenorrhea.

EVALUATION

Doctors determine whether amenorrhea is primary or secondary. This information can help them identify the cause.

WARNING SIGNS

Certain symptoms are cause for concern:

- Delayed puberty
- Development of masculine characteristics, such as excess body hair, a deepened voice, and increased muscle size
- New or unusual headaches
- Vision problems

WHEN TO SEE A DOCTOR

Girls should see a doctor within a few weeks if

- They have no signs of puberty (such as breast development or a growth spurt) by age 13.
- Pubic hair has not appeared by age 14.
- Periods have not started by age 16 or by 2 years after girls develop secondary sexual characteristics.

Such girls may have primary amenorrhea.

If women of childbearing age have had menstrual periods that have stopped, they should do a home pregnancy test. If the test is negative and if they have headaches or changes in vision, they should see a doctor within a week. Otherwise, they should see a doctor within a few weeks if

- They are not pregnant and have missed 3 menstrual periods.
- They have fewer than 9 periods a year.
- The pattern of periods suddenly changes.

Such women may have secondary amenorrhea.

WHAT THE DOCTOR DOES

Doctors first ask about the medical history, including the menstrual history. Doctors then do a physical examination. What they find during the history and physical examination often suggests a cause of amenorrhea and the tests that may need to be done (see Table on pages 261 to 262).

For the menstrual history, doctors determine whether amenorrhea is primary or secondary by asking the girl or woman whether she has ever had a menstrual period. If she has, she is asked how old she was when the periods started and when the last period occurred. She is also asked to describe the periods:

- How long they lasted
- How often they occurred
- Whether they were ever regular
- How heavy they were
- Whether her breasts were tender or she had mood changes related to periods

If a girl has never had a period, doctors ask whether breasts have started to develop, whether she has had a growth spurt, and whether pubic and underarm hair (signs of puberty) has appeared. This information enables doctors to rule out some causes. Information about delayed puberty and genetic disorders in family members can help doctors determine whether the cause is a genetic disorder.

Doctors ask about other symptoms that may suggest a cause and about use of drugs, exercise, eating habits, and other conditions that can cause amenorrhea.

During the physical examination, doctors determine whether secondary sexual characteristics have developed. A breast examination is done. A pelvic examination is done to determine

SOME CAUSES AND FEATURES OF AMENORRHEA

Cause*	Common Features†	Tests
Hormonal disorders		
Hyperthyroidism (an overactive thyroid gland)	Warm, moist skin, difficulty tolerating heat, excessive sweating, an increased appetite, weight loss, bulging eyes, double vision, shakiness (tremor), and frequent bowel movements	Blood tests to measure thyroid hormone levels
	Sometimes an enlarged thyroid gland (goiter)	
Hypothyroidism (an underactive thyroid gland)	Difficulty tolerating cold, a decreased appetite, weight gain, coarse and thick skin, loss of eyebrow hair, a puffy face, drooping eyelids, fatigue, sluggishness, slow speech, and constipation	Blood tests to measure thyroid hormone levels
Pituitary disorders, including tumors that produce prolactin‡ and injuries	Vision problems and headaches, particularly at night	Blood test to measure prolactin levels
	Sometimes production of breast milk in men or in women who are not breastfeeding (galactorrhea)	MRI of the brain
Polycystic ovary syndrome	Development of masculine characteristics (such as excess body hair, a deepened voice, and increased muscle size)	Blood tests to measure hormone levels
	Irregular or no menstrual periods, acne, excess fat in the torso, and dark, thick skin in the underarm, on the nape of the neck, and in skinfolds	Ultrasonography of the pelvis
Premature menopause	Symptoms of menopause, including hot flashes, night sweats, and vaginal dryness and thinning (atrophic vaginitis)	Blood tests to measure levels of estrogen and other hormones
	Risk factors such as removal of the ovaries, chemotherapy, or radiation therapy directed at the pelvis (the lowest part of the torso)	For women under 35, examination of chromosomes in a sample of tissue (such as blood)
Tumors that produce male hormones (androgens), usually in the ovaries or adrenal glands	Development of masculine characteristics, acne, and genitals that are not clearly male or female (ambiguous genitals)	CT, MRI, or ultrasonography

(continued)

SOME CAUSES AND FEATURES OF AMENORRHEA (continued)

Cause*	Common Features†	Tests
Structural disorders		
Birth defects:	Primary amenorrhea	A doctor's examination
▪ Cervical stenosis (narrowing of the passageway through the cervix) ▪ Imperforate hymen (an abnormal hymen that completely blocks the vagina's opening) ▪ Transverse vaginal septum (a wall of tissue across the vagina, which prevents menstrual blood from flowing out) ▪ Absence of reproductive organs	Normal development of breasts and secondary sexual characteristics Abdominal pain that occurs in cycles and bulging of the vagina or uterus (because menstrual blood is blocked and accumulates)	Hysterosalpingography (x-rays taken after a dye is injected into the uterus and fallopian tubes) or hysteroscopy (insertion of a viewing tube through the vagina to view the uterus)
Asherman syndrome (scarring of the lining of the uterus due to an infection or surgery)	Secondary amenorrhea Often repeated miscarriages and infertility	Ultrasonography, sonohysterography (ultrasonography after fluid is infused into uterus), or hysterosalpingography Sometimes if results are unclear, MRI
Fibroids	Secondary amenorrhea Pain, vaginal bleeding, constipation, repeated miscarriages, and an urge to urinate frequently or urgently	Ultrasonography
Polyps	Secondary amenorrhea Vaginal bleeding	Ultrasonography
Conditions that cause the hypothalamus to malfunction		
Excessive exercise	Often a low body weight and body fat	A doctor's examination
Mental disorders (such as depression or obsessive-compulsive disorder)	Withdrawal from usual activities Sluggishness or sadness Sometimes weight gain or weight loss, difficulty sleeping or too much sleep	A doctor's examination
Poor nutrition (as may result from poverty, eating disorders, or excessive dieting)	Often low body weight and body fat	A doctor's examination
Stress	A stressful life event, difficulty concentrating, worry, and sleep problems (too much or too little)	A doctor's examination

*Drugs can also cause amenorrhea (see Table on page 263).
†Features include symptoms and results of the doctor's examination. Features mentioned are typical but not always present.
‡High levels of prolactin (a hormone that stimulates the breasts to produce milk) can result in no periods.
CT = computed tomography; MRI = magnetic resonance imaging.

whether genital organs are developing normally and to check for abnormalities in reproductive organs. Doctors also check for symptoms that may suggest a cause such as

■ A milky discharge from both nipples: Possible causes include pituitary disorders and drugs that increase levels of prolactin (a hormone that stimulates milk production).

■ Headaches and partial loss of vision or double vision: Possible causes include tumors of the pituitary gland or hypothalamus.

■ Development of masculine characteristics, such as excess body hair, a deepened voice, and increased muscle size: Possible causes include polycystic ovary syndrome, tumors that produce male hormones, and use of drugs such as synthetic male hormones (androgens), antidepressants, or high doses of synthetic female hormones called progestins.

DRUGS THAT CAN CAUSE MENSTRUAL PERIODS TO STOP

Type	Examples	Symptoms
Drugs that can increase the production of prolactin		
Antihypertensive drugs	Methyldopa	Production of breast milk in men or in women who are not breastfeeding
	Reserpine	
	Verapamil	
Antipsychotic drugs	Haloperidol	
	Molindone	
	Olanzapine	
	Phenothiazines	
	Pimozide	
	Risperidone	
Illegal or recreational drugs	Cocaine	
	Hallucinogens	
Estrogen	—	
Drugs used to treat digestive disorders	Cimetidine	
	Metoclopramide	
Opioids	Codeine	
	Morphine	
Tricyclic antidepressants	Clomipramine	
	Desipramine	
Drugs that affect the balance of female and male hormones		
Synthetic androgens	Danazol	Development of masculine characteristics (such as excess body hair, a deepened voice, and increased muscle size)
Antidepressants (infrequently)	Paroxetine	Irregular bleeding
	Selegiline	
	Sertraline	

- Hot flashes, vaginal dryness, and night sweats: Possible causes include premature menopause, a disorder that causes the ovaries to malfunction, radiation therapy, and use of a chemotherapy drug.

TESTING

In girls or women of childbearing age, the first test is a pregnancy test. If pregnancy is ruled out, other tests are done based on results of the examination and the suspected cause.

Tests are usually done in a certain order, and causes are identified or eliminated in the process. Whether additional tests are needed and which tests are done depend on results of the previous tests. Typical tests include

- Blood tests to measure levels of prolactin (to check for conditions that cause high levels), thyroid hormones (to check for thyroid disorders), follicle-stimulating hormone (to check for pituitary or hypothalamus malfunction), and male hormones (to check for disorders that cause masculine characteristics to develop)
- Imaging tests of the abdomen and pelvis using computed tomography (CT), magnetic resonance imaging (MRI), or ultrasonography to look for a tumor in the ovaries or adrenal glands
- Examination of chromosomes in a sample of tissue (such as blood) to check for genetic disorders
- Imaging of the uterus and usually fallopian tubes (hysteroscopy or hysterosalpingography) to check for blockages in these organs
- Use of hormones (estrogen and a progestin) to try and trigger menstrual bleeding

If hormones trigger menstrual bleeding, the cause is not a disorder of the uterus or a structural abnormality preventing menstrual blood from flowing out.

If symptoms suggest a specific disorder, tests for that disorder may be done first. For example, if women have headaches and vision problems, MRI of the brain is done to check for a pituitary tumor.

TREATMENT

When amenorrhea results from another disorder, that disorder is treated if possible. With such treatment, menstrual periods sometimes resume. For example, if an abnormality is blocking the flow of menstrual blood, it is usually surgically repaired, and periods resume. Some disorders, such as Turner syndrome and other genetic disorders, cannot be cured.

If a girl's periods never started and all test results are normal, she is examined every 3 to 6 months to check on the progression of puberty. She may be given a progestin and sometimes estrogen to start her periods and to stimulate the development of secondary sexual characteristics, such as breasts.

Problems associated with amenorrhea may require treatment, such as

- Taking hormones if pregnancy is desired
- Treating symptoms and long-term effects of an estrogen deficiency (for example, by taking vitamin D and bisphosphonates for osteoporosis)
- Reducing excess body hair (see page 179)

KEY POINTS

- Various conditions can disrupt the complex hormonal system that regulates the menstrual cycle, causing menstrual periods to stop.
- Doctors distinguish between primary amenorrhea (periods have never started) and secondary amenorrhea (periods started, then stopped).
- The first test is a pregnancy test.
- Unless a woman is pregnant, other testing is usually required to determine the cause of amenorrhea.
- Problems related to amenorrhea (such as a low estrogen level) may also require treatment.

MENSTRUAL PERIODS, PAINFUL (MENSTRUAL CRAMPS)

Menstrual cramps (also called dysmenorrhea) are pains in the lowest part of the torso (pelvis) a few days before, during, or after a menstrual period. The pain tends to be most intense about 24 hours after periods begin and to subside after 2 to 3 days. The pain is usually crampy or sharp and comes and goes, but it may be a dull, constant ache. It sometimes extends to the lower back and legs.

Many women also have a headache, nausea (sometimes with vomiting), and constipation or diarrhea. They may need to urinate frequently. Symptoms of premenstrual syndrome (such as irritability, nervousness, depression, fatigue, and abdominal bloating) may persist during part or all of the menstrual period. Sometimes menstrual blood contains clots. The clots, which may appear bright red or dark, may contain tissue and fluid from the lining of the uterus, as well as blood.

Symptoms tend to be more severe if

- Menstrual periods started at an early age.
- Periods are long or heavy.
- Women smoke.
- Family members also have dysmenorrhea.

CAUSES

Menstrual cramps may have no identifiable cause (called primary dysmenorrhea) or may result from another disorder (called secondary dysmenorrhea). Primary dysmenorrhea usually starts during adolescence and may become less severe with age and after pregnancy. Secondary dysmenorrhea usually starts during adulthood.

COMMON CAUSES

More than 50% of women with dysmenorrhea have

- **Primary dysmenorrhea**

In about 5 to 15% of these women, cramps are severe enough to interfere with daily activities and may result in absence from school or work.

Experts think that primary dysmenorrhea may be caused by release of substances called prostaglandins during menstruation. Prostaglandin levels are high in women with primary

dysmenorrhea. Prostaglandins may cause the uterus to contract (as occurs during labor), reducing blood flow to the uterus. These contractions can cause pain and discomfort. Prostaglandins also make nerve endings in the uterus more sensitive to pain. Lack of exercise and anxiety about menstrual periods may also contribute to the pain.

Secondary dysmenorrhea is commonly caused by

- Endometriosis: Tissue that normally occurs only in the lining of the uterus (endometrial tissue) appears outside the uterus. Endometriosis is the most common cause of secondary dysmenorrhea.
- Fibroids: These noncancerous tumors are composed of muscle and fibrous tissue and grow in the uterus.
- Adenomyosis: Endometrial tissue grows into the wall of the uterus, causing it to enlarge and swell during menstrual periods.

LESS COMMON CAUSES

There are many less common causes of secondary dysmenorrhea. They include birth defects, cysts and tumors in the ovaries, pelvic inflammatory disease, and use of an intrauterine device (IUD) that releases copper or a progestin (a synthetic form of the female hormone progesterone—see Table on pages 267 to 268). IUDS that release a progestin cause less cramping than those that release copper.

In a few women, pain occurs because the passageway through the cervix (cervical canal) is narrow. A narrow cervical canal (cervical stenosis) may develop after a procedure, as when a polyp in the uterus is removed or a precancerous condition (dysplasia) or cancer of the cervix is treated. A growth (polyp or fibrosis) can also narrow the cervical canal.

EVALUATION

Doctors usually diagnose dysmenorrhea when a woman reports that she regularly has bothersome pain during menstrual periods. They then determine whether dysmenorrhea is primary or secondary.

Doctors must distinguish dysmenorrhea from two serious disorders that can also cause pelvic pain (see page 324).

- An abnormally located (ectopic) pregnancy—that is, one not in its usual location in the uterus
- Pelvic inflammatory disease—infection of the uterus and/or fallopian tubes and sometimes the ovaries

Doctors can usually identify these disorders because the pain and the other symptoms they cause typically differ from those of dysmenorrhea.

An ectopic pregnancy usually causes sudden pain that begins in a specific spot and is constant (not crampy). It may or may not be accompanied by vaginal bleeding. The pain may become severe. If the ectopic pregnancy ruptures, women may feel light-headed, faint, have a racing heart, or go into shock.

In pelvic inflammatory disease, the pain may become severe and may be felt on one or both sides. Women may also have a foul-smelling, puslike discharge from the vagina, vaginal bleeding, or both. Sometimes women have a fever, nausea or vomiting, or pain during sexual intercourse or urination.

WARNING SIGNS

In women with dysmenorrhea, certain symptoms are cause for concern:

- Severe pain that began suddenly
- Fever
- A puslike discharge from the vagina

WHEN TO SEE A DOCTOR

Women with any warning sign should see a doctor that day. If women without warning signs have more severe cramps than usual or have pain that lasts longer than usual, they should see a doctor within a few days. Other women who have menstrual cramps should call their doctor. The doctor can decide how quickly they need to be seen based on their other symptoms, age, and medical history.

WHAT THE DOCTOR DOES

Doctors or other health care practitioners ask about the pain and the medical history, including the menstrual history. Practitioners then do a physical examination. What they find during the history and physical examination may suggest a cause of the cramps and the tests that may need to be done (see Table on pages 267 to 268).

For the menstrual history, practitioners ask the woman

- How old she was when menstrual periods started
- How long they last
- How heavy they are
- How long the interval between periods is
- Whether periods are regular
- When symptoms occur in relation to periods

Practitioners also ask the woman how old she was when symptoms began and what other symptoms she has. She is asked to describe the pain, including how severe it is, what relieves or worsens symptoms, and how symptoms interfere with her daily activities. Whether she has pelvic pain unrelated to periods is also important.

The woman is asked whether she has or has had disorders and other conditions that can cause cramps, including use of certain drugs (such as birth control pills) or an IUD.

A pelvic examination is done. Doctors check the vagina, vulva, cervix, uterus, and the area around the ovaries for abnormalities, including polyps and fibroids.

TESTING

Testing is done to rule out disorders that may be causing the pain. For most women, tests include

- A pregnancy test
- Ultrasonography of the pelvis to check for fibroids, endometriosis, adenomyosis, and cysts in the ovaries

If pelvic inflammatory disease is suspected, a sample of secretions is taken from the cervix, examined under a microscope, and sent to a laboratory to be tested.

If these tests are inconclusive and symptoms persist, other tests are done:

- Hysterosalpingography or sonohysterography to identify polyps, fibroids, and birth defects
- Magnetic resonance imaging (MRI) to identify other abnormalities or, if surgery is planned, to provide more information about previously identified abnormalities

SOME CAUSES AND FEATURES OF MENSTRUAL CRAMPS

Cause	Common Features*	Tests
Adenomyosis (growth of tissue that normally lines the uterus—called endometrial tissue—into the wall of the uterus)	Heavy, painful periods, vaginal bleeding between periods, pain in the lowest part of the torso (pelvis), and a feeling of pressure on the bladder and rectum Sometimes pain during sexual intercourse	Ultrasonography or MRI of the pelvis In women with abnormal vaginal bleeding, sometimes a biopsy
Birth defects of the reproductive tract	Sometimes genitals that feel or look abnormal or a lump in the pelvis	Sometimes hysterosalpingography (x-rays taken after a dye is injected into the uterus and fallopian tubes) or sonohysterography (ultrasonography after fluid is infused into the uterus)
Cervical stenosis (narrowing of the passageway through the cervix)	Irregular or no menstrual periods, vaginal bleeding between periods, infertility, and abdominal pain that occurs in cycles Possibly bulging of the vagina or uterus	A doctor's examination Sometimes ultrasonography of the pelvis
Cysts and tumors in the ovaries (cancerous or not)	Often no other symptoms Sometimes abnormal vaginal bleeding If cancer is advanced, sometimes indigestion, bloating, and backache	Transvaginal ultrasonography (using a handheld device inserted into the vagina) If cancer is suspected, blood tests to measure substances produced by certain tumors
Endometriosis (patches of endometrial tissue that are abnormally located outside the uterus)	Sharp or crampy pain that occurs before and during the first days of menstrual periods Infertility Often pain during sexual intercourse, bowel movements, or urination	A doctor's examination Sometimes laparoscopy (insertion of a viewing tube through a small incision just below the navel) Sometimes ultrasonography of the pelvis
Fibroids	Often no other symptoms With large fibroids, sometimes pain, pressure, abnormal vaginal bleeding, or a feeling of heaviness in the pelvic area	Ultrasonography Sometimes sonohysterography If results are unclear, MRI
Intrauterine devices (IUDs) that release copper or, less often, a progestin (a synthetic form of the female hormone progesterone)	Pain and vaginal bleeding that often subside several months after insertion of the IUD	A doctor's examination Usually ultrasonography of the pelvis to determine whether the IUD is correctly placed in the uterus
Pelvic congestion syndrome (chronic pain due to accumulation of blood in veins of the pelvis)	Pain that is ■ Typically dull and aching but sometimes sharp or throbbing ■ Worse at the end of the day and relieved by lying down ■ Worse during or after sexual intercourse	A doctor's examination Ultrasonography Sometimes laparoscopy

(continued)

SOME CAUSES AND FEATURES OF MENSTRUAL CRAMPS (continued)

Cause	Common Features*	Tests
Pelvic congestion syndrome (continued)	Often low back pain, aches in the legs, and abnormal vaginal bleeding	
	Occasionally a clear or watery discharge from the vagina	
	Sometimes fatigue, mood swings, headaches, and bloating	
Polyps in the cervix	Vaginal bleeding or discharge	A doctor's examination
		Sometimes ultrasonography of the pelvis

*Features include symptoms and results of the doctor's examination. Features mentioned are typical but not always present. MRI = magnetic resonance imaging.

For hysterosalpingography, x-rays are taken after a dye that can be seen on x-rays (radiopaque dye) is injected through the cervix into the uterus and fallopian tubes. For sonohysterography, ultrasonography is done after fluid is infused in the uterus through a thin tube inserted through the vagina and cervix. The fluid makes abnormalities easier to identity.

If results of these tests are inconclusive, hysteroscopy or laparoscopy can be done, enabling doctors to directly view structures in the pelvis. A viewing tube is inserted into the uterus through the vagina and cervix for hysteroscopy or through a small incision just below the navel for laparoscopy.

TREATMENT

When menstrual cramps result from another disorder, that disorder is treated if possible. For example, a narrow cervical canal can be widened surgically. However, this operation usually relieves the pain only temporarily. If needed, fibroids or misplaced endometrial tissue (due to endometriosis) is surgically removed.

When doctors diagnose primary dysmenorrhea, they reassure women that no other disorder is causing the pain and recommend general measures to relieve symptoms.

GENERAL MEASURES

Measures that may help relieve the pain include

- Adequate rest and sleep
- Regular exercise
- Heat applied to the pelvic area
- A low-fat diet
- Sometimes nutritional supplements such as omega-3 fatty acids, flaxseed, magnesium, vitamin E, zinc, and vitamin B_1

DRUGS

If pain persists, nonsteroidal anti-inflammatory drugs (NSAIDs), such as ibuprofen or mefenamic acid, may help. NSAIDs should be started 24 to 48 hours before a period begins and continued 1 or 2 days after the period begins.

If NSAIDs are ineffective, doctors may recommend birth control pills that contain a progestin and a low dose of estrogen. These pills prevent the ovaries from releasing an egg (ovulation). Other hormone treatments may also help relieve symptoms. They include danazol (a synthetic male hormone), progestins (such as levonorgestrel, etonogestrel, or medroxyprogesterone), gonadotropin-releasing hormone agonists (synthetic forms of a hormone produced by the body), and an IUD that releases a progestin.

OTHER TREATMENTS

Some alternative treatments have been suggested but have not been studied well. They include acupuncture, acupressure, chiropractic therapy, and transcutaneous electrical nerve stimulation (application of a gentle electric current through electrodes placed on the skin). Hypnosis is being studied as treatment.

If women have severe pain that persists despite treatment, surgery may be recommended. For

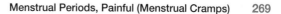

example, the nerves to the uterus may be cut to prevent pain signals from being transmitted and perceived. However, this operation occasionally injures other organs in the pelvis, such as the ureters.

O━ᴛ KEY POINTS

- Usually, menstrual cramps have no identifiable cause (called primary dysmenorrhea).
- Pain is typically crampy or sharp, starts a few days before a menstrual period, and subsides after 2 or 3 days.
- For most women, evaluation includes a pregnancy test, a doctor's examination, and ultrasonography (to check for abnormal structures or growths in the pelvis).
- For primary dysmenorrhea, general measures, such as adequate sleep, regular exercise, heat, and a low-fat diet, may help relieve symptoms.
- If such measures do not help, NSAIDs or low-dose birth control pills may be used.

MOUTH, DRY

Dry mouth (xerostomia) is caused by a reduced or absent flow of saliva. This condition can cause discomfort, interfere with speech and swallowing, make wearing dentures difficult, cause bad breath (halitosis—see page 22), and worsen oral hygiene by causing a decrease in the acidity of the mouth and an increase in bacterial growth. Longstanding dry mouth can result in severe tooth decay and candidiasis of the mouth. Dry mouth is a common complaint among older people.

CAUSES

Dry mouth occurs when the salivary glands (glands in the mouth that produce saliva) malfunction and thus decrease saliva production. There are many causes (see Table on page 271).

The **most common causes** of dry mouth are

- Drugs
- Radiation to the head and neck (for cancer treatment)

Drugs are the most common cause overall. About 400 prescription drugs and many nonprescription (over-the-counter) drugs cause a decrease in saliva production. The most common classes of drugs include the following:

- Drugs that have anticholinergic effects (drugs that block acetylcholine)
- Antiparkinsonian drugs (drugs used to treat Parkinson disease)
- Cancer chemotherapy drugs

Many commonly used drugs have anticholinergic effects. Dry mouth is only one among many anticholinergic side effects.

Chemotherapy drugs cause severe dryness and mouth sores (stomatitis—see page 276) while they are being taken. These problems usually end after the drugs are stopped.

Other common drugs that cause dry mouth include certain antihypertensives (drugs used to lower high blood pressure), anxiolytics (drugs used to treat anxiety disorders), and antidepressants (drugs used to treat depression).

Illegal methamphetamine use has resulted in a disorder called "meth mouth," which is severe tooth decay caused by methamphetamine-induced dry mouth. The damage is worsened by the tooth grinding and clenching caused by the drug and by the heat of the inhaled vapor. This combination causes very rapid destruction of teeth and a lifetime of dental problems for younger people.

Tobacco use usually decreases saliva production.

Radiation therapy for head and neck cancer can severely damage the salivary glands, often causing permanent dryness. Even low doses of radiation can cause temporary drying.

Bodywide (systemic) disorders are less common causes of dry mouth, although dry mouth is very common among people with the rare disorder Sjögren syndrome. Some people with diabetes or HIV infection have problems with dry mouth.

EVALUATION

Not all people with a dry mouth need to be immediately evaluated by a doctor. The following information can help people decide whether a doctor's evaluation is needed and help them know what to expect during the evaluation.

WARNING SIGNS

In people with dry mouth, certain symptoms and characteristics are cause for concern. They include

- Extensive tooth decay
- Dry eyes, dry skin, rash, or joint pain
- Risk factors for HIV infection

WHEN TO SEE A DOCTOR

People who have warning signs should see a doctor right away. People with extensive tooth decay should have a dental examination. People with a dry mouth but no warning signs and who otherwise feel well may see their doctor within a week or so.

WHAT THE DOCTOR DOES

Doctors first ask questions about the person's symptoms and medical history. Symptoms of dry or irritated eyes, dry skin, skin rash, and/or joint pain raise the possibility of Sjögren syndrome. Doctors also ask about a history of past or current radiation treatment, head and neck trauma, and a diagnosis of or risk factors for HIV infection. Doctors need to know all the drugs a person is taking to find out whether any are causing the dry mouth.

Doctors then do a physical examination. The physical examination is focused on the mouth, to see the degree of dryness. If the degree of dryness is unclear, doctors can hold a tongue depressor against the inside of the cheek for 10 seconds. If the tongue depressor falls off immediately when released, the flow of saliva is considered normal. If there is difficulty removing the tongue depressor, the flow of saliva is not normal. In women, the lipstick sign, where lipstick sticks to the front teeth, may be a useful indicator of dry mouth. Doctors also examine the mouth for the presence of any sores caused by the fungus *Candida albicans* and check the condition of the teeth (for instance, whether there are any cavities).

SOME CAUSES OF DRY MOUTH

Cause	Examples
Drugs	
Drugs with anticholinergic effects	Antidepressants
	Antiemetics
	Antihistamines
	Antipsychotics
	Anxiolytics
Recreational/illegal	Marijuana (cannabis)
	Methamphetamines
	Tobacco
Other	Antihypertensive drugs
	Antiparkinsonian drugs
	Bronchodilators
	Chemotherapy drugs
	Decongestants
	Diuretics
	Meperidine, methadone, and other opioids
Systemic disorders	
—	Amyloidosis
	HIV infection
	Leprosy
	Sarcoidosis
	Sjögren syndrome
	Tuberculosis
Other	
—	Breathing through the mouth too much
	Head and neck trauma (causing nerve injury)
	Radiation therapy to the head and neck area
	Viral infections

What doctors find during the history and physical examination often suggests a cause of the dry mouth (see Table on page 271) and the tests that may need to be done. If the dry mouth began shortly after a new drug was started, doctors often try stopping the drug to see whether symptoms go away.

TESTING

Sometimes, doctors test how well the salivary glands are functioning by measuring the flow of saliva (sialometry). People chew paraffin or apply citric acid to the tongue to stimulate the flow of saliva, and then doctors collect the saliva. Measuring the flow of saliva can help doctors determine whether the dry mouth is getting better or worse.

If doctors are unable to determine the cause of dry mouth, people should usually undergo a biopsy (removal of a sample of tissue for examination under a microscope) of a minor salivary gland on the lower lip to detect Sjögren syndrome, sarcoidosis, amyloidosis, tuberculosis, or cancer. They may also consider HIV testing.

TREATMENT

When possible, the cause of dry mouth is treated. For people with drug-related dry mouth whose current drug cannot be changed to another drug, drug schedules should be modified to achieve maximum drug effect during the day, because nighttime dry mouth is more likely to cause cavities. For all drugs, easy-to-take formulations, such as liquids, should be considered. Drugs that need to be placed under the tongue should be avoided. People should drink water before swallowing capsules and tablets or before placing nitroglycerin under the tongue. People also should avoid decongestants and antihistamines.

SYMPTOM CONTROL

Treatment that helps control the symptoms of dry mouth consists of measures that

- Increase existing saliva
- Replace saliva with other liquid
- Control cavities

Drugs that increase saliva production include cevimeline and pilocarpine. The main side effect of cevimeline is nausea. The main side effects of pilocarpine include sweating, flushing, and excreting large volumes of diluted urine (polyuria).

Sipping sugarless fluids frequently and chewing gum that contains xylitol helps stimulate saliva flow. Using an over-the-counter saliva substitute containing carboxymethylcellulose, hydroxyethylcellulose, or glycerin may also help.

Petroleum jelly can be applied to the lips and under dentures to relieve drying, cracking, soreness, and trauma of the lining of the mouth. A cold-air humidifier may aid mouth breathers who typically have their worst symptoms at night.

Meticulous oral hygiene is essential. People should brush and floss regularly (including just before bedtime) and use fluoride rinses or gels daily. Newer toothpastes with added calcium and phosphorous also may help prevent cavities. People should see their dentist more often for preventive dental care and plaque removal. The most effective way to prevent cavities is to use custom-fitted mouth guards for at-home fluoride application. In addition, a dentist can apply a sodium fluoride varnish 2 to 4 times per year.

People should avoid sugary or acidic foods and beverages and any irritating foods that are dry, spicy, or excessively hot or cold. People should especially avoid sugar near bedtime.

ESSENTIALS FOR OLDER PEOPLE

Dry mouth is more common among older people, but this is probably due to the many drugs typically used by older people rather than aging itself.

⊙━π KEY POINTS

- Drugs are the most common cause, but systemic diseases (most commonly Sjögren syndrome or HIV infection) and radiation therapy can also cause dry mouth.
- Saliva flow can be increased by chewing gum that contains xylitol or sucking on sugarless candy, by taking certain drugs, and by using artificial saliva replacement.
- Because people with dry mouth are at high risk of tooth decay, meticulous oral hygiene, additional preventive measures at home, and dentist-applied fluorides are essential.

MOUTH GROWTHS

Growths can originate in any type of tissue in and around the mouth, including connective tissues, bone, muscle, and nerve. Most commonly, growths form on the lips, the sides of the tongue, the floor of the mouth, and the back portion of the roof of the mouth (soft palate). Some growths cause pain or irritation.

CAUSES

Mouth growths can be

- Noncancerous (benign)
- Precancerous (dysplastic)
- Cancerous (malignant)

NONCANCEROUS GROWTHS

Most mouth growths are noncancerous.

A variety of noncancerous growths may occur in and around the mouth. A persistent lump or raised area on the gums (gingiva) should be evaluated by a dentist. Such a lump may be caused by a gum or tooth abscess or by irritation. Noncancerous growths due to irritation are relatively common and, if necessary, can be removed by surgery. In 10 to 40% of people, noncancerous growths on the gums reappear because the irritant remains. Occasionally such irritation, particularly if it persists over a long period of time, can lead to cancerous changes. Because any unusual growths in or around the mouth can be cancer, the growths should be checked by a doctor or dentist without delay.

Ordinary warts (verrucae vulgaris) can infect the mouth if a person sucks or chews one that is growing on a finger. A different type of wart—a genital wart—may be transmitted through oral sex. A doctor may remove an ordinary wart using one of several methods.

Thrush is a yeast infection of the skin and moist areas (such as the mouth and vagina) that often appears as whitish, cheese-like patches in the mouth. Thrush sticks tightly to the mucus membranes and, when the material is wiped away, leaves a red patch. Thrush is most common among people with diabetes or a suppressed immune system and in those who are taking antibiotics.

A torus, which is a slow-growing, rounded projection of bone, may form in the middle of the roof of the mouth or on the lower jaw by the side of the tongue. This hard growth is both common and harmless. Even a large growth can be left alone unless it gets scraped during eating or the person needs a denture that covers the area. Multiple bony growths in the mouth may indicate familial adenomatous polyposis, a hereditary disorder of the digestive tract where the person has numerous polyps in the colon that often become cancerous.

Keratoacanthomas are growths that form on the lips and other sun-exposed areas, such as the face, forearms, and hands. A keratoacanthoma usually reaches its full size of ½ to 1 inch (about 1 to 3 centimeters) or more in diameter within 1 or 2 months, then begins to shrink after another few months and may eventually disappear without treatment. Once, all keratoacathomas were considered to be noncancerous, but many experts now consider them to be cancerous.

Many kinds of cysts (hollow, fluid-filled swellings) cause jaw pain and swelling. Often they are next to an impacted wisdom tooth and can destroy considerable areas of the jawbone as they expand. Certain types of cysts are more likely to recur after surgical removal. Various types of cysts may also develop in the floor of the mouth. Often, these cysts are surgically removed because they make swallowing uncomfortable or because they are unattractive.

Odontomas are overgrowths of tooth-forming cells that look like small, misshapen extra teeth. In children, they may get in the way of normal teeth coming in. In adults, they may push teeth out of alignment. They are usually removed surgically.

Most (75 to 80%) salivary gland tumors are noncancerous, slow-growing, and painless. They usually occur as a single, soft, movable lump beneath normal-looking skin or under the lining (mucosa) of the inside of the cheek. Occasionally, when hollow and fluid-filled, they are firm. The most common type (called a mixed tumor or pleomorphic adenoma) occurs mainly in women older than 40. This type can become cancerous and is removed surgically. Unless completely removed, this type of tumor is likely to grow back. Other types of noncancerous tumors are also removed surgically but are much less likely to become cancerous or to grow back once removed.

PRECANCEROUS CHANGES

White, red, or mixed white-red areas that are not easily wiped away, persist for more than 2 weeks, and are not definable as some other condition may be precancerous. The same risk factors are involved in precancerous changes as in cancerous growths, and precancerous changes may become cancerous if not removed.

Leukoplakia is a flat white spot that may develop when the moist lining of the mouth (oral mucosa) is irritated for a long period. The irritated spot appears white because it has a thickened layer of keratin—the same material that covers the skin and normally is less abundant in the lining of the mouth.

Erythroplakia is a red and flat or worn away area that results when the lining of the mouth thins. The area appears red because the underlying capillaries are more visible. Erythroplakia is a much more ominous predictor of oral cancer than leukoplakia.

ORAL CANCER

People who use tobacco, alcohol, or both are at much greater risk (up to 15 times) of oral cancer. For those who use chewing tobacco and snuff, the insides of the cheeks and lips are common sites of oral cancer. In other people, the most common sites for oral cancer include the sides of the tongue, the floor of the mouth, and the throat. Rarely, cancers found in the mouth region have spread there from other parts of the body, such as the lungs, breast, or prostate.

Oral cancer can have many different appearances but typically resembles precancerous lesions. For example, white, red, or mixed white-red areas that are not easily wiped away.

EVALUATION

The following information can help people decide when a doctor's evaluation is needed and help them know what to expect during the evaluation.

WARNING SIGNS

Certain symptoms and characteristics are cause for concern. They include

- Weight loss
- Firm lump in the neck

WHEN TO SEE A DOCTOR

People with a mouth growth that does not go away in a week or two should see their doctor or dentist when convenient. Warning signs suggest a higher risk of cancer, and although evaluation is not urgent, people with warning signs (particularly those who use tobacco) should not put off being evaluated.

Because oral cancer often causes no symptoms early on, it is important for people to have a yearly examination of the mouth. Such an examination can be done during an annual dental check-up.

WHAT THE DOCTOR DOES

Doctors first ask questions about the person's symptoms and medical history. Doctors then do a physical examination. What they find during the history and physical examination can help suggest a cause of the mouth growth.

Doctors ask people about how long the growth has been present, whether it is painful, and whether there was any injury to the area (for example, biting a cheek or scraping by a sharp tooth edge or dental restoration). Other things they ask about include

- The amount and duration of use of alcohol and tobacco
- Risk factors for thrush, including use of antibiotics and a history of diabetes or HIV infection
- Whether the person has lost weight or been feeling generally ill

The physical examination focuses on the mouth and neck. Doctors look carefully at all areas of the mouth and throat, including under the tongue. They feel the sides of the neck for swollen glands (lymph nodes), which indicate possible cancer or chronic infection.

TESTING

If a growth has the appearance of thrush, doctors examine scrapings under a microscope. For other growths that have lasted longer than a few weeks, most doctors recommend removing all or part of the growth for examination in a laboratory (biopsy). Biopsy is often necessary to make sure a growth is noncancerous.

TREATMENT

Treatment differs depending on the cause of the growth.

🔑 KEY POINTS

- Most mouth growths are noncancerous.
- Warts, yeast infections, and repeated trauma (such as biting or rubbing against a sharp tooth edge) are common causes of noncancerous growths.
- Use of alcohol and tobacco is a risk factor for oral cancer.
- Because cancerous growths are difficult to recognize by their appearance, doctors frequently recommend a biopsy.

MOUTH SORES

Mouth sores and inflammation (stomatitis) vary in appearance and size and can affect any part of the mouth, inside and outside. People may have swelling and redness of the lining of the mouth or individual, painful ulcers. An ulcer is a hole that forms in the lining of the mouth when the top layer of cells breaks down. Many ulcers appear red, but some are white because of dead cells and food debris inside the center portion. Some sores are raised and filled with fluid, similar to blisters (in which case they are called vesicles or bullae, depending on size). Rarely, the mouth looks normal even though people have symptoms of mouth inflammation (burning mouth syndrome).

Noncancerous (benign) ulcers are usually painful until healing is well under way. The pain makes eating difficult, which sometimes leads to dehydration and undernutrition. Some sores go away but recur.

CAUSES

There are many types and causes of mouth sores. Mouth sores may be caused by an infection, a bodywide (systemic) disease, a physical or chemical irritant, or an allergic reaction (see Table on page 278). Often the cause is unknown. In general, because the normal flow of saliva helps protect the lining of the mouth, any condition that decreases saliva production makes mouth sores more likely (see page 270).

The most common specific causes of mouth sores are

- Recurrent aphthous stomatitis (canker sores)
- Viral infections (particularly herpes simplex and herpes zoster)
- Other infections (caused by fungi or bacteria)
- Injury or irritating food or chemicals
- Tobacco use
- Drugs (particularly chemotherapy drugs) and radiation therapy
- Systemic disorders

VIRAL INFECTIONS

Viruses are the most common infectious causes of mouth sores. Cold sores of the lip and, less commonly, ulcers on the palate caused by the herpes simplex virus are perhaps the most well known. However, many other viruses can cause mouth sores. Herpes zoster, the virus responsible for chickenpox as well as the painful skin disorder called shingles, can cause multiple sores to form on one side of the mouth. These sores are the result of a flare-up of the virus, which, just like herpes simplex virus, never leaves the body. Occasionally, the mouth remains painful for months or years or even permanently after the sores have healed.

OTHER INFECTIONS

A bacterial infection can lead to sores and swelling in the mouth. Infections may be caused by an overgrowth of organisms normally present in the mouth or by newly introduced organisms, such as the bacteria that cause syphilis or gonorrhea. Bacterial infections from teeth or gums can spread to form a pus-filled pocket of infection (abscess) or cause widespread inflammation (cellulitis).

Syphilis may produce a red, painless sore (chancre) that develops in the mouth or on the lips during the early stage of infection. The sore usually heals after several weeks. About 4 to 10 weeks later, a white area (mucous patch) may form on the lip or inside the mouth if the syphilis has not been treated. Both the chancre and the mucous patch are highly contagious, and kissing may spread the disease during these stages. In late-stage syphilis, a hole (gumma) may appear in the palate or tongue. The disease is not contagious at this stage.

The yeast *Candida albicans* is a normal resident of the mouth. However, it can overgrow in people who have taken antibiotics or corticosteroids or who have a weak immune system, such as people with AIDS. *Candida* can cause whitish, cheese-like patches that destroy the top layer of the lining of the mouth when wiped off. Sometimes only flat, red areas appear.

INJURY OR IRRITATION

Any type of damage or injury to the mouth, for instance, when the inside of the cheek is accidentally bitten or scraped by jagged teeth or poor-fitting dentures, can cause blisters (vesicles or bullae) or ulcers to form in the mouth. Typically, the surface of a blister breaks down quickly (ruptures), forming an ulcer.

Many foods and chemicals can be irritating or trigger a type of allergic reaction, causing mouth sores. Acidic foods, cinnamon flavoring, or astringents may be particularly irritating, as can certain ingredients in common substances such as toothpaste, mouthwash, candy, and gum.

TOBACCO

Tobacco use can cause mouth sores. The sores most likely result from exposure to the irritants, toxins, and carcinogens found naturally in tobacco products but may also result from the drying effects on the lining of the mouth, the high temperatures in the mouth, changes to the acid-base balance of the mouth, or decreased resistance to viral, bacterial, and fungal infections.

DRUGS AND RADIATION THERAPY

The most common drugs causing mouth sores include certain cancer chemotherapy drugs and drugs containing gold (sometimes used to treat rheumatoid arthritis). Radiation therapy is also a common cause of mouth sores. Rarely, people may develop mouth sores after taking antibiotics.

SYSTEMIC DISORDERS

Many diseases affect the mouth along with other parts of the body. Behçet syndrome, an inflammatory disease affecting many organs, including the eyes, genitals, skin, joints, blood vessels, brain, and gastrointestinal tract, can cause recurring, painful mouth sores. Stevens-Johnson syndrome, a type of allergic reaction, causes skin blisters and mouth sores. Some people with inflammatory bowel disease also develop mouth sores. People with severe celiac disease, which is caused by an intolerance to gluten (a component of wheat and some other grains), often develop mouth sores. Lichen planus, a skin disease, can rarely cause mouth sores, although usually these sores are not as uncomfortable as those on the skin. Pemphigus vulgaris and bullous pemphigoid, both skin diseases, can also cause blisters to form in the mouth.

EVALUATION

Not all mouth sores require immediate evaluation by a doctor. The following information can help people decide whether a doctor's evaluation is needed and help them know what to expect during the evaluation.

WARNING SIGNS

In people with mouth sores, certain symptoms and characteristics are cause for concern for systemic disorders. They include

- Fever
- Blisters on the skin
- Inflammation of the eye
- Any sores in people with a weakened immune system (such as people with HIV infection)

WHEN TO SEE A DOCTOR

People who have warning signs should see a doctor right away. Those who have no warning signs but have a lot of pain, feel generally ill, and/or have trouble eating should see a doctor within several days. All people with a sore that lasts for 10 days or more must be examined by a dentist or doctor to ensure that it is not cancerous or precancerous.

WHAT THE DOCTOR DOES

Doctors first ask questions about the person's symptoms and medical history. Doctors ask people about their consumption of or exposure to food, drugs, and other substances (such as tobacco, chemicals, metals, fumes, or dust). Doctors need to know about all currently known conditions that might cause mouth sores (such as herpes simplex, Behçet syndrome, or inflammatory bowel disease), conditions that are risk factors for mouth sores (such as a weakened immune system, cancer, or HIV infection), and the person's sexual history.

Doctors then do a physical examination. The mouth is inspected, noting the location and nature of any sores. Doctors then do a general examination to look for signs of systemic disorders that could affect the mouth. The skin, eyes, and genitals are examined for any sores, blisters, or rashes.

What doctors find during the history and physical examination often suggests a cause of the mouth sores and the tests that may need to be done (see Table on pages 278 to 279).

SOME CAUSES OF MOUTH SORES

Category	Examples
Bacterial infections	Trench mouth (acute necrotizing ulcerative gingivitis)
	Gonorrhea
	Syphilis
Fungal infections	Candidal infections (most common)
Viral infections	Chickenpox (varicella zoster)
	Herpes simplex infection (primary or secondary)
	Shingles (reactivation of varicella zoster)
	Others (such as infection by coxsackievirus, cytomegalovirus, Epstein-Barr virus, or HIV, as well as genital warts, influenza, and measles)
Systemic disorders	Behçet syndrome
	Celiac disease
	Cyclic neutropenia
	Erythema multiforme
	Inflammatory bowel disease
	Iron deficiency
	Kawasaki disease
	Leukemia
	Pemphigoid or pemphigus vulgaris
	Platelet disorders
	Stevens-Johnson syndrome
	Thrombotic thrombocytopenia
	Vitamin B deficiency (pellagra)
	Vitamin C deficiency (scurvy)
Drugs	Antibiotics*
	Anticonvulsants*
	Barbiturates*
	Chemotherapy drugs
	Gold
	Iodides*
	Nonsteroidal anti-inflammatory drugs (NSAIDs)*
Physical irritation	Biting the mouth
	Dentures that fit poorly
	Jagged teeth
Irritants and allergies	Acidic foods
	Allergic reaction to ingredients in toothpaste, mouthwash, candy, gum, dyes, or lipstick
	Aspirin, when applied to tissues inside the mouth
	Dental appliances containing nickel or palladium
	Occupational exposure to dyes, heavy metals, acid fumes, or metal or mineral dust
	Tobacco (chewing and/or smoking) *(continued)*

SOME CAUSES OF MOUTH SORES *(continued)*

Category	Examples
Other	Burning mouth syndrome
	Canker sores (recurrent aphthous stomatitis)
	Lichen planus
	Radiation therapy to the head and neck

*Rare causes of mouth sores.

TESTING

The need for tests depends on what doctors find during the history and physical examination, particularly whether warning signs are present. People with a brief episode of mouth sores and no symptoms or risk factors for a systemic illness probably require no testing. In people with several episodes of mouth sores, viral and bacterial cultures and various blood tests are done. A biopsy may be done for persistent sores that do not have an obvious cause.

Systematically eliminating foods from the diet can be useful, as can changing brands of toothpaste, chewing gum, or mouthwash.

TREATMENT

Doctors treat the cause, if known. For example, people are given antibiotics for bacterial infections. Avoiding any substances or drugs that are causing the mouth sores is recommended. Frequent, gentle toothbrushing with a soft brush and salt-water rinses may help keep sores from becoming infected.

Pain can be helped by avoiding acidic or highly salty foods and any other substances that are irritating.

TOPICAL TREATMENTS

Topical treatments are substances applied directly to an affected part of the body. Topical treatments for mouth sores include

- Anesthetics
- Protective coatings
- Corticosteroids
- Burning with a laser or chemicals

An anesthetic such as dyclonine or lidocaine may be used as a mouth rinse. However, because these mouth rinses numb the mouth and throat and thus may make swallowing difficult, children using them should be watched to ensure that they do not choke on their food. Lidocaine in a thicker preparation (viscous lidocaine) can also be swabbed directly on the mouth sore.

Protective coatings containing sucralfate and aluminum-magnesium antacids can be soothing when applied as a rinse. Many doctors add other ingredients such as lidocaine and/or diphenhydramine (an antihistamine). Amlexanox paste is another alternative.

Once doctors are sure that the sore is not caused by an infection, they may prescribe a corticosteroid rinse or a corticosteroid gel to be applied to each sore.

Some mouth sores can be treated with a low-powered laser, which relieves pain immediately and often prevents sores from returning. Chemically burning the sore with a small stick coated with silver nitrate may similarly relieve pain but is not as effective as a laser.

KEY POINTS

- A mouth sore that lasts more than 10 days should be evaluated by a doctor or dentist.
- Isolated mouth sores in people with no other symptoms or risk factors for a systemic illness are usually caused by a viral infection or recurrent aphthous stomatitis.
- Symptoms outside the mouth, skin rash, or both suggest a more immediate need for a diagnosis.

MUSCLE CRAMPS

A cramp is a sudden, brief, unintended (involuntary), and usually painful contraction of a muscle or group of muscles.

CAUSES

The **most common** causes of muscle cramps are

- Benign leg cramps that occur for no known reason, typically at night
- Exercise-associated muscle cramping (cramping during or immediately after exercise)

Muscle cramps (also called charley horses) often occur in healthy people, usually in middle-aged and older people but sometimes in younger people. Cramps tend to occur during or after vigorous exercise but sometimes occur during rest. Some people have leg cramps during sleep. These painful cramps usually affect the calf and foot muscles, causing the foot and toes to curl downward. Although painful, these cramps are usually not serious and are thus called benign leg cramps.

Having tight calf muscles is a common cause of leg cramps. Muscles become tight when they are not stretched, when people are inactive, or sometimes when fluid repeatedly accumulates (called edema) in the lower leg.

Low levels of electrolytes (such as potassium, magnesium, or calcium) in the blood can also cause cramps. Low electrolyte levels may result from use of some diuretics, alcoholism, certain endocrine disorders, vitamin D deficiency, or conditions that cause loss of fluids (and thus electrolytes). Electrolyte levels may become low late in pregnancy.

Cramps can occur shortly after dialysis, possibly because dialysis removes too much fluid from the body, removes the fluid to quickly, and/or lowers electrolyte levels.

Other causes include nerve disorders, an underactive thyroid gland (hypothyroidism), and use of certain drugs.

DISORDERS THAT CAUSE SIMILAR SYMPTOMS

Some disorders cause symptoms that resemble muscle cramps.

Dystonias are involuntary muscle contractions, but they usually last longer than cramps. Also, they tend to affect other muscles and may affect many other muscles, including any limb muscles as well as those of the back, neck, and voice. In contrast, benign leg cramps and exercise-associated muscle cramping tend to affect the calf muscles.

Tetany is continuous or periodic spasms of muscles throughout the body. These spasms last much longer than muscle cramps and are more widespread. The muscles may also twitch.

Some people feel as if they are having cramps but no muscle contraction occurs (called illusory muscle cramps).

Hardening of the arteries in the legs (peripheral arterial disease) may cause calf pain during physical activity such as walking. This pain is due to inadequate blood flow to muscles, not to muscle contraction as occurs with cramps.

EVALUATION

The following information can help people decide whether a doctor's evaluation is needed and help them know what to expect during the evaluation.

WARNING SIGNS

In people with muscle cramps, the following symptoms and characteristics are of particular concern:

- Cramps in the arms or trunk
- Muscle twitching
- Alcoholism
- Weakness
- Cramps that occur after loss of body fluids (dehydration) or use of diuretics
- Loss of sensation or pain unless they occur at the same time as the cramping

If people have cramps in the arms or trunk or muscle twitching, the cause is more likely to be a disorder (such as an electrolyte or endocrine disorder) or a drug than benign leg cramps or exercise-related muscle cramps.

CONDITIONS THAT CAUSE OR CONTRIBUTE TO MUSCLE CRAMPS

Category	Examples
Drugs	
Use of certain drugs	Angiotensin II receptor blockers, bronchodilators, cisplatin, clofibrate, diuretics, donepezil, lovastatin, birth control pills (oral contraceptives), pyrazinamide, raloxifene, synthetic parathyroid hormone (teriparatide), tolcapone, or vincristine
	Stimulants, such as amphetamines, caffeine, cocaine, ephedrine, nicotine, or pseudoephedrine
Sudden stopping of a drug	Sedatives, such as alcohol, barbiturates, or benzodiazepines
	Drugs used to treat insomnia or anxiety
Disorders	
Electrolyte and endocrine disorders	Low levels of potassium, magnesium, or calcium in the blood
	Alcoholism
	Hypothyroidism (an underactive thyroid gland)
Musculoskeletal disorders	Tight calf muscles
	Myopathies (disorders that affect muscle)
	Structural disorders, such as flat feet or genu recurvatum (a deformity of the knee joint that causes the knee to bend backward)
Nerve disorders	Motor neuron disease (nerve disorders that affect voluntary muscles—those controlled by conscious effort)
	Peripheral neuropathies (damage to nerves outside the brain and spinal cord)
	Compression of a spinal nerve root
Water balance disorders	Dehydration
	Excessive sweating with inadequate replacement of salt or potassium
	Effects of dialysis—for example, if too much fluid is removed from the body or if fluid is removed too quickly
Other conditions	
Exercise and lifestyle	Cramping during or soon after exercise
	Sitting for a long time

WHEN TO SEE A DOCTOR

People with muscle cramps should consult a doctor as soon as possible if they also have alcoholism, sudden weakness or loss of sensation, or severe symptoms or if they have lost body fluids (for example, through vomiting, diarrhea, or excessive sweating). Otherwise, people should call their doctor in a day or two to discuss how soon the doctor needs to see them.

WHAT THE DOCTOR DOES

Doctors first ask questions about the person's symptoms and medical history and then does a physical examination. What doctors find during the history and physical examination often suggests a cause and the tests that may need to be done.

Doctors ask the person to describe the cramps, including how long they last, how frequent they are, where they are, whether any event seems to trigger them, and whether any other symptoms are present. They ask about symptoms that suggest clues to the cause:

- Lack of menstrual periods or menstrual irregularities—symptoms that suggest pregnancy-related leg cramps
- Vomiting, diarrhea, use of diuretics, excessive exercise, and sweating— symptoms that suggest loss of body fluids or electrolytes
- Difficulty tolerating cold, weight gain, and coarse, thick skin—symptoms that may indicate hypothyroidism
- Weakness, pain, or loss of sensation— symptoms that suggest a nerve disorder

The person is also asked about use of drugs and alcohol, recent dialysis treatment, and any association between past dialysis treatments and muscle cramps.

The physical examination focuses first on the nervous system (neurologic examination), including assessment of muscles and reflexes. Doctors also inspect the skin for signs of alcoholism, hypothyroidism (such as a puffy face and loss of eyebrow hair), and dehydration.

TESTING

No tests are routinely done.

PREVENTION

Preventing cramps is the best approach. The following measures can help:

- Not exercising immediately after eating
- Gently stretching the muscles before exercising or going to bed
- Drinking plenty of fluids (particularly sports beverages that contain potassium) after exercise
- Not consuming caffeine (for example, in coffee or chocolate)
- Not smoking
- Avoiding drugs that are stimulants, such as ephedrine or pseudoephedrine (a decongestant contained in many products that do not require a prescription but are available only behind the pharmacy counter)

Stretching makes muscles and tendons more flexible and less likely to contract involuntarily. The runner's stretch is the best stretch for preventing calf cramps. A person stands with one leg forward and bent at the knee and the other leg behind with the knee straight—a lunge position. The hands can be placed on the wall for balance. Both heels remain on the floor. The knee of the front leg is bent further until a stretch is felt along the back of the other leg. The greater the distance between the two feet and the more the front knee is bent, the greater the stretch. The stretch is held for 30 seconds and repeated 5 times. Then the set of stretches is repeated on the other side.

Most of the drugs prescribed to prevent cramps from recurring (including calcium supplements, magnesium carbonate, and benzodiazepines such as diazepam) have not proved to be effective, and they can have side effects. Whether quinine is effective is unclear, but it does have side effects, such as vomiting, vision problems, ringing in the ears, and headaches. Mexiletine (used to treat abnormal heart rhythms) sometimes helps but has many side effects, such as nausea, vomiting, tremors (rhythmic shaking of a body part), and seizures.

TREATMENT

If a cramp occurs, stretching the affected muscle often relieves the cramp. For example, for a calf cramp, the person could use a hand to pull the foot and toes upward or could do the runner's stretch.

O—π KEY POINTS

- Leg cramps are common.
- The most common causes are benign leg cramps and exercise-associated cramping.
- Stretching and not consuming caffeine can help prevent muscle cramps.
- Drug therapy is not usually recommended to prevent muscle cramps.

NASAL CONGESTION AND DISCHARGE

Nasal congestion and discharge (runny nose, rhinorrhea) are extremely common problems that commonly occur together but occasionally occur alone.

CAUSES

COMMON CAUSES

The most common causes (see Table on page 285) are the following:

- Viral upper respiratory infections (colds)
- Allergic reactions

LESS COMMON CAUSES

Less common causes include

- Sinus infection (sinusitis)
- Foreign object (body) in the nose
- Overuse of decongestant sprays

Fluid sometimes drains from an infected sinus. Children sometimes put a foreign object in their nose. If adults do not see them do this, the first sign may be a foul-smelling nasal discharge due to infection and irritation from the foreign object. Rarely, adults with mental disorders put objects in their nose.

People who use nasal decongestant sprays for more than 1 or 2 days often experience significant rebound congestion (the return of congestion that is worse than before) when the effects of the drug wear off. People then continue using the decongestant in a vicious circle of persistent, worsening congestion. This situation (rhinitis medicamentosa) may persist for some time, and people may misinterpret it as a continuation of the original problem rather than a consequence of treatment.

EVALUATION

Not all episodes of nasal congestion and discharge require immediate evaluation by a doctor. The following information can help people decide whether a doctor's evaluation is needed and help them know what to expect during the evaluation.

WARNING SIGNS

In people with nasal congestion and discharge, certain symptoms and characteristics are cause for concern. They include

- Discharge from only one side of the nose, particularly if it contains pus or blood
- Face pain, tenderness, or both

WHEN TO SEE A DOCTOR

People who have warning signs and those whose caretakers think may have put something in their nose should see a doctor right away. People who have nasal congestion and discharge but no warning signs should call their doctor. They may not need to be seen, particularly if they have typical cold symptoms and are otherwise healthy.

WHAT THE DOCTOR DOES

Doctors first ask questions about the person's symptoms and medical history and then do a physical examination. What doctors find during the history and physical examination often suggests a cause of the nasal congestion and discharge and the tests that may need to be done (see Table).

During the medical history, doctors ask about the following:

- The nature of the discharge (such as whether it is watery, sticky, pus-filled, or bloody) and whether it is present most or all of the time (chronic) or comes and goes
- Symptoms of possible causes, including fever and face pain (sinusitis); watery, itchy eyes (allergies); and sore throat, a general feeling of illness (malaise), fever, and cough (viral upper respiratory infection)
- Whether people have allergies, diabetes, or a weakened immune system and whether they have been using decongestant sprays

If the discharge comes and goes, doctors try to determine whether it relates to where the person lives, the season, or exposure to potential triggers (such as pets or dust).

During the physical examination, doctors look at the following:

- The nose and the area over the sinuses

- The face for redness over the sinuses just above the eyebrows (frontal sinuses) and the sinuses in the cheekbones (maxillary sinuses)
- The membranes lining the nose (nasal mucosa) for color (whether they are red or pale), swelling, color and nature of the discharge, and (particularly in children) whether there is any foreign object

Doctors also tap their finger over the sinuses to look for tenderness.

TESTING

Testing is generally not needed for acute nasal symptoms unless severe sinusitis is suspected in a person with diabetes or a weakened immune system. These people usually should have a computed tomography (CT) scan.

TREATMENT

The best way to treat nasal congestion and discharge is to treat the underlying disorder. There are two basic approaches to relieving the symptoms:

- Decongestants (spray or pills)
- Antihistamines (pills)

Decongestant sprays typically contain oxymetazoline. Decongestants taken by mouth include pseudoephedrine. Decongestant sprays should not be used for more than a day or 2 to avoid the problem of rebound congestion.

Antihistamines can be taken for symptoms due to viral infection and allergic reactions. Doctors often recommend diphenhydramine

SOME CAUSES AND FEATURES OF NASAL CONGESTION AND DISCHARGE

Cause	Common Features*	Tests
Acute sinusitis (a sinus infection that just started)	A mucus- and pus-filled discharge, often from only one side of the nose Sometimes a foul or metallic taste in the mouth, facial pain or headache, and redness or tenderness over the cheeks or above the eyebrows No itching and no eye or throat irritation	A doctor's examination Possibly CT if people have diabetes, a weakened immune system, or signs of a serious illness
Allergies	A watery discharge, sneezing, and watery, itchy eyes Pale, soft, swollen membranes lining the nose (nasal mucosa), seen during the examination Symptoms that often occur during certain seasons or after exposure to possible triggers	A doctor's examination
Decongestant sprays if overused	Congestion that returns when the decongestant wears off (rebound congestion) Pale, extremely swollen nasal mucosa No discharge	A doctor's examination
A foreign object in the nose, mainly in children	Often a foul-smelling, sometimes blood-tinged discharge from one side of the nose	A doctor's examination
Vasomotor rhinitis	A recurring watery discharge, sneezing, and red, swollen nasal mucosa No identifiable triggers	A doctor's examination
Viral upper respiratory infections	A discharge that may be watery or sticky, a sore throat, a general feeling of illness (malaise), and red nasal mucosa	A doctor's examination

*Features include symptoms and the results of the doctor's examination. Features mentioned are typical but not always present.
CT = computed tomography.

for people with colds. For people with allergies, other antihistamines that have fewer side effects, such as fexofenadine, are used. Nasal corticosteroid sprays (such as mometasone) also help allergic conditions.

Decongestants and antihistamines are not recommended for children under 6 years of age.

ESSENTIALS FOR OLDER PEOPLE

The main concerns with older people involve treatment. Antihistamines can have sedating and anticholinergic effects (such as confusion, blurred vision, and loss of bladder control). These effects are more common among and more troublesome in older people. Antihistamines should be avoided or used in decreased dosages. Pseudoephedrine, a decongestant, stimulates the heart rate and increases blood pressure. If pseudoephedrine is needed, it should be taken at the lowest effective dose.

⚬━π KEY POINTS

- Most nasal congestion and discharge are caused by an upper respiratory infection or allergies.
- In children, doctors consider the possibility of a foreign object in the nose.
- Doctors also consider the possibility of rebound congestion in people who overuse decongestant sprays.

NAUSEA AND VOMITING IN ADULTS

Nausea is an unpleasant feeling of needing to vomit. People also may feel dizziness, vague discomfort in the abdomen, and an unwillingness to eat.

Vomiting is a forceful contraction of the stomach that propels its contents up the esophagus and out the mouth. Vomiting empties the stomach and often makes people with nausea feel considerably better, at least temporarily. Vomiting is quite uncomfortable and can be violent. Severe vomiting can project stomach contents many feet (projectile vomiting). Vomiting is not the same as regurgitation, which is the spitting up of stomach contents without forceful abdominal contractions or nausea. For instance, people with achalasia or Zenker diverticulum may regurgitate undigested food without nausea.

Vomitus—the material that is vomited up—usually reflects what was recently eaten. Sometimes it contains chunks of food. When blood is vomited, the vomitus is usually red (hematemesis), but if the blood has been partly digested, the vomitus looks like coffee grounds. When bile is present, the vomitus is bitter and yellow-green.

COMPLICATIONS

In addition to being uncomfortable, vomiting can cause complications:

- Inhaled vomitus (aspiration)
- Torn esophagus (Mallory-Weiss tear)
- Dehydration and electrolyte abnormalities
- Undernutrition and weight loss

People who are unconscious or only partly conscious can inhale their vomitus. The acid in the vomitus can severely irritate the lungs.

Vomiting greatly increases pressure within the esophagus, and severe vomiting can tear the lining of the esophagus. A small tear causes pain and sometimes bleeding, but a large tear can be fatal.

Because people lose water and minerals (electrolytes) in vomitus, severe vomiting can cause dehydration and electrolyte abnormalities. Newborns and infants are particularly susceptible to these complications.

Chronic vomiting can cause undernutrition, weight loss, and metabolic abnormalities.

CAUSES

Nausea and vomiting result when the vomiting center in the brain is activated. Causes typically involve disorders of the digestive tract or the brain, or ingested substances.

COMMON CAUSES

The most common causes of nausea and vomiting are

- Gastroenteritis (infection of the digestive tract)
- Drugs
- Toxins

Nausea and vomiting commonly occur with any dysfunction of the digestive tract but are particularly common with gastroenteritis. A less common digestive tract disorder is obstruction of the intestine, which causes vomiting because food and fluids back up into the stomach because of the obstruction. Many other abdominal disorders that cause vomiting also cause significant abdominal pain (see page 1). In such disorders (for example, appendicitis or pancreatitis), it is typically the pain rather than the vomiting that causes people to seek medical care.

Many drugs, including alcohol, opioid analgesics (such as morphine), and chemotherapy drugs, can cause nausea and vomiting. Toxins, such as lead or those found in some foods and plants, can cause severe nausea and vomiting.

LESS COMMON CAUSES

Less common causes of nausea and vomiting include

- Brain or central nervous system disorders
- Motion sickness
- Metabolic changes or bodywide (systemic) illness
- Psychologic disorders

The vomiting center also can be activated by certain brain or central nervous system disorders, including infections (such as meningitis and encephalitis), migraines, and disorders that increase pressure inside the skull (intracranial pressure). Disorders that increase intracranial pressure include brain tumors, brain hemorrhage, and severe head injuries.

The balance organs of the inner ear (vestibular apparatus) are connected to the vomiting center. This connection is why some people become nauseated by the movement of a boat, car, or airplane and by certain disorders of the inner ear (such as labyrinthitis and positional vertigo).

Nausea and vomiting may also occur when there are metabolic changes in the body, such as during early pregnancy, or when people have diabetes that is severely out of control or severe liver failure or kidney failure.

Psychologic problems also can cause nausea and vomiting (known as functional or psychogenic vomiting). Such vomiting may be intentional. For instance, people who have bulimia make themselves vomit to lose weight. Or it may be unintentional. For instance, children who are afraid of going to school vomit as a response to their psychologic distress.

EVALUATION

Not every episode of nausea and vomiting requires immediate evaluation by a doctor. The following information can help people decide whether a doctor's evaluation is needed and help them know what to expect during the evaluation.

WARNING SIGNS

Certain symptoms and characteristics are cause for concern. They include

- Signs of dehydration (such as thirst, dry mouth, little or no urine output, and feeling weak and tired)
- Headache, stiff neck, confusion, or decreased alertness
- Constant abdominal pain
- Tenderness when the abdomen is touched
- Distended (swollen) abdomen

WHEN TO SEE A DOCTOR

People who have warning signs should see a doctor right away, as should people who vomited any blood or who recently had a head injury.

People who have nausea and vomiting but no warning signs should see a doctor if vomiting continues for more than 24 to 48 hours or if they are unable to tolerate more than a few sips of liquid. People who have a few episodes of vomiting (with or without diarrhea) but are able to tolerate at least some liquids should call their doctor. Depending on their age, other symptoms, and known medical conditions (such as cancer or diabetes), the doctor may suggest that people be seen for an evaluation or stay home and try simple remedies.

WHAT THE DOCTOR DOES

Doctors first ask questions about the person's symptoms and medical history. Doctors then do a physical examination. What they find during the history and physical examination often suggests a cause of the vomiting and the tests that may need to be done (see Table on pages 289 to 290).

During the history, doctors ask whether the person is pregnant or has diabetes, migraines, liver or kidney disease, or cancer (including the timing of any chemotherapy or radiation therapy). All recently ingested drugs and substances are noted because certain substances may not be toxic until several days after ingestion (such as acetaminophen and some mushrooms).

During the physical examination, doctors look for the following:

- Signs of dehydration (such as a rapid heart rate, low blood pressure, and dry mouth)
- Signs of a serious abdominal disorder (such as a distended abdomen and/or severe tenderness to the touch)
- Decreased alertness or any other neurologic abnormalities suggesting a brain disorder

Doctors note any previous abdominal surgery, because fibrous bands of scar tissue (adhesions) may have formed and caused an intestinal obstruction.

Although people with previously known disorders that cause vomiting (such as migraine) may simply be having a recurrence of that disorder, doctors thoroughly look for signs of a new, different problem.

TESTING

The need for tests depends on what doctors find during the history and physical examination, particularly whether warning signs are present and whether findings suggest a particular disorder (see Table).

Possible tests include

- Pregnancy test
- Blood and urine tests

SOME CAUSES AND FEATURES OF NAUSEA AND VOMITING

Cause	Common Features*	Tests†
Digestive tract disorders		
Appendicitis or another sudden, severe disorder within the abdomen (such as a perforated intestine, gallbladder inflammation, or pancreatitis)	Significant abdominal pain Abdomen that is tender to the touch	Abdominal imaging tests (such as x-rays, ultrasonography, and/or CT)
Intestinal obstruction	No bowel movements and no flatus Cramping abdominal pain that comes and goes Distended abdomen Usually in people who are known to have a hernia or who have had abdominal surgery	Abdominal x-rays taken with the person in flat and upright positions
Gastroenteritis	Vomiting and diarrhea Little or no abdominal pain (except during vomiting) Rarely fever or blood in stool Normal abdominal examination	A doctor's examination
Hepatitis	Mild to moderate nausea for many days and sometimes vomiting A general feeling of illness (malaise) Yellowing of the skin and whites of the eyes (jaundice) Loss of appetite Mild discomfort in the upper right part of the abdomen	Blood tests
Ingestion of a toxin (there are many that cause vomiting—common examples include alcohol, aspirin, iron, lead, or insecticides)	Ingestion usually clear based on the person's history Various other symptoms depending on the substance ingested	Depends on the substance ingested but may include blood tests and liver function tests
Brain and nervous system disorders		
Head injury (such as caused by a recent motor vehicle crash, sports injury, or fall)	Injury clear based on the person's history Often headache, confusion, and difficulty remembering recent events	CT of the head
Brain hemorrhage	Sudden, often severe headache Confusion	CT of the head Spinal tap if CT results are normal
Brain infection (such as meningitis)	Gradual headache and confusion Often fever and pain with tilting head forward May cause a reddish purple rash of tiny dots on the skin (petechiae) if due to meningococcal meningitis‡	Spinal tap (sometimes preceded by CT of the head)
Increased pressure within the skull (such as caused by a blood clot or tumor)	Headache, confusion, and sometimes problems with nerve, spinal cord, or brain function	CT of the head

(continued)

SOME CAUSES AND FEATURES OF NAUSEA AND VOMITING (continued)

Cause	Common Features*	Tests†
Labyrinthitis (inflammation of the inner ear)	A false sensation of movement (vertigo), rhythmic jerking movement of the eyes (nystagmus), and symptoms worsened by motion of the head Sometimes ringing in the ears (tinnitus)	A doctor's examination Sometimes MRI
Migraine	Usually a moderate to severe headache Headache sometimes preceded by seeing flashing lights and blind spots (aura) Sometimes sensitivity to light (photophobia) or temporary disturbances in balance or muscle strength Often a history of repeated similar attacks	A doctor's examination Sometimes CT or MRI of the head and spinal tap (if results of the examination unclear)
Motion sickness	Trigger clear based on the person's history	A doctor's examination
Psychologic disorders	No diarrhea or abdominal pain Vomiting that often occurs with stress Consumption of food considered repulsive	A doctor's examination
Systemic (bodywide) conditions		
Diabetic ketoacidosis	An increased volume of urine excreted each day (polyuria), excessive thirst (polydipsia), and often significant dehydration	Blood tests
Drug side effects or toxicity	Ingestion or a drug or substance clear based on the person's history	Depends on the substance ingested but may include blood tests
Liver failure or kidney failure	Often jaundice in advanced liver disease Ammonia odor to the breath in kidney failure Often in people known to have the disorder	Blood and urine tests to evaluate liver and kidney function
Pregnancy	Nausea and/or vomiting often in the morning or triggered by food Normal examination (except the person may be dehydrated) Often a missed or late menstrual period	Pregnancy test
Radiation exposure	Exposure usually clear based on the person's history Severe nausea, vomiting, and diarrhea	A doctor's examination

*Features include symptoms and the results of the doctor's examination. Features mentioned are typical but not always present.
†Doctors usually do a urine pregnancy test for all girls and women of childbearing age.
‡Sometimes forceful vomiting (caused by any disorder or condition) causes petechiae on the upper torso and face, which may resemble petechiae caused by meningococcal meningitis, a particularly dangerous form of meningitis. People with meningococcal meningitis are usually very ill, whereas people with petechiae caused by vomiting are often otherwise quite well.
CT = computed tomography; MRI = magnetic resonance imaging.

Girls and women of childbearing age typically should have a pregnancy test.

Otherwise healthy adults and older children who have only a few episodes of vomiting (with or without diarrhea) and no other symptoms typically do not require any testing.

People whose vomiting is severe or has lasted more than 1 day or who have signs of dehydration need laboratory tests of blood (particularly electrolyte levels and sometimes liver tests) and urine.

TREATMENT

Specific conditions are treated. If there is no serious underlying disorder and the person is not dehydrated, small amounts of clear liquids may be given 30 minutes or so after the last bout of vomiting. Typically an ounce (30 milliliters) or two are given at first. Plain water is an appropriate liquid, but broth or weak, sweetened tea may be given. Sports drinks have no particular advantage but are not harmful. Carbonated beverages and alcohol should be avoided. If these liquids are tolerated, the amounts are increased gradually. When these increases are tolerated, the person may resume eating normal foods.

Even when people are slightly dehydrated, doctors usually recommend oral rehydration solutions as long as people can tolerate some liquids by mouth. People with significant dehydration or electrolyte abnormalities, people who are actively vomiting, and people who cannot tolerate any liquids by mouth usually require fluids and/or drugs given by vein (intravenously).

For some adults and adolescents, doctors give drugs to relieve nausea (antiemetic drugs) depending on the cause and the severity of the vomiting:

- For vomiting caused by motion sickness: Antihistamines (such as dimenhydrinate), scopolamine patches, or both
- For mild to moderate symptoms: Prochlorperazine or metoclopramide
- For severe vomiting (including vomiting caused by chemotherapy): Dolasetron, ondansetron, or granisetron, or sometimes aprepitant

O—π KEY POINTS

- People whose nausea and vomiting have an obvious cause and who have a normal examination only need treatment of their symptoms.
- Doctors look for signs of severe, sudden changes to the abdomen or disorders within the skull.
- Girls and women of childbearing age are tested for pregnancy.

NAUSEA AND VOMITING DURING EARLY PREGNANCY

Up to 80% of pregnant women have nausea and vomiting to some extent. Nausea and vomiting are most common and most severe during the 1st trimester. Although commonly called morning sickness, such symptoms may occur at any time during the day. Symptoms vary from mild to severe.

Hyperemesis gravidarum is a severe, persistent form of pregnancy-related vomiting. Women with hyperemesis gravidarum vomit so much that they lose weight and become dehydrated. Such women may not consume enough food to provide their body with energy. Then the body breaks down fats, resulting in a buildup of waste products (ketones) called ketosis. Ketosis can cause fatigue, bad breath, dizziness, and other symptoms. Women with hyperemesis gravidarum often become so dehydrated that the balance of electrolytes, needed to keep the body functioning normally, is upset.

If women vomit occasionally but gain weight and are not dehydrated, they do not have hyperemesis gravidarum. Morning sickness and hyperemesis gravidarum tend to resolve during the 2nd trimester.

CAUSES

Usually, nausea and vomiting during pregnancy are related to the pregnancy. However, sometimes they result from a disorder unrelated to the pregnancy.

COMMON CAUSES

The most common causes of nausea and vomiting are

- Morning sickness (most common)
- Hyperemesis gravidarum
- Gastroenteritis (infection of the digestive tract)

Why morning sickness and hyperemesis gravidarum occur during pregnancy is unclear. However, these symptoms may occur because during pregnancy, levels of two hormones increase: human chorionic gonadotropin (hCG), which is produced by the placenta early in pregnancy, and estrogen, which helps maintain the pregnancy. Estrogen levels are particularly high in women with hyperemesis gravidarum. Also, hormones such as progesterone (produced continuously during pregnancy) may slow the movement of the stomach's contents, possibly contributing to nausea and vomiting. Psychologic factors may also be involved.

LESS COMMON CAUSES

Occasionally, prenatal vitamins with iron cause nausea. Rarely, severe, persistent vomiting results from a hydatidiform mole (overgrowth of tissue from the placenta).

Causes unrelated to the pregnancy include

- Disorders of the abdomen such as appendicitis, a blockage in the intestine (bowel obstruction), or inflammation of the gallbladder (cholecystitis)
- Brain disorders such as migraine, bleeding within the brain (intracranial hemorrhage), and increased pressure within the brain (increased intracranial pressure)

However, these disorders usually cause other symptoms that are more prominent, such as abdominal pain or headaches.

EVALUATION

Doctors first try to determine whether nausea and vomiting are caused by a serious disorder. Morning sickness and hyperemesis gravidarum are diagnosed only after other causes are ruled out.

WARNING SIGNS

In pregnant women who are vomiting, the following symptoms are cause for concern:

- Abdominal pain
- Signs of dehydration, such as decreased urination, decreased sweating, increased thirst, a dry mouth, a racing heart, and dizziness when standing up
- Fever

- Vomit that is bloody, black (resembling coffee grounds), or green
- No movement of the fetus if the fetus is older than 24 weeks
- Confusion, weakness or numbness of one side of the body, speech or vision problems, or sluggishness—symptoms that suggest bleeding within the brain

WHEN TO SEE A DOCTOR

Women with warning signs should see a doctor right away, as should those with vomiting that is particularly severe or is worsening. Women without warning signs should talk to their doctor. The doctor can help them decide whether and how quickly they need to be seen based on the nature and severity of their symptoms. Women who have mild to moderate nausea and vomiting, have not lost weight, and are able to keep some liquids down may not need to see a doctor unless their symptoms worsen.

WHAT THE DOCTOR DOES

Doctors ask about symptoms and the medical history. Doctors then do a physical examination. What they find during the history and physical examination often suggests a cause and the tests that may need to be done (see Table on page 294).

Doctors ask about the vomiting:

- When it started
- How long it lasts
- How many times a day it occurs
- Whether anything relieves or makes it worse
- What the vomit looks like
- How much there is

The woman is asked whether she has other symptoms, particularly abdominal pain, diarrhea, and constipation, and how her symptoms have affected her and her family—whether she can work and care for her children. The woman is also asked about vomiting in previous pregnancies, about previous abdominal surgery, and use of drugs that may contribute to vomiting.

During the physical examination, doctors first look for signs of serious disorders, such as blood pressure that is too low or too high, fever, confusion, and sluggishness. A pelvic examination is done to check for evidence of a hydatidiform mole and other abnormalities.

This information helps doctors determine whether vomiting results from the pregnancy or another, unrelated disorder. For example, vomiting probably results from the pregnancy if it

- Began during the 1st trimester
- Lasts or recurs over several days to weeks
- Is not accompanied by abdominal pain

Vomiting probably results from another disorder if it

- Began after the 1st trimester
- Is accompanied by abdominal pain, diarrhea, or both

TESTING

Doctors often use a handheld Doppler ultrasound device, placed on the woman's abdomen, to check for a heartbeat in the fetus. If no heartbeats are detected by the time they should be (at about 11 weeks), a hydatidiform mole is possible. If the woman is vomiting often or appears dehydrated or if a hydatidiform mole is possible, tests are usually done. Which tests are done depend on the cause doctors suspect:

- Hyperemesis gravidarum: Urine tests (to measure ketone levels) and possibly blood tests (to measure electrolyte levels and other substances)
- A hydatidiform mole: Ultrasonography of the pelvis
- A disorder unrelated to the pregnancy: Tests specific for that disorder

TREATMENT

If vomiting is due to a disorder, that disorder is treated. If vomiting is related to pregnancy, some changes in diet or eating habits may help:

- Drinking or eating small amounts more frequently (5 or 6 small meals a day)
- Eating before getting hungry
- Eating only bland foods, such as bananas, rice, applesauce, and dry toast (called the BRAT diet)
- Keeping crackers by the bed and eating one or two before getting up
- Drinking carbonated drinks (sodas)

If vomiting results in dehydration, the woman may be given fluids intravenously. If vomiting persists, she may be hospitalized. She may be

SOME CAUSES AND FEATURES OF NAUSEA AND VOMITING DURING EARLY PREGNANCY

Cause	Common Features*	Tests
Related to the pregnancy (obstetric)		
Morning sickness	Mild nausea and vomiting that comes and goes and that occurs at varying times throughout the day, primarily during the 1st trimester	A doctor's examination
Hyperemesis gravidarum	Frequent, persistent nausea and vomiting Inability to consume enough fluids, food, or both Usually signs of dehydration, such as decreased urination, decreased sweating, a dry mouth, increased thirst, a racing heart, and dizziness when standing up Weight loss	Blood tests to check for signs of dehydration and chemical imbalances by measuring levels of electrolytes, blood urea nitrogen (BUN), and creatinine Urine tests to measure ketones (produced when not enough food is consumed and the body breaks down fats for energy) If vomiting persists, possibly blood tests to evaluate the liver (liver function tests) and ultrasonography of the pelvis
A hydatidiform mole (overgrowth of tissue from the placenta)	A uterus that is larger than expected No heartbeat or movement detected in the fetus during the 2nd trimester Sometimes high blood pressure, swelling of the feet or hands, vaginal bleeding, or passage of tissue that resembles a bunch of grapes	Measurement of blood pressure Blood tests to measure human chorionic gonadotropin (hCG—a hormone produced by the placenta early in pregnancy) Ultrasonography of the pelvis A biopsy if no pregnancy is seen in the uterus
Not related to the pregnancy		
Gastroenteritis	Vomiting that began suddenly, often accompanied by diarrhea Sometimes recent contact with infected people or animals or recent consumption of undercooked, contaminated food or contaminated water	A doctor's examination Sometimes examination and culture of stool
A blockage in the intestine (bowel obstruction)	Symptoms that begin suddenly, usually in women who have had abdominal surgery in the past Crampy pain and a swollen abdomen	X-rays and ultrasonography of the abdomen Possibly CT (if x-ray and ultrasound results are unclear)
A urinary tract infection or kidney infection (pyelonephritis)	An urge to urinate often (frequency), a compelling need to urinate immediately (urgency), or difficulty starting to urinate (hesitancy) With kidney infection, pain in the side and fever	Urine tests (urinalysis) and culture

*Features include symptoms and results of the doctor's examination. Features mentioned are typical but not always present. CT = computed tomography.

given sugar (glucose), electrolytes, and occasionally vitamins intravenously with the fluids. After vomiting has subsided, she is given fluids by mouth. If she can keep these fluids down, she can begin eating frequent, small portions of bland foods. The size of the portions is increased as the woman can tolerate more food.

If needed, drugs to relieve nausea (antiemetic drugs) are given. Doctors choose drugs that appear to be safe during early pregnancy. Vitamin B_6 is used first. If it is ineffective, another drug (doxylamine, metoclopramide, ondansetron, or promethazine) is also given.

Ginger, acupuncture, motion sickness bands, and hypnosis may help, as may switching from prenatal vitamins to children's chewable vitamins with folate.

Rarely, weight loss continues and symptoms persist despite treatment. Then the woman is fed through a tube passed through the nose and down the throat to the small intestine. Tube feeding is continued for as long as necessary.

O—π KEY POINTS

- Usually, nausea and vomiting during pregnancy do not cause weight loss or other problems, and they resolve before or during the 2nd trimester.
- Hyperemesis gravidarum, a severe, persistent form of pregnancy-related vomiting, is less common and can cause dehydration and weight loss.
- Nausea and vomiting may be due to disorders not related to pregnancy, such as gastroenteritis, a urinary tract infection, or, rarely, a blockage in the intestine.
- Modifying the diet may help relieve mild nausea and vomiting that are related to pregnancy.
- If women with hyperemesis gravidarum become dehydrated, they may need to be given fluids intravenously.

NAUSEA AND VOMITING IN INFANTS AND CHILDREN

Vomiting is the uncomfortable, involuntary, forceful throwing up of food. In infants, vomiting must be distinguished from spitting up. Infants often spit up small amounts while being fed or shortly afterward—typically while being burped. Spitting up may occur because infants feed rapidly, swallow air, or are overfed, although it may occur for no apparent reason. Vomiting is typically caused by a disorder. Experienced parents can usually tell the difference between spitting up and vomiting, but first-time parents may need to talk to a doctor or nurse.

Vomiting can cause dehydration because fluid is lost. Sometimes children cannot drink enough to make up for lost fluid—either because they are continuing to vomit or because they do not want to drink. Children who are vomiting usually do not want to eat, but this lack of appetite rarely causes a problem.

CAUSES

Vomiting can be beneficial by getting rid of toxic substances that have been swallowed. However, vomiting is most often caused by a disorder. Usually, the disorder is relatively harmless, but occasionally vomiting is a sign of a serious problem, such as a blockage in the stomach or intestine or increased pressure within the skull (intracranial hypertension).

COMMON CAUSES

Likely causes of vomiting depend on the child's age. In **newborns and infants,** the most common causes include

- Gastroenteritis (infection of the digestive tract) due to a virus
- Gastroesophageal reflux disease

  In **older children,** the most common cause is

- Gastroenteritis due to a virus

LESS COMMON CAUSES

In **newborns and infants,** some causes, although less common, are important because they may be life threatening:

- Narrowing or blockage of the passage out of the stomach (pyloric stenosis) in infants aged 3 to 6 weeks
- A blockage of the intestine caused by birth defects, such as twisting (volvulus) or narrowing (stenosis) of the intestine
- Sliding of one segment of intestine into another (intussusception) in infants aged 3 to 36 months

Food intolerance, allergy to cow's milk protein, and certain uncommon hereditary metabolic disorders may also cause vomiting in newborns and infants.

In **older children and adolescents,** rare causes include serious infections (such as a kidney infection or meningitis), acute appendicitis, or a disorder that increases pressure within the skull (such as a brain tumor or a serious head injury). In adolescents, causes also include gastroesophageal reflux disease or peptic ulcer disease, food allergies, cyclic vomiting, a slowly emptying stomach (gastroparesis), pregnancy, eating disorders, and ingestion of a toxic substance.

EVALUATION

For doctors, the first goal is to determine whether children are dehydrated and whether the vomiting is caused by a life-threatening disorder.

WARNING SIGNS

The following symptoms and characteristics are cause for concern:

- Lethargy and listlessness
- In infants, inconsolability or irritability and bulging of the soft spots (fontanelles) between the skull bones
- In older children, a severe headache, stiff neck that makes lowering the chin to the chest difficult, sensitivity to light, and fever
- Abdominal pain, swelling, or both
- Persistent vomiting in infants who have not been growing or developing as expected
- Bloody stools

Children with warning signs should be immediately evaluated by a doctor, as should all newborns; children whose vomit is bloody, resembles coffee grounds, or is bright green; and children with a recent (within a week) head injury. Not every tummy ache counts as abdominal pain (the warning sign). However, if children appear uncomfortable even when not vomiting and their discomfort lasts more than a few hours, they should probably be evaluated by a doctor.

For other children, signs of dehydration, particularly decreased urination, and the amount they are drinking help determine how quickly they need to be seen. The urgency varies somewhat by age because infants and young children can become dehydrated more quickly than older children. Generally, infants and young children who have not urinated for more than 8 hours or who have been unwilling to drink for more than 8 hours should be seen by a doctor.

The doctor should be called if children have more than 6 to 8 episodes of vomiting, if the vomiting continues more than 24 to 48 hours, or if other symptoms (such as cough, fever, or rash) are present.

Children who have had only a few episodes of vomiting (with or without diarrhea), who are drinking at least some fluids, and who otherwise do not appear very ill rarely require a doctor's visit.

Doctors first ask questions about the child's symptoms and medical history. Doctors then do a physical examination. A description of the child's symptoms and a thorough examination usually enable doctors to identify the cause of vomiting (see Table on pages 298 to 301).

Doctors ask

- When the vomiting started
- How often it occurs
- What the vomit looks like (including its color)
- Whether it is forceful (projectile)
- How much is vomited

Determining whether there is a pattern—occurring at certain times of the day or after eating certain foods—can help doctors identify

possible causes. Information about other symptoms (such as fever and abdominal pain), bowel movements (frequency and consistency), and urination can also help doctors identify a cause.

Doctors also ask about recent travel, injuries, and, for sexually active adolescents, use of birth control.

A physical examination is done to check for clues to possible causes. Doctors note whether children are growing and developing as expected.

Doctors choose tests based on suspected causes suggested by results of the examination. Most children do not require testing. However, if abnormalities in the abdomen are suspected, imaging tests are typically done. If a hereditary metabolic disorder is suspected, blood tests specific for that disorder are done.

If dehydration is suspected, blood tests to measure electrolytes (minerals necessary to maintain fluid balance in the body) are sometimes done.

TREATMENT

If a specific disorder is the cause, it is treated. Vomiting caused by gastroenteritis usually stops on its own.

Making sure children are well-hydrated is important. Fluids are usually given by mouth. Oral rehydration solutions that contain the right balance of electrolytes are used. In the United States, these solutions are widely available without a prescription from most pharmacies and from supermarkets. *Sports drinks, sodas, juices, and similar drinks have too little sodium and too much carbohydrate and should not be used.*

Even children who are vomiting frequently may tolerate small amounts of solution that are given often. Typically, 1 teaspoon (5 milliliters) is given every 5 minutes. If children keep this amount down, the amount is gradually increased. Older children can be given popsicles or gelatin, although red versions of these foods can be confused with blood if children vomit again. With patience and encouragement, most children can take enough fluid by mouth to avoid the need for intravenous (IV) fluids.

SOME CAUSES AND FEATURES OF VOMITING IN INFANTS, CHILDREN, AND ADOLESCENTS

Cause (listed from most to least common)	Common Features*	Tests
In infants		
Gastroenteritis	Usually with diarrhea (which rarely is bloody) Sometimes a fever Sometimes recent contact with infected people (as at a day care center), with animals at a petting zoo (where *Escherichia [E.] coli* may be acquired), or with reptiles (which may be infected with *Salmonella* bacteria) or recent consumption of undercooked, contaminated food or contaminated water	A doctor's examination Sometimes examination and culture of stool
Gastroesophageal reflux disease	Symptoms that occur after feeding, including fussiness, spitting up, arching of the back, crying, or a combination Sometimes a cough when lying down, poor weight gain, or both	A doctor's examination Sometimes treatment with drugs to suppress acid production (if symptoms are relieved, the cause is probably gastroesophageal reflux disease) Sometimes x-rays of the upper digestive tract after barium is given by mouth (upper GI series) Sometimes endoscopy
Pyloric stenosis (narrowing or blockage of the passage out of the stomach)	Forceful (projectile) vomiting that occurs immediately and after all feedings in infants aged 3–6 weeks Signs of dehydration, an emaciated appearance, or both In infants, appearing hungry and feeding eagerly More common among boys, especially first-born boys	Ultrasonography of the stomach If ultrasonography is unavailable or inconclusive, upper GI series
Birth defects that cause narrowing (stenosis) or blockage (atresia) of the digestive tract	Delayed passage of the first BM (called meconium) A swollen abdomen Bright green or yellow vomit, indicating bile, during the first 24–48 hours of life (if the digestive tract is blocked) or somewhat later (if it is only narrowed) More common among infants who have Down syndrome or whose mother had too much amniotic fluid in the uterus during pregnancy	An x-ray of the abdomen Upper GI series or x-rays of the lower digestive tract after insertion of barium into the rectum (barium enema), depending on the suspected location of the problem

(continued)

SOME CAUSES AND FEATURES OF VOMITING IN INFANTS, CHILDREN, AND ADOLESCENTS (continued)

Cause (listed from most to least common)	Common Features*	Tests
Intussusception (sliding of one segment of intestine into another)	Crying that occurs in bouts every 15–20 minutes, with children often drawing their legs up to their chest Later tenderness of the abdomen when it is touched and bowel movements that look like currant jelly (because they contain blood) Typically in children 3–36 months old	Insertion of air into the rectum (air enema) Sometimes ultrasonography of the abdomen
Malrotation (abnormal development of the intestine, resulting in its being abnormally located and increasing the likelihood it will twist on itself)	Bright green or yellow vomit (indicating bile), a swollen abdomen, and blood in stool Often in newborns	An x-ray of the abdomen Upper GI series or barium enema
Sepsis	Fever and lethargy	A complete blood cell count Culture of blood, urine, and cerebrospinal fluid A chest x-ray if children have breathing problems
Allergy to cow's milk protein	Diarrhea or constipation Poor feeding Weight loss, poor growth, or both Blood in stools	Symptoms that lessen when the formula is changed Possibly endoscopy, colonoscopy, or both
Hereditary metabolic disorders	Poor feeding and not growing or developing as expected (failure to thrive) Sluggishness (lethargy) Other features depending on the disorder, such as ■ Jaundice ■ Cataracts ■ Unusual body and urine odors	Screening all newborns using a small sample of blood obtained by pricking the heel Blood tests to measure levels of electrolytes (minerals necessary to maintain fluid balance in the body), ammonia, and glucose Other tests based on the suspected cause
In children and adolescents		
Gastroenteritis	Usually with diarrhea (which rarely is bloody) Sometimes fever Sometimes recent contact with infected people (as at a day care center, at a camp, or on a cruise), with animals at a petting zoo (where Escherichia [E.] coli may be acquired), or with reptiles (which may be infected with Salmonella bacteria) or recent consumption of undercooked, contaminated food or contaminated water	A doctor's examination Sometimes examination or culture of stool

(continued)

SOME CAUSES AND FEATURES OF VOMITING IN INFANTS, CHILDREN, AND ADOLESCENTS *(continued)*

Cause (listed from most to least common)	Common Features*	Tests
Gastroesophageal reflux disease or peptic ulcer disease	Heartburn	A doctor's examination
	Pain in the chest or upper abdomen	Symptoms that lessen or are relieved after treatment with drugs to suppress acid production
	Symptoms that worsen when lying down or after eating	
	Sometimes a nighttime cough	Sometimes upper GI series
		Sometimes endoscopy
Gastroparesis or delayed gastric emptying (the stomach empties slowly)	Feeling of fullness after eating only small amounts	A doctor's examination
	Sometimes a recent viral illness	Upper GI series or x-rays taken after formula or food is given by mouth (gastric emptying scan)
Food allergy	Vomiting that occurs immediately after eating certain food	A doctor's examination
		Sometimes allergy testing
	Often hives, lip or tongue swelling, difficulty breathing, wheezing, abdominal pain, diarrhea, or a combination	Avoidance of a particular food to see whether symptoms stop
Infections in parts of the body other than the digestive tract	Fever	A doctor's examination
	Often symptoms that suggest the location of the infection, such as headache, ear pain, sore throat, swollen lymph nodes in the neck, pain during urination, pain in the side (flank), or a runny nose	Sometimes tests based on the suspected cause
Appendicitis	Initially a general feeling of illness and discomfort in the middle of the abdomen, followed by pain moving to the lower right part of the abdomen	Ultrasonography or CT of the abdomen
	Then vomiting, loss of appetite, and fever	
Increased pressure within the skull (intracranial hypertension), caused by a tumor or an injury	Waking up because of a headache during the night or waking in the morning with a headache	CT of the brain
	Headaches that become progressively worse and are made worse by coughing or BMs	
	Sometimes changes in vision and difficulty walking, talking, or thinking	
Cyclic vomiting	Recurring episodes of vomiting separated by periods of wellness	A doctor's examination
	Often headaches associated with vomiting	Sometimes tests to rule out other causes of recurring episodes of vomiting
	Often a family history of migraines	

(continued)

SOME CAUSES AND FEATURES OF VOMITING IN INFANTS, CHILDREN, AND ADOLESCENTS *(continued)*

Cause (listed from most to least common)	Common Features*	Tests
Eating disorders	Purposefully eating too little to lose weight or eating too much (bingeing) followed by purposefully vomiting or taking laxatives (purging) Erosion of enamel on teeth and scars on the hands from using them to trigger vomiting A distorted body image	A doctor's examination
Pregnancy	No menstrual periods Morning sickness, bloating, and tender breasts Sexual activity (although many adolescents deny it) with no or inadequate use of birth control	A urine pregnancy test
Ingestion of a toxin such as large amounts of acetaminophen, iron, or alcohol	Various features depending on the substance Often a history of taking the substance	Blood tests to measure levels of the substance

*Features include symptoms and results of the doctor's examination. Features mentioned are typical but not always present.
BM = bowel movement; CT = computed tomography; GI = gastrointestinal.

However, children with severe dehydration and those who do not take enough fluid by mouth may need IV fluids.

DRUGS TO REDUCE VOMITING

Drugs frequently used in adults to reduce nausea and vomiting are less often used in children because their usefulness has not been proved. Also, these drugs may have side effects.

DIET

As soon as children have received enough fluid and are not vomiting, they should be given an age-appropriate diet. Infants may be given breast milk or formula.

⊶ KEY POINTS

- Usually, vomiting is caused by gastroenteritis due to a virus and causes no long-lasting or serious problems.
- Sometimes, vomiting is a sign of a serious disorder.
- If diarrhea accompanies vomiting, the cause is probably gastroenteritis.
- Children should be evaluated by a doctor immediately if vomiting persists or they have any warning signs (such as lethargy, irritability, a severe headache, abdominal pain or swelling, vomit that is bloody or bright green or yellow, or bloody stools).

NECK LUMP

People may discover an abnormal lump (mass) in their neck. Sometimes, doctors discover a neck lump during an examination. Neck lumps may be painful or painless depending on what has caused them. Painless neck lumps may be present for a long time before people notice them.

CAUSES

Most neck lumps are enlarged lymph nodes (see also Swollen Lymph Nodes on page 383). Sometimes, the lump is a congenital cyst, an enlarged salivary gland, or an enlarged thyroid gland.

ENLARGED LYMPH NODES

The most common causes of enlarged lymph nodes include the following:

- Reaction to nearby infection (such as a cold or a throat infection)
- Direct bacterial infection of a lymph node
- Certain bodywide (systemic) infections

One or more neck lymph nodes often enlarge in response to an upper respiratory infection, throat infection, or dental infection. These nodes are soft, not tender, and typically return to normal shortly after the infection goes away.

Sometimes, bacteria can directly infect a lymph node (lymphadenitis). Such infected nodes are quite tender to the touch.

Certain systemic infections typically cause multiple lymph nodes to enlarge, including some in the neck. The most common of these infections are mononucleosis, human immunodeficiency virus (HIV), and tuberculosis.

A much less common but more serious cause of enlarged lymph nodes is

- Cancer

Cancerous (malignant) neck lumps are more common among older people, but they may occur in younger people. The cancer most often is one that has spread (metastasized) from a nearby structure, such as the mouth or throat. However, cancerous lymph nodes may also be due to a cancer in a more distant part of the body, or be a cancer of the lymphatic system itself (lymphoma). Cancerous lumps are not painful or tender to the touch and often are stone-hard.

OTHER CAUSES

Cysts are hollow, fluid-filled masses that are usually harmless unless they become infected. Some cysts in the neck are present from birth because of abnormalities that occurred during fetal development. Sometimes cysts develop in the skin (sebaceous cyst), including in the skin of the neck.

A salivary gland under the jaw (submandibular gland) can enlarge if it is blocked by a stone, becomes infected, or develops a cancer.

The thyroid gland, which is in the middle of the neck just above the breastbone, can enlarge. The most common type of enlargement is goiter, which is noncancerous (benign). Cancers and thyroid inflammation (thyroiditis) are less common.

EVALUATION

The following information can help people decide whether a doctor's evaluation is needed and help them know what to expect during the evaluation.

WARNING SIGNS

In people with a neck lump, certain symptoms and characteristics are cause for concern. They include

- A very hard lump
- Sores or growths in the mouth
- Difficulty swallowing and/or hoarseness
- A new lump or lumps in an older person

In general, painless lumps are somewhat more worrisome than painful ones.

WHEN TO SEE A DOCTOR

People who have any type of neck lump for more than a few days should see a doctor, particularly people with warning signs. Typically they can be seen within about a week unless they have other symptoms (such as fever) that warrant an earlier visit.

WHAT THE DOCTOR DOES

Doctors ask questions about the person's symptoms and medical history and do a physical examination. What doctors find during the history and physical examination helps decide what, if any, tests need to be done.

During the medical history, doctors ask about the following:

- Symptoms of colds and throat or dental infections
- Symptoms of cancer in the neck (such as difficulty speaking or swallowing) as well as risk factors for cancer, particularly smoking and alcohol drinking
- Risk factors for HIV and tuberculosis infection

During the physical examination, doctors focus on the ears, nose, and throat (including the tonsils, base of the tongue, and thyroid and salivary glands). They look for signs of infection or abnormal growths, including looking down the throat with a mirror or a thin flexible viewing tube (laryngoscopy). They also feel the neck lump to determine whether it is soft, rubbery or hard and whether or not it is tender.

TESTING

If there is an obvious source of infection, such as a cold or a sore throat, or the person is young and healthy and has a tender lump present for only a few days, no tests are needed immediately. Such people are watched closely to see whether the lump goes away without treatment. If it does not go away, tests are needed.

Most other people should have a blood count and a chest x-ray. For younger people without risk factors for or findings that suggest cancer (such as mouth growths), doctors often take a tissue sample (biopsy). For older people, particularly those with warning signs or risk factors for cancer, doctors often do several tests to look for a source of cancer before doing a biopsy. Such tests often include a needle biopsy of the lump, but some doctors start with computed tomography (CT) or magnetic resonance imaging (MRI) of the head and neck. Children, in whom lumps are caused most often by infection, are usually first given a trial of antibiotics.

To look for cancer originating in other parts of the body, doctors usually take x-rays of the upper digestive tract, do a thyroid scan, and do a CT scan of the chest. Direct examination of the larynx (laryngoscopy), lungs (bronchoscopy), and esophagus (esophagoscopy) may be needed.

TREATMENT

When cancer cells are found in an enlarged lymph node in the neck and there are no signs of cancer anywhere else, the entire lymph node containing the cancer cells is removed along with additional lymph nodes and fatty tissue within the neck. If the tumor is large enough, doctors may also remove the internal jugular vein, along with nearby muscles and nerves. Radiation therapy is often given as well.

O—π KEY POINTS

- Most neck lumps are enlarged lymph nodes.
- Painless lumps are somewhat more worrisome than painful ones.
- Usually testing is not needed unless the doctor suspects cancer.
- Cancerous neck lumps are removed surgically.

NECK PAIN

The neck's flexibility makes it susceptible to wear and tear and to injuries that overstretch it, such as whiplash. Also, the neck has the critical job of holding up the head. Poor posture makes that job more difficult. Thus, neck pain, like back pain (see page 12), is common and becomes more common as people age. For pain located in the front of the neck, see Sore Throat on page 367.

The part of the spine in the neck (cervical spine) consists of seven back bones (vertebrae), which are separated by disks made of jelly-like material and cartilage. The spine contains the spinal cord. Along the length of the spinal cord, spinal nerves emerge through spaces between the vertebrae to connect with nerves throughout the body. The part of the spinal nerve nearest the spinal cord is the spinal nerve root. Muscles and ligaments in the neck support the spine.

Neck pain can involve damage to bones, muscles, disks, or ligaments, but pain can also be caused by damage to nerves or the spinal cord. A spinal nerve root can be compressed when the spine is injured, resulting in pain and sometimes weakness, numbness, and tingling in an arm. Compression of the spinal cord can cause numbness and weakness of both arms and both legs and sometimes loss of bladder and bowel control (incontinence).

CAUSES

Most of the disorders that can cause low back pain can also cause neck pain, and most involve the spine, the tissues that support it, or both.

COMMON CAUSES

The most common cause of neck pain is

- Muscle strains and ligament sprains

In such cases, neck pain usually resolves completely.

Other common causes include

- Muscle spasms
- Arthritis (usually osteoarthritis)
- Cervical spondylosis
- A ruptured or herniated disk
- Fibromyalgia

Spasms of the neck muscles are common and may occur on their own or after an injury, even a minor injury.

In cervical spondylosis, the vertebrae in the neck and the disks between them degenerate, usually because of osteoarthritis. As a result, the nerves that emerge through the vertebrae may be pinched. Sometimes the spinal canal is narrowed (cervical spinal stenosis), and the spinal cord is compressed.

The disks between each of the vertebrae have a tough covering and a soft, jelly-like interior. If a disk is suddenly squeezed by the vertebrae above and below it, the covering may tear (rupture), causing pain. The interior of the disk can bulge out through the tear (herniate). The bulging disk can push on or even damage the spinal nerve root next to it. Rarely, the disk compresses the spinal cord.

Fibromyalgia is a common cause of pain sometimes including neck pain. This disorder causes chronic widespread pain in muscles and other soft tissues in areas besides the neck.

LESS COMMON CAUSES

Less common causes that are serious include

- A tear in the lining of a neck artery (dissection)
- Meningitis
- A spinal tumor or infection
- A heart attack or angina (chest pain due to an inadequate blood supply to the heart muscle)

Spasmodic torticollis is also a less common cause but is not as serious as some causes. It is a severe type of spasm that causes the head to tilt and rotate into an abnormal position. Sometimes the spasms are rhythmic, causing the head to jerk. The cause may be unknown or may be due to certain drugs or hereditary disorders.

EVALUATION

The following information can help people decide whether a doctor's evaluation is needed and help them know what to expect during the evaluation. In the evaluation, doctors first try to identify serious disorders.

WARNING SIGNS

In people with neck pain, certain signs are cause for concern. They include

- Loss of strength or sensation—possibly a symptom of nerve damage
- Fever
- Night sweats
- Headache
- Lethargy or confusion
- Chest discomfort
- Sudden sweating or difficulty breathing
- Pain that is triggered by exertion or worsens during exertion

WHEN TO SEE A DOCTOR

People with warning signs or difficulty or pain when swallowing should see a doctor immediately. If people without warning signs have severe pain (particularly if it is not relieved by acetaminophen or a nonsteroidal anti-inflammatory drug [NSAID]), they should see a doctor within a day or so. Other people can wait a few days or call their doctor to discuss how soon they need to be seen.

WHAT THE DOCTOR DOES

Doctors first ask questions about the person's symptoms and medical history. Doctors then do a physical examination. What they find during the history and examination often suggests a cause and the tests that need to be done (see Table on pages 306 to 307).

The physical examination focuses on the spine and nervous system (neurologic examination) to look for signs of nerve root or spinal cord compression. Signs of nerve root compression include muscle weakness, abnormal reflexes (tested by tapping the tendons around the elbow, below the knee, and behind the ankle), decreased sensation in parts of the body other than the head, inability to urinate, and incontinence of urine or stool. Doctors may ask the person to move the neck in certain ways.

With information about the pain, the person's medical history, and results of a physical examination, doctors may be able to determine the most likely causes:

- Loss of strength or sensation may indicate damage to the spinal cord or nerves or a tear in the lining of a neck artery.

- Pain on the front or one side of the neck usually is not caused by a problem with the spinal cord.
- Pain that radiates down an arm is usually caused by cervical spondylosis with compression of the spinal nerve root.
- Pain that is constant, severe, progressively worse, and unrelieved by rest, particularly if it keeps the person awake at night and is accompanied by sweating, may indicate cancer or an infection.

TESTING

Often, testing is not necessary because most neck pain is caused by sprains and strains, which doctors can typically diagnose based on the examination. Testing is usually done if doctors suspect certain other disorders (see Table). If people have symptoms of nervous system malfunction (neurologic symptoms), such as weakness or numbness, magnetic resonance imaging (MRI) or computed tomography (CT) is usually done. MRI provides clearer images of soft tissues (including disks and nerves) than CT. MRI and CT provide better images of bones than plain x-rays. However, plain x-rays can often identify common abnormalities in bone (such as arthritis), so if doctors suspect such an abnormality, x-rays may be done first.

Occasionally, electromyography and nerve conduction studies are done to evaluate possible nerve root compression.

TREATMENT

Specific disorders are treated. For example, if the spinal cord or a spinal nerve is compressed, surgery is usually needed.

Most often, a sprain, strain, or other musculoskeletal injury is the cause and an over-the-counter analgesic, such as acetaminophen or an NSAID, to relieve the pain is all that is needed. Symptoms usually resolve completely. If inflammation is not contributing to the pain (as with sprains, strains, and other injuries), acetaminophen is usually recommended because it is thought to be safer than NSAIDs. Ice or heat may also help. People are taught how to stand, sit, and sleep in ways that do not strain the neck.

Avoiding aggravating activities, such as sitting for extended periods of time (particularly when also using a computer, phone, or other

SOME CAUSES AND FEATURES OF NECK PAIN

Cause	Common Features*	Tests
More common but less serious causes		
Sprains and strains	Pain that ■ Usually occurs off to one side of the spine ■ Worsens with movement and lessens with rest	A doctor's examination
Muscle spasms	Constant pain and stiffness, causing difficulty or pain when the head is turned one way or the other (sometimes both ways) No symptoms of nervous system malfunction (neurologic symptoms)	A doctor's examination
Osteoarthritis (without compression of the spinal nerve root)	Pain that ■ Is sometimes constant ■ Worsens with motion Often arthritis in the joints of fingers, hips, and/or knees	A doctor's examination Sometimes neck x-rays
Cervical spondylosis (with compression of the spinal nerve root)	Pain that ■ Often extends down the arm, sometimes to the hand ■ Usually occurs in the neck itself Sometimes weakness and/or numbness in the arms	MRI of the neck
A herniated disk (typically with compression of the spinal nerve root)	Same as for Cervical spondylosis, above	MRI of the neck
Fibromyalgia	Aching and stiffness in many areas of the body (not just the neck) Sore areas that are tender to the touch Often poor sleep Most common among women aged 20 to 50	A doctor's examination
Less common but more serious causes		
A tear in the lining of a neck artery	Usually constant head, neck, or facial pain Usually neurologic symptoms such as loss of balance or taste, confusion, weakness of an arm and leg on the same side of the body, and difficulty swallowing, speaking, and/or seeing	MRA
A bone tumor in the spine	Progressively worsening, constant pain (even at night), regardless of position or movement Sometimes night sweats or weight loss	MRI Sometimes biopsy
Infection of bone or nearby tissues	Progressively worsening, constant pain (even at night) regardless of position or movement Sometimes night sweats, fever, and/or weight loss	MRI Usually culture of a sample of infected tissue

(continued)

SOME CAUSES AND FEATURES OF NECK PAIN *(continued)*

Cause	Common Features*	Tests
Meningitis	Severe headache	A spinal tap (lumbar puncture) and analysis of spinal fluid
	Neck pain that worsens when the head is bent forward, but not when rotated side-to-side	
	Usually fever, lethargy, and/or confusion	
A heart attack or angina	Sudden and sometimes recurring sweating, difficulty breathing, and/or chest discomfort	Electrocardiography, blood tests to measure substances called cardiac markers to check for heart damage, and/or imaging tests such as cardiac catheterization or stress testing
	Usually risk factors for heart disease	

*Features include symptoms and results of the doctor's examination. Features mentioned are typical but not always present.
MRA = magnetic resonance angiography; MRI = magnetic resonance imaging.

electronic device), may help. People should use good posture and body mechanics when standing, sitting, lying down, or doing any activity. People who sleep on their side should use a pillow to support the head and neck in a neutral position (not tilted down toward the bed or up toward the ceiling). People who sleep on their back should use a pillow to support, but not raise, the head and neck. People should avoid sleeping on their stomach. Doctors or physical therapists may suggest stretching and strengthening exercises, including strengthening exercises for the upper back.

If more pain relief is needed, doctors may prescribe opioid analgesics. Muscle relaxants, such as carisoprodol, cyclobenzaprine, diazepam, metaxalone, or methocarbamol, are sometimes used, but their usefulness is controversial. Muscle relaxants are not recommended for older people, who are more likely to have side effects.

For spasmodic torticollis, physical therapy or massage can sometimes temporarily stop the spasms. Drugs (including the anticonvulsant carbamazepine and some mild sedatives such as clonazepam, taken by mouth or injected) can usually relieve the pain. But drugs control spasms in only up to one third of people. If the pain is severe or if posture is distorted, botulinum toxin (a bacterial toxin used to paralyze muscles) may be injected into the affected muscles.

> ### O—ᴛᴛ KEY POINTS
>
> - Most neck pain is caused by sprains and strains and resolves completely.
> - Most of the disorders that can cause low back pain can cause neck pain.
> - People with warning signs, such as nerve damage, should see a doctor immediately.
> - Most neck pain can be relieved by over-the-counter analgesics and modification of activities.

NIPPLE DISCHARGE

Fluid that leaks from one or both nipples is called a nipple discharge. Each breast has several (15 to 20) milk ducts. A discharge can come from one or more of these ducts.

Nipple discharge can occur normally during the last weeks of pregnancy and after childbirth when breast milk is produced. Nipple discharge is also common among women who are not pregnant or breastfeeding, especially during the reproductive years. For example, in women, fondling, suckling, irritation from clothing, or sexual arousal can stimulate a nipple discharge, as can stress.

A normal nipple discharge is a usually thin, cloudy, whitish, or almost clear fluid that is not sticky. However, the discharge may be other colors, such as gray, green, yellow, or brown. During pregnancy or breastfeeding, a normal discharge is sometimes slightly bloody. Abnormal discharges vary in appearance depending on the cause. An abnormal discharge may be accompanied by other abnormalities, such as dimpled skin, swelling, redness, crusting, sores, and a retracted nipple. (A nipple is retracted if it pulls inward and does not return to its normal position when it is stimulated.)

CAUSES

Several disorders can cause an abnormal discharge. A discharge from one milk duct or from one breast is likely to be caused by a problem with that breast, such as a noncancerous (benign) or cancerous breast tumor. A discharge from both breasts or from several milk ducts in one breast is more likely to be caused by a problem outside the breast, such as a hormonal disorder or use of certain drugs.

COMMON CAUSES

Usually, the cause is a benign disorder of the milk ducts:

- A benign tumor in a milk duct (intraductal papilloma)
- Dilated milk ducts (mammary duct ectasia)
- Fibrocystic changes, including pain, cysts, and general lumpiness
- An abscess or infection

Intraductal papilloma is the most common cause. It is also the most common cause of a bloody nipple discharge when there is no lump in the breast.

LESS COMMON CAUSES

Certain disorders stimulate the production of breast milk in women who are not pregnant or breastfeeding. In most of these disorders, the level of prolactin (a hormone that stimulates production of breast milk) is elevated. Taking certain drugs can have the same effect.

Cancer causes fewer than 10% of cases.

EVALUATION

The following information can help people decide whether a doctor's evaluation is needed and help them know what to expect during the evaluation.

WARNING SIGNS

Nipple discharge is a cause for concern when it

- Occurs without the nipple being squeezed or stimulated by other means
- Occurs in women aged 40 or older
- Comes from only one breast
- Is bloody or pink
- Is accompanied by a lump that can be felt
- Occurs in a boy or man

WHEN TO SEE A DOCTOR

If a nipple discharge continues for more than one menstrual cycle or if any of the warning signs are present, women should see a doctor. Delay of a week or so is not harmful unless there are signs of infection such as redness, swelling, and/or a discharge of pus. Women with such symptoms should see a doctor within 1 or 2 days.

WHAT THE DOCTOR DOES

Doctors first ask questions about the woman's symptoms and medical history. Doctors then do a physical examination. What they find during the history and physical examination often suggests a cause of the discharge and the tests that may need to be done (see Table on pages 309 to 310).

SOME CAUSES AND FEATURES OF NIPPLE DISCHARGE

Cause	Common Features*	Tests
Benign breast disorders		
Intraductal papilloma (a benign tumor in a milk duct)—the most common cause	A bloody or pink discharge from one breast	Usually ultrasonography Additional tests depending on the results (as for breast lumps—see page 26)
Mammary duct ectasia (dilated milk ducts)	A bloody, pink, or multicolored (puslike, gray, or milky) discharge from one or both breasts	Same as for intraductal papilloma
Fibrocystic changes (including pain, cysts, and general lumpiness)	A lump, often rubbery and tender, usually developing before menopause Possibly a history of having breast lumps	Same as for intraductal papilloma
An abscess or infection	Pain, tenderness, redness, warmth, or a combination that begins suddenly in a breast Often fever With an abscess, a tender lump and possibly a puslike discharge that smells foul	Physical examination (infection is usually obvious) If the discharge does not resolve with treatment, evaluation as for intraductal papilloma
Breast cancer		
Usually intraductal carcinoma or invasive ductal carcinoma	Possibly a palpable lump, changes in the skin, or enlarged lymph nodes, most often in the armpit Sometimes a bloody or pink discharge	Same as for intraductal papilloma
Increased levels of prolactin†		
Various disorders, including the following: ■ Hypothyroidism (an underactive thyroid gland) ■ Disorders of the pituitary gland or hypothalamus (part of the brain) ■ Chronic kidney or liver disorders	A milky (not bloody) discharge, usually from both breasts No lumps Possibly menstrual irregularities or no menstrual periods (amenorrhea) *In hypothyroidism*: Intolerance of cold, sluggishness, constipation, or weight gain *In pituitary or hypothalamus disorders*: Possibly hormonal abnormalities, changes in vision, or headaches *In kidney or liver disorders*: With liver disorders, ascites or jaundice In people known to have a kidney or liver disorder	Blood tests to measure prolactin and thyroid-stimulating hormone levels A review of drugs being taken If the prolactin or thyroid-stimulating level is elevated, MRI of the head

(continued)

SOME CAUSES AND FEATURES OF NIPPLE DISCHARGE *(continued)*

Cause	Common Features*	Tests
Certain drugs including ▪ Opioids ▪ Oral contraceptives	Use of causative drug	Blood tests to measure prolactin and thyroid-stimulating hormone levels
▪ Some drugs used to treat stomach disorders (such as cimetidine, ranitidine, and metoclopramide) ▪ Some antidepressants and drugs used to treat nausea or psychosis ▪ Some antihypertensives (such as methyldopa, reserpine, and verapamil)		A review of drugs being taken If the prolactin or thyroid-stimulating level is elevated, MRI of the head

*Features include symptoms and the results of the doctor's examination. Features mentioned are typical but not always present.
†A hormone that stimulates production of breast milk.
MRI = magnetic resonance imaging.

To help identify the cause, doctors ask about the discharge and about other symptoms that may suggest possible causes. Women are also asked whether they have had disorders or take drugs that can increase prolactin levels.

Doctors examine the breast, looking for abnormalities, including lumps (see page 25). If the discharge does not occur spontaneously, the area around the nipples is gently pressed to try to stimulate a discharge.

TESTING

If doctors suspect that a hormonal disorder is the cause, blood tests are done to measure the levels of prolactin and thyroid-stimulating hormone.

If a pituitary or brain disorder is suspected, magnetic resonance imaging (MRI) or computed tomography (CT) of the head is done.

If the discharge is not obviously bloody, it is analyzed to determine whether it contains small amounts of blood. If blood is present, a sample of the discharge is examined under a microscope (called cytology) to look for cancer cells.

If a lump can be felt, ultrasonography is done. Testing is similar to that for any breast lump (see page 26). Cysts are drained (by aspiration), and the fluid is tested. If cysts remain after aspiration or if lumps are solid, mammography is done, followed by a biopsy.

When there is no lump but cancer is still suspected or when other test results are unclear, mammography is done.

If no lump can be felt and the mammogram is normal, cancer is highly unlikely. Sometimes a specific cause cannot be identified.

TREATMENT

If a disorder is identified, it is treated. If a noncancerous tumor or disorder is causing a discharge from one breast, the duct that the discharge is coming from may be removed. This procedure requires only a local anesthetic and does not require an overnight stay in the hospital.

KEY POINTS

▪ Usually, the cause of nipple discharge is not cancer.
▪ If the discharge comes from both breasts or from several milk ducts and is not bloody or pink, the cause is usually a noncancerous hormonal disorder.
▪ If the discharge comes from only one breast or one milk duct and is bloody or pink, cancer is possible, especially in women aged 40 or older.

NOSEBLEEDS

Some people get nosebleeds (epistaxis) rather often, and others rarely get them. There may be just a trickle of blood or a strong stream. If people swallow the blood, they often vomit it because blood is irritating to the stomach.

Nosebleeds usually come from the front part of the nose (anterior nosebleed) from small blood vessels on the cartilage that separates the two nostrils. This cartilage is the nasal septum, which contains many blood vessels. Most anterior nosebleeds are more frightening than serious. However, bleeding from blood vessels in the back part of the nose (posterior nosebleed), although uncommon, is more dangerous and difficult to treat. Posterior nosebleeds usually involve larger blood vessels than anterior nosebleeds. Because these vessels are in the back of the nose, they are hard for doctors to reach for treatment. Posterior nosebleeds tend to occur in people who have atherosclerosis (which reduces or blocks blood flow in arteries), who have bleeding disorders, who are taking drugs that interfere with blood clotting, or who have had nasal or sinus surgery.

CAUSES

Nosebleeds occur when the moist inner lining of the nose is irritated or when blood vessels in the nose are broken. There are many causes (see Table on page 312). In all cases, people who take aspirin or other drugs that interfere with blood clotting (anticoagulants), people with clotting disorders, and people with hardening of the arteries (arteriosclerosis) are more likely to develop nosebleeds.

COMMON CAUSES

The most common causes of nosebleeds are

- Trauma (such as nose blowing and picking)
- Drying of the moist inner lining of the nose (such as occurs in winter)

LESS COMMON CAUSES

Less common causes of nosebleeds include

- Nasal infections
- Bodywide (systemic) disorders

- Foreign objects (bodies)
- Rendu-Osler-Weber syndrome
- Tumors of the nose or sinuses
- Bleeding disorders (coagulopathies)

High blood pressure (hypertension) may help keep a nosebleed going that has already begun but is unlikely to be the actual cause.

EVALUATION

The following information can help people decide whether a doctor's evaluation is needed and help them know what to expect during the evaluation.

WARNING SIGNS

In people with a nosebleed, certain symptoms and characteristics are cause for concern. They include

- Signs of excessive blood loss (such as weakness, fainting, or dizziness when standing up)
- Use of drugs that interfere with blood clotting
- Signs of a bleeding disorder or a known bleeding disorder (such as hemophilia)
- Several recent episodes of nosebleeds, particularly with no clear cause

The most common drugs that interfere with blood clotting include aspirin, clopidogrel, and warfarin.

Signs of a bleeding disorder include numerous small, purplish spots on the skin (petechiae), many large bruises, easily bleeding gums, bloody or tarry stools, coughing up blood, blood in the urine, and excess bleeding while brushing the teeth, having blood tests, or suffering minor cuts.

WHEN TO SEE A DOCTOR

People who cannot get the nosebleed to stop by pinching the nose should go to the hospital right away. Even if the bleeding has stopped, people who have warning signs also should go to the hospital right away. People without warning signs who had a nosebleed that stopped (with or without treatment) and otherwise feel well should call their doctor. They may not need to be seen.

WHAT THE DOCTOR DOES

Doctors first ask questions about the person's symptoms and medical history and then do a physical examination. What doctors find during the history and physical examination often suggests a cause of the nosebleed and the tests that may need to be done (see Table, below).

During the medical history, doctors ask about the following:

- Obvious triggers (such as sneezing, nose blowing or picking, and recent upper respiratory infections)

SOME CAUSES AND FEATURES OF NOSEBLEEDS

Cause*	Common Features†	Tests
Common		
Blowing or picking the nose	In people who report such behavior or injuries	A doctor's examination
A blow or other injury to the nose		
Drying of the moist membranes lining the nose, as may occur in cold weather	Usually dryness that is seen during the examination	A doctor's examination
Less common		
Nasal infections (such as a cold or sinusitis)	Crusting in the nostrils	A doctor's examination
	Often pain and drying of the moist membranes lining the nose	
Systemic disorders, such as severe liver disease or AIDS	In people who are known to have such disorders	A doctor's examination
A foreign object (body) in the nose, mainly in children	Often recurring nosebleeds and/or a foul-smelling discharge from one side of the nose	A doctor's examination
Arteriosclerosis	Usually in older people	A doctor's examination
Rendu-Osler-Weber syndrome	Dilated small blood vessels (telangiectasias) on the face, lips, membranes lining the mouth and nose, and tips of the fingers and toes	A doctor's examination
	Usually in people with family members who have the disorder	
Tumors (noncancerous or cancerous) of the nose or sinuses	Sometimes a mass that can be seen inside the nose	CT
	Bulging of the side of the nose	
A hole (perforation) in the nasal septum (which divides the interior of the nose in two)	A hole that can be seen during the examination	A doctor's examination
	Sometimes in people who snort cocaine frequently	
Bleeding disorders (coagulopathies)	In people who have had nosebleeds or other bleeding in other areas, such as the gums	Blood tests, such as a complete blood cell count and tests to measure how quickly blood clots

*Conditions that can cause nosebleeds are more likely to cause nosebleeds in people who also have a bleeding disorder or who take drugs that interfere with blood clotting. In such people, bleeding is often more severe and difficult to treat.
†Features include symptoms and results of the doctor's examination. Features mentioned are typical but not always present.
CT = computed tomography.

- The time and number of previous nose-bleeding episodes and how they were stopped
- Whether the person (or a family member) has a bleeding disorder or other disorders that sometimes cause problems with blood clotting
- Whether the person takes any drugs that interfere with blood clotting

Disorders that can cause problems with clotting include severe liver disease (such as cirrhosis or hepatitis) and certain cancers.

During the physical examination, doctors focus on the nose, looking for the bleeding site. They also check the person's skin for signs of bleeding disorders, including petechiae, large bruises, and dilated small blood vessels in and around the mouth and on the tips of the fingers and toes.

An anterior bleeding site is usually easy for the doctor to see with a handheld light. To see a posterior bleeding site, doctors need to use a flexible viewing scope. However, an actively bleeding posterior site produces too much blood for the doctor to see anything, even with a viewing scope.

TESTING

Routine laboratory testing is not required. People with symptoms of a bleeding disorder and/or signs of significant blood loss and people with severe or recurring nosebleeds should have blood tests. Computed tomography (CT) may be done if a foreign object, a tumor, or sinusitis is suspected.

TREATMENT

Doctors initially treat all nosebleeds as they would treat an anterior nosebleed. The few people who have lost a large amount of blood are given fluids by vein (intravenously) and rarely blood transfusions. Any known or identified bleeding disorders are treated.

ANTERIOR NOSEBLEED

Bleeding usually can be controlled at home by pinching the nostrils together for 10 minutes while the person sits upright. People should not pinch over the bony upper part of the nose. It is important to hold the nose with a firm pinch and not let go even once during the 10 minutes. Other at-home techniques, such as ice packs to the nose, wads of tissue paper in the nostrils, and placing the head in various positions, are not effective.

If the pinch technique does not stop the bleeding, it can be repeated once for another 10 minutes. If the bleeding does not stop after the 10 minutes, the person should see a doctor. The doctor typically places several pieces of cotton in the bleeding nostril. The cotton is saturated with a numbing drug (such as lidocaine) along with a drug that causes blood vessels in the nose to close (such as phenylephrine). Then the nose is pinched for 10 minutes or so and the cotton is removed. For minor bleeds, often nothing more is done. Alternatively, doctors sometimes place a special foam sponge (nasal tampon) in the bleeding side. The sponge swells to stop the bleeding. The sponge is removed after 2 to 4 days.

For more severe or recurring bleeding, sometimes the doctor seals (cauterizes) the bleeding source with a chemical, silver nitrate, or an electrical current (electrocautery). If these methods are ineffective, various commercial nasal balloons can be used to compress bleeding sites. Rarely, the doctor may need to pack the entire nasal cavity on one side with a long strip of gauze. Nasal packing is usually removed after 3 days.

POSTERIOR NOSEBLEED

Bleeding in this area is very difficult to stop and can be life threatening. For a posterior nosebleed, the pinch technique does not stop the bleeding. Pinching simply makes the blood run down the throat instead of out the nose. For a posterior nosebleed, doctors may place a specially shaped balloon in the nose and inflate it to compress the bleeding site. However, this and other types of posterior nasal packing are very uncomfortable and interfere with the person's breathing. Doctors usually give people sedatives by vein before inserting this kind of balloon and packing. Also, people who have had this type of packing are admitted to the hospital and given oxygen and antibiotics to prevent an infection of the sinuses or the middle ear. The packing remains in place for 4 to 5 days.

If the balloon does not work, doctors need to directly close the bleeding vessel. Doctors typically do a surgical procedure in which a fiberoptic endoscope is placed through the wall of the sinus. The endoscope allows the doctor to reach and close off (typically with a clip) the larger artery that feeds the bleeding vessel. Occasionally, doctors use x-ray techniques to pass a small catheter through the person's blood vessels to the bleeding site and inject material to block the bleeding vessel (embolization).

O—ㅠ KEY POINTS

- Most nosebleeds occur from the front part of the nose and are easily stopped by pinching the nostrils together.
- If pinching the nostrils does not stop the bleeding, people should seek medical attention.
- During the history and physical examination, doctors ask people about bleeding disorders and their use of drugs that affect blood clotting, such as warfarin, clopidogrel, and aspirin and other nonsteroidal anti-inflammatory drugs (NSAIDs).
- People should try the 10-minute pinch technique to stop a nosebleed.

NUMBNESS

Numbness refers to the partial or complete loss of sensation. People with numbness may be unable to feel light touch, pain, temperature, or vibration or to know where parts of their body are (position sense). When people do not know where parts of their body are, they have problems with balance, coordination, and walking.

Many people mistakenly use the term numbness when they have abnormal sensations such as tingling, prickling, or a pins-and-needles sensation or when a limb feels weak or is paralyzed—perhaps partly because people with numbness often also have such abnormal sensations and symptoms. The presence of other symptoms depends on what is causing numbness.

If numbness has been present a long time, particularly in the feet, it can lead to other problems. People may have difficulty walking and driving and may be more likely to fall. They may not notice infections, foot sores (ulcers), and injuries because they cannot sense pain as well. In such cases, treatment may be delayed.

PATHWAY FOR SENSATION

For a person to feel sensations normally, sensory receptors (specialized ends of sensory nerve fibers in the skin) must detect information in and around the body. These receptors must then send a signal along the following pathway:

- Through sensory nerves (nerves from the skin to the spinal cord)
- Through spinal nerve roots, formed by sensory nerves joined together into thick short branches that pass through the backbones (vertebrae) to connect with the spinal cord
- Up the spinal cord
- Through the brain stem
- To the part of the brain that perceives and interprets these signals (in the cerebrum)

For some parts of the body, the pathway includes a plexus or the cauda equina.

Plexuses are networks of sensory nerve fibers and motor nerve fibers (which carry signals from the brain and spinal cord to muscles and other body parts). In plexuses, these nerve fibers are combined and sorted to serve a particular area of the body. The fibers then branch off from the plexus to become peripheral nerves. There are four plexuses in the torso.

The cauda equina is a bundle of spinal nerve root fibers at the bottom of the spinal cord. This structure resembles a horse's tail, which is what its name means in Latin. It supplies sensation to the thighs, buttocks, genitals, and the area between them, which are called the saddle area because they are the area of the body that would touch a saddle.

CAUSES

Numbness results when one part of the pathway for sensation malfunctions, usually because of a disorder or drug. Many conditions can cause numbness in various ways. For example, they may

- Reduce or block the blood supply to nerves in the body, as occurs in vasculitis, or in the brain, as results from stroke
- Damage part of the pathway for sensation, as may result from injuries or from hereditary disorders that affect nerves (neuropathies), such as Friedreich ataxia
- Put pressure on (compress) part of the pathway
- Infect a nerve, as occurs in leprosy, HIV infection, or Lyme disease
- Cause nerves in part of the pathway to become inflamed and lose their outer layer (called demyelination), as occurs in multiple sclerosis or Guillain-Barré syndrome
- Cause metabolic abnormalities, as may occur in diabetes, vitamin B_{12} deficiency, or arsenic poisoning or with use of chemotherapy drugs

Pressure on different parts of the pathway has various causes (see Table on pages 317 to 318), as in the following:

- On nerves: Repeating specific movements over and over, causing swelling, as occurs in carpal tunnel syndrome, or remaining in one position too long, as when people sit with their legs crossed a long time
- On spinal nerve roots: Rupture or herniation of a disk in the spine, osteoarthritis, or

narrowing of the passageway for the spinal canal (spinal stenosis)

- On the spinal cord: A tumor, an injury, or a pocket of blood (hematoma) or pus (abscess) near the spinal cord

- Both sides of the body below a specific level of the body: Spinal cord malfunction
- Both sides, mainly in the hands and feet: Simultaneous malfunction of many peripheral nerves throughout the body (a polyneuropathy)

EVALUATION

Because so many disorders can cause numbness, doctors ask questions systematically, focusing on more likely causes.

WARNING SIGNS

In people with numbness, the following symptoms are cause for concern:

- Numbness that begins suddenly (within minutes or hours)
- Weakness that begins suddenly or rapidly (within hours or days)
- Numbness or weakness that rapidly spreads up or down the body, involving more and more parts of the body
- Difficulty breathing
- Numbness in the thighs, buttocks, genitals, and the area between them (saddle area) and loss of bladder and bowel control (incontinence)
- Numbness on both sides below a specific level of the body (such as below the midchest)
- Numbness of an entire leg or arm
- Loss of sensation in the face and torso

WHEN TO SEE A DOCTOR

People who have warning signs should go to a hospital immediately. People without warning signs should call their doctor. The doctor can decide how rapidly they need to be seen based on their symptoms.

WHAT THE DOCTOR DOES

Doctors begin by asking which body parts are affected. The pattern of body parts affected by numbness often indicates which part of the nerve pathway is malfunctioning:

- Part of a limb: Peripheral nerve or sometimes spinal nerve root malfunction
- Arm and leg on the same side of the body: Brain malfunction

Then doctors ask about the person's other symptoms and medical history. Doctors also do a physical examination. What they find during the history and physical examination often suggests a cause and the tests that may need to be done (see Table on pages 317 to 318).

Doctors first ask the person to describe the numbness. Then doctors may ask specific questions:

- When numbness began
- How quickly it began
- Whether the person also has other symptoms such as abnormal sensations, weakness or paralysis, loss of bowel or bladder control, retention of urine, vision problems, difficulty swallowing, or deterioration of mental function
- Whether any event, such as pressure on a limb, an injury, sleeping in an awkward position, or an infection, triggered the symptoms

Knowing how quickly numbness and other symptoms began helps doctors determine the type of disorder.

The person is asked about symptoms that may suggest a cause. For example, back and/or neck pain suggests osteoarthritis, a ruptured disk, or another disorder that puts pressure on the spinal cord. Doctors also ask whether the person has had a disorder that can cause numbness, particularly diabetes, chronic kidney disease, infections (such as HIV infection or Lyme disease), a stroke, or arthritis. Doctors may ask whether any family members have had similar symptoms or have a hereditary disorder that affects the nervous system. They ask the person about use of drugs, including recreational drugs, and about possible exposure to toxins.

The physical examination includes a complete evaluation of the nervous system (neurologic examination), focusing on testing sensation (whether the person can feel stimuli, such as touch and temperature, normally), as well as reflexes and muscle function.

SOME CAUSES AND FEATURES OF NUMBNESS

Cause	Common Features*	Tests
Numbness in both limbs (arm and leg) on one side of the body		
Disorders that affect the part of the brain above the brain stem such as	Loss of sensation on the same side of the face and body and loss of the ability to recognize items by touch	MRI or CT of the brain
■ Stroke ■ Tumor ■ Multiple sclerosis ■ Degenerative brain disorders	Usually weakness, loss of coordination, and other symptoms indicating malfunction of the nervous system	
Disorders that affect the upper part of the brain stem, such as	Loss of sensation on the same side of the face and body	MRI or CT of the brain
■ Stroke ■ Tumors	Often double vision	
Disorders that affect the lower part of the brain stem, such as	Loss of sensation on one side of the face and on the opposite side of the body	MRI of the brain
■ Stroke ■ Tumors ■ Degenerative brain disorders	Often vision problems and difficulty chewing, swallowing, and speaking	
Numbness in the limbs or torso on both sides		
Disorders that affect the width of the spinal cord, such as ■ Compression of the spinal cord by injuries, tumors, a ruptured or herniated disk, hematomas (pockets of blood), or abscesses (pockets of pus) ■ Acute transverse myelitis (sudden inflammation of the spinal cord)	Loss of sensation and usually weakness below a certain level of the body No loss of sensation in the face Usually retention of urine, loss of bowel and bladder control (incontinence), and/or reduced sexual response, including erectile dysfunction in men	MRI of the spinal cord
Cauda equina syndrome, caused by pressure, as may result from ■ A ruptured or herniated disk ■ Spread of cancer to the spine	Numbness mainly in the thighs, buttocks, bladder, genitals, and the area between them (saddle area) Usually pain in the lower back Often retention of urine, loss of bowel and bladder control, and/or reduced sexual response, including erectile dysfunction in men	MRI of the spinal cord
Polyneuropathies (simultaneous malfunction of many peripheral nerves throughout the body), as may result from ■ Use of certain drugs ■ Diabetes ■ Chronic kidney disease ■ Metabolic disorders, such as diabetes, uremia (build up of toxic substances in blood due to kidney failure), and vitamin B_{12} deficiency ■ Infections, such as HIV infection or Lyme disease	Numbness and abnormal sensations in about the same areas on both sides of the body, mainly in the feet and hands Sometimes weakness and loss of reflexes	Nerve conduction studies (measuring how fast nerves transmit signals) and electromyography (stimulating muscles and recording their electrical activity) Other tests depending on the disorder suspected

(continued)

SOME CAUSES AND FEATURES OF NUMBNESS *(continued)*

Cause	Common Features*	Tests
Disorders that cause nerves to become inflamed and lose their outer layer (myelin sheath), such as ■ Multiple sclerosis	Often weakness or clumsiness Sometimes changes in vision or speech	MRI of the brain and spinal cord Spinal tap (lumbar puncture) to examine a sample of cerebrospinal fluid
Numbness in part of one limb		
Disorders that affect a spinal nerve root such as ■ A ruptured or herniated disk ■ Collapse of the backbones (vertebrae) due to arthritis or osteoporosis	Pain that ■ Sometimes shoots down an arm or a leg ■ May feel like an electric shock ■ May be worsened by moving the spine, coughing, or doing a Valsalva maneuver (forcefully trying to exhale without letting air escape through the nose or mouth) Often weakness and/or reduced or absent reflexes in the area supplied by the nerve root	A doctor's examination Sometimes MRI or CT of the spinal cord Sometimes nerve conduction studies and electromyography
Disorders that affect a plexus (a network of nerve fibers), such as ■ Thoracic outlet compression syndrome ■ An injury such as a stabbing ■ Cancer that spreads to organs near a plexus ■ Brachial neuritis (sudden malfunction of the plexus in the neck and shoulder)	Numbness, pain, and/or weakness in a relatively large area of a limb	Nerve conduction studies and electromyography MRI unless the cause is an injury or brachial neuritis is suspected
Mononeuropathy (malfunction of one peripheral nerve), as occurs in ■ Carpal tunnel syndrome ■ Peroneal nerve palsy (affecting a nerve near the knee)	Numbness with or without pain Often weakness and reduced or absent reflexes in an area supplied by one nerve	A doctor's examination Sometimes nerve conduction studies and electromyography

*Features include symptoms and results of the doctor's examination. Features mentioned are typical but not always present.
CT = computed tomography; MRI = magnetic resonance imaging.

TESTING

Tests are done based on where doctors think the problem is:

■ For sensory nerves, plexuses, or spinal nerve roots: Nerve conduction studies and electromyography

■ For plexuses: Sometimes magnetic resonance imaging (MRI) after a contrast agent is injected into a vein

■ For the brain or spinal cord: MRI

Nerve conduction studies and electromyography are often done at the same time. Nerve conduction studies use electrodes or small needles to stimulate a nerve. Then doctors measure how fast the nerve transmits signals. For electromyography, small needles are inserted into a muscle to record its electrical activity when the muscle is at rest and when it is contracting.

Other tests are then done to identify the specific disorder. For example, if results suggest a polyneuropathy, doctors do blood tests to check for its various causes (such as diabetes or kidney disorders).

TREATMENT

The condition causing numbness is corrected or treated when possible.

General measures can help relieve symptoms and prevent additional problems. Precautions to prevent injury are needed because people with numbness are less likely to feel discomfort. If their feet are numb, particularly if circulation is impaired, they should wear socks and shoes that fit well and should check their shoes for pebbles or other foreign material before putting their shoes on. People should inspect their feet frequently for sores and signs of infection, such as redness. If hands or fingers are numb, people should be careful when handling objects that could be hot or sharp.

If people are having difficulty walking or have lost their sense of position (where body parts are), physical therapy can help them learn to walk more safely and to prevent falls. People should be aware that they may have problems driving, and if they do, they should talk to their doctor about the problems.

KEY POINTS

- Numbness refers to partial or complete loss of sensation and is often accompanied by abnormal sensations, such as tingling.
- Numbness, which has many causes, occurs when one part of the pathway from sensory receptors in the skin to the brain malfunctions.
- If people have any warning sign, they should see a doctor immediately.
- Telling doctors which parts of the body are affected and how quickly symptoms develop helps doctors identify the location and cause of the malfunction.
- Testing usually starts with nerve conduction studies and electromyography if the sensory nerves, plexuses, or spinal nerve roots are thought to be affected or with MRI if the brain or spinal cord is thought to be affected.

PALPITATIONS

Palpitations are the awareness of heartbeats. The sensation may feel like pounding, fluttering, racing, or skipping beats. Other symptoms—for example, chest discomfort or shortness of breath—may be present depending on the cause of the palpitations.

Palpitations are common. Some people find them unpleasant and alarming, but they rarely indicate a life-threatening heart disorder. Many people without heart disease also have palpitations.

CAUSES

Ordinarily, people do not notice the beating of their heart. However, many people can feel their heart beating when something causes it to beat more forcefully or rapidly than usual. Such rapid, forceful beats are a normal response by the heart (sinus tachycardia). Causes include the following:

- Exercise
- Strong emotions (such as anxiety, fear, pain)
- Low blood count (anemia)
- Low blood pressure
- Fever
- Dehydration

In other cases, palpitations result from a disturbance of heart rhythm (arrhythmia).

TYPES OF ARRHYTHMIAS

Arrhythmias range from harmless to life threatening.

The **most common arrhythmias** include

- Atrial premature beats
- Ventricular premature beats

Both of these arrhythmias usually occur in people without a heart disorder and are harmless. The premature beat itself is not felt. What is felt is the following normal heartbeat, which occurs after a slight delay and is slightly stronger than usual. Although people feel as if their heart skipped a beat, it actually did not.

Other arrhythmias that cause palpitations include

- Paroxysmal supraventricular tachycardia (PSVT)
- Atrioventricular nodal reentrant tachycardia
- Atrial fibrillation or flutter
- Ventricular tachycardia

These other arrhythmias involve the heart beating much faster than normal. Arrhythmias in which the heart beats too slowly rarely cause palpitations, although some people do feel the slow rate.

CAUSES OF ARRHYTHMIAS

Some arrhythmias (for example, atrial premature beats, ventricular premature beats, or PSVT) often occur in people who have no serious underlying disorders. Others are often caused by a serious heart disorder or a disorder elsewhere in the body.

Serious heart disorders include angina, heart attack (acute coronary syndrome), congenital heart diseases, disorders of heart valves, and conduction system disturbances (for example, Wolff-Parkinson-White syndrome).

Disorders not related to the heart that may cause arrhythmias include

- Overactive thyroid gland (hyperthyroidism)
- Low level of oxygen in the blood (hypoxia)
- Low level of potassium in the blood (hypokalemia)
- Low level of magnesium in the blood (hypomagnesemia)
- Certain drugs, including alcohol, caffeine, digoxin, nicotine, and some stimulant drugs (such as albuterol, amphetamines, cocaine, epinephrine, ephedrine, and theophylline)

COMPLICATIONS

Arrhythmias that cause the heart to beat too fast can cause complications (particularly in older people). If the heart goes too fast, it may not be able to pump blood adequately, and people may feel faint or pass out or develop heart failure. Heart failure occurs mainly in people who have previously had heart failure or a heart attack, although it can occur in other people if the heart rate is very fast or if the heart beats too fast for a long time. A rapid heart rate also increases the oxygen needs of the heart muscle.

People who have narrowing of the arteries to the heart muscle (coronary artery disease) can develop chest pain due to angina or a heart attack (which may be fatal).

Some arrhythmias, particularly ventricular tachycardia, are unstable and can lead directly to cardiac arrest.

EVALUATION

Although not all palpitations are caused by a heart disorder, the consequences of some heart disorders are so serious that people with palpitations should usually be evaluated by a doctor. The following information can help people decide when to see a doctor and help them know what to expect during the evaluation.

WARNING SIGNS

In people with palpitations, certain symptoms and characteristics are cause for concern. They include

- Light-headedness or fainting
- Chest pain or pressure
- Shortness of breath
- Pulse rate over 120 per minute
- Having heart disease or a family history of sudden death

WHEN TO SEE A DOCTOR

People who have palpitations and any warning signs should go to an emergency department right away, as should those who have continuous, ongoing palpitations. Those who have fainting, chest pain, or shortness of breath should call emergency services.

People without warning signs who have occasional palpitations or had an episode that stopped should call their doctor. The doctor will determine how quickly they need to be seen based on their age, underlying conditions, and other symptoms. Typically a delay of a day or two is not harmful.

WHAT THE DOCTOR DOES

Doctors first ask questions about the person's symptoms and medical history. Doctors then do a physical examination. What they find during the history and physical examination helps determine the possible cause.

Doctors ask

- How often palpitations occur

- How long palpitations last
- What factors (for example, emotional distress, activity, or intake of caffeine or other drugs) trigger or worsen palpitations
- What drugs, including caffeine, the person is taking

Sometimes doctors ask the person to tap out the rate and cadence of palpitations because the pattern of beats can help them determine the cause.

The physical examination begins with the doctor checking the vital signs (pulse, temperature, and blood pressure). The pulse rate and whether the pulse is regular or irregular help suggest causes. An elevated temperature suggests fever is the cause. A low blood pressure does not suggest a cause but indicates extreme urgency.

Doctors listen to the heart for abnormal sounds that might indicate a valve disorder or heart inflammation. They listen to the lungs for sounds that indicate heart failure. They look at and feel the front of the neck to see if the thyroid gland is enlarged or inflamed.

Palpitations that occur with other symptoms, such as shortness of breath, chest pain, weakness, fatigue, or fainting, are more likely to result from an abnormal heart rhythm or a serious disorder.

TESTING

Even though most causes of palpitations are not serious, testing typically is done.

- Electrocardiography (ECG), sometimes with ambulatory monitoring
- Laboratory testing
- Sometimes imaging studies, stress testing, or both
- Sometimes electrophysiologic testing

ECG is done. If the ECG is done while the person is having palpitations or an abnormal pulse rate, the diagnosis is usually clear. However, only a few of the possible causes produce an abnormal ECG when people are not having palpitations. Thus, people who have intermittent palpitations may need to wear an ECG monitor for a day or two (Holter monitoring) or for a longer period (event recorder) to detect brief or irregularly occurring abnormal rhythms.

Laboratory testing is needed. Doctors do a complete blood count and measure serum

SOME FEATURES AND CAUSES OF PALPITATIONS

Feature*	Possible Cause
Perception of an occasional skipped heartbeat	Atrial premature beats or ventricular premature beats
Sudden episodes of rapid heartbeats that abruptly slow to the normal rate; often in people who have had previous episodes of rapid heartbeats	PSVT or Wolff-Parkinson-White syndrome Less often ventricular tachycardia or congenital long QT syndrome
A constant sensation of rapid, irregular heartbeats	Atrial fibrillation
Fainting during palpitations	Ventricular tachycardia, congenital long QT syndrome, inherited hypertrophic cardiomyopathy, or Brugada syndrome
Palpitations during exercise or an emotional situation	*In healthy people*: Sinus tachycardia (the heart's normal response to stress) *In people with coronary artery disease*: Sometimes arrhythmia caused by a decrease in blood flow triggered by exercise
In people with a family history of fainting or sudden death	Brugada syndrome, congenital long QT syndrome, or inherited dilated or hypertrophic cardiomyopathy
In people who are bleeding, have a fever, are in pain, or have lost fluids (as may result from vomiting or diarrhea)	Sinus tachycardia
Intolerance of heat, weight loss, bulging eyeballs, and tenderness and/or swelling in the front of the neck	Sinus tachycardia or atrial fibrillation due to hyperthyroidism

*Features include symptoms and the results of the doctor's examination. Features mentioned are typical but not always present.
PSVT = paroxysmal supraventricular tachycardia.

electrolytes, including potassium, magnesium, and calcium. Doctors may measure other substances in the blood (cardiac markers) if the person has other symptoms that suggest a possible acute coronary syndrome. Doctors measure levels of thyroid hormone in the blood if they suspect an overactive thyroid and measure levels of other hormones in people who may have pheochromocytoma.

Imaging is often needed. In people with ECG findings that suggest heart disease, doctors do echocardiography and sometimes magnetic resonance imaging (MRI) of the heart. People with symptoms on exertion require stress testing sometimes with stress echocardiography or nuclear scanning.

Electrophysiologic testing is done when people's symptoms are severe and doctors suspect a dangerous heart rhythm problem that was not found with other tests. In this test, doctors pass small electrodes through a vein into the heart. The electrodes record the heart's electrical activity in more detail than an ECG does.

TREATMENT

Drugs and substances such as caffeine that are known to worsen a person's palpitations are stopped. If dangerous or debilitating arrhythmias are caused by a necessary therapeutic drug, doctors try a different drug.

Doctors usually simply provide reassurance for people with atrial premature beats or ventricular premature beats that are not caused by a heart disorder. If such harmless palpitations are very bothersome, doctors sometimes give a beta-blocker (a type of antiarrhythmic drug). Other identified rhythm disturbances and underlying disorders are investigated and treated. Doctors often first give rhythm-controlling drugs (such as digoxin, flecainide, verapamil, diltiazem, or amiodarone). However, many of these drugs can themselves cause rhythm disturbances as well as other side effects. If drugs are not effective or if people have certain dangerous rhythm disturbances, doctors may use more invasive treatments such as direct current cardioversion, radioablation, or implantation of a combination pacemaker and defibrillator. The choice of procedure depends on the specific condition causing the disturbance.

ESSENTIALS FOR OLDER PEOPLE

Older people are at particular risk of side effects due to antiarrhythmic drugs. Older people are likely to have several health problems and take several drugs, and these drug combinations may put them at risk of side effects. In older people, the kidneys are less effective at filtering drugs from the blood, which contributes to the risk of side effects. Some older people may even need a pacemaker before they can take antiarrhythmic drugs.

O—ᴨ KEY POINTS

- Palpitations are common, and they have many causes that range from harmless to life-threatening.
- People who have other symptoms such as light-headedness, chest pain or pressure, or shortness of breath may have a serious problem and should see a doctor quickly.
- ECG and certain blood tests are done.
- Treatment depends on the cause.

PELVIC PAIN

Pelvic pain is discomfort that occurs in the lowest part of the torso, the area below the abdomen and between the hipbones. It does not include pain that occurs externally in the genital area (vulva). Many women have pelvic pain. Pain is considered chronic if it continues to occur for more than 4 to 6 months.

The pain may be sharp or crampy (like menstrual cramps—see page 265) and may come and go. It may be sudden and excruciating, dull and constant, or some combination. The pain may gradually increase in intensity, sometimes occurring in waves. Often, pelvic pain occurs in cycles that coordinate with the menstrual cycle. That is, pain may occur every month just before or during menstrual periods or in the middle of the menstrual cycle, when the egg is released (during ovulation).

The pelvic area may feel tender when touched. Depending on the cause, women may have bleeding or a discharge from the vagina. The pain may also be accompanied by fever, nausea, vomiting, sweating, and/or light-headedness.

CAUSES

Usually, pelvic pain is not caused by a serious disorder. It is often related to the menstrual cycle. However, several disorders that cause pelvic pain can lead to peritonitis (inflammation and usually infection of the abdominal cavity), which is a serious disorder (see page 1).

Disorders that can cause pelvic pain include

- Gynecologic disorders—those that affect the reproductive organs (vagina, cervix, uterus, fallopian tubes, and ovaries)
- Disorders that affect other organs in the pelvis, such as the bladder, rectum, or appendix
- Disorders that affect organs near but outside the pelvis, such as the abdominal wall, intestine, kidneys, ureters, or lower part of the aorta

Often doctors cannot identify a disorder.

GYNECOLOGIC DISORDERS

Gynecologic disorders may be related to the menstrual cycle or not. The most common causes include

- Menstrual cramps (dysmenorrhea)
- Pain in the middle of the menstrual cycle (mittelschmerz), occurring during ovulation
- Endometriosis (abnormally located patches of tissue that is normally located only in the lining of the uterus)

Many other gynecologic disorders can cause pelvic pain (see Table on pages 326 to 328).

OTHER DISORDERS

Common causes include

- Digestive tract disorders: Irritable bowel syndrome, gastroenteritis, inflammatory bowel disease, appendicitis, diverticulitis, constipation, a blockage or tear (perforation) in the intestine, collections of pus (abscesses), and tumors (cancerous or not), such as colon cancer
- Urinary disorders: Infections (such as cystitis), stones in the urinary tract (such as kidney stones), and inflammation of the bladder without infection (such as interstitial cystitis)
- Musculoskeletal disorders: Separation of the pubic bones after delivery of a baby, fibromyalgia, and strained abdominal muscles
- Other disorders: Abscesses in the pelvis and a bulge in the lower part of the aorta (abdominal aortic aneurysm)

Psychologic factors, especially stress and depression, may contribute to any kind of pain, including pelvic pain, but, by themselves, rarely cause pelvic pain.

Many women with chronic pelvic pain have been physically, psychologically, or sexually abused. Young girls who have been sexually abused may have pelvic pain. In such women and girls, psychologic factors may contribute to the pain.

EVALUATION

When a woman has new, sudden, very severe pain in the lower abdomen or pelvis, doctors must quickly decide whether emergency surgery is required. Disorders that require emergency surgery include appendicitis, a ruptured ectopic pregnancy (an abnormally located pregnancy— not in its usual place in the uterus), twisting of an ovary, a ruptured abscess in the pelvis, a tear in the intestine, and an abdominal aortic aneurysm.

Doctors check for pregnancy in all girls and women of childbearing age.

WARNING SIGNS

In women with pelvic pain, certain symptoms are cause for concern:

- Light-headedness, sudden loss of consciousness however brief (fainting, or syncope), or dangerously low blood pressure (shock)
- Vaginal bleeding after menopause
- Fever or chills
- Sudden, severe pain, especially when accompanied by nausea, vomiting, excessive sweating, or agitation

WHEN TO SEE A DOCTOR

Women with warning signs should see a doctor immediately. However, if the only warning sign is vaginal bleeding after menopause, women can see a doctor within a week or so.

If women without warning signs have new pain that is constant and steadily worsening, they should see a doctor that day. If such women have new pain that is not constant and is not worsening, they should schedule a visit when practical, but a delay of several days is usually not harmful.

Recurring or chronic pelvic pain should be evaluated by a doctor at some point. Mild cramping and pain associated with menstrual periods is normal and does not require evaluation unless it is very painful (see Menstrual Periods, Painful on page 265).

WHAT THE DOCTORS DOES

After making sure that the woman does not require emergency surgery, doctors ask the woman questions about her symptoms and medical history. Doctors then do a physical examination. What they find during the history and physical examination often suggests a cause and the tests that may need to be done (see Table on pages 326 to 328).

Doctors ask about the pain:

- Whether it begins suddenly or gradually

- Whether it is sharp or dull
- How severe it is
- When it occurs in relation to the menstrual cycle, eating, sleeping, sexual intercourse, physical activity, urination, and bowel movements
- Whether any other factors worsen or ease the pain

The woman is asked about other symptoms, such as vaginal bleeding, a discharge, and light-headedness.

The woman is asked to describe past pregnancies and menstrual periods. Doctors also ask whether she has had any disorders that can cause pelvic pain and whether she has had abdominal or pelvic surgery.

Doctors may ask about stress, depression, and other psychologic factors to determine whether these factors may be contributing to the pain, especially if the pain is chronic.

Certain groups of symptoms suggest a type of disorder. For example, fever and chills suggest an infection. A vaginal discharge suggests pelvic inflammatory disease. Loss of appetite, nausea, vomiting, or relief or worsening of the pain during a bowel movement suggests a digestive tract disorder. Vaginal bleeding suggests menstrual cramps, an ectopic pregnancy, or a possible miscarriage. Menstrual cramps are diagnosed only after other, more serious causes are ruled out.

The physical examination focuses on the abdomen and pelvis. Doctors gently feel the abdomen and do a pelvic examination. This evaluation helps doctors determine which organs are affected and whether an infection is present. Often, doctors also check the rectum for abnormalities.

TESTING

The following tests are done:

- Urine tests (urinalysis)
- A urine test for pregnancy if women are of childbearing age

If a urine pregnancy test indicates that the woman is pregnant, ultrasonography is done to rule out an ectopic pregnancy. If results of ultrasonography are unclear, other tests, such as laparoscopy or a series of blood tests, are done to rule out ectopic pregnancy. For laparoscopy, doctors make a small incision just

SOME GYNECOLOGIC CAUSES OF PELVIC PAIN

Cause	Common Features*	Tests†
Related to the menstrual cycle		
Menstrual cramps (dysmenorrhea)	Sharp or crampy pain that ■ Occurs a few days before or during menstrual periods ■ Is most intense about 24 hours after periods begin and subsides after 2–3 days Often headache, nausea, constipation, diarrhea, or an urge to urinate often (frequency)	A doctor's examination
Endometriosis (abnormally located patches of tissue that is normally located only in the lining of the uterus)	Sharp or crampy pain that occurs before and during the first days of menstrual periods Often pain during sexual intercourse and/or bowel movements May eventually cause pain unrelated to the menstrual cycle Sometimes infertility	A doctor's examination Sometimes laparoscopy (insertion of a thin viewing tube into the abdomen) to check for abnormal tissue and to obtain a sample
Mittelschmerz (pain in the middle of the menstrual cycle)	Severe, sharp pain that ■ Begins suddenly ■ Can occur on either side but on only one side at a time ■ Occurs at the same time during the menstrual cycle, usually midway between the start of menstrual periods (when the egg is released) ■ Is most intense when it begins, then subsides over 1–2 days Often light spotty bleeding	A doctor's examination
Related to the reproductive system but not the menstrual cycle		
Pelvic inflammatory disease	Aching pelvic pain that may be felt on one or both sides Usually a vaginal discharge that sometimes has a foul odor and, as infection worsens, can become puslike and yellow-green Sometimes pain during urination and/or sexual intercourse, fever or chills, nausea, or vomiting	Tests to detect sexually transmitted diseases using a sample of secretions taken from the cervix Sometimes ultrasonography of the pelvis
A ruptured ovarian cyst	Pain that ■ Begins suddenly ■ Is most severe when it begins ■ Often rapidly decreases over a few hours Sometimes light-headedness, fainting, slight vaginal bleeding, nausea, or vomiting	A doctor's examination Sometimes ultrasonography of the pelvis
A ruptured ectopic pregnancy (an abnormally located pregnancy—not in its usual place in the uterus)	Constant (not crampy) pain that ■ Begins suddenly ■ Is at first confined to one area of the lower abdomen Often slight vaginal bleeding Sometimes light-headedness, fainting, a racing heart, or dangerously low blood pressure (shock)	Urine or blood tests to measure a hormone produced by the placenta (called human chorionic gonadotropin, or hCG) Ultrasonography of the pelvis Sometimes laparoscopy or laparotomy (a large incision into the abdomen enabling doctors to directly view organs)

(continued)

SOME GYNECOLOGIC CAUSES OF PELVIC PAIN (continued)

Cause	Common Features*	Tests†
Sudden degeneration of a fibroid in the uterus	Pain that begins suddenly Most common during the first 12 weeks of pregnancy or after delivery or termination of a pregnancy Vaginal bleeding	Ultrasonography of the pelvis
Adnexal torsion (twisting) of an ovary	Severe pain that ■ Begins suddenly ■ Occurs on one side ■ Peaks quickly Occasionally pain that comes and goes (as the ovary twists and untwists) Often occurs when women are pregnant, after drugs are used to treat infertility, or when ovaries are enlarged	Ultrasonography of the pelvis Sometimes laparoscopy or laparotomy
Cancer of the ovaries or the lining of the uterus (endometrium)	Pain that develops gradually Abnormal vaginal bleeding (bleeding after menopause or bleeding between menstrual periods) or a brown or bloody discharge Sometimes weight loss	A Papanicolaou (Pap) test Ultrasonography of the pelvis A biopsy Sometimes imaging tests of the pelvis such as ultrasonography, MRI, or CT
Adhesions (bands of scar tissue between normally unconnected structures in the uterus or pelvis)	Pelvic pain that ■ Develops gradually ■ Often becomes chronic Pain during sexual intercourse No vaginal bleeding or discharge Sometimes nausea and vomiting (suggesting a blockage of the intestine) In women who have had abdominal surgery (usually) or pelvic infections (sometimes)	A doctor's examination Sometimes x-rays of the abdomen
A miscarriage (spontaneous abortion) or one that may occur (threatened abortion)	Crampy pain in the pelvis or back Vaginal bleeding that accompanies the pain Other symptoms of early pregnancy such as breast tenderness, nausea, and absence of periods Sometimes passage of tissue through the vagina	A pregnancy test Ultrasonography of the pelvis to determine whether a miscarriage has occurred and, if not, whether the pregnancy can continue
Not related to the reproductive system		
Appendicitis	Pain that usually settles in the right lower part of the abdomen Loss of appetite and usually nausea and vomiting Often fever	A doctor's examination Sometimes CT or ultrasonography of the abdomen
Bladder infection	Pain just above the pubic bone Sometimes an urgent need to urinate, more frequent urination, or burning during urination	A urine test

(continued)

SOME GYNECOLOGIC CAUSES OF PELVIC PAIN *(continued)*

Cause	Common Features*	Tests†
Diverticulitis	Pain or tenderness in the lower left part of the abdomen Fever	Sometimes CT of the abdomen Often colonoscopy after the infection subsides
Inflammatory bowel disease including ■ Crohn disease ■ Ulcerative colitis	Crampy abdominal pain Diarrhea, which in ulcerative colitis is often bloody Loss of appetite and weight	CT of the small and large intestine (CT enterography) to check for Crohn disease Endoscopy (usually colonoscopy or sigmoidoscopy) Sometimes x-rays of the upper digestive tract after barium is given by mouth (barium swallow) or of the lower digestive tract after insertion of barium into the rectum (barium enema)
Stones in the urinary tract	Excruciating intermittent pain in the lower abdomen, side, or lower back, depending on the stone's location Nausea and vomiting Blood in the urine	Urine tests (urinalysis) Imaging tests, such as CT or ultrasonography

*Features include symptoms and results of the doctor's examination. Features mentioned are typical but not always present.
†If women are of childbearing age, a pregnancy test is always done, regardless of the cause suspected. If symptoms have begun suddenly, recur, or are severe, ultrasonography of the pelvis is usually done. Typically, doctors also do a urine test to look for a urinary tract infection.
CT = computed tomography; MRI = magnetic resonance imaging.

below the navel and insert a viewing tube (laparoscope) to look for an ectopic pregnancy directly. For the blood tests, doctors measure levels of a hormone produced by the placenta (human chorionic gonadotropin, or hCG). If hCG levels are low, the pregnancy may be too early for ultrasonography to detect. If levels are high and ultrasonography does not detect a pregnancy, ectopic pregnancy is possible.

If a very early pregnancy is possible and the urine test is negative, a blood test for pregnancy is done. The blood test is more accurate than the urine test when a pregnancy is less than 5 weeks.

Ultrasonography of the pelvis is usually done when doctors think a gynecologic disorder may be the cause and symptoms have begun suddenly, recur, or are severe. Ultrasonography is also done when a tumor is suspected. Doctors use a handheld ultrasound device that is placed on the abdomen or inside the vagina.

Other tests depend on which disorders are suspected. Tests may include

■ Examination and culture of samples of urine or a discharge to check for infections that can cause pelvic pain
■ Computed tomography (CT) or magnetic resonance imaging (MRI) of the abdomen and pelvis
■ If other tests do not identify a cause, laparoscopy

TREATMENT

If the disorder causing pelvic pain is identified, that disorder is treated if possible. Pain relievers may also be needed.

Initially, pain is treated with nonsteroidal anti-inflammatory drugs (NSAIDs), such as ibuprofen. Women who do not respond well to one NSAID may respond to another. If NSAIDs are ineffective, other pain relievers or hypnosis may be tried. If the pain involves muscles, rest, heat, or physical therapy may help.

Rarely, when women have severe pain that persists despite treatment, surgery to cut the nerves to the uterus may be done. However, this operation occasionally injures other organs in the pelvis, such as the ureters. If pain still persists, hysterectomy (surgery to remove the uterus) can be done, but it may be ineffective or even worsen the pain.

ESSENTIALS FOR OLDER WOMEN

In older women, common causes of pelvic pain may be different because some disorders that cause pelvic pain become more common as women age, particularly after menopause. These disorders include

- Bladder problems, including infections
- Constipation
- Diverticulosis
- Pelvic floor disorders
- Many cancers of the reproductive tract, including cancers of the lining of the uterus (endometrial cancer), fallopian tubes, ovaries, and vagina

After menopause, estrogen levels decrease, weakening many tissues, including bone, muscles (such as those of the bladder), and tissues around the vagina and urethra. As a result, fractures and bladder infections become more common. Also, this weakening may contribute to pelvic floor disorders, which may cause symptoms only when women become older. In these disorders, weakened or damaged tissues in the pelvis can no longer hold the uterus, vagina, or other organs in the pelvis in place. As a result, one or more of these organs may drop down.

Older women are more likely to take drugs that can increase the risk of some causes of pelvic pain, such as constipation and diverticulosis. Obviously, disorders related to menstrual periods are no longer possible causes.

EVALUATION

Evaluation is similar to that for younger women, except doctors pay particular attention to symptoms of urinary and digestive tract disorders. Older women should see a doctor promptly if they

- Suddenly lose weight or their appetite
- Suddenly start having indigestion
- Have a sudden change in bowel movements

The doctor then does an examination to make sure that the cause is not ovarian or endometrial cancer.

Sexual intercourse may cause pain in older women (because the lining of the vagina thins and dries after menopause), and women may describe or experience this pain as pelvic pain. To check for this cause, doctors ask the woman questions to determine whether she is sexually active. If so, doctors may recommend a break from sexual intercourse until symptoms subside.

KEY POINTS

- Many women have pelvic pain.
- Many disorders (related to reproductive organs or other nearby organs) can cause pelvic pain.
- Doctors can determine likely causes based on a description of the pain, its relationship to the menstrual cycle, and results of a physical examination.
- If women are of childbearing age, a pregnancy test is always done.
- Urine tests and usually other tests, such as blood tests and ultrasonography of the pelvis, are done to confirm the suspected diagnosis.
- Menstrual cramps are a common cause of pelvic pain but are diagnosed only after other causes have been ruled out.

PELVIC PAIN DURING EARLY PREGNANCY

Early in pregnancy, many women have pelvic pain. Pelvic pain refers to pain in the lowest part of the torso, in the area below the abdomen and between the hipbones (pelvis). The pain may be sharp or crampy (like menstrual cramps) and may come and go. It may be sudden and excruciating, dull and constant, or some combination. Usually, temporary pelvic pain is not a cause for concern. It can occur normally as the bones and ligaments shift and stretch to accommodate the fetus.

If caused by a disorder, pelvic pain may be accompanied by other symptoms, including vaginal bleeding (see page 429). In some disorders, such bleeding can be severe, sometimes leading to dangerously low blood pressure (shock).

Pelvic pain differs from abdominal pain, which occurs higher in the torso, in the area of the stomach and intestine. However, sometimes women have trouble discerning whether pain is mainly in the abdomen or pelvis. Causes of abdominal pain during pregnancy are usually not related to the pregnancy.

CAUSES

During early pregnancy, pelvic pain may result from disorders that are related to

- The pregnancy (obstetric disorders)
- The female reproductive system (gynecologic disorders) but not the pregnancy
- Other organs, particularly the digestive tract and urinary tract

Sometimes no particular disorder is identified. The **most common obstetric causes** during early pregnancy are

- The normal changes of pregnancy
- A miscarriage that has occurred or is occurring (spontaneous abortion)
- A miscarriage that may occur (threatened abortion)

In a miscarriage that has occurred, all of the contents of the uterus (fetus and placenta) may be expelled (complete abortion) or not (incomplete abortion).

The **most common serious obstetric cause** is

- Rupture of an abnormally located (ectopic) pregnancy—one that is not in its usual place in the uterus, for example, one that is in a fallopian tube

When an ectopic pregnancy ruptures, blood pressure may drop very low, the heart may race, and blood may not clot normally. Immediate surgery may be required.

Pelvic pain may also occur when an ovary twists around the ligaments and the tissues that support it, cutting off the ovary's blood supply. This disorder, called adnexal torsion, is not related to the pregnancy but is more common during pregnancy. During pregnancy, the ovaries enlarge, making an ovary more likely to twist.

Digestive and urinary tract disorders, which are common causes of pelvic pain in general, are also common causes during pregnancy. These disorders include

- Gastroenteritis (infection of the digestive tract) due to a virus
- Irritable bowel syndrome
- Appendicitis
- Inflammatory bowel disease
- Urinary tract infections (UTIs)
- Kidney stones

Pelvic pain during late pregnancy may result from labor or from a disorder unrelated to the pregnancy.

RISK FACTORS

Various characteristics (risk factors) increase the risk of some obstetric disorders that cause pelvic pain.

For **miscarriage,** risk factors include

- Age over 35
- One or more miscarriages in previous pregnancies
- Cigarette smoking
- Use of drugs such as cocaine, consumption of alcohol, or consumption of a lot of caffeine
- Abnormalities in the uterus, such as fibroids or scars, as may be caused by surgery,

dilation and curettage (D and C), radiation therapy, or infections

For ectopic pregnancy, risk factors include

- A previous ectopic pregnancy (the most important risk factor)
- Previous abdominal surgery, especially surgery to sterilize the woman (tubal ligation)
- A previous infection with a sexually transmitted disease or pelvic inflammatory disease
- Cigarette smoking
- Use of an intrauterine device (IUD)
- Age over 35
- A history of infertility, use of fertility drugs, or use of assisted reproductive techniques
- Several sex partners
- An abortion in a previous pregnancy
- Douching

EVALUATION

If a pregnant woman has sudden, very severe pain in the lower abdomen or pelvis, doctors must quickly try to determine whether prompt surgery is required—as is the case when the cause is an ectopic pregnancy or appendicitis.

WARNING SIGNS

In pregnant women with pelvic pain, the following symptoms are cause for concern:

- Fainting, light-headedness, or a racing heart—symptoms that suggest very low blood pressure
- Fever, particularly if accompanied by a vaginal discharge that contains pus
- Vaginal bleeding
- Pain that is severe and is made worse with movement

WHEN TO SEE A DOCTOR

Women with warning signs should see a doctor immediately. Women without warning signs should try to see a doctor within a day or so if they have pain or burning during urination or pain that interferes with daily activities. Women with only mild discomfort and no other symptoms should call the doctor. The doctor can help them decide whether and how quickly they need to be seen.

WHAT THE DOCTOR DOES

To determine whether emergency surgery is needed, doctors first check blood pressure and temperature and ask about key symptoms, such as vaginal bleeding. Doctors then ask about other symptoms and the medical history. They also do a physical examination. What they find during the history and physical examination often suggests a cause and the tests that may need to be done (see Table on pages 332 to 333).

Doctors ask about the pain:

- Whether it begins suddenly or gradually
- Whether it occurs in a specific spot or is more widespread
- Whether moving or changing positions worsens the pain
- Whether it is crampy and whether it is constant or comes and goes

Doctors also ask about other symptoms, such as vaginal bleeding, a vaginal discharge, a need to urinate often or urgently, vomiting, diarrhea, and constipation. They ask particularly about previous pregnancy-related events (obstetric history), including past pregnancies, miscarriages, and intentional terminations of pregnancy (induced abortions) for medical or other reasons, as well as risk factors for miscarriage and ectopic pregnancy.

The physical examination focuses on the pelvic examination. Doctors gently press on the abdomen to see whether pressing causes any pain.

TESTING

Doctors use a handheld Doppler ultrasound device, placed on the woman's abdomen, to check for a heartbeat in the fetus.

A pregnancy test using a urine sample is almost always done. If the pregnancy test is positive, ultrasonography of the pelvis is done to confirm that the pregnancy is normally located—in the uterus—rather than somewhere else (an ectopic pregnancy). For this test, a handheld ultrasound device is placed on the abdomen, inside the vagina, or both.

Blood tests are usually done. If a woman has vaginal bleeding, testing usually includes a complete blood cell count and blood type plus Rh status (positive or negative) in case the woman needs a transfusion. Knowing Rh status also helps doctors prevent problems in subsequent pregnancies. If doctors suspect an ectopic pregnancy, testing also includes a blood test to measure a hormone produced by the placenta early during pregnancy (human chorionic gonadotropin, or hCG). If symptoms (such as

SOME CAUSES AND FEATURES OF PELVIC PAIN DURING EARLY PREGNANCY

Cause	Common Features*	Tests†
Pregnancy-related (obstetric) disorders		
An ectopic pregnancy (an abnormally located pregnancy—not in its usual place in the uterus)	Abdominal or pelvic pain that ■ Is often sudden and constant (not crampy) ■ Begins in a specific spot ■ May or may not be accompanied by vaginal bleeding If the ectopic pregnancy has ruptured, possibly fainting, light-headedness, or a racing heart	A blood test to measure a hormone produced by the placenta (human chorionic gonadotropin, or hCG) Ultrasonography of the pelvis Sometimes laparoscopy (insertion of a viewing tube through an incision in the abdomen) or laparotomy (surgery involving an incision into the abdomen)
A miscarriage that ■ Has occurred or is occurring (spontaneous abortion) ■ May occur (threatened abortion)	Crampy pain in the pelvis and often throughout the abdomen Often vaginal bleeding, sometimes with passage of tissue from the fetus	Tests as for ectopic pregnancy
Septic abortion (infection of the contents of the uterus before, during, or after a miscarriage)	Usually in women who have had an abortion (often done by untrained practitioners or by the women themselves) Fever and chills, constant abdominal or pelvic pain, and a vaginal discharge that contains pus	Cultures of a sample taken from the cervix (the lower part of the uterus)
Normal changes of pregnancy, including stretching and growth of the uterus during early pregnancy	A crampy or burning sensation in the lower abdomen, pelvis, and/or lower back	Ultrasonography of the pelvis
Gynecologic disorders unrelated to the pregnancy		
Degeneration of a fibroid in the uterus	Pelvic pain that ■ Begins suddenly ■ Is often accompanied by nausea, vomiting, and fever Sometimes vaginal bleeding	Ultrasonography of the pelvis
Adnexal torsion (twisting) of an ovary	Pelvic pain that ■ Begins suddenly ■ May be colicky and is often mild if the ovary untwists on its own Often nausea or vomiting	Doppler ultrasonography (to evaluate blood flow to and from the ovary) Sometimes laparoscopy or laparotomy
Rupture of a corpus luteum cyst (which develops in the structure that releases the egg after the egg is released)	Abdominal or pelvic pain that ■ Occurs in a specific spot ■ Sometimes resembles pain due to a twisted ovary ■ Usually begins suddenly Vaginal bleeding	Ultrasonography of the pelvis Sometimes laparoscopy or laparotomy

(continued)

SOME CAUSES AND FEATURES OF PELVIC PAIN DURING EARLY PREGNANCY *(continued)*

Cause	Common Features*	Tests†
Pelvic inflammatory disease (which is uncommon during pregnancy)	Pelvic pain that ■ Is continuous ■ Usually develops gradually ■ Usually occurs on both sides A vaginal discharge that contains pus Sometimes fever or chills More common among women who have sexual intercourse with new partners and do not use condoms or diaphragms	Cultures of a sample taken from the cervix Sometimes ultrasonography of the pelvis
Other disorders		
Appendicitis	Usually continuous pain and tenderness in the lower right part of the abdomen Possibly pain in a different location (for example, higher in the abdomen) or a different kind of pain (milder and crampy) from that in people who are not pregnant	Ultrasonography of the pelvis and abdomen Possibly CT if ultrasonography is inconclusive
Urinary tract infections	Discomfort felt in the area over the pubic bone Often burning during urination, an urge to urinate often (frequency), and a need to urinate immediately (urgency) Sometimes blood in urine	Urine tests (urinalysis) and culture
Inflammatory bowel disease including ■ Crohn disease ■ Ulcerative colitis	Pain that ■ May be crampy or constant ■ Can occur in various locations Often diarrhea that sometimes contains mucus or blood Usually in women known to have the disease	Sometimes endoscopy of the upper digestive tract, lower digestive tract (sigmoidoscopy or colonoscopy), or both
A blockage in the intestine (intestinal obstruction)	Cramping pain that comes and goes Vomiting No bowel movements or gas (flatulence) A swollen abdomen Usually in women who have had abdominal surgery	Ultrasonography of the pelvis and abdomen Possibly CT if ultrasonography is inconclusive
Gastroenteritis	Usually vomiting and diarrhea	A doctor's examination

*Features include symptoms and results of the doctor's examination. Features mentioned are typical but not always present.
†A urine pregnancy test is typically done if women have had only a home pregnancy test. Because an ectopic pregnancy can be very dangerous, tests are done to look for ectopic pregnancy in most pregnant women with pelvic pain, unless symptoms clearly point to another disorder (such as gastroenteritis).
CT = computed tomography.

very low blood pressure or a racing heart) suggest that an ectopic pregnancy may have ruptured, blood tests are done to determine whether the woman's blood can clot normally.

Other tests are done depending on which disorders are suspected. Doppler ultrasonography, which shows the direction and speed of blood flow, helps doctors identify a twisted ovary, which can cut off the ovary's blood supply. Other tests can include cultures of blood, urine, or a discharge from the vagina and urine tests (urinalysis) to check for infections.

If pain is persistently troublesome and the cause remains unknown, doctors make a small incision just below the navel and insert a viewing tube (laparoscope) to directly view the uterus and thus identify the cause of the pain. Rarely, a larger incision (a procedure called laparotomy) is required.

TREATMENT

Specific disorders are treated. If pain relievers are needed, acetaminophen is the safest one for pregnant women, but if it is ineffective, an opioid may be necessary.

PAIN DUE TO NORMAL CHANGES DURING PREGNANCY

Women may be advised to

- Limit how much they move, but move often.
- Avoid heavy lifting or pushing.
- Maintain good posture.
- Sleep with a pillow between their knees.
- Rest as much as possible with their back well-supported.
- Apply heat to painful areas.
- Do Kegel exercises (squeezing and releasing the muscles around the vagina, urethra, and rectum).
- Use a maternity support belt.
- Possibly try acupuncture.

O—ᴛᴛ KEY POINTS

- Pelvic pain during early pregnancy usually results from changes that occur normally during pregnancy.
- Sometimes it results from disorders, which may be related to the pregnancy, to female reproductive organs but not the pregnancy, or to other organs.
- Doctors' first priority is to identify disorders that require emergency surgery, such as an ectopic pregnancy or appendicitis.
- Ultrasonography is usually done.
- General measures (such as resting and applying heat) can help relieve pain due to the normal changes during pregnancy.

PERSONALITY AND BEHAVIOR CHANGES

Healthy people differ significantly in their overall personality, mood, and behavior. Each person also varies from day to day, depending on the circumstances. However, a sudden, major change in personality and/or behavior, particularly one that is not related to an obvious event (such as taking a drug or losing a loved one), often indicates a problem.

Changes in personality and behavior can be roughly categorized as one of the following:

- Confusion or delirium
- Delusions
- Disorganized speech or behavior
- Hallucinations
- Mood extremes (such as depression)

These categories are not disorders. They are just one way doctors organize different types of abnormal thought, speech, and behavior.

People may have more than one type of change. For example, people with confusion due to Alzheimer disease sometimes become depressed, and people with delirium may have disorganized speech or hallucinations.

Confusion and delirium refer to a disturbance of consciousness. That is, people are less aware of their environment and, depending on the cause, may be excessively agitated and belligerent or drowsy and sluggish. Some people alternate between being less alert and being overly alert. Their thinking appears cloudy and slow or inappropriate. They have trouble focusing on simple questions and are slow to respond. Speech may be slurred. Often, people do not know what day it is, and they may not be able to say where they are. Some cannot give their name.

Delusions are fixed false beliefs that people hold despite evidence against those beliefs. Some delusions are based on a misinterpretation of actual perceptions and experiences. For example, people may feel persecuted, thinking that a person behind them on the street is following them or that an ordinary accident is purposeful sabotage. Other people think that song lyrics or newspaper articles contain messages that refer specifically to them. Some beliefs seem more plausible and can be difficult to identify as delusions because they could occur or have occurred in real life. For example, people occasionally are followed by government investigators or have their work sabotaged by coworkers. In such cases, a belief can be identified as a delusion by how strongly people hold the belief despite evidence against it. Other delusions are easier to identify. For example, in religious or grandiose delusions, people may believe they are Jesus or the president of the country. Some delusions are quite bizarre. For example, people may think that their organs have all been replaced by machine parts or that their head contains a radio that receives messages from the government.

Disorganized speech refers to speech that does not contain the expected logical connections between thoughts or between questions and answers. For example, people may jump from one topic to another without ever finishing a thought. The topics may be slightly related or entirely unrelated. In other cases, people respond to simple questions with long, rambling answers, full of irrelevant detail. Answers may be illogical or completely incoherent. Occasionally misspeaking or intentionally being evasive, rude, or humorous is not considered disorganized speech.

Disorganized behavior refers to doing quite unusual things (such as undressing or masturbating in public or shouting and swearing for no apparent reason) or to being unable to behave normally. People with disorganized behavior typically have trouble doing normal daily activities (such as maintaining good personal hygiene or obtaining food).

Hallucinations refers to hearing, seeing, smelling, tasting, or feeling things that are not there. That is, people perceive things, seemingly through their senses, that are not caused by an outside stimulus. Any sense can be involved. The most common hallucinations involve hearing things (auditory hallucinations), usually voices. The voices often make derogatory comments about the person or command the person to do something. Not all hallucinations are caused by a mental disorder. Some types of hallucinations are more likely to be caused by a neurologic disorder. For example, before a seizure occurs, people may smell something when there is no smell (an olfactory hallucination).

Mood extremes include outbursts of rage, periods of extreme elation (mania) or depression, and, conversely, constant expression of little or no emotion (appearing unresponsive or apathetic).

CAUSES

Although people sometimes assume that changes in personality, thinking, or behavior are all due to a mental disorder, there are many possible causes. All causes ultimately involve the brain, but dividing them into four categories can be helpful:

- Mental disorders
- Drugs (including drug intoxication, withdrawal, and side effects)
- Disorders that affect mainly the brain
- Bodywide (systemic) disorders that also affect the brain

Of these causes, drugs are the most common cause overall, followed by mental disorders.

Drugs may affect personality or behavior when they cause

- Intoxication: Particularly alcohol (when consumed for a long time), amphetamines, cocaine, hallucinogens (such as LSD), and phencyclidine (PCP)
- Withdrawal: Alcohol, barbiturates, and benzodiazepines
- Side effects: Drugs intended to affect brain function (including anticonvulsants, antidepressants, antipsychotics, sedatives, and stimulants), drugs with anticholinergic effects (such as antihistamines), opioid pain relievers, and corticosteroids

Rarely, certain antibiotics and drugs used to treat high blood pressure cause changes in personality and behavior.

Mental disorders include

- Bipolar disorder
- Depression
- Schizophrenia
- Posttraumatic stress disorder

Disorders affecting mainly the brain include

- Alzheimer disease
- Brain infections, such as meningitis, encephalitis, and human immunodeficiency virus (HIV) infection that involves the brain (HIV-associated encephalopathy)
- Brain tumors
- Head injuries, such as a concussion and postconcussion syndrome
- Multiple sclerosis
- Parkinson disease
- Seizure disorders
- Stroke

Bodywide disorders that also affect the brain include

- Kidney failure
- Liver failure
- Low blood sugar (hypoglycemia)
- Systemic lupus erythematosus (lupus)
- Thyroid disorders, such as an underactive thyroid gland (hypothyroidism) or an overactive thyroid gland (hyperthyroidism)

Less commonly, Lyme disease, sarcoidosis, syphilis, or a vitamin deficiency causes personality and behavior changes.

EVALUATION

During the initial evaluation, doctors try to determine whether symptoms are due to a mental or physical disorder.

The following information can help people decide when a doctor's evaluation is needed and help them know what to expect during the evaluation.

WARNING SIGNS

In people with changes in personality or behavior, certain symptoms and characteristics are cause for concern. They include

- Symptoms that appear suddenly
- Attempts to harm themselves or others or threats to do so
- Confusion or delirium
- Fever
- Headache
- Symptoms that suggest malfunction of the brain, such as difficulty walking, balancing, or speaking or vision problems
- A recent head injury (within several weeks)

WHEN TO SEE A DOCTOR

People who have warning signs should be taken to the hospital right away. Law enforcement may need to be called if people are violent or belligerent.

If people take drugs for diabetes, a fingerstick test to check their blood sugar level should be done if possible. For this test, the finger is pricked to obtain a small sample of blood. If this test cannot be done or if the blood sugar level is low, people should be taken to the hospital right away.

People who have no warning signs should see a doctor within a day or two if the personality or behavior change was recent. If the change occurred gradually over a period of time, people should see a doctor as soon as is practical, but a delay of a week or so is not harmful.

WHAT THE DOCTOR DOES

Doctors first ask questions about the person's symptoms and medical history. Doctors then do a physical examination, including a neurologic examination. What they find during the history and physical examination often suggests a cause of the changes and the tests that need to be done (see Table, below).

Doctors ask when symptoms began. Many mental disorders begin in a person's teens or 20s. If a mental disorder begins during middle age or later, especially if there is no obvious trigger (such as loss of a loved one), the cause is more likely to be a physical disorder. A physical disorder is also more likely to be the cause when mental symptoms change significantly during middle age or later in people with a chronic mental disorder. If changes began recently and suddenly in people of any age, doctors ask about conditions that can trigger such changes. For example, they ask whether people have just started or stopped taking a prescription drug or a recreational (usually illegal) drug.

SOME CAUSES AND FEATURES OF PERSONALITY AND BEHAVIOR CHANGES

Cause	Common Features*	Tests
Mental disorders†		
Schizophrenia	Usually symptoms that develop slowly, with mildly disorganized thinking and difficulty coping with daily routines Later symptoms: ■ Delusions and/or hallucinations ■ Often lack of emotion and disinterest ■ Increasingly disorganized thinking and behavior ■ Difficulty maintaining relationships and employment	A doctor's examination
Bipolar disorder	Symptoms that occur in episodes lasting a few weeks to a few months and that include mania, depression, or both Episodes of mania: ■ Elation or irritability ■ Grandiosity ■ Talkativeness ■ Racing thoughts, jumping from one idea to another ■ Sometimes hallucinations or delusions of persecution Episodes of depression: ■ Sluggishness ■ Sadness, despair, and a pessimistic mood ■ Loss of interest in typical pleasures ■ Lack of energy ■ Difficulty sleeping ■ Thoughts of death or suicide	A doctor's examination
Depression	Episodes of depression as described in bipolar disorder (see above) but that last longer	A doctor's examination *(continued)*

SOME CAUSES AND FEATURES OF PERSONALITY AND BEHAVIOR CHANGES *(continued)*

Cause	Common Features*	Tests
Drugs		
Use of a drug, particularly ■ Alcohol ■ Amphetamines ■ Cocaine ■ Hallucinogens ■ Phencyclidine (PCP)	Agitation and sometimes panic or aggression Sometimes hallucinations With long-term use of alcohol: 　■ Sometimes balance problems 　■ Twitching eyes 　■ An abnormal way of walking With long-term use of amphetamines: 　■ Sometimes paranoia With short-term excessive use of amphetamines or cocaine: 　■ An increased heart rate 　■ Sometimes fever Usually in people known to use the drug	A doctor's examination Sometimes blood or urine tests to detect the drug Sometimes EEG
Withdrawal of a drug, particularly ■ Alcohol ■ Barbiturates ■ Benzodiazepines	Typically significant confusion and delirium Shaking (tremors), headache, sweating, fever, and a rapid heart rate or palpitations Sometimes seizures, hallucinations, and sleep disturbances Usually in people known to use the drug	A doctor's examination
Side effects	Vary, depending on the drug Drugs with anticholinergic effects: 　■ Constipation 　■ Blurred vision 　■ Light-headedness 　■ Difficulty starting and stopping urination 　■ Dry mouth Usually in people known to use the drug	A doctor's examination Sometimes stopping the drug to see whether the symptom goes away
Brain disorders		
Alzheimer disease	Symptoms that progress slowly Loss of short-term memory, difficulty finding the right words, and poor judgment Difficulty with daily activities (such as balancing a checkbook or finding their way around their neighborhood) Usually in people over 60	A doctor's examination Often CT , MRI, or PET of the brain Detailed testing of mental function involving a series of simple questions and tasks (neuropsychologic testing)
Brain infections such as ■ Encephalitis ■ Herpes simplex encephalitis ■ Meningitis	Headache Usually confusion and fever Pain and/or stiffness when the doctor bends the neck forward (more common in people with meningitis) With herpes simplex encephalitis, hallucinations of bad odors and sometimes seizures	A spinal tap (lumbar puncture) Often CT or MRI of the brain Culture of samples of blood, urine, and material from the throat EEG　　*(continued)*

SOME CAUSES AND FEATURES OF PERSONALITY AND BEHAVIOR CHANGES *(continued)*

Cause	Common Features*	Tests
Head injuries (such as postconcussion syndrome)	Forgetfulness and headaches Emotional instability in the weeks after a significant head injury	CT or MRI of the brain Testing of IQ and executive functions such as the ability to plan and solve problems (neurocognitive testing)
Brain tumors or bleeding (hemorrhage) in the brain	With brain tumors, a headache that develops gradually and is often worse during the night or early morning and when lying flat With hemorrhage, a headache that starts suddenly (called a thunderclap headache) Often confusion and drowsiness Sometimes seizures	CT or MRI of the brain
Multiple sclerosis	Weakness and/or numbness that comes and goes in different parts of the body Sometimes partial loss of vision or double vision Sometimes symptoms that are worsened by heat (such as a warm bath or hot weather)	MRI of the brain and spinal cord Sometimes a spinal tap Nerve conduction studies (measuring how fast nerves transmit signals) and electromyography (stimulating muscles and recording their electrical activity)
Parkinson disease	Tremors of the hands and fingers while they are at rest Stiffness and difficulty moving and maintaining balance Slowed speech and limited facial expressions	A doctor's examination
Seizure disorders (typically complex partial seizures)	Episodes of abnormal behavior Usually confusion and staring Sometimes involuntary chewing, smacking of the lips, and purposeless movements of the limbs Typically no loss of consciousness and no general shaking of the body (convulsions) Sometimes hallucinations of odor or taste	MRI of the brain EEG
Stroke	Symptoms that appear suddenly Usually weakness or paralysis on one side of the body and unsteadiness when walking	CT or MRI of the brain
Bodywide (systemic) disorders		
Hypoglycemia (a low level of blood sugar)	Weakness, sweating, and confusion Almost always in people taking drugs for diabetes	Tests to measure the blood sugar (glucose) level
Kidney failure	Swelling of the legs, loss of appetite, and nausea Weakness that typically develops over several weeks	Blood and urine tests to evaluate how well the kidneys are functioning

(continued)

SOME CAUSES AND FEATURES OF PERSONALITY AND BEHAVIOR CHANGES (continued)

Cause	Common Features*	Tests
Liver failure	Yellow color of the skin and/or whites of the eyes (jaundice)	Blood tests to evaluate how well the liver is functioning (liver function tests)
	Usually swelling of legs and/or abdomen	
	A reddish purple rash of tiny dots (petechiae)	
	Usually in people already known to have a liver disorder	
Systemic lupus erythematosus (lupus)	Usually painful, swollen joints	Blood tests to check for certain antibodies
	Often a rash, particularly on the face or areas exposed to sunlight	
	Sometimes a headache	
Thyroid disorders, including ■ Hyperthyroidism (an overactive thyroid gland) ■ Hypothyroidism (an underactive thyroid gland)	*Typically in hyperthyroidism*: Palpitations, excessive sweating, difficulty tolerating heat, an increased appetite, weight loss, shakiness (tremor), and sometimes bulging eyes *Typically in hypothyroidism*: Fatigue, constipation, difficulty tolerating cold, decreased appetite, weight gain, slow speech, sluggishness, a puffy face, drooping eyelids, coarse and thick dry skin, and loss of eyebrow hair	Blood tests to evaluate how well the thyroid gland is functioning
Vitamin deficiency, such as deficiency of thiamin or vitamin B_{12}	Disorientation, an impaired memory, and irritability	Blood tests to measure vitamin levels
	Abnormal sensations in the hands and feet	
	Other symptoms, depending on which vitamin is deficient	

*Features include symptoms and results of the doctor's examination. Features mentioned are typical but not always present.
†These disorders typically begin in a person's teens to mid-20s. People are usually alert and are not confused or delirious. Results of their physical examination (including the neurologic examination) are normal.
CT = computed tomography; EEG = electroencephalography; IQ = intelligence quotient; MRI = magnetic resonance imaging; PET = positron emission tomography.

Doctors ask about other symptoms that may suggest a cause, such as

■ Palpitations: Possibly an overactive thyroid gland or use or withdrawal of a drug
■ Tremors: Parkinson disease or withdrawal of a drug
■ Difficulty walking or speaking: Multiple sclerosis, Parkinson disease, stroke, or intoxication from an opioid or a sedative
■ Headache: Brain infection, brain tumor, or bleeding in the brain (hemorrhage)
■ Numbness or tingling: A stroke, multiple sclerosis, or a vitamin deficiency

People are also asked whether they have previously been diagnosed and treated for a mental or seizure disorder. If they have been treated, doctors ask whether they have stopped taking

their drugs or decreased the dose. However, because people with mental disorders may also develop physical disorders, doctors do not automatically assume that any new abnormal behavior is caused by the mental disorder.

During the physical examination, doctors look for signs of physical disorders, particularly

■ Fever (suggesting an infection, alcohol withdrawal, or use of amphetamines or cocaine in high doses)
■ A rapid heart rate
■ Confusion or delirium
■ Abnormalities during the neurologic examination

Confusion and delirium are more likely to result from a physical disorder. People with mental disorders are rarely confused or delirious.

However, many physical disorders that cause changes in behavior do not cause confusion or delirium, but they often cause other symptoms that may appear to be a mental disorder.

Doctors bend the person's neck forward. If doing so is difficult or painful, meningitis may be the cause. Doctors check the legs and abdomen for swelling, which may result from kidney or liver failure. If the skin or whites of the eyes look yellow, the cause may be liver failure.

TESTING

Typically, doctors clip a sensor to the person's fingertip to measure the oxygen level in the blood (called pulse oximetry). They also measure blood sugar (glucose) levels and blood levels of any anticonvulsants the person is taking.

For most people known to have a mental disorder, no further testing is needed if their only symptoms are worsening of their typical symptoms, if they are awake and alert, and if results of their physical examination are normal. For most other people, the following additional tests are usually done.

- Blood tests to measure the alcohol level
- Urine tests to check for drugs
- Blood tests to check for HIV infection

Some doctors also routinely do blood tests to measure electrolyte levels and to evaluate kidney function.

Other tests are done based mainly on the symptoms and examination results (see Table on pages 337 to 340). They include

- Computed tomography (CT) or magnetic resonance imaging (MRI) of the brain: If symptoms of mental dysfunction have just appeared or if people have delirium, a headache, a recent head injury, or any abnormality detected during the neurologic examination
- A spinal tap (lumbar puncture): If people have symptoms of meningitis or if results of CT are normal in people with a fever, a headache, or delirium
- Blood tests to evaluate thyroid function: If people are taking lithium, have symptoms of a thyroid disorder, or are over 40 years old and have personality or behavior changes that have

just started (particularly women and people with a family history of thyroid disorders)
- Chest x-ray, urinalysis and culture, a complete blood count, and blood cultures: If people have a fever
- Blood tests to evaluate liver function: If people have symptoms of a liver disorder or a history of alcohol or drug abuse or if specific information about them is not available

TREATMENT

The underlying condition is corrected or treated when possible. Whatever the cause, people who are a danger to themselves or others typically need to be hospitalized and treated whether they are willing or not. Many states require that such decisions be made by someone appointed to make health care decisions for the mentally ill person. If the person has not appointed a decision maker, doctors may contact the next of kin, or a court may appoint an emergency guardian. People who are not dangerous to themselves or others can refuse evaluation and treatment, despite the difficulties their refusal may create for themselves and their family.

O—π KEY POINTS

- Not all changes in personality and behavior are due to mental disorders.
- Other causes include drugs (including withdrawal and side effects), brain disorders, and bodywide disorders that affect the brain.
- Doctors are particularly concerned about people with confusion or delirium, fever, headache, symptoms that suggest brain malfunction, or a recent head injury and about people who want to harm themselves or others.
- Typically, doctors do blood tests to measure the levels of oxygen, sugar (glucose), and any drugs (such as anticonvulsants) the person is taking, and they may do other tests based on the symptoms and results of the examination.

PUPILS, UNEQUAL

The pupil is the black center part of the eye. Pupils get larger (dilate) in dim light and smaller (constrict) in bright light. Usually both pupils are about the same size and respond to light equally. Unequal pupil size is called anisocoria.

If pupil sizes are very unequal, a person may notice the discrepancy. More often, unequal pupils are noticed only during a doctor's examination. Unequal pupils themselves usually cause no symptoms, but, occasionally, a person may have trouble focusing on near objects. Also, the underlying disorder sometimes causes other symptoms such as eye pain and redness, loss of vision, drooping eyelid, double vision, or headache. These more noticeable symptoms are often the reason people seek medical care rather than the unequal pupils.

CAUSES

The **most common cause** of unequal pupils is

- Physiologic anisocoria

Physiologic anisocoria is pupils that are naturally different in size. No disorder is present. About 20% of people have this lifelong condition, which is considered a normal variation. In such people, both pupils react normally to light and darkness and there are no symptoms.

Less commonly, people have unequal pupils because of

- Eye disorders
- Nervous system disorders

Either the larger or the smaller pupil may be the abnormal one depending on the cause. Often, the larger pupil is unable to constrict normally. However, sometimes, as in Horner syndrome, the smaller pupil is unable to widen. If the larger pupil is abnormal, the difference between pupil sizes is greater in bright light. If the smaller pupil is abnormal, the difference is greater in the dark.

Eye disorders that cause unequal pupils include birth defects and eye injury. Also, certain drugs that get into the eye may affect the pupil. Such drugs may be drops intended to treat eye disorders (for example, homatropine

used for certain inflammatory disorders or injuries or pilocarpine used for glaucoma), or they may be drugs or other substances that accidentally get into the eye (for example, scopolamine used as a patch for motion sickness, plants such as jimsonweed, or certain insecticides). Inflammation of the iris (iritis) and certain types of glaucoma cause unequal pupils, but this finding is usually overshadowed by severe eye pain.

Nervous system disorders that cause unequal pupils are those that affect the 3rd cranial nerve or certain parts of the sympathetic or parasympathetic nervous system (the autonomic nervous system). These pathways carry nerve impulses to the pupil and to the muscles that control the eye and eyelid. Thus, people with nervous system disorders that affect the pupil often also have a drooping eyelid, double vision, and/or visibly misaligned eyes. Brain disorders that can affect these pathways include strokes, brain hemorrhage (spontaneous or due to head injury), and, less commonly, certain tumors or infections. Disorders outside the brain that affect the sympathetic nervous system include tumors and injuries that involve the neck or upper part of the chest. Horner syndrome refers to the combination of a constricted pupil, drooping eyelid, and loss of sweating around the affected eye. Horner syndrome is caused by interruption of the sympathetic nerves to an eye from any cause.

EVALUATION

Doctors' first goal is to determine whether the pupils have always been unequal or whether there is another cause such as a drug or disorder. Then, the goal is to decide whether the larger or the smaller pupil represents the problem. The following information can help people decide when a doctor's evaluation is needed and help them know what to expect during the evaluation.

WARNING SIGNS

In people with unequal pupils, certain symptoms and characteristics are cause for concern. They include

- Drooping eyelid (ptosis)
- Double vision
- Loss of vision
- Headache or neck pain
- Eye pain
- Recent head or eye injury

WHEN TO SEE A DOCTOR

People with warning signs should see a doctor right away. People without warning signs but who have any other symptoms should call the doctor. The doctor can decide how quickly they need to be seen based on their symptoms.

People who simply happen to have noticed unequal pupils and feel well can usually wait a week or two to see a doctor.

WHAT THE DOCTOR DOES

Doctors first ask questions about the person's symptoms and medical history, including questions about smoking. Doctors then do a physical examination. What they find during the history and physical examination often suggests a cause of the unequal pupils (see Table, below) and the tests that may need to be done.

SOME CAUSES AND FEATURES OF UNEQUAL PUPILS

Cause	Common Features*
Adie (tonic) pupil (a pupil that does not constrict normally in response to light)	One or both pupils are too wide, do not fully constrict in response to light, and widen slowly after being constricted by light No other symptoms
Birth defects of the iris	Features that are present lifelong Usually other birth defects
Chemicals and drugs (including scopolamine patches, drugs in animal flea collars or sprays, certain aerosol drugs for asthma or COPD such as ipratropium or tiotropium, and organophosphate insecticides) if they contact the eye and some eye drops	In people who use or have been exposed to these substances Sometimes difficulty focusing, particularly on nearby objects
Horner syndrome (disruption of certain nerve fibers that connect the eye and the brain)	On one side of the face, a drooping eyelid, a small pupil that is slow to widen in response to darkness, and decreased sweating If the cause is a disorder (such as migraines or a lung tumor) or an injury, other symptoms
An eye injury or eye surgery	In people who have had an eye injury or eye surgery Sometimes pain with exposure to bright light and/or eye redness
Physiologic anisocoria (pupils that are normally different sizes)	Present for a long time No symptoms or abnormalities found during the examination A difference of less than 1/16 inch (about 1 millimeter) in pupil size and pupils that constrict normally in response to light
Third cranial nerve paralysis	Double vision and a drooping eyelid Sometimes in people who have had a head injury or who have a bulge (aneurysm) in an artery supplying the brain, bleeding in the brain, a brain tumor, or diabetes

*Features include symptoms and the results of the doctor's examination. Features mentioned are typical but not always present.
COPD = chronic obstructive pulmonary disease.

Doctors ask when the person noticed the unequal pupils, whether vision is blurred in the light or dark, and whether the person has any other symptoms. Other important symptoms involving the eyes include a droopy eyelid, double vision, pain with bright light, loss of vision, and eye pain. Other important symptoms that do not involve the eyes include headache, dizziness or loss of balance, cough, chest pain, or shortness of breath. Doctors ask whether the person has recently had a head or eye injury, what eye drops the person has used, and whether the person has ever had an eye disorder or eye surgery.

The physical examination focuses on the head and eyes. Doctors examine the person's pupils in light and dark rooms. Doctors examine whether the eyes move normally when the person follows a doctor's finger moving up, down, left, right, and toward the eyes. Doctors examine the entire eye, usually using a slit lamp (an instrument that enables a doctor to examine the eye under high magnification). Other eye symptoms are evaluated as necessary. Doctors may use eye drops to test how the pupils respond to drugs that cause the pupils to constrict or widen.

Sometimes doctors examine an old photograph of the person (for example, on the person's driver's license) to see whether pupils were previously unequal.

Typically, people with eye symptoms such as pain, redness, blurry vision, or light sensitivity have an eye disorder. People who have a droopy eyelid, double vision, headache, or balance difficulties have Horner syndrome or a 3rd cranial nerve paralysis (possibly due to a brain disorder). People whose only symptom is recent blurry vision, particularly when focusing on near objects, may have a pupil that has been widened by a drug. People with no other symptoms or abnormalities often have chronic conditions such as physiologic anisocoria, birth defects of the iris, or Adie (tonic) pupil (see Table on page 343).

TESTING

Testing is usually unnecessary unless people have other symptoms. People with Horner syndrome or 3rd cranial nerve paralysis usually require magnetic resonance imaging (MRI) or computed tomography (CT).

TREATMENT

Treatment of unequal pupils is unnecessary. However, the underlying disorder may need to be treated.

KEY POINTS

- Unequal pupils are very common and are often only a normal variation.
- Doctors examine the pupils in light and dark rooms to help determine the cause.
- People with a drooping eyelid or double vision may have a serious disorder.

SCROTAL PAIN

Pain in the scrotum (the sac that surrounds and protects the testes) can occur in males of any age, from newborns to older men. The testes are very sensitive, so even minor injuries may cause pain or discomfort.

CAUSES

Pain may be directly related to the testes or be caused by disorders in the scrotum, groin, or abdomen.

COMMON CAUSES

The most common causes of sudden scrotal pain include

- Twisting of a testis (testicular torsion)
- Twisting of the testicular appendage (a small piece of tissue attached to the testis)
- Inflammation of the epididymis (epididymitis)

Testicular torsion occurs when a testis twists on its spermatic cord. The twisting blocks blood flow to the testis, causing pain and sometimes death of the testis. Testicular torsion is more common in newborns and after puberty. Torsion can also occur in the testicular appendage, a small piece of basically functionless tissue that is left over from development of the embryo. Like testicular torsion, the twisting of the testicular appendage can block blood flow, causing pain. Torsion of the testicular appendage is more common among boys aged 7 to 14.

Epididymitis is inflammation of the coiled tube on top of the testis in which sperm mature. Epididymitis is the most common cause of scrotal pain in adults. Epididymitis is usually caused by an infection, typically a sexually transmitted one. However, sometimes there is no infection. In such cases, doctors believe the epididymis becomes inflamed by reverse flow of urine into the epididymis, perhaps because of straining (as when people lift something heavy).

LESS COMMON CAUSES

There are a number of less common causes. Less common causes include

- A hernia in the groin (inguinal hernia)

- Infection of the testis (orchitis), usually caused by mumps or another virus
- Pain from a disorder in the abdomen (such as a kidney stone or appendicitis)
- Injury

Dangerous disorders that sometimes cause scrotal pain include a ruptured abdominal aortic aneurysm and necrotizing infection of the perineum—the area between the genitals and anus—called Fournier gangrene. Cancer of a testis only rarely causes pain.

EVALUATION

The following information can help people decide when immediate medical attention is necessary and help them know what to expect during the evaluation.

WARNING SIGNS

In men with pain in the scrotum, certain symptoms and characteristics are cause for concern. They include

- Sudden, severe pain
- Swelling in the scrotum or groin area, particularly one that cannot be pushed down and that is accompanied by severe pain or vomiting
- Blisters and/or red or black discoloration of the scrotum or the area between the penis and the anus
- Symptoms of severe illness, such as high fever, difficulty breathing, sweating, dizziness, or confusion

WHEN TO SEE A DOCTOR

Men or boys who have warning signs or are in severe pain should see a doctor immediately because some causes of pain can lead to loss of a testis or other severe complications. People without warning signs should see a doctor in a day or two.

WHAT THE DOCTOR DOES

Doctors first ask questions about the person's symptoms and medical history and then do a

SOME CAUSES AND FEATURES OF SCROTAL PAIN

Cause	Common Features*	Tests
Testicular torsion (twisting of a testis)	Severe, constant pain that begins suddenly in one testis	Ultrasonography
	A testis that may be pulled up closer to the body than the other testis	
	Most often occurring in newborns and boys after puberty but sometimes in adults	
Torsion of the testicular appendage (twisting of a small piece of tissue attached to the testis)	Pain that usually develops over several days and that occurs in the top part of the testis	Ultrasonography
	Sometimes swelling around the testis	
	Typically occurring in boys aged 7–14 years	
Epididymitis (inflammation of the epididymis) or epididymo-orchitis (inflammation of an epididymis and testis)	Pain that begins gradually or suddenly in the epididymis and sometimes the testis	Urinalysis and urine culture
	Possibly frequent urination or pain or burning during urination	Sometimes tests for sexually transmitted diseases
	Possibly in men who have recently been doing heavy lifting or straining	
	Often swelling of the scrotum	
	Sometimes a discharge from the penis	
	Typically occurring in boys after puberty and in men	
Injury	In men who have had an injury to the genitals	Ultrasonography
	Often swelling of the scrotum	
Inguinal hernia (a hernia in the groin)	Typically in men who have had painless bulge in the groin for a long time, often in those already known to have a hernia	Only a doctor's examination
	A bulge that	
	■ Feels soft and balloon-like ■ Typically enlarges when men are in an upright position or pressure within the abdomen increases (for example, when bearing down as if having a bowel movement or when doing heavy lifting) ■ Sometimes disappears when lying down ■ Can sometimes be pushed back into the abdomen	
	Pain that begins gradually or suddenly, typically when the bulge cannot be pushed back into the abdomen	
Referred pain (for example, pain that comes from an abdominal aortic aneurysm, stones in the urinary tract, pressure on spinal nerve roots in the lower part of the spine, appendicitis, or a tumor or pain that occurs after a hernia is repaired)	Normal results detected during examination of the scrotum	Depends on examination findings and the suspected cause
	Sometimes abdominal tenderness	
Orchitis (infection of the testis), usually due to a virus, such as the mumps virus	Pain in the scrotum and abdomen, nausea, and fever	Repeated blood tests to measure antibodies to the virus suspected to be the cause
	Swelling and sometimes redness of the scrotum	

(continued)

SOME CAUSES AND FEATURES OF SCROTAL PAIN (continued)

Cause	Common Features*	Tests
Necrotizing infection of the perineum (the area between the genitals and anus), called Fournier gangrene	Severe pain, an ill appearance, fever, and sometimes confusion, difficulty breathing, sweating, or dizziness Redness of the scrotum or blistering or dead tissue in the genital area Sometimes in men who have recently had abdominal surgery More common among older men with diabetes, peripheral arterial disease, or both	Usually only a doctor's examination Sometimes imaging tests

*Features include symptoms and the results of the doctor's examination. Features mentioned are typical but not always present.

physical examination. What they find during the history and physical examination often suggests a cause of the scrotal pain and the tests that may need to be done (see Table, above).

Doctors ask

- Where the pain is located
- How long pain has been present
- Whether there are injuries to the groin area
- About the man's sexual history
- Whether there are any problems urinating (such as burning or discharge)
- Whether there are any disorders that may cause pain to travel to the groin

Although the physical examination concentrates on the genitals, the groin area, and the abdomen, doctors also look for signs of disorders elsewhere that may cause pain to be felt in the scrotum. Doctors first look to identify disorders that require immediate treatment. The onset and nature of the pain and the age of the person can provide clues to the cause.

TESTING

The need for tests depends on what doctors find during the history and physical examination. However, some testing is typically done.

- Urinalysis and urine culture
- Testing for sexually transmitted diseases
- Color Doppler ultrasonography if testicular torsion seems possible

Timely surgery for testicular torsion is critical, so when doctors are very concerned about testicular torsion they may do surgery immediately instead of testing.

TREATMENT

The best treatment of scrotal pain is treatment of the cause of pain. For example, testicular torsion, strangulated hernias, and necrotizing infection require prompt surgery.

Doctors may give analgesics, such as nonsteroidal anti-inflammatory drugs or opioids, to relieve severe pain.

ESSENTIALS FOR OLDER PEOPLE

Testicular torsion is uncommon in older men. When it occurs, the symptoms may be unusual, making the diagnosis more difficult. Epididymitis and orchitis are more common in older men. Sexually transmitted diseases are less often the cause of epididymitis. Occasionally, inguinal hernia, perforation of the colon, or kidney stones (renal colic) may cause scrotal pain in older men.

⊙━┰ KEY POINTS

- Testicular torsion is the first consideration in males with sudden onset of scrotal pain, particularly in children and adolescents.
- Epididymitis is the most common cause of scrotal pain in men, particularly those with discharge or burning or pain during urination.
- Doctors may do surgery instead of imaging tests if they are particularly concerned about testicular torsion.
- Scrotal pain can be caused by pain that is referred from the abdomen.

SCROTAL SWELLING

The scrotum (the sac that surrounds and protects the testes) may swell on one or both sides. Swelling can be small and detectable only by carefully feeling the scrotum, or it may be very large and easily visible. Some disorders that cause swelling of the scrotum are painful (see page 345).

CAUSES

Painless swelling of the scrotum can be caused by generally harmless conditions or can be a sign of cancer. There are several causes.

COMMON CAUSES

The most common causes are

- A collection of fluid in the scrotum (hydrocele)
- A hernia in the groin (inguinal hernia)
- Widening of the veins that carry blood from a testis (varicocele)

A hydrocele is a disorder in which fluid collects between layers of tissue that surround the testis. Hydrocele and inguinal hernia are the most common causes among boys. Up to 20% of men have a varicocele, which can cause infertility.

LESS COMMON CAUSES

Less common causes include

- A cyst in the epididymis (spermatocele)
- A collection of blood in the scrotum (hematocele)
- Accumulation of excess fluid in the body (edema)
- Cancer of a testis

Cancer of a testis is the most concerning cause of painless scrotal swelling. Most often swelling does not turn out to be cancer. But cancer of a testis is the most common solid cancer in men younger than 40 years and it also can occur in younger and older men, so any testicular swelling or lump should be checked by a doctor.

EVALUATION

The following information can help men know how quickly to see a doctor and what to expect during the evaluation.

WARNING SIGNS

In men with a lump in the scrotum, the most concerning signs are

- A solid lump that is attached to or part of the testis
- A balloon-like bulge that extends from the abdomen into the scrotum and cannot be pushed back

WHEN TO SEE A DOCTOR

Men who have a balloon-like swelling that extends from the abdomen into the scrotum and cannot be pushed back could have an inguinal hernia that has become trapped (incarcerated). They should see a doctor right away. If a painless swelling suddenly becomes painful, men should also see a doctor right away because the cause may be an inguinal hernia that has become trapped and the blood supply shut off (strangulated hernia). Other men should see a doctor when an office appointment is available. A delay of a week or so is not harmful.

WHAT THE DOCTOR DOES

Doctors first ask questions about the man's symptoms and then do a physical examination. What they find during the history and physical examination often suggests a cause of the swelling and the tests that may need to be done (see Table on pages 349 to 350).

Doctors ask how long the swelling has been present and whether there is any change in the swelling when the man stands up or lies down or when abdominal pressure increases (such as with coughing or straining to lift something). Doctors also ask about the man's medical history because disorders in other parts of the body (for example, edema related to heart failure or liver failure) may contribute to scrotal swelling.

The physical examination is done with the man standing and lying down. The doctor carefully feels the testis, epididymis, and spermatic

SOME CAUSES AND FEATURES OF SCROTAL SWELLING

Cause	Common Features*	Tests
Edema (accumulation of excess fluid in the body)	Swelling that ■ Feels spongy ■ Occurs on both sides throughout the scrotum ■ Remains indented after pressure is applied and removed (called pitting edema) Often in men with swelling in the legs and sometimes abdomen In men with disorders that can cause swelling such as heart failure or a severe liver or kidney disorder	A doctor's examination Sometimes ultrasonography
Hematocele (a collection of blood in the scrotum)	Swelling that ■ Is painful and tender ■ Develops after an injury	A doctor's examination Sometimes ultrasonography
Hydrocele (a collection of fluid in the scrotum)	Swelling that ■ Feels soft ■ Does not disappear when lying down ■ Cannot be pushed back into the abdomen	A doctor's examination Sometimes ultrasonography
Inguinal hernia (a hernia in the groin)	Typically in men who have had a painless bulge in the groin for a long time, often in those already known to have a hernia A bulge that ■ Feels soft and balloon-like ■ Often can also be felt above the scrotum ■ Typically enlarges when men are in an upright position or when pressure within the abdomen increases (for example, when bearing down as if having a bowel movement or when doing heavy lifting) ■ Sometimes disappears when lying down ■ Can sometimes be pushed back into the abdomen Sometimes pain that begins gradually or suddenly, typically when the bulge cannot be pushed back into the abdomen	Only a doctor's examination
Lymphedema (accumulation of lymph fluid)—for example, due to a tropical worm infection called filariasis or present from birth	Rubbery swelling throughout the scrotum No indentations when the area is pressed	A doctor's examination Sometimes ultrasonography

(continued)

SOME CAUSES AND FEATURES OF SCROTAL SWELLING *(continued)*

Cause	Common Features*	Tests
Spermatocele (a cyst in the epididymis)	A lump near the top of the testis	A doctor's examination Sometimes ultrasonography
Testicular cancer	A hard lump attached to or in the testis Possibly dull, aching pain or, if the cancer bleeds, sudden sharp pain	Ultrasonography Blood tests Sometimes CT of the abdomen, pelvis, and chest
Varicocele (widening of the veins that carry blood from a testis)	Swelling that ■ Feels like a bag of worms ■ Usually occurs on the left side Possibly pain and a feeling of fullness when standing Possibly a shrunken testis (testicular atrophy)	Only a doctor's examination

*Features include symptoms and the results of the doctor's examination. Features mentioned are typical but not always present.
CT = computed tomography.

---

cord to detect the exact location of the swelling or lump, and whether the swelling is tender. Sometimes the doctor shines a bright light behind the scrotum to see if light passes through (transillumination). Light can often pass through a collection of fluid (such as a hydrocele) but not through a solid lump (such as a cancer).

TESTING

Sometimes the doctor can determine the cause of the swelling based on the symptoms and the results of the physical examination. If the symptoms and physical examination do not reveal the cause, testing is usually needed. Often the first test is ultrasonography. Ultrasonography is done when

■ Doctors are unsure of the diagnosis
■ Doctors detect a hydrocele during the examination (ultrasonography may show the source of the fluid)
■ Transillumination does not show fluid in the area of swelling

Depending on the results of ultrasonography, further testing may be done for cancer of a testis.

Testing for testicular cancer includes blood tests and sometimes computed tomography (CT) of the abdomen, pelvis, and chest.

TREATMENT

The best way to treat scrotal swelling is to treat the cause of the swelling. Treatment is not always needed. Sometimes doctors try to reduce an inguinal hernia by pushing gently against the protruding intestine and forcing it back into place.

O—π KEY POINTS

■ Men and boys with scrotal swelling, even if it does not cause pain, should see a doctor.
■ Cancer of a testis is a concern in all boys and men, especially those who are younger than 40.
■ The diagnosis is usually evident from the symptoms, physical examination findings, and ultrasonography.

SEMEN, BLOOD IN

Blood in semen (called hematospermia, because sperm are mixed with blood in the semen) can be a frightening symptom, but it is usually not a sign of a serious problem. Blood in semen is not usually a sign of cancer and does not affect sexual function.

Semen is composed of sperm from the epididymis and fluids from the seminal vesicles, prostate, and small mucous glands that provide fluids to nourish sperm. Thus, blood could come from injury to any of these structures.

CAUSES

Most cases of blood in semen are

- Idiopathic, that is they arise without warning and doctors cannot find a cause

Such cases resolve on their own within a few days to a few months.

The most common known cause is

- Prostate biopsy

Bleeding can last a few weeks or so after a prostate biopsy. Bleeding can also occur during the first week or two after a vasectomy.

Less common causes include benign prostatic hyperplasia (a benign enlargement of the prostate gland), infections (for example, prostatitis, urethritis, or epididymitis), and prostate cancer (in men over 35 to 40 years). Occasionally, blood in semen occurs in men who have tumors of the seminal vesicles and testes. A mass of abnormal blood vessels (hemangioma) in the urethra or the ducts that connect the testes to the urethra (spermatic ducts) may cause quite a bit of blood to appear in semen.

Schistosoma haematobium, a parasitic worm that commonly causes infections in Africa (and to a lesser extent India and parts of the Middle East), can invade the urinary tract, causing blood to appear in the urine and often in semen. Schistosomiasis is unlikely in men who have not spent time in these areas. Tuberculosis may cause blood in semen.

EVALUATION

Although blood in semen can be alarming, it is not usually serious, and it does not require an immediate evaluation. The following information can help men decide when a doctor's evaluation is needed and help them know what to expect during the evaluation.

WARNING SIGNS

Certain symptoms and characteristics are cause for concern. They include

- Bleeding lasting longer than 1 month
- A lump that can be felt in the scrotum
- Travel to a region where schistosomiasis is prevalent

WHEN TO SEE A DOCTOR

Men who have warning signs should see a doctor. Timing is not critical, and a delay of a week or so is not harmful. Men who do not have warning signs and are younger than age 35 do not need to see a doctor unless they have other symptoms, such as pain in the scrotum or groin or pain during urination. Men who do not have warning signs and are over 35 should see a doctor within a few weeks.

WHAT THE DOCTOR DOES

Doctors first ask questions about the man's symptoms and medical history. Doctors then do a physical examination. What they find during the history and physical examination often suggests a cause of the blood and the tests that may need to be done.

Doctors ask

- When the man first noticed the blood
- Whether he has recently had a biopsy of the prostate gland
- Whether he has any symptoms that might suggest a urinary tract infection (for example, blood in the urine, difficulty starting or stopping urine flow, burning during urination, or a discharge from the penis)
- Whether he has a tendency to bleed excessively or a disorder that causes bleeding

■ Whether he has a prostate disorder (for example, benign prostatic hyperplasia)

Doctors examine the genitals for redness, a lump, or tenderness. A digital rectal examination is done to examine the prostate for enlargement, tenderness, or a lump.

Doctors can often determine what causes are likely after taking a history and doing an examination. For example, the following kinds of information can provide clues. In men with an abnormal prostate detected during a digital rectal examination, a prostate disorder is likely, such as prostate cancer, benign prostatic hyperplasia, or prostatitis. In men with urethral discharge, urethritis is likely. In men with tenderness of the epididymis, epididymitis is likely. However, such abnormalities may not be the cause of blood in semen. For example, most older men have benign prostatic hyperplasia, yet few of them have blood in semen.

In men who have bleeding that lasted less than a month, have not been in areas where schistosomiasis is prevalent, and have no warning signs or abnormalities on examination, a cause cannot usually be found.

TESTING

In most cases, especially in men younger than 35 to 40 years, and men who recently had a prostate biopsy, blood in semen is not serious and resolves on its own. Urinalysis and urine culture are usually done. Further testing is not usually needed unless there are urinary symptoms that suggest an infection or other disorder.

However, if the doctor suspects certain potentially serious disorders, further testing is done, for example, some doctors typically do tests for prostate cancer on men over 40.

Testing includes prostate-specific antigen (PSA) testing and transrectal ultrasonography (TRUS). Occasionally, magnetic resonance imaging (MRI) and cystoscopy (which involves inserting a thin, flexible viewing tube through the urethra to enable doctors to see inside the urethra and bladder) are needed. Semen inspection and analysis are rarely done.

TREATMENT

Treatment is directed at the cause if known. Often no treatment is needed, and the blood goes away on its own.

KEY POINTS

■ In most cases, a cause cannot be found or bleeding occurs after a prostate biopsy.
■ Blood in semen is not usually a sign of cancer and does not affect sexual function.
■ More detailed evaluation is needed mainly for men with symptoms that last longer than a month, who are over 40, or who have abnormal findings.
■ Doctors may need to test for schistosomiasis in men who have traveled to Africa, India, or certain parts of the Middle East.

SHORTNESS OF BREATH (DYSPNEA)

Shortness of breath—what doctors call dyspnea—is the unpleasant sensation of having difficulty breathing. People experience and describe shortness of breath differently depending on the cause.

The rate and depth of breathing normally increase during exercise and at high altitudes, but the increase seldom causes discomfort. Breathing is also increased at rest in people with many disorders, whether of the lungs or other parts of the body. For example, people with a fever generally breathe faster.

With dyspnea, faster breathing is accompanied by the sensation of running out of air. People feel as if they cannot breathe fast enough or deeply enough. They may notice that more effort is needed to expand the chest when breathing in or to expel air when breathing out. They may also have the uncomfortable sensation that inhaling (inspiration) is urgently needed before exhaling (expiration) is completed and have various sensations often described as tightness in the chest.

Other symptoms, such as cough or chest pain, may be present depending on the cause of dyspnea.

CAUSES

Dyspnea is usually caused by disorders of the lungs or heart (see Table on pages 355 to 357). The most common causes overall include

- Asthma
- Pneumonia
- Chronic obstructive pulmonary disease (COPD)
- A heart attack or angina (chest pain due to inadequate blood flow and oxygen to the heart—called myocardial ischemia)
- Physical deconditioning (weakening of muscles and the heart due to inactivity)
- Pulmonary embolism (sudden blockage of an artery of the lung, usually by a blood clot)

The most common cause in people with a chronic lung or heart disorder is

- Worsening of their disease

However, such people may also develop another disorder. For example, people with long-standing asthma may have a heart attack, or people with chronic heart failure may develop pneumonia.

LUNG DISORDERS

People who have lung disorders often experience dyspnea when they physically exert themselves. During exercise, the body makes more carbon dioxide and uses more oxygen. The respiratory center in the brain speeds up breathing when blood levels of oxygen are low or blood levels of carbon dioxide are high. If the heart or lungs are not functioning normally, even a little exertion can dramatically increase the breathing rate and dyspnea. Dyspnea is so unpleasant that people avoid exertion. As the lung disorder becomes more severe, dyspnea may occur even at rest.

Dyspnea may result from restrictive or obstructive lung disorders.

In restrictive lung disorders (such as idiopathic pulmonary fibrosis), lungs become stiff and require more effort to expand during inhalation. Severe curvature of the spine (scoliosis) can also restrict breathing because it reduces movement of the rib cage.

In obstructive disorders (such as COPD or asthma), resistance to airflow is increased because the airways are narrowed. Because airways widen during inhalation, air can usually be pulled in. However, because airways narrow during exhalation, air cannot be exhaled from the lungs as fast as normal, and people wheeze and breathing is labored. Dyspnea results when too much air is left in the lungs after exhaling.

People with asthma have dyspnea when they have an attack. Doctors typically advise people to keep an inhaler on hand to use during an attack. The drug in the inhaler helps open the airways.

HEART FAILURE

The heart pumps blood through the lungs. If the heart is pumping inadequately (called heart failure), fluid may accumulate in the lungs—a disorder called pulmonary edema. This disorder causes dyspnea that is often accompanied by a feeling of smothering or heaviness in the chest. The fluid accumulation in the lungs may also narrow the airways and cause wheezing—a disorder called cardiac asthma.

Some people with heart failure have orthopnea, paroxysmal nocturnal dyspnea, or both. Orthopnea is shortness of breath that occurs when people lie down and is relieved by sitting up. Paroxysmal nocturnal dyspnea is a sudden, often terrifying attack of dyspnea during sleep. People awaken gasping and must sit or stand to take a breath. This disorder is an extreme form of orthopnea and a sign of severe heart failure.

ANEMIA

When people have anemia or have lost a large amount of blood because of an injury, they have fewer red blood cells. Red blood cells carry oxygen to the tissues, so in these people, the amount of oxygen that blood can deliver is decreased. Most people with anemia are comfortable sitting still. However, they often feel dyspnea during physical activity because the blood cannot deliver the increased oxygen the body requires. Thus, they breathe rapidly and deeply in a reflex effort to try to increase the amount of oxygen in the blood.

OTHER CAUSES

If a large amount of acid accumulates in the blood (called metabolic acidosis), people may feel out of breath and begin to pant quickly. Severe kidney failure, sudden worsening of diabetes mellitus, and ingestion of certain drugs or poisons can cause metabolic acidosis. Anemia and heart failure may contribute to dyspnea in people with kidney failure.

In hyperventilation syndrome, people feel that they cannot get enough air, and they breathe heavily and rapidly. This syndrome is commonly caused by anxiety rather than a physical problem. Many people who experience it are frightened, may have chest pain, and may believe they are having a heart attack. They may have a change in consciousness, usually described as feeling that events occurring around them are far away, and they may feel tingling in their hands and feet and around their mouth.

EVALUATION

The following information can help people decide whether a doctor's evaluation is needed and help them know what to expect during the evaluation.

WARNING SIGNS

In people with dyspnea, the following symptoms are of particular concern:

- Shortness of breath at rest
- A decreased level of consciousness, agitation, or confusion
- Chest discomfort or the feeling the heart is pounding or racing or has skipped a beat (palpitations)
- Weight loss
- Night sweats

WHEN TO SEE A DOCTOR

People who have shortness of breath at rest, chest pain, palpitations, a decreased level of consciousness, agitation, or confusion or have difficulty moving air in or out of their lungs should go to the hospital right away. Such people may need immediate testing, treatment, and sometimes admission to the hospital. Other people should call a doctor. The doctor can determine how rapidly they need to be evaluated based on the nature and severity of their symptoms, their age, and any underlying medical conditions. Typically, they should be evaluated within a few days.

WHAT THE DOCTOR DOES

Doctors first ask questions about the person's symptoms and medical history. Doctors then do a physical examination. What doctors find during the history and physical examination often suggests a cause and the tests that may need to be done (see Table on pages 355 to 357).

Doctors ask questions to determine

- When shortness of breath started
- Whether it started abruptly or gradually
- How long the person has felt short of breath
- Whether any conditions (such as cold, exertion, exposure to allergens, or lying down) trigger it or make it worse

The person is also asked questions about past medical history (including any lung or heart disorders), a history of smoking, any family

SOME CAUSES AND FEATURES OF SHORTNESS OF BREATH

Cause	Common Features*	Tests†
Acute (develops within minutes or hours)		
Anxiety disorder—hyperventilation	Shortness of breath related to a specific situation, often accompanied by agitation and tingling or numbness in the fingers and/or around the mouth Normal results on the heart and lung examination	A doctor's examination
Asthma‡	Wheezing that starts spontaneously or after exposure to specific stimuli (such as pollen or another allergen, an upper respiratory infection, cold air, or exercise) Usually a history of asthma	A doctor's examination Sometimes one or more of the following tests: ■ Tests to evaluate how well the lungs are functioning (pulmonary function testing), or measurement of peak air flow (how fast air can be exhaled) ■ Measurement of lung function before and after exercise or administration of methacholine (a drug that narrows airways) ■ Sometimes use of bronchodilators (drugs that widen airways) to see whether symptoms go away
A foreign object that has been inhaled	A cough or high-pitched wheezing that starts suddenly in people (typically infants or young children) without any symptoms of an upper respiratory infection or other illness	A chest x-ray or CT Sometimes bronchoscopy
A heart attack or acute myocardial ischemia (inadequate blood flow and oxygen supply to the heart)	Deep chest pressure that may or may not radiate to the arm or jaw, particularly in people with risk factors for coronary artery disease	Electrocardiography Blood tests to measure substances called cardiac markers, which are released into the blood when the heart is damaged
Heart failure§	Often swelling (edema) of the legs Shortness of breath that worsens while lying flat (orthopnea) or that appears 1–2 hours after falling asleep (paroxysmal nocturnal dyspnea) Sounds suggesting fluid in the lungs, heard through a stethoscope Frothy, pink sputum, sometimes with blood streaks	A chest x-ray Sometimes a blood test to measure brain natriuretic peptide (BNP), a substance that is produced when the heart is strained Sometimes echocardiography
Papillary muscles (muscles holding the heart valves) that malfunction or tear	Chest pain that occurs suddenly A new, loud heart murmur and lung congestion detected during a doctor's examination Often in people who have had a recent heart attack	Echocardiography

(continued)

SOME CAUSES AND FEATURES OF SHORTNESS OF BREATH *(continued)*

Cause	Common Features*	Tests†
Pneumothorax (a collapsed lung)	Sharp chest pain and rapid breathing that start suddenly May follow an injury or occur spontaneously, especially in tall, thin people and in people with COPD	A chest x-ray
Pulmonary embolism (sudden blockage of an artery in a lung, usually by a blood clot)	Sudden appearance of sharp chest pain that usually worsens when inhaling A rapid heart rate and a rapid breathing rate Often risk factors for pulmonary embolism, such as cancer, immobility (as results from being bedbound), blood clots in the legs, pregnancy, use of birth control pills (oral contraceptives) or other drugs that contain estrogen, recent surgery or hospitalization, or a family history of the disorder	Specialized lung imaging tests, such as CT angiography or ventilation/perfusion (V/Q) scanning
Subacute (develops over hours or days)		
Angina or coronary artery disease	Deep chest pressure that may or may not radiate to the arm or jaw, often triggered by physical exertion Often in people with risk factors for coronary artery disease	Electrocardiography Stress testing Sometimes cardiac catheterization
A chronic obstructive pulmonary disease (COPD) flare-up	Often a cough that may or may not produce sputum (productive or nonproductive) Wheezing and breathing through pursed lips In people who already have COPD	A doctor's examination Sometimes a chest x-ray
Pneumonia	Fever, a feeling of illness, and a productive cough Sudden appearance of sharp chest pain when taking deep breaths Certain abnormal breath sounds, heard through a stethoscope	A chest x-ray
Chronic (present for many weeks to years)		
Anemia	Shortness of breath during exertion, progressing to shortness of breath at rest Normal lung examination results and oxygen levels in the blood	A complete blood cell count
Interstitial lung disease	Abnormal lung sounds called crackles, heard through a stethoscope	High-resolution CT of the chest

(continued)

SOME CAUSES AND FEATURES OF SHORTNESS OF BREATH (continued)

Cause	Common Features*	Tests†
Obstructive lung disease	A history of extensive smoking, a barrel-shaped chest, and difficulty moving air in and out of the lungs Usually in people who already have COPD	A chest x-ray Pulmonary function testing (at the initial evaluation)
Physical deconditioning	Shortness of breath only during exertion In older people with a sedentary lifestyle	A doctor's examination
Pleural effusion (fluid in the chest cavity)	Sometimes a history of cancer, heart failure, rheumatoid arthritis, systemic lupus erythematosus (lupus), or acute pneumonia	A chest x-ray Often CT of the chest and thoracentesis
Restrictive lung disease	Progressive dyspnea in people known to have been exposed to inhaled irritants at work (occupational exposure) or to have a disorder of the nervous system	A chest x-ray Pulmonary function testing (at the initial evaluation)
Stable angina or coronary artery disease	Deep chest pressure that may or may not radiate to the arm or jaw, often triggered by physical exertion Often in people with risk factors for coronary artery disease	Electrocardiography Stress testing Sometimes cardiac catheterization

*Features include symptoms and results of the doctor's examination. Features mentioned are typical but not always present.
†Doctors almost always measure the oxygen level in the blood and, unless symptoms are clearly a mild flare-up of an already diagnosed chronic disorder, take a chest x-ray.
‡Asthma can also be a subacute cause of dyspnea.
§Heart failure can also be chronic cause of dyspnea.
COPD = chronic obstructive pulmonary disease; CT = computed tomography.

members who have had high blood pressure or high cholesterol levels, and risk factors for pulmonary embolism (such as recent hospitalization, surgery, or long-distance travel).

The physical examination focuses on the heart and lungs. Doctors listen to the lungs for congestion, wheezing, and abnormal sounds called crackles. They listen to the heart for murmurs (suggesting a heart valve disorder). Swelling of both legs suggests heart failure, but swelling of only one leg is more likely to result from a blood clot in the leg. A blood clot in the leg may break off and travel to the blood vessels in the lungs, causing pulmonary embolism.

TESTING

To help determine the severity of the problem, doctors measure oxygen levels in the blood with a sensor placed on a finger (pulse oximetry). Typically, they also take a chest x-ray unless the person clearly appears to be having a mild flare-up of an already diagnosed chronic disorder, such as asthma or heart failure. The chest x-ray can show evidence of a collapsed lung, pneumonia, and many other lung and heart abnormalities. For most adults, electrocardiography (ECG) is done to check for inadequate blood flow to the heart.

Other tests are done based on results of the examination (see Table). Tests to evaluate how well the lungs are functioning (pulmonary function testing) are done when the doctor's examination suggests a lung disorder but the chest x-ray does not provide a diagnosis. Pulmonary function tests can measure the degree of restriction or obstruction and the ability of the lungs to transport oxygen from the air to the blood. A lung problem may include restrictive and obstructive abnormalities as well as abnormal oxygen transport.

For people at moderate or high risk of pulmonary embolism, specialized imaging tests, such as computed tomography (CT) angiography or ventilation/perfusion scanning, are done. For people at low risk of pulmonary embolism, a D-dimer test may be done. This blood test helps identify or rule out a blood clot. Other tests may be necessary to diagnose and further evaluate anemia, heart problems, and certain specific lung problems.

TREATMENT

Treatment of dyspnea is directed at the cause. People with a low blood oxygen level are given supplemental oxygen using plastic nasal prongs or a plastic mask worn over the face. In severe cases, particularly if people cannot breathe deeply or rapidly enough, breathing may be assisted by mechanical ventilation using a breathing tube inserted in the windpipe or a tight-fitting face mask.

Morphine may be given intravenously to reduce anxiety and the discomfort of dyspnea in people with various disorders, including a heart attack, pulmonary embolism, and a terminal illness.

O—π KEY POINTS

- Shortness of breath (dyspnea) is usually caused by lung or heart disorders.
- In people with a chronic lung or heart disorder (such as asthma), the most common cause of dyspnea is a flare-up of the chronic disorder, but these people can also develop a new problem (such as a heart attack) that contributes to or causes dyspnea.
- People who have dyspnea at rest, a decreased level of consciousness, or confusion should go to the hospital immediately for emergency evaluation.
- To determine the severity of the problem, doctors measure oxygen levels in the blood with a sensor placed on a finger (pulse oximetry).
- Doctors evaluate people for inadequate delivery of blood and oxygen to the heart (myocardial ischemia) and for pulmonary embolism, but sometimes symptoms of these disorders are vague.

SMELL, LOSS OF (ANOSMIA)

Anosmia is complete loss of smell. Hyposmia is partial loss of smell. Most people with anosmia can recognize salty, sweet, sour, and bitter substances but cannot tell the difference between specific flavors. The ability to tell the difference between flavors actually depends on smell, not the taste receptors on the tongue. Therefore, people with anosmia often complain of losing their sense of taste and of not enjoying food.

CAUSES

Anosmia occurs when swelling or another blockage of the nasal passages prevents odors from reaching the olfactory area or when parts of the olfactory area or its connections to the brain are destroyed (see Table on page 361). The olfactory area is where odors are detected and is located high in the nose (see art box on page 360).

COMMON CAUSES

The most common causes include

- Head injury (young adults)
- Viral infections and Alzheimer disease (older adults)

A common cause of permanent loss of smell is a head injury, as may occur in a car accident. Head injury can damage or destroy fibers of the olfactory nerves (the pair of cranial nerves that connect smell receptors to the brain) where they pass through the roof of the nasal cavity. Sometimes the injury involves a fracture of the bone (cribriform plate) that separates the brain from the nasal cavity. Damage to the olfactory nerves can also result from infections (such as abscesses) or tumors near the cribriform plate.

Another common cause is an upper respiratory infection, especially influenza (flu). Flu may be the cause in up to one quarter of people with hyposmia or anosmia. Alzheimer disease and some other degenerative brain disorders (such as multiple sclerosis) can damage the olfactory nerves, commonly causing loss of smell.

LESS COMMON CAUSES

Drugs can contribute to anosmia in susceptible people. Polyps, tumors, other infections in the nose, and seasonal allergies (allergic rhinitis) may interfere with the ability to smell. Occasionally, serious infections of the nasal sinuses or radiation therapy for cancer causes a loss of smell or taste that lasts for months or even becomes permanent. These conditions can damage or destroy smell receptors. The role of tobacco is uncertain. A very few people are born without a sense of smell.

EVALUATION

The following information can help people decide whether a doctor's evaluation is needed and help them know what to expect during the evaluation.

WARNING SIGNS

The following findings are of particular concern:

- Recent head injury
- Symptoms of nervous system dysfunction, such as weakness, trouble with balance, or difficulty seeing, speaking, or swallowing
- Sudden start of symptoms

WHEN TO SEE A DOCTOR

People who have warning signs should see a doctor within a day or two. Other people should see a doctor when possible, but a doctor's evaluation is not urgent unless other symptoms develop.

WHAT THE DOCTOR DOES

Doctors first ask questions about the person's symptoms and medical history and then do a physical examination. What doctors find during the history and physical examination often suggests a cause and the tests that may need to be done (see Table on page 361).

Doctors ask about onset and duration of anosmia and its relation to any cold, bout of flu, or head injury. They note other symptoms such

HOW PEOPLE SENSE FLAVORS

To distinguish most flavors, the brain needs information about both smell and taste. These sensations are communicated to the brain from the nose and mouth. Several areas of the brain integrate the information, enabling people to recognize and appreciate flavors.

A small area on the mucous membrane that lines the nose (the olfactory epithelium) contains specialized nerve cells called smell receptors. These receptors have hairlike projections (cilia) that detect odors. Airborne molecules entering the nasal passage stimulate the cilia, triggering a nerve impulse in nearby nerve fibers. The fibers extend upward through the bone that forms the roof of the nasal cavity (cribriform plate) and connect to enlargements of nerve cells (olfactory bulbs). These bulbs form the cranial nerves of smell (olfactory nerves). The impulse travels through the olfactory bulbs, along the olfactory nerves, to the brain. The brain interprets the impulse as a distinct odor. Also, the area of the brain where memories of odors are stored—the smell and taste center in the middle part of the temporal lobe—is stimulated. The memories enable a person to distinguish and identify many different odors experienced over a lifetime.

Thousands of tiny taste buds cover most of the tongue's surface. A taste bud contains several types of taste receptors with cilia. Each type detects one of the five basic tastes: sweet, salty, sour, bitter, or savory (also called umami, the taste of monosodium glutamate). These tastes can be detected all over the tongue, but certain areas are more sensitive for each taste. Sweetness is most easily identified by the tip of the tongue, whereas saltiness is best appreciated at the front sides of the tongue. Sourness is best perceived along the sides of the tongue, and bitter sensations are readily detected in the back one third of the tongue. Food placed in the mouth stimulates the cilia, triggering a nerve impulse in nearby nerve fibers, which are connected to the cranial nerves of taste (the facial and glossopharyngeal nerves). The impulse travels along these cranial nerves to the brain, which interprets the combination of impulses from the different types of taste receptors as a distinct taste. Sensory information about the food's smell, taste, texture, and temperature is processed by the brain to produce a distinct flavor when food enters the mouth and is chewed.

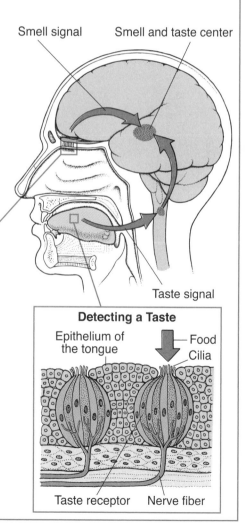

Smell signal   Smell and taste center

Taste signal

Detecting a Taste

Epithelium of the tongue   Food
Cilia

Taste receptor   Nerve fiber

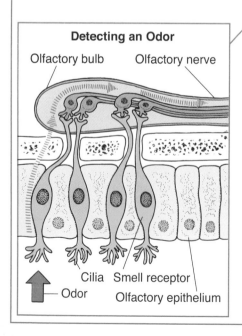

Detecting an Odor

Olfactory bulb   Olfactory nerve

Cilia   Smell receptor
Odor   Olfactory epithelium

SOME CAUSES AND FEATURES OF ANOSMIA

Cause	Common Features*	Tests
Blockage within the nose		
Nasal allergies	In people who have chronic allergy symptoms (such as nasal congestion and a clear discharge) No pain Symptoms that often occur during certain seasons or after exposure to specific substances	A doctor's examination
Nasal polyps	Polyps that are usually seen during the examination	A doctor's examination
Destruction of smell receptors		
Chronic sinusitis	A thick, foul-smelling nasal discharge most or all of the time Previous sinus infections	A doctor's examination Usually CT
Some viral upper respiratory infections (such as influenza)	Loss of smell that occurs after an infection	A doctor's examination
Tumors (a rare cause)	Possibly vision problems or only loss of smell	CT MRI
Drugs (such as amphetamines, enalapril, estrogen, naphazoline, phenothiazines, and reserpine or use of decongestants for a long time)	Usually in people who report taking such drugs	A doctor's examination
Toxins (such as cadmium and manganese)	Usually in people who report exposure to such toxins	A doctor's examination
Destruction of olfactory pathways in the brain		
Alzheimer disease	Progressive confusion and loss of recent memory	MRI Sequential memory tests
Head injuries	In people who have had a head injury	CT
Degenerative neurologic disorders (such as multiple sclerosis)	Intermittent episodes of other symptoms of nervous system dysfunction, such as weakness, numbness, or difficulty speaking, seeing, or swallowing	MRI Sometimes a spinal tap
Brain surgery or infection	In people who have had brain surgery or a brain infection	CT or MRI
Brain tumors	Sometimes headache and/or symptoms of nervous system dysfunction	CT or MRI

*Features include symptoms and results of the doctor's examination. Features mentioned are typical but not always present.
CT = computed tomography; MRI = magnetic resonance imaging.

as a runny or stuffy nose and whether any nasal discharge is watery, bloody, thick, or foul-smelling. Doctors seek out any neurologic symptoms, especially those that involve a change in mental status (for example, difficulty with short-term memory) or the cranial nerves (for example, double vision or difficulty speaking or swallowing). Questions about the person's medical history involve sinus disorders, head injury or surgery, allergies, drugs used, and exposure to chemicals or fumes.

During the physical examination, doctors inspect the nasal passages for swelling, inflammation, discharge, and polyps. Doctors also do a complete neurologic examination that is particularly focused on mental status and the cranial nerves.

TESTING

To test smell, doctors hold common fragrant substances (such as soap, a vanilla bean, coffee, and cloves) under the person's nose, one nostril at a time. The person is then asked to identify the smell. Smell can also be tested more formally using standardized commercial smell test kits. One kit requires the person to scratch and sniff many different smell samples and try to identify them. Another kit contains diluted samples of a smelly chemical. Doctors see how dilute the sample can be before the person can no longer smell the chemical.

If there is no clear cause of anosmia, computed tomography (CT) or magnetic resonance imaging (MRI) of the head (including the sinuses) is done to look for structural abnormalities (such as a tumor, an abscess, or a fracture).

TREATMENT

Doctors treat the cause of the anosmia. For example, people with sinus infections and irritation may be treated with steam inhalation, nasal sprays, antibiotics, and sometimes surgery. However, the sense of smell does not always return even after successful treatment of sinusitis. Tumors are surgically removed or treated with radiation, but such treatment usually does not restore the sense of smell. Polyps in the nose are removed, sometimes restoring the ability to smell. People who smoke tobacco should stop.

There are no treatments for anosmia itself. People who retain some sense of smell may find that adding concentrated flavoring agents to food improves their enjoyment of eating. Smoke alarms, important in all homes, are even more essential for people with anosmia because they cannot smell smoke. Doctors recommend that people with anosmia use caution before consuming stored food and using natural gas for cooking or heating, because they may have difficulty detecting food spoilage or gas leaks.

ESSENTIALS FOR OLDER PEOPLE

The ability to smell decreases as people age. The decrease is caused by a loss of smell receptors. People typically notice changes in smell by age 60. After age 70, changes are substantial.

KEY POINTS

- Anosmia may be part of normal aging.
- Common causes include upper respiratory infection, sinusitis, and head injury.
- An imaging test such as CT or MRI is typically needed unless the cause is obvious to the doctor.

SNORING

Snoring is a raspy noise produced in the nose and throat during sleep. It is quite common and becomes more common as people age. About 57% of men and 40% of women snore. However, what qualifies as snoring depends on the person listening to it, and how loudly and how much a person snores vary from night to night. Thus, the percentage of people who snore is only an estimate.

A few people snore quietly, but snoring is usually noticeable and is sometimes loud enough to be heard in another room. Snoring is distressing only to other people, typically a bed partner or roommate trying to sleep. People seldom know that they snore unless others tell them.

Snoring can have significant social consequences. It frequently causes stress between the snorer and bed partner or roommates. Snorers have been assaulted and rarely even murdered because of their snoring.

Other symptoms such as waking up frequently, gasping or choking during sleep, excessive daytime sleepiness, and morning headache may also be present, depending on what is causing the snoring.

Snoring results from fluttering of soft tissues in the nose and throat, particularly the soft palate (the back part of the roof of the mouth). The fact that people do not snore when they are awake suggests that relaxation of muscles during sleep is the cause. This relaxation is thought to decrease the stiffness of tissue, making it more likely to flutter (just as a cloth flag is more likely to flutter in a breeze than a similar-sized sheet of metal). Also, tissue relaxation probably narrows parts of the upper airway, making flutter more likely.

CAUSES

Primary snoring is snoring that does not cause people to wake up more often than normal during the night. During sleep, the amount of airflow into the lungs and oxygen level in the blood are normal. Because these factors are normal, people do not have excessive daytime sleepiness.

SLEEP-DISORDERED BREATHING

Snoring is often a symptom of sleep-disordered breathing. Sleep-disordered breathing ranges from upper airway resistance syndrome to obstructive sleep apnea (OSA). These forms differ mainly in how much of the airway is blocked (degree of airway obstruction) and what the effects of the blockage are. The effects involve mainly disturbances of sleep and/or airflow.

People with OSA stop breathing briefly more than 5 times per hour during sleep and have one or more of the following:

- Daytime sleepiness, episodes of unintentionally falling asleep, unrefreshing sleep, fatigue, or insomnia
- Waking up with breath holding, gasping, or choking
- Reports by a bed partner of loud snoring, interruptions in breathing, or both during the person's sleep

People with upper airway resistance syndrome have excessive daytime sleepiness or other symptoms but do not have all the features required for doctors to diagnose OSA.

COMPLICATIONS

Although snoring itself has no adverse effects, people who have OSA have an increased risk of high blood pressure, stroke, and heart disorders.

RISK FACTORS

Risk factors for snoring include

- Older age (over 50)
- Obesity, particularly fat distributed around the neck or midriff
- Use of alcohol or other sedatives
- Long-term (chronic) nasal congestion
- A small jaw or a jaw that is farther back than normal
- Menopause
- Male sex
- Black race
- Pregnancy

Snoring also appears to run in families.

EVALUATION

For doctors, the main goal is identifying people who are at high risk of OSA. Most people who snore do not have OSA. However, most people with OSA do snore.

WARNING SIGNS

The following symptoms are cause for concern:

- Episodes of not breathing or of choking during sleep (as witnessed by a bed partner)
- Headaches when waking up in the morning
- Extreme sleepiness during the day
- Obesity
- Very loud, constant snoring

WHEN TO SEE A DOCTOR

People with warning signs should see a doctor at some point because testing may be needed. Timing of the appointment is not critical and can be when mutually convenient.

People without warning signs are unlikely to need testing and may wish to try general measures to help reduce snoring before they call a doctor. If these measures are unsuccessful and snoring is very bothersome to their bed partner, people should see their doctor.

WHAT THE DOCTOR DOES

Doctors first ask questions about the snoring and other symptoms and then about the person's other medical history. Because several important findings are noticed mainly by others, doctors try to interview the bed partner or roommates when possible. Doctors then do a physical examination. What they find during the history and physical examination helps them decide whether tests for OSA need to be done.

Doctors ask how severe the snoring is. For example, they may ask the bed partner

- Whether the person snores every night and, if not, how many nights
- Whether the person snores all night long and, if not, how much of the night
- How loud the snoring is

The person and bed partner are also asked to describe

- How often the person seems to wake up during the night

- Whether the person stopped breathing or had episodes of gasping or choking
- Whether sleep seems nonrefreshing or the person has morning headaches
- How sleepy the person is during the day

Doctors also ask about disorders that may be associated with OSA, particularly high blood pressure, heart disorders, stroke, acid reflux, atrial fibrillation (an abnormal heart rhythm), depression, and diabetes. They ask about the amount of alcohol the person drinks, including how close to bedtime the person drinks it. Whether the person takes any sedating or muscle-relaxing drugs is also important.

During the physical examination, doctors measure the person's height and weight in order to calculate body mass index (BMI). The higher the person's BMI, the greater the risk of OSA. Doctors may measure the neck. OSA is more likely when the neck is larger than about 16 inches for women and about 17 inches for men.

Doctors also inspect the nose and mouth for signs of airway obstruction and risk factors for snoring—for example, nasal polyps, chronic nasal congestion, a high and arched palate, a jaw that is small or farther back than normal, and an enlarged tongue, tonsils, or uvula (the structure that hangs down at the back of the throat). Doctors measure blood pressure because OSA is more likely when blood pressure is high.

Although doctors are not able to predict risk precisely, the more risk factors and warning signs people have, the greater their risk of OSA.

TESTING

When doctors suspect OSA, they typically do tests to confirm the diagnosis.

Testing consists of polysomnography. For this test, people sleep overnight in a laboratory while their breathing and other functions are monitored. However, because snoring is so common and polysomnography is costly and time-consuming, polysomnography is usually done only when doctors strongly suspect OSA. Thus, they typically test only people who have warning signs (particularly those with episodes of not breathing witnessed by another person and those with several risk factors).

If people without warning signs do not appear to have any sleep disturbance other than snoring, they typically do not need tests.

However, they should schedule regular follow-ups so that their doctor can check for the development of such problems.

TREATMENT

Causes of snoring, such as chronic nasal obstruction and OSA, are treated.

For snoring itself, treatment includes general measures to eliminate risk factors and physical methods to open the airways.

GENERAL MEASURES

Several general measures may help reduce primary snoring. None are effective in everyone, but some people may benefit. Measures include

- Avoiding alcohol and sedating drugs for several hours before bedtime
- Sleeping with the head elevated
- Losing weight
- Using earplugs
- Having alternate sleeping arrangements (such as a separate room)

The best way to elevate the head is to put blocks under two of the bed's legs to raise the head of the bed or to use a wedge pillow that slants the whole upper body. People should not use pillows to raise only the head.

ORAL APPLIANCES

Oral appliances are worn only during sleep. They include mandibular advancement splints and tongue-retaining devices. These appliances, which must be fitted by specially trained dentists, can help keep the airway open during sleep in people with mild to moderate OSA and may help reduce snoring.

Mandibular advancement splints are small plastic devices that fit in the mouth like a mouth guard or orthodontic retainer. They push the lower jaw (mandible) and tongue forward and thus help keep the airway open during sleep. Some of these devices can be adjusted in small increments to ensure the best results. Adjustable devices are more effective than those that cannot be adjusted.

Tongue-retaining devices use suction to keep the tongue forward. If the tongue moves back in the mouth, it can block the airway. These devices are more uncomfortable and probably less effective than mandibular advancement devices.

Oral appliances may be used alone or with other treatments for sleep-related breathing disorders, such as weight management, surgery, or continuous positive airway pressure. Oral appliances can cause discomfort and excess salivation, and teeth may be pushed out of alignment. But most people tolerate them well.

CONTINUOUS POSITIVE AIRWAY PRESSURE (CPAP)

With CPAP, people breathe through a small mask applied to the nose or to the nose and mouth. The mask is attached to a device that supplies air at a pressure that helps prevent the airway from narrowing or collapsing when people breathe in (which is when most snoring occurs). CPAP provides very effective relief of OSA and helps reduce snoring. However, many people find CPAP devices uncomfortable and inconvenient. People with OSA tend to be more motivated to use CPAP than those whose only problem is snoring because untreated OSA can cause significant symptoms and increase the risk of serious disorders.

SURGERY

Some airway obstructions that contribute to snoring, such as nasal polyps, enlarged tonsils, and a deviated septum, can be treated surgically. But whether and how well such procedures reduce snoring have not been proved.

In addition, a number of surgical procedures have been developed specifically to treat OSA, and some can help reduce snoring. These procedures reshape tissues of the palate and/or uvula or stiffen the palate using implants or injections. They include uvulopalatopharyngoplasty, laser-assisted uvuloplasty, injection snoreplasty, radiofrequency ablation, and palatal implants.

In uvulopalatopharyngoplasty, tissues of the palate and uvula are surgically reshaped. Excess tissue is removed, and the airway is widened. This procedure requires a general anesthetic and a stay in the hospital. It can reduce snoring, but its effects may last only a few years.

For laser-assisted uvuloplasty, a laser or high-energy microwave device is used to reshape tissue, so this procedure is less invasive than uvulopalatopharyngoplasty. However, whether it can reduce snoring has not been proved, although some people seem to benefit from it.

For **injection snoreplasty** (a form of sclerotherapy), a substance that irritates the tissues and causes fibrous scar tissue to form is injected into the soft palate. As a result, the soft palate and uvula become stiffer and less likely to vibrate. Whether this procedure can reduce snoring requires further study.

For **radiofrequency ablation,** a probe is used to deliver heat (from an electrical current) into the soft palate. This procedure shrinks and stiffens tissues. It can reduce snoring, but further study is needed.

Palatal implants, made of polyethylene, can be placed into the soft palate to stiffen it. Three small implants are used. Whether these implants are useful for snoring alone has not been proved.

KEY POINTS

- Only a few people who snore have OSA, but most people who have OSA snore.
- Warning signs, such as episodes of not breathing or of choking during sleep, daytime sleepiness, and obesity, help identify people at risk of OSA and thus in need of testing with polysomnography.
- General measures to reduce snoring include avoiding alcohol and sedating drugs before bedtime, sleeping with the head elevated, losing weight, and, for the bed partner, using earplugs and having alternative sleeping arrangements.
- Specific treatments include CPAP, mandibular advancement devices, and surgery.

SORE THROAT (PHARYNGITIS)

Sore throat is pain in the back of the throat. The pain can be severe and is usually worsened by swallowing. Many people with sore throat refuse to eat or drink. Sometimes pain is also felt in the ear (nerves to the back of the throat run very close to nerves from the ear).

CAUSES

A sore throat results from infection (see Table on page 369). The most common infection is

- Tonsillopharyngitis

Much less common, but more serious, causes of sore throat are

- Abscess
- Infection of the epiglottis (epiglottitis)

Abscess and epiglottitis are of particular concern because they may block the airway.

TONSILLOPHARYNGITIS

Tonsillopharyngitis is infection of the tonsils (patches of lymphoid tissue at the back of the throat) and the throat (pharynx). Doctors may use the term tonsillitis when the tonsils are particularly inflamed or the term pharyngitis when the tonsils are not particularly inflamed or when people who have no tonsils have a sore throat.

Tonsillopharyngitis is usually caused by a virus, typically one of the same viruses that causes the common cold. Most common colds begin with a mild sore throat. A less common viral cause is acute mononucleosis (caused by the Epstein-Barr virus), which occurs mainly in children and young adults. Rarer still, sore throat can be part of the initial infection with human immunodeficiency virus (HIV).

About 10% of sore throats in adults (and slightly more in children) are caused by *Streptococcus* bacteria (streptococci). Such streptococcal infections are often termed strep throat. Strep throat is unusual in children younger than 2 years.

Rare bacterial causes include gonorrhea and diphtheria (in countries with low vaccination rates).

ABSCESS

A collection of pus (abscess) may form beneath or near one of the tonsils (peritonsillar abscess). The usual cause is a streptococcal infection that has spread from the tonsils into deeper tissue. In young children, an abscess can form in the tissue at the back of the throat (retropharyngeal abscess).

EPIGLOTTITIS

The epiglottis is a small flap of tissue that closes the entrance to the voice box and windpipe during swallowing. The epiglottis can become infected by certain bacteria. This infection causes severe pain and swelling. The swelling can close off the windpipe, particularly in infants and children. Epiglottitis used to occur mainly in children and usually was caused by *Haemophilus influenzae* type B (HiB) bacteria. Now that most children are vaccinated against HiB, epiglottitis is quite rare in children, and most cases occur in adults.

EVALUATION

Not every sore throat requires immediate evaluation by a doctor. The following information can help people decide whether a doctor's evaluation is needed and help them know what to expect during the evaluation.

WARNING SIGNS

In people with a sore throat, certain symptoms and characteristics are cause for concern. They include

- Squeaking sound when breathing in (stridor)
- Any sign of difficulty breathing (particularly the tripod position, in which children sit upright, leaning forward, with their neck tilted back and jaw thrust forward)
- Drooling
- Muffled, "hot potato" voice (speaking as if a hot object is being held in the mouth)
- Visible bulge in the back of the throat

People who have warning signs should go to the hospital right away.

People with a sore throat but no warning signs should call their doctor. People who have typical cold symptoms and mild to moderate discomfort may be advised to stay at home and treat their symptoms with over-the-counter (OTC) remedies. People with severe pain and/or other symptoms (such as fever, extreme fatigue, or a productive cough) typically should be seen within a day or two.

Doctors first ask questions about the person's symptoms and medical history and then do a physical examination. What doctors find during the history and physical examination helps them decide what, if any, tests need to be done (see Table on page 369).

During the medical history, doctors ask about the following:

- Symptoms of a runny nose, cough, and difficulty swallowing, speaking, or breathing
- Whether the person has had any general feeling of severe weakness before the sore throat (suggests mononucleosis)
- Whether the person has had a previous episode of mononucleosis (people rarely get mononucleosis twice)
- Whether people have any risk factors for gonorrhea (such as recent oral-genital sexual contact) or HIV infection (such as unprotected sex, multiple sex partners, or intravenous drug abuse)

During the physical examination, doctors focus on the nose and throat. However, if doctors suspect epiglottitis in children (because there are warning signs and no evidence of a cold), they do not examine the throat in their office because inserting a tongue depressor may cause a spasm that triggers complete airway blockage.

If epiglottitis is not suspected, doctors do the following:

- Look in the mouth to see whether the throat and/or tonsils are red, whether there are white patches (exudate) on the tonsils, and whether there are any bulges suggesting an abscess
- Examine the neck for enlarged, tender lymph nodes
- Feel the abdomen for an enlarged spleen

The need for tests depends on what doctors find during the history and physical examination, particularly whether warning signs are present.

Possible tests include

- Flexible fiberoptic laryngoscopy
- X-rays of the neck
- Rapid strep screening (for children)
- Throat culture (for adults)

A doctor's first concern is to recognize which people might have epiglottitis. Stridor and drooling are warning signs, particularly in people who appear ill or with difficulty breathing. In such cases, people should not have x-rays. Instead, the doctor looks down the throat with a thin, flexible viewing tube inserted through the nose (flexible fiberoptic laryngoscopy). Because children are more likely to have sudden, complete blockage of their airway when their throat is examined, doctors minimize this danger by doing this examination only in the operating room, where advanced airway equipment and personnel are available. Adults who do not appear seriously ill and have no respiratory symptoms may have neck x-rays to look for a swollen epiglottis or have flexible fiberoptic laryngoscopy done in the emergency department or a specialist's office.

An abscess is often noticeable during the doctor's examination. The doctor can both diagnose and treat the abscess by inserting a small needle into the swollen area after spraying the throat with an anesthetic. If pus comes out, an abscess is confirmed, and the doctor removes as much pus as possible. If the location and extent of an abscess are unclear, doctors do a computed tomography (CT) scan of the neck.

Despite what many people think, it is difficult for doctors to distinguish a strep throat from a sore throat caused by a virus based only on appearance. Both may cause a very red throat with white patches. Thus, unless people clearly have just a cold, doctors usually do tests to diagnose strep throat. There are two types of test, a rapid strep antigen test and a throat culture. Both tests are done on a sample taken from the back of the throat with a swab. The rapid strep antigen test can be done in the doctor's office in about 20 minutes. The rapid test is usually done only in children. If results are positive, children are treated for strep throat with antibiotics. If

SOME CAUSES AND FEATURES OF SORE THROAT

Cause	Common Features*	Tests
Viral tonsillopharyngitis (infection of the tonsils and throat caused by a virus)	Mild to moderate throat pain and little or no fever Usually a runny nose and/or cough Throat and tonsils that are slightly to very red and that may be coated with a white discharge or pus Sometimes one or two enlarged lymph nodes in the neck	A doctor's examination
Strep throat	Often severe throat pain and fever Rarely a runny nose or cough Often a very red throat and tonsils that are coated with a white discharge or pus Usually one or two tender, enlarged lymph nodes in the neck	Testing of a sample taken from the throat with a swab
Mononucleosis (caused by the Epstein-Barr virus)	Moderate to severe throat pain, high fever, and constant fatigue but no cold symptoms Usually in adolescents or young adults who have never had mononucleosis Often a very red throat and tonsils, coated with a white discharge or pus Typically many enlarged lymph nodes on both sides of the neck and sometimes an enlarged spleen detected during a doctor's examination	A blood test for antibodies to Epstein-Barr virus
Abscess†	Severe throat pain, often fever, and no cold symptoms Sometimes a muffled voice that sounds as if a hot object is being held in the mouth ("hot potato" voice) Throat and tonsils that may be slightly to very red Typically substantial swelling on one side of the throat detected during the examination	Usually removal of pus with a needle (for diagnosis and treatment) Sometimes CT of the neck
Epiglottitis† (infection of the epiglottis—the small flap of tissue that covers the opening to the voice box, or larynx)	Severe throat pain and difficulty swallowing that begin abruptly In children, often drooling and signs of severe illness (such as little or no eye contact, failure to recognize parents, and irritability) Sometimes (more often in children) respiratory symptoms, including ■ Breathing rapidly (tachypnea) ■ Squeaking when breathing in (stridor) ■ Sitting upright and leaning forward, with the neck tilted back and jaw thrust forward (to try to increase the amount of air reaching the lungs) A throat that typically appears normal seen during the examination (however, examination may not be advisable)	For most children and for adults who appear seriously ill, flexible fiberoptic laryngoscopy (insertion of a thin flexible tube into the throat to directly view the epiglottis), done in operating room Sometimes for people who do not have all the symptoms of epiglottitis and who do not appear seriously ill, x-rays of the neck

*Features include symptoms and the results of the doctor's examination. Features mentioned are typical but not always present.
†These causes are rare.
CT = computed tomography.

results are negative, another sample is sent to the laboratory for culture (growing microorganisms on a special gel so that there are enough to identify). If adults need testing for strep throat, doctors usually do only a throat culture because adults may have another bacterial infection that would not be identified by the rapid antigen test.

Doctors do blood tests for mononucleosis or HIV only when they suspect people have one of these infections.

TREATMENT

Doctors treat any specific or underlying conditions. For example, people with strep throat or other bacterial infections are given antibiotics.

It is important to relieve the pain of sore throat so that people can eat and drink. Ibuprofen or acetaminophen helps relieve pain and fever. People in severe pain may require the short-term use of opioids (such as oxycodone or hydrocodone). Warm saltwater gargles and throat lozenges or throat sprays (such as those containing benzocaine, lidocaine, or dyclonine) may temporarily help relieve pain. Providing soup is a good way to keep children well hydrated and nourished when swallowing is painful and before their appetite has returned.

KEY POINTS

- Most sore throats are caused by viral tonsillopharyngitis and resolve without treatment.
- Occasionally, sore throats are caused by certain bacteria (particularly streptococci) and result in strep throat.
- It is difficult for doctors to distinguish viral from bacterial causes of tonsillopharyngitis without testing.
- Abscess and epiglottitis are rare but serious causes.

SWALLOWING DIFFICULTY

Some people have difficulty swallowing (dysphagia). In dysphagia, foods and/or liquids do not move normally from the throat (pharynx) to the stomach. People feel as though food or liquids become stuck on the way down the tube that connects the throat to the stomach (esophagus). Dysphagia should not be confused with lump in throat (globus sensation—see page 251), in which people have the sensation of a lump in their throat but have no difficulty swallowing.

COMPLICATIONS

Dysphagia can cause people to inhale (aspirate) mouth secretions and/or material they eat or drink. Aspiration can cause acute pneumonia. If aspiration occurs over a long period of time, people may develop chronic lung disease. People who have had dysphagia for a long time are often inadequately nourished and lose weight.

CAUSES

Although most people take swallowing for granted, it is actually a complicated process. For swallowing to take place normally, the brain must unconsciously coordinate the activity of numerous small muscles of the throat and the esophagus. These muscles must contract strongly and in the proper sequence to push food from the mouth to the back of the throat and then down the esophagus. Finally, the lower part of the esophagus must relax to allow food to enter the stomach. Thus, swallowing difficulty can result from the following:

- Disorders of the brain or nervous system
- Disorders of the muscles in general
- Disorders of the esophagus (a physical blockage or a motility [movement] disorder)

Brain and nervous system disorders that cause difficulty swallowing include stroke, Parkinson disease, multiple sclerosis, and amyotrophic lateral sclerosis (ALS). People with these disorders typically have other symptoms in addition to difficulty swallowing. Many have already been diagnosed with these disorders.

General muscle disorders that cause difficulty swallowing include myasthenia gravis, dermatomyositis, and muscular dystrophy.

A physical blockage can result from cancer of the esophagus, rings or webs of tissue across the inside of the esophagus, and scarring of the esophagus from chronic acid reflux or from swallowing a caustic liquid. Sometimes the esophagus is compressed by a nearby organ or structure such as an enlarged thyroid gland, a bulge in the large artery in the chest (aortic aneurysm), or a tumor in the middle of the chest.

Esophageal motility disorders include achalasia (in which the rhythmic contractions of the esophagus are greatly decreased and the lower esophageal muscle does not relax normally to allow food to pass into the stomach) and esophageal spasm. Systemic sclerosis (scleroderma) may also cause a motility disorder.

EVALUATION

Not every episode of dysphagia requires immediate evaluation by a doctor. The following information can help people decide when a doctor's evaluation is needed and help them know what to expect during the evaluation.

WARNING SIGNS

In people with dysphagia, certain symptoms and characteristics are cause for concern. They include

- Symptoms of a complete physical blockage (such as drooling or inability to swallow anything at all)
- Dysphagia resulting in weight loss
- Painful swallowing (odynophagia)
- A new problem in nerve, spinal cord, or brain function, particularly any weakness

WHEN TO SEE A DOCTOR

People who have warning signs should see a doctor right away unless the only warning sign is weight loss. In such cases, a delay of a week or so is not harmful.

People with dysphagia but no warning signs should see their doctor within a week or so.

However, people who cough or choke whenever they eat or drink should be evaluated sooner.

WHAT THE DOCTOR DOES

Doctors first ask questions about the person's symptoms and medical history. Doctors then do a physical examination. What they find during the history and physical examination often suggests a cause of the dysphagia and the tests that may need to be done (see Table on pages 373 to 374).

During the history, doctors ask about the following:

- Any difficulty swallowing solids, liquids, or both
- Food coming out the nose
- Drooling or food spilling from the mouth
- Coughing or choking while eating

People with equal difficulty swallowing liquids and solids are more likely to have a motility disorder. People who have gradually increasing difficulty swallowing first solids and then liquids may have a worsening physical blockage, such as a tumor. Food unintentionally coming out of the nose or mouth suggests a neurologic or muscular problem rather than a problem with the esophagus.

Doctors look for symptoms that suggest neuromuscular, gastrointestinal, and connective tissue disorders. Major neuromuscular symptoms include weakness, either constant weakness of a body part (such as an arm or leg) or off-and-on weakness that occurs during activity and is relieved by rest; walking (gait) or balance disturbance; involuntary, rhythmic, shaking movements (tremors); and difficulty speaking. Doctors also need to know whether the person has a known disease that causes dysphagia (see Table).

Doctors then do a physical examination. The physical examination is focused on the neurologic examination, but doctors also pay attention to the person's nutritional status and any abnormalities of the skin and/or muscles. During the physical examination, doctors look at the following:

- Tremors present while the person is at rest
- Muscle strength (including muscles of the eyes, mouth, and face)
- The performance of a repetitive action (such as blinking or counting aloud) by people who become weak with activity (to see how rapidly their performance worsens)

- The way people walk and their balance
- The skin for rash and thickening or texture changes, particularly on the fingertips
- Muscles, to see whether any are wasting away or visibly twitching under the skin (fasciculations) or feel tender
- The neck for an enlarged thyroid gland or other mass

TESTING

Possible tests include

- Upper endoscopy
- Barium swallow

For people who have symptoms of a complete or nearly complete blockage, doctors immediately look in the esophagus with a flexible tube (upper endoscopy).

For people whose symptoms do not suggest a complete blockage, doctors usually take x-rays while the person swallows barium liquid (which shows up on x-rays). Typically, people first swallow plain barium liquid and then barium liquid mixed with some material such as a marshmallow or cracker. If the barium swallow suggests blockage, doctors usually then do upper endoscopy to look for the cause (particularly to rule out cancer). If the barium test is negative or suggests a motility disorder, doctors do esophageal motility tests. In motility tests, people swallow a thin tube containing many pressure sensors. As people swallow, the pressure sensors show whether the esophagus is contracting normally and whether the lower part of the esophagus is relaxing normally.

TREATMENT

The best way to treat dysphagia is to treat the specific cause.

To help relieve symptoms, doctors usually advise people to take small bites and chew food thoroughly.

People with dysphagia caused by a stroke may benefit from treatment by a rehabilitation specialist. Rehabilitation measures may involve changing head position while eating, retraining the swallowing muscles, doing exercises that improve the ability to accommodate a lump of food in the mouth, or doing strength and coordination exercises for the tongue.

SOME CAUSES AND FEATURES OF SWALLOWING DIFFICULTY

Cause	Common Features*	Tests
Neurologic disorders		
Stroke	Usually a previous diagnosis of a stroke Weakness or paralysis on one side of the body, difficulty speaking, difficulty walking, or a combination	CT or MRI of the brain
Parkinson disease	Involuntary, rhythmic, shaking movements (tremors), incoordination (ataxia), and balance disturbance	A doctor's examination Sometimes CT or MRI
Multiple sclerosis	Come-and-go symptoms involving various parts of the body, including vision problems, muscle weakness, and/or abnormal sensations Sometimes weak, clumsy movements	MRI Often a spinal tap
Some motor neuron disorders, such as ▪ Amyotrophic lateral sclerosis ▪ Progressive bulbar palsy ▪ Pseudobulbar palsy	Muscle twitching, wasting, and weakness Progressive difficulty with chewing, swallowing, and talking	Electrodiagnostic tests (such as needle electromyography, which involves stimulating muscles then recording their electrical activity) Laboratory tests MRI of the brain
Muscle disorders		
Myasthenia gravis	Weak, drooping eyelids and weak eye muscles Excessive weakness of muscles after they are used	Use of a drug (given intravenously) that temporarily improves strength if the cause is myasthenia Electromyography Blood tests
Dermatomyositis	Muscle weakness Fever, fatigue, and weight loss Sometimes joint pain and/or swelling Sometimes a dusky, red rash	Blood tests Electromyography Muscle biopsy
Muscular dystrophy	Muscle weakness beginning in childhood	Muscle biopsy Genetic testing
Motility (movement) disorders of the esophagus		
Achalasia (rhythmic contractions of the esophagus are greatly decreased, and the lower esophageal muscle does not relax normally)	Difficulty swallowing (dysphagia) solids and liquids that worsens over months to years Sometimes regurgitation (spitting up) of undigested food while sleeping Discomfort in the chest Fullness after a small meal (early satiety), nausea, vomiting, bloating, and symptoms that are worsened by food	Barium swallow Measurements of pressure produced during contractions of the esophagus (esophageal manometry)

(continued)

SOME CAUSES AND FEATURES OF SWALLOWING DIFFICULTY *(continued)*

Cause	Common Features*	Tests
Diffuse esophageal spasm	Chest pain	Barium swallow
	Swallowing difficulty comes and goes	Esophageal manometry
Systemic sclerosis (scleroderma)	Raynaud phenomenon	A doctor's examination
	Joint pain and/or swelling	Usually blood tests
	Swelling, thickening, and tightening of the skin of the fingers and sometimes of the face and other areas	
	Occasionally heartburn, difficulty swallowing, and shortness of breath	
Physical blockage of the esophagus		
Narrowing by scar tissue resulting from exposure to stomach acid (peptic stricture)	A long history of gastrointestinal reflux symptoms (such as heartburn)	Endoscopy (examination of internal structures with a flexible viewing tube)
Esophageal cancer	Constant difficulty swallowing foods and liquids that worsens rapidly	Endoscopy
		Biopsy
	Weight loss	
	Chest pain	
Lower esophageal rings	Swallowing difficulty comes and goes	Barium swallow
Compression of the esophagus, as may be caused by ■ A bulge in the large artery in the chest (aortic aneurysm) ■ An enlarged thyroid gland ■ A tumor in the chest	Sometimes an enlarged thyroid gland	Barium swallow X-rays taken after a radiopaque dye (which is visible on x-rays) is injected into an artery (arteriography)
Ingestion of a caustic substance, such as strong acids and alkalis	Swallowing difficulty occurs weeks to months after a known ingestion	Endoscopy

*Features include symptoms and the results of the doctor's examination. Features mentioned are typical but not always present.
CT = computed tomography; MRI = magnetic resonance imaging.

People who cannot swallow without a high risk of choking may need to stop eating and be fed through a feeding tube placed through the wall of their abdomen into their stomach or small intestine.

ESSENTIALS FOR OLDER PEOPLE

Chewing, swallowing, tasting, and communicating require intact, coordinated neurologic and muscular function in the mouth, face, and neck. Oral motor function in particular declines measurably with age, even in healthy people. Decline in function may occur in several ways:

■ As people age, the muscles required for chewing decrease in strength and coordination, especially among people with partial or complete dentures. This decrease may lead to a tendency to swallow larger food particles, which can increase the risk of choking or aspiration.

■ With increased age, it takes longer to move food from the mouth to the throat, which increases the likelihood of aspiration.

After age-related changes, the most common causes of oral motor disorders are neuromuscular disorders (such as cranial neuropathies caused by diabetes, stroke, Parkinson disease, amyotrophic lateral sclerosis, or multiple sclerosis). Sometimes, treatments can contribute to oral motor disorders. For example, drugs (such as anticholinergics or diuretics), radiation therapy to the head and neck, and chemotherapy can greatly impair saliva production. Reduced saliva production (hyposalivation) is a major cause of delayed and impaired swallowing.

In addition to their regular doctor, people with oral motor disorders or dysfunction are also treated by specialists in prosthetic dentistry, rehabilitative medicine, speech pathology, otolaryngology, and gastroenterology.

KEY POINTS

- People who have dysphagia typically need upper endoscopy or a barium swallow test.
- If the endoscopy and barium test are normal or if they suggest a motility disorder, doctors do esophageal motility tests.
- Treatment is aimed at the cause.

SWELLING
(EDEMA)

Swelling is due to excess fluid in the tissues. The fluid is predominantly water.

Swelling may be widespread or confined to a single limb or part of a limb. Swelling is often in the feet and lower legs. However, people who are required to remain in bed for extended periods (bed rest) sometimes develop swelling in the buttocks, genitals, and back of the thighs. Women who lie on only one side may develop swelling in the breast they lie on. Rarely, a hand or an arm swells.

Sometimes a limb suddenly swells. More often, swelling develops slowly, beginning with weight gain, puffy eyes upon awakening in the morning, and tight shoes at the end of the day. Swelling may develop so gradually that people do not notice until the swelling is considerable. Sometimes people have a feeling of tightness or fullness. Other symptoms may be present depending on the cause of the swelling and may include shortness of breath or pain in the affected limb.

Swelling is sometimes described as pitting. When pressure is applied to the swollen area, an indentation that persists for some time is left after the pressure is released. Any form of pressure (for example, a finger or the elastic in socks) can cause pitting. Edema is described as nonpitting if no indentation is left.

CAUSES

Swelling that occurs throughout the body has different causes than swelling that is confined to a single limb or part of a limb.

Widespread swelling is most commonly caused by

- Heart failure
- Liver failure
- Kidney disorders (especially nephrotic syndrome)

These disorders all cause fluid retention, which is the cause of the swelling.

Another cause of swelling of the lower legs is pooling of blood in the legs. Many obese, middle-aged or older people normally have a small amount of swelling at the end of the day due to blood pooling. This swelling typically goes away by morning. Blood can also pool in the legs if the valves in the veins are widened or damaged (chronic venous insufficiency) such as may occur in people who previously had blood clots in the legs. In such people, the swelling usually does not go away overnight.

Many women normally have some swelling during the later stages of pregnancy (see page 380). However, women who have a large amount of swelling, particularly if swelling also involves the hands and face and is accompanied by high blood pressure, may have preeclampsia, which can be dangerous.

Swelling that is confined to a single limb or part of a limb is most commonly caused by

- A blood clot in a deep-lying vein in a limb (deep vein thrombosis)
- Skin infection (cellulitis)
- Blockage of a lymph vessel

Many disorders increase risk of blood clots in a vein. Most often, these clots develop in a leg vein but sometimes they occur in an arm vein. Blood clots in a vein can be dangerous if the clot breaks off and travels to the lungs, blocking an artery there (called pulmonary embolism).

Cellulitis typically causes swelling of the skin over only part of a limb. Much less often, an infection deep under the skin or in the muscles can cause the whole limb to swell.

Lymph vessels, which occur throughout the body, help drain fluid from tissues. If a tumor pushes on the lymph vessels or surgery is done to remove some lymph vessels or nodes (for example, when women with breast cancer have lymph nodes removed from the armpit), a limb can swell. In many tropical countries, certain parasites can block lymph vessels and cause swelling (lymphatic filariasis).

Sometimes, an allergic reaction causes swelling around the mouth (angioedema). Angioedema can also be a hereditary disorder in which swelling comes and goes at irregular intervals.

SOME CAUSES AND FEATURES OF SWELLING

Cause	Common Features*	Tests†
Angioedema (allergic, idiopathic, or hereditary)	Painless swelling of the face, lips, and sometimes tongue Sometimes itching or tight sensation Swelling that does not remain indented after being pressed (nonpitting swelling)	Only a doctor's examination
A blood clot in a deep-lying vein in a leg (typically), an arm, or the pelvis (deep vein thrombosis)	Sudden, nonpitting swelling Usually pain, redness, warmth, and/or tenderness in the affected area If the clot travels and blocks an artery to the lung (pulmonary embolism), usually shortness of breath and sometimes coughing up blood Sometimes in people who have risk factors for blood clots, such as recent surgery, an injury, bed rest, a cast on a leg, hormone therapy, or cancer	Ultrasonography
Chronic venous insufficiency (causing blood to pool in the legs)	Swelling in one or both ankles or legs Chronic mild discomfort, aching, or cramps in the legs but no pain Sometimes reddish brown, leathery areas on the skin and shallow sores on the lower legs Often varicose veins	Only a doctor's examination
Drugs (such as minoxidil, nonsteroidal anti-inflammatory drugs, estrogens, fludrocortisone, and some calcium channel blockers)	Painless swelling that remains slightly indented after being pressed (slight pitting) in both legs and feet	Only a doctor's examination
Heart failure	Painless swelling that remains indented after being pressed (pitting) in both legs and feet Often shortness of breath during exertion or while lying down and during sleep Often in people known to have heart disease and/or high blood pressure	Chest x-ray ECG Usually echocardiography
Infection of the skin (cellulitis)	An irregular area of redness, warmth, and tenderness on part of one limb Nonpitting swelling Sometimes fever	Only a doctor's examination
Infection deep under the skin or in the muscles (rare)	Deep, constant pain in one limb Redness, warmth, tenderness, and nonpitting swelling that feels tight Signs of severe illness (such as fever, confusion, and a rapid heart rate) Sometimes a foul discharge, blisters, or areas of blackened, dead skin	Blood and tissue cultures X-rays Sometimes MRI
Kidney disease (mainly nephrotic syndrome)	Widespread, painless, pitting swelling Often fluid within the abdomen (ascites) Sometimes puffiness around the eyes or frothy urine	Measurement of protein in a urine specimen *(continued)*

SOME CAUSES AND FEATURES OF SWELLING (continued)

Cause	Common Features*	Tests†
Liver disease if chronic	Widespread, painless, pitting swelling	Measurement of albumin in the blood
	Often fluid within the abdomen (ascites)	
	Causes that are often apparent based on history (such as alcohol abuse or hepatitis)	Other blood tests to evaluate liver function
	Sometimes small spiderlike blood vessels that are visible in the skin (spider angiomas), reddening of the palms and, in men, breast enlargement and a decrease in the size of the testes	
Lymphatic vessel obstruction due to surgery or radiation therapy for cancer	Painless, nonpitting swelling of one limb	Only a doctor's examination
	A cause (surgery or radiation therapy) that is apparent based on history	
Lymphatic filariasis (a lymph vessel infection due to certain parasitic worms)	Painless, nonpitting swelling of one limb and sometimes the genitals	Examination of a blood sample under a microscope
	In people who have been in a developing country where filariasis is common	
Normal swelling	A small amount of pitting swelling of both feet and/or ankles that occurs at the end of the day and resolves by morning	Only a doctor's examination
	No pain, redness, or other symptoms	
Pregnancy or a normal premenstrual symptom	Painless, pitting swelling in both legs and feet	Only a doctor's examination
	Usually relieved to some extent by rest and leg elevation	
	In women known to be pregnant or about to have a menstrual period	
Pregnancy, with preeclampsia	Painless, pitting swelling in both legs and feet	Measurement of protein in urine
	High blood pressure (often new)	
	Occurring during the 3rd trimester of pregnancy	
Pressure on a vein (for example, by a tumor, pregnancy, or extreme abdominal obesity)	Painless swelling that develops slowly	Ultrasonography or CT if a tumor is suspected

*Features include symptoms and the results of the doctor's examination. Features mentioned are typical but not always present.

†In most people with swelling, doctors do a complete blood count, other blood tests, and urinalysis (to check for protein in the urine).

CT = computed tomography; ECG = electrocardiography; MRI = magnetic resonance imaging.

EVALUATION

Although swelling may seem like a minor irritation, especially if it does not cause discomfort and goes away while a person is sleeping, it can be a symptom of a serious disorder. The following information can help people decide when a doctor's examination is needed and to know what to expect during the evaluation.

WARNING SIGNS

In people with swelling, certain symptoms and characteristics are cause for concern. They include

- Sudden onset
- Swelling of only one leg
- Significant pain or tenderness
- Shortness of breath
- Coughing up blood

WHEN TO SEE A DOCTOR

People who have warning signs should see a doctor right away. People without warning signs who have a history of heart, lung, or kidney disease or who are pregnant should see a doctor within a few days. Other people without warning signs should schedule a doctor's appointment when convenient. Typically a delay of a week or so is not harmful.

WHAT THE DOCTOR DOES

Doctors first ask questions about the person's symptoms and medical history. Doctors then do a physical examination. What they find during the history and physical examination often suggests a cause of the swelling and the tests that may need to be done.

Doctors ask about the location and duration of the swelling and presence and degree of pain or discomfort. Women are usually asked whether they are pregnant or whether swelling seems related to menstrual periods. Doctors also ask whether the person has any disorders (for example, heart, liver, or kidney disorders) or takes any drugs (for example, minoxidil, nonsteroidal anti-inflammatory drugs, or amlodipine and other calcium channel blockers) that are known to cause swelling. Doctors also ask about the amount of salt used in cooking and at the table because excess salt can make swelling worse, particularly in people with heart or kidney disorders.

Doctors look for symptoms that may indicate the cause of swelling. For example, people with heart failure may have shortness of breath during exertion or may wake at night with shortness of breath. People with swelling and easy bruising may have a liver disorder, and people who have recently had surgery or a cast on their leg may have deep vein thrombosis.

Doctors may ask people with swelling that is long lasting to keep a record of their daily weight so that increases in swelling are detected quickly.

During the physical examination, doctors pay particular attention to the area of swelling, but they also carefully examine the person for other signs. Doctors listen to the heart and lungs with the stethoscope because swelling may be a sign of a heart disorder.

TESTING

For most people with widespread swelling, blood tests are done to evaluate the function of the heart, kidneys, and liver. Urinalysis is usually also done to check for large amounts of protein, which can indicate nephrotic syndrome or, in pregnant women, preeclampsia. Other tests are done based on the suspected cause. For example, in people with isolated leg swelling, doctors may do ultrasonography to look for blockage of a vein in the leg.

TREATMENT

Specific causes are treated (for example, anticoagulants [blood thinners] are given to people with blood clots in the legs). Any drugs that caused the swelling are stopped or changed if possible.

Because swelling itself is not harmful, doctors do not give water pills (diuretics) to people unless they are needed to treat the cause of the swelling (such as heart failure). However, some simple general measures, such as sitting with the legs elevated or limiting the amount of salt in the diet, sometimes help relieve swelling.

KEY POINTS

- Swelling may be widespread or confined to a single area.
- Not all swelling is harmful.
- The main causes of widespread swelling are heart, liver, and kidney disorders.
- The main causes of swelling of a single limb are blood clots in a vein and an infection.
- Sudden onset of swelling may indicate a serious disorder, so people should see a doctor right away.

SWELLING DURING LATE PREGNANCY

As pregnancy progresses, fluid may accumulate in tissues, usually in the feet, ankles, and legs, causing them to swell and appear puffy. This condition is called edema. Occasionally, the face and hands also swell. Some fluid accumulation during pregnancy is normal, particularly during the 3rd trimester. It is called physiologic edema.

Fluid accumulates during pregnancy because the adrenal glands produce more of the hormones that make the body retain fluids (aldosterone and cortisol). Fluid also accumulates because the enlarging uterus interferes with blood flow from the legs to the heart. As a result, fluid backs up in the veins of the legs and seeps out into the surrounding tissues.

CAUSES

COMMON CAUSES

Usually during pregnancy, swelling is

- Physiologic edema

LESS COMMON CAUSES

Less commonly, swelling during pregnancy results from a disorder (see Table on page 381). However, such disorders are often serious. They include

- Deep vein thrombosis
- Preeclampsia
- Cellulitis

In deep vein thrombosis, blood clots form in veins located deep within part of the body, often in the legs. Pregnancy increases the risk of this disorder in several ways. During pregnancy, the body produces more of the proteins that help blood clot (clotting factors), probably intended to prevent too much bleeding during childbirth. Also, changes during pregnancy cause blood to back up in veins, making clots more likely to form. If the pregnant woman is less mobile, blood is even more likely to back up in leg veins and clot. The clots may interfere with blood flow. If a blood clot breaks loose, it can travel through the bloodstream to the lungs, blocking

blood flow there. This blockage (called pulmonary embolism) is life threatening.

In preeclampsia, blood pressure and protein levels in urine increase during pregnancy. Fluids may accumulate, causing swelling in the face, hands, or feet and weight gain. If severe, preeclampsia can damage organs, such as the brain, kidneys, lungs, or liver, and cause problems in the baby.

In cellulitis, bacteria infect the skin and tissues under the skin, sometimes causing swelling with redness and tenderness. Cellulitis most commonly affects the legs but may occur anywhere.

RISK FACTORS

The risk of deep vein thrombosis and preeclampsia is increased by various conditions (risk factors).

For deep vein thrombosis, risk factors include

- A recent leg injury
- A previous episode of deep vein thrombosis
- A disorder that makes blood more likely to clot, such as cancer or sometimes systemic lupus erythematosus (lupus)
- Cigarette smoking
- Immobility, as may occur after an illness or surgery

For preeclampsia, risk factors include

- High blood pressure that was present before pregnancy
- Preeclampsia during a previous pregnancy or a family member who has had preeclampsia
- Age under 17 or over 35
- A first pregnancy
- A pregnancy with more than one fetus
- Diabetes

EVALUATION

Doctors must rule out deep vein thrombosis, preeclampsia, cellulitis, and other possible causes before they can diagnose physiologic edema.

In pregnant women with swollen legs, the following symptoms are cause for concern:

- Blood pressure that is 140/90 mm Hg or higher
- Swelling in only one leg or calf, particularly if the area is warm, red, and/or tender or fever is present
- Swelling in the hands
- Swelling that suddenly increases
- Confusion, difficulty breathing, changes in vision, shaking (tremor), a seizure, sudden abdominal pain, or a sudden headache—symptoms that may be caused by preeclampsia

Women should go to the hospital immediately if they have

- Symptoms that suggest preeclampsia

Women with other warning signs should see a doctor that day. Women without warning signs should see a doctor, but a delay of several days is usually not harmful.

Doctors first ask questions about the swelling and other symptoms and about the medical history. Doctors then do a physical examination. What they find during the history and

SOME CAUSES AND FEATURES OF SWELLING DURING LATE PREGNANCY

Cause	Common Features*	Tests
Normal (physiologic) edema	Similar and equal painless swelling (edema) in both legs that usually decreases when the woman lies on her left side	A doctor's examination
Deep vein thrombosis	Swelling and pain in only one leg or calf	Doppler ultrasonography of the affected leg to check for a blockage in the veins
	Often tenderness, redness, and warmth in the affected area	
	Sometimes risk factors for deep vein thrombosis	Sometimes a blood test to measure a substance released from blood clots (called D-dimer)
	If a blood clot travels to the lungs and blocks a blood vessel there (causing pulmonary embolism), chest pain and difficulty breathing	If the woman has chest pain and difficulty breathing, CT of the chest or ventilation/perfusion (nuclear lung) scanning
Preeclampsia	Swelling in both feet and sometimes in the face and/or hands	Measurement of blood pressure and the amount of protein in urine
	No tenderness, redness, or warmth in the swollen areas	
	Sometimes headache, confusion, blurred vision, nausea or vomiting, or a reddish purple rash of tiny dots (which indicates bleeding in the skin)	
	Sometimes risk factors for preeclampsia	
Cellulitis	Swelling in one leg or calf and tenderness, redness, and warmth in the affected area	A doctor's examination
	Possibly pitting of the affected skin (resembling an orange peel)	
	Often affecting a relatively small area	
	Sometimes fever	

*Features include symptoms and results of the doctor's examination. Features mentioned are typical but not always present.

physical examination often suggests a cause of the swelling and the tests that may need to be done (see Table).

Doctors ask when the swelling started, how long it has been present, and whether any activity (such as lying on the left side) lessens or worsens it. Lying on the left side decreases physiologic edema. Doctors also ask about conditions that increase the risk of developing deep vein thrombosis and preeclampsia.

Women are asked about other symptoms, which may suggest a cause. They are asked whether they have ever had deep vein thrombosis, pulmonary embolism, preeclampsia, or high blood pressure.

During the physical examination, doctors look for evidence of a serious cause. To check for symptoms of preeclampsia, doctors measure blood pressure and may check the woman's reflexes and look at the back of her eyes with an ophthalmoscope (a handheld device that resembles a small flashlight).

TESTING

If deep vein thrombosis is suspected, Doppler ultrasonography of the affected leg is done. This test can show disturbances in blood flow caused by blood clots in the leg veins.

If preeclampsia is suspected, the protein level is measured in a urine sample. High blood pressure plus a high protein level in urine indicates preeclampsia. If the diagnosis is unclear, the woman is asked to collect her urine for 24 hours, and protein is measured in that volume of urine. This measurement is more accurate.

TREATMENT

When swelling results from a disorder, that disorder is treated.

The swelling that occurs normally during pregnancy can be reduced by doing the following:

- Lying on the left side, which moves the uterus off the large vein that returns blood to the heart (inferior vena cava)
- Resting frequently with the legs elevated
- Wearing elastic support stockings
- Wearing loose clothing that does not restrict blood flow, particularly in the legs (for example, not wearing socks or stockings that have tight bands around the ankles or calves)

KEY POINTS

- Some swelling in the legs and ankles is normal (physiologic) during pregnancy and occurs during the 3rd trimester.
- Doctors can identify serious causes of swelling based on results of a physical examination, blood pressure measurement, urine tests, and sometimes ultrasonography.
- If pregnancy itself is the cause, swelling can be reduced by lying on the left side, elevating the legs periodically, and wearing support stockings.

SWOLLEN LYMPH NODES (SWOLLEN GLANDS)

Lymph nodes are tiny, bean-shaped organs that filter lymph fluid. They are located throughout the body, but particular collections are found just under the skin in the neck, under the arms, and in the groin area. Lymph nodes are part of the lymphatic system, which is one of the body's defense mechanisms against the spread of infection and cancer.

Lymph is clear fluid that is made up of water, white blood cells, proteins, and fats that have filtered out of blood vessels into the spaces between cells. Some of the fluid is reabsorbed by the blood vessels but the rest enters the lymphatic vessels. Lymph then passes through the lymph nodes, which are specific collection points where damaged cells, infectious organisms, and cancer cells are filtered from the fluid and destroyed. If many infectious organisms or cancer cells are present, the lymph nodes swell. Sometimes, organisms cause infection within a lymph node.

A few small nodes often can be felt in healthy people. Lymph nodes that are larger and easily felt may be a sign of a disorder. Some people use the term "swollen glands" to refer to swollen lymph nodes, especially when the nodes in the neck are swollen. However, lymph nodes are not glands. Doctors use the term lymphadenopathy to refer to swollen lymph nodes.

Lymph nodes in only one body area may be swollen, or nodes in two or more body areas can be swollen. When swollen lymph nodes are painful or have signs of inflammation (for example, redness or tenderness), the condition is termed lymphadenitis. Other symptoms, such as sore throat, runny nose, or fever, may be present depending on the cause. Sometimes swollen lymph nodes are discovered when the person is being examined because of another symptom.

CAUSES

Because lymph nodes participate in the body's immune response, a large number of infections, inflammatory disorders, and cancers are potential causes. Only the more common causes are discussed here.

The most common causes are

- Upper respiratory infections (URI)
- Infections in tissues near the swollen lymph node

Sometimes doctors cannot determine the cause of the swelling, but swelling goes away on its own without causing the person any harm.

The most dangerous causes are cancer, human immunodeficiency virus (HIV) infection, and tuberculosis. However, probably less than 1% of people with swollen lymph nodes have cancer.

EVALUATION

Not every person with swollen lymph nodes requires immediate evaluation by a doctor. The following information can help people decide when a doctor's evaluation is needed and help them know what to expect during the evaluation.

WARNING SIGNS

In people with swollen lymph nodes, certain symptoms and characteristics are cause for concern. They include

- A node that is an inch or more in diameter
- A node that is draining pus
- A node that feels hard
- Risk factors for HIV infection (such as occupational exposure, high-risk sexual activities, injecting street drugs) or tuberculosis (such as living or working with a person who has tuberculosis or having recently moved from an area where tuberculosis is prevalent)
- Fever or unexplained weight loss

WHEN TO SEE A DOCTOR

If a lymph node is very painful or draining pus or other material, people should see a doctor right away. Other people should call their doctor. The doctor will decide how quickly they need to be seen based on the presence of warning signs and other symptoms. For people who have no warning signs and otherwise feel well, a delay of a week or so is not harmful.

The doctor first asks questions about the person's symptoms and medical history. Doctors then do a physical examination. What they find during the history and physical examination often suggests a cause of the swollen lymph nodes and the tests that may need to be done (see Table, below).

Doctors ask

- Where the swollen nodes are located
- How long nodes have been swollen
- Whether the person has pain
- Whether the person has recently had an injury (particularly cat scratches and rat bites)
- Whether the person has an infection or symptoms of an infection (for example, a runny nose, cough, fever, sore throat, unexplained weight loss, or tooth or gum pain)

Doctors then do a physical examination. Doctors check for fever and examine areas where lymph nodes are found. Doctors check the person for any signs of infection or lump elsewhere in the body. People who have swollen lymph nodes throughout the body usually have a disorder that affects the entire body. However, people who have swollen lymph nodes in only one area may have a disorder that affects only that area (for example, an infection) or more widespread disease.

Sometimes the history and physical examination suggest the cause, as for example when the person has an upper respiratory infection or a dental infection. In other cases, findings do not point to a single cause. People with warning signs are more likely to have a serious disorder, but people with lymph node swelling and no other symptoms may also have a serious disorder.

Nodes that are hard, very enlarged, and do not move when pushed may indicate cancer. Tenderness, redness, and warmth in a single enlarged lymph node may indicate an infection of the node.

SOME CAUSES AND FEATURES OF SWOLLEN LYMPH NODES

Cause	Common Features*	Tests
Infections		
Upper respiratory infection (including sore throat)	Neck nodes are affected with only little or no tenderness	Only a doctor's examination
	Sore throat, runny nose, or cough	
Dental infection	Neck nodes on one side are affected (often tender)	Only a doctor's examination
	Painful tooth	
Mononucleosis	Swelling on both sides, typically in the neck but sometimes under the arms or in the groin	Blood test for mononucleosis
	Fever, sore throat, and severe fatigue	
	Typically in an adolescent or a young adult	
Tuberculosis affecting the lymph nodes	Usually swelling of nodes in the neck or above the collarbone	Tuberculin skin testing
	Sometimes lymph nodes inflamed or draining	Usually lymph node aspiration or biopsy
	Often in a person who has HIV infection	
HIV (immediately after the person became infected—the primary infection)	Generalized lymph node swelling	HIV blood testing
	Usually fever, malaise, rash, and joint pain	
	Often in a person known to have been exposed to HIV or to having exposure to a high-risk activity (such as occupational exposure, high-risk sexual activities, injecting street drugs)	

(continued)

SOME CAUSES AND FEATURES OF SWOLLEN LYMPH NODES (continued)

Cause	Common Features*	Tests
STDs (particularly herpes simplex, chlamydia, and syphilis)	Except for secondary syphilis, only swollen nodes in the groin Often urinary symptoms (such as pain during urination) and urethral or vaginal discharge Sometimes sores on the genitals For secondary syphilis, often widespread sores on the mucous membranes and widespread lymph node swelling	STD testing
Skin and soft tissue infections (for example, cellulitis, abscess, cat-scratch disease), including direct lymph node infection	Usually a visible cut or infection of the skin near the swollen node	Usually only a doctor's examination Sometimes blood tests to identify antibodies to the infecting organism
Toxoplasmosis	Swollen nodes on both sides of the neck and under both arms Sometimes flu-like symptoms and an enlarged liver and spleen Often history of exposure to cat feces	Blood tests
Cancers		
Leukemias (typically chronic and sometimes acute lymphocytic leukemia)	Fatigue, fever, and weight loss With acute leukemia, often easy bruising and/or bleeding	Complete blood count and peripheral smear (examination of a blood sample with a microscope to determine characteristics of the cells) Bone marrow examination
Lymphomas	Painless lymph node swelling (local or widespread) Nodes often rubbery and sometimes clumped together Often fever, night sweats, and weight loss	Lymph node biopsy
Metastatic cancers (often of the head and neck, thyroid, breast, or lung)	One or several painless nodes in the neck Nodes often hard, sometimes unable to be moved when pushed	Tests to identify the primary tumor, often including looking in the throat, esophagus, and trachea with a flexible tube
Connective tissue disorders		
Systemic lupus erythematosus (SLE)	Widespread node swelling Typically painful and sometimes swollen joints Sometimes red rash affecting the nose and the cheeks and other skin sores	A doctor's examination plus blood tests

(continued)

SOME CAUSES AND FEATURES OF SWOLLEN LYMPH NODES (continued)

Cause	Common Features*	Tests
Sarcoidosis	Painless lymph node swelling that may be widespread	Chest imaging (plain x-ray or CT)
	Often cough and/or shortness of breath, fever, malaise, muscle weakness, weight loss, and joint pains	Sometimes lymph node biopsy
Kawasaki disease	Tender swollen nodes in the neck in a child	Only a doctor's examination
	Fever, usually higher than 102° F (39° C), rash on the trunk, prominent red bumps on the tongue, peeling skin on the palms, soles, and around the nails	
Other		
Drugs: Common drugs include allopurinol, antibiotics (for example, cephalosporins, penicillin, and sulfonamides), atenolol, captopril, carbamazepine, phenytoin, pyrimethamine, and quinidine	History of using a causative drug

Except for phenytoin, rash, joint and muscle pain, and fever | Only a doctor's examination |
| Silicone breast implants | Node swelling under the arms in a woman with breast implants | A doctor's examination and often tests for other causes of node swelling |

*Features include symptoms and the results of the doctor's examination. Features mentioned are typical but not always present.

CT = computed tomography; HIV = human immunodeficiency virus; STD = sexually transmitted disease.

TESTING

If doctors suspect a specific disorder (for example, mononucleosis in a young person with fever, sore throat and an enlarged spleen), initial testing is directed at that condition (see Table).

If history and physical examination do not show a likely cause, further testing depends on the nodes involved and the other findings present.

People with warning signs and those with widespread lymph node swelling should have a complete blood count and chest x-ray. Doctors may also test for tuberculosis, HIV infection, and mononucleosis. Sometimes blood tests are needed to detect toxoplasmosis and syphilis. In people with joint pain or stiffness or a rash, blood tests are done for systemic lupus erythematosus (lupus).

If doctors suspect cancer or lymphoma, the person has a lymph node biopsy. Biopsy may also be needed when widespread lymph node swelling does not resolve within 3 to 4 weeks.

TREATMENT

Primary treatment is directed at the cause. Swollen lymph nodes are not treated.

KEY POINTS

- In most cases, the cause is an obvious nearby skin or tissue infection or a harmless viral infection that goes away on its own.
- Testing is usually needed when there are warning signs, when other symptoms or risk factors suggest a specific disorder, or when widespread lymph node swelling has no apparent cause.
- When lymph node swelling does not resolve within 3 or 4 weeks, a biopsy may be needed.

TOOTHACHE

Pain in and around the teeth is a common problem, particularly among people with poor oral hygiene. Pain may be constant, felt after stimulation (from heat, cold, sweet food or drink, chewing, or brushing), or both.

CAUSES

The most common causes of toothache are

- Cavities
- Pulpitis
- Periapical abscess
- Trauma
- Wisdom tooth pushing through the gum tissue (causing pericoronitis)

Toothaches are usually caused by tooth decay and its resulting consequences, such as pulpitis and abscess. Tooth decay can be largely prevented by good oral hygiene, which helps remove plaque. Removing plaque helps because the bacteria in plaque produce acid which can damage tooth enamel and dentin.

Cavities (tooth decay) cause pain when they extend through the outer surface of the tooth (enamel) into the hard tissue beneath the enamel (dentin). Pain usually occurs only after stimulation from cold, heat, sweet food or drink, or brushing. The pulp, the living center of a tooth, is likely not irreversibly affected if the pain stops immediately after the stimulus is removed.

Pulpitis (inflammation of the tooth pulp) is typically caused by advanced cavities but also may be due to pulp damage from extensive or defective previous dental work or trauma. Pulpitis may be reversible or irreversible. If heat or cold is applied, the pain may linger for a minute or longer. Pain also may be present without stimulation. Pulp inflammation frequently causes the pulp to die. Once the pulp dies, pain ends briefly (for hours to weeks). Then, pain may come back as the tissue surrounding the root of the tooth becomes inflamed (apical periodontitis) or if a collection of pus (abscess) develops.

A **periapical abscess** (a collection of pus around the root of the tooth) may occur when infection develops around the root of the tooth

after untreated cavities or pulpitis. The tooth is extremely sensitive to tapping with a metal dental probe or tongue blade (percussion) and to chewing. The periapical abscess may come to a head and drain on its own or spread into nearby tissues (cellulitis).

Trauma includes broken or loosened teeth. Tooth trauma can damage the pulp and cause pulpitis and sometimes discoloration of the tooth, which may begin soon after the injury or up to decades later.

Pericoronitis is inflammation and infection of the gum around the crown of a tooth, usually a tooth that is just breaking through the gum (erupting) or cannot break through (impacted). It usually occurs around an erupting wisdom tooth (almost always a lower one) but can involve any tooth.

In young children, **teething** is often a cause of discomfort as the tooth erupts through the gum.

COMPLICATIONS

The main serious complications of disorders that cause toothache involve spread of infection from the area next to the tooth to nearby tissues. Infection can spread to the nasal sinuses (from an upper tooth), to a large vein at the base of the brain, to the cavernous sinus or under the tongue. Infection under the tongue is called Ludwig angina and can cause enough swelling to close off the person's airway. Cavernous sinus thrombosis and Ludwig angina are life threatening and require immediate treatment.

More commonly, pain from a sinus infection is mistakenly perceived as originating in the (unaffected) teeth—especially if the toothache develops while the person has or recently has had a cold. Additional symptoms suggesting sinusitis are headache and tenderness and swelling of the skin above the affected sinus.

EVALUATION

People with tooth pain should see a dentist. The following information can help people decide when a dentist's examination is needed and help them know what to expect during the evaluation.

In people with a toothache, certain symptoms and characteristics are cause for concern. These signs are warnings that a dental infection may have spread and include

- Headache and/or confusion
- Fever
- Swelling or tenderness of the floor of the mouth
- Difficulty seeing or double vision

WHEN TO SEE A DOCTOR OR A DENTIST

People who have warning signs and those with swelling around an eye should go to the hospital right away. People who do not have warning signs but who have swelling over the jaw, very severe pain, or drainage of pus from the base of a tooth should see a dentist as soon as possible. Other people who have a toothache should see a dentist at some point, but a delay of several days is not harmful.

WHAT THE DENTIST DOES

Dentists first ask questions about the person's symptoms and medical history. Dentists then examine the face, mouth, and teeth. What they find during the history and physical examination often suggests a cause of the toothache and the tests that may need to be done (see Table, below).

TESTING

The need for tests depends on what dentists or doctors find during the history and physical examination, particularly whether warning

SOME CAUSES AND FEATURES OF TOOTHACHE

Cause	Common Features*	Tests
Apical abscess (a collection of pus around the tooth's root)	Constant pain that worsens when chewing or biting Normally, the person can precisely identify the involved tooth Tooth tender when tapped with a metal probe or tongue blade (percussed) Sometimes visible swelling of the gum over the affected root and painful swelling of the adjacent cheek and/or lip	A dentist's examination†
Apical periodontitis (inflammation of tissues around the tooth's root)	Features similar to those of apical abscess but less severe and without swelling over the affected root	A dentist's examination†
Cavities	Pain that - Occurs mainly after brushing or after chewing or swallowing hot, cold, or sweet food or drink - Is isolated to a single tooth - Usually stops when the stimulus is removed Usually a visible cavity or a root surface exposed by gum recession or an abrasion	A dentist's examination†
Fracture of a tooth	Sharp pain when chewing Marked sensitivity to cold	A dentist's examination†

(continued)

SOME CAUSES AND FEATURES OF TOOTHACHE (continued)

Cause	Common Features*	Tests
Pericoronitis (usually involving an erupting or partially impacted wisdom tooth)	Constant dull pain, especially when chewing Visible swelling, redness, and sometimes pus around the affected tooth Commonly spasms of the chewing muscles (trismus) may occur and limit opening	A dentist's examination†
Pulpitis (inflammation of the tooth pulp)	Pain that occurs without stimulation and/or that lingers for more than a few seconds after stimulation May have difficulty identifying the affected tooth	A dentist's examination†
Sinusitis	Pain in several upper teeth on one side, especially molars and premolars	A doctor's examination, sometimes with CT of the sinuses
	Sensitivity when chewing and when teeth are tapped (percussed)	A dentist's examination if no sinusitis is detected
	Often a nasal discharge and tenderness when the sinus is tapped	
	Pain when changing positions, especially lowering the head (as when bending down to tie shoe laces)	
Teething	Discomfort and fussiness during tooth eruption in young children Commonly drooling and chewing on things (such as the crib rail)	A doctor's examination

*Features include symptoms and the results of the doctor's examination. Features mentioned are typical but not always present.
†Dental x-rays are usually taken.
CT = computed tomography.

signs are present. However, dental x-rays are usually done. If cavernous sinus thrombosis or Ludwig angina is suspected, an imaging study—typically computed tomography (CT) or magnetic resonance imaging (MRI)—is done.

TREATMENT

Nonprescription pain relievers (analgesics) such as acetaminophen or ibuprofen can be taken while people await dental evaluation.

Antibiotics such as penicillin or clindamycin are given for disorders such as abscesses, pericoronitis, or cellulitis.

Specific disorders are treated. An **abscess** is typically drained through an incision with a scalpel blade. A rubber drain, held in place by a stitch, may be placed.

Pericoronitis is treated by rinsing the mouth 3 or 4 times a day with the antiseptic chlorhexidine or salt water (1 tablespoon of salt mixed in a glass of hot water—no hotter than the coffee or tea a person normally drinks). The salt water is held in the mouth on the affected side until it cools and then is spit out and immediately replaced with another mouthful.

Teething pain in young children may be treated with acetaminophen or ibuprofen (dosed by the child's weight). Other options include chewing hard crackers (such as biscotti), applying a benzocaine gel 4 times a day (provided there is no family history of methemoglobinemia, which can make use of benzocaine dangerous), and chewing on anything cold (such as gel-containing teething rings).

The rare person with cavernous sinus thrombosis or Ludwig angina requires immediate hospitalization, removal of the infected tooth, and antibiotics given by vein (intravenously).

ESSENTIALS FOR OLDER PEOPLE

Older people are more prone to cavities of the root surfaces, usually because of receding gums. Periodontitis often begins in young adulthood. If untreated, tooth pain and loss are common in old age.

KEY POINTS

- Most toothaches involve cavities or the resulting complications (such as pulpitis or an abscess).
- Treatment of symptoms and referral to a dentist are usually adequate.
- Antibiotics are given if people have an abscess, a tooth with pulp that has died, or more severe conditions.
- A dental infection that has spread to the floor of the mouth or to the cavernous sinus is a very rare but serious complication.
- Dental infections rarely cause sinusitis, but a sinus infection may cause pain that feels as though it originates in the teeth.

TREMOR

A tremor is an involuntary, rhythmic, shaking movement of part of the body, such as the hands, head, vocal cords, trunk, or legs. Tremors occur when muscles repeatedly contract and relax.

TYPES OF TREMORS

Tremors are usually classified based on when they occur:

- Resting tremor: Occurring mainly at rest
- Intention tremor: Triggered by movement toward a target (for example, reaching for a glass)
- Postural tremor: Triggered by holding a limb outstretched in one position

Tremors can also be classified by what causes them. Examples include the following:

- Physiologic (the normal tremors that everyone has to some degree)
- Essential (a common disorder that rarely causes any other symptoms)
- Cerebellar (caused by damage to part of the brain called the cerebellum)
- Secondary (caused by a disorder or drug)

Other important characteristics of tremors are

- How fast the shaking is (frequency): Slow to fast
- How wide the movement is (amplitude): Fine to coarse
- How often the tremor occurs: Intermittent to constant
- How severe it is
- How rapidly it appears: Sudden to gradual

RESTING TREMOR

This tremor occurs when muscles are at rest. An arm or a leg shakes even when a person is completely relaxed. The tremor becomes less noticeable or disappears when the person moves the affected muscles. Resting tremors are often slow and coarse.

These tremors develop when nerve cells in the part of the brain called the basal ganglia are disturbed. Such disturbances usually result from Parkinson disease. However, they can result from use of drugs that can affect this part of the brain, such as antipsychotic drugs and some drugs used to relieve nausea.

Resting tremors may be socially embarrassing, but because they go away when people try to do something (such as drinking a glass of water), they typically do not interfere with daily activities.

INTENTION TREMOR

This tremor occurs during a purposeful movement, as when reaching for an object with the hand. People may miss the object because of the tremor. Intention tremors worsen as people get closer to the targeted object. These tremors are relatively slow and coarse.

Intention tremors may result from damage to the cerebellum, the part of the brain responsible for balance and coordination. Thus, cerebellar tremor and intention tremor may be used as synonyms.

Certain hereditary disorders that affect the cerebellum (called spinocerebellar ataxias) are a common cause of intention tremors, as is multiple sclerosis. Stroke, a tumor, alcoholism, and overuse of sedatives or anticonvulsants can also cause the cerebellum to malfunction, resulting in an intention tremor.

POSTURAL TREMOR

This type of tremor is most obvious when a limb is held in a position that requires resisting the pull of gravity, as when people hold their arms outstretched. The most common postural tremors are essential tremor and physiologic (normal) tremor.

COMPLEX TREMOR

Complex tremor is a tremor that has features of more than one type of tremor. Common causes of complex tremors are psychologic factors and widespread nerve damage such as that caused by diabetes or Guillain-Barré syndrome.

CAUSES

Tremors can be normal (physiologic) or abnormal. Many disorders can cause tremor (see Table on pages 393 to 394).

Most commonly, tremors are

- Physiologic tremor (most common overall)
- Essential tremor
- Due to Parkinson disease
- Due to a stroke or multiple sclerosis affecting parts of the brain that control movement
- Due to hereditary disorders involving the cerebellum, such as Friedreich ataxia and spinocerebellar ataxias
- Psychogenic tremor (due to psychologic factors)

Physiologic tremor is the normal tremor that everyone has to some degree. For example, most people's hands, when held outstretched, usually tremble slightly. Such slight, rapid tremor reflects the precise moment-by-moment control of muscles by nerves. In most people, the tremor is barely noticeable. However, a normal tremor may become more noticeable under certain conditions and may worry people. For example, the tremor may be more noticeable when people

- Feel stressed, anxious, tired, or sleepy
- Stop drinking alcohol or taking a sedative (such as a benzodiazepine) or an opioid
- Consume caffeine
- Take certain drugs, including theophylline and albuterol (which are used to treat asthma and COPD), corticosteroids, and recreational drugs (such as cocaine or amphetamines)

Essential tremor results from a problem in the nervous system, but people with this tremor rarely have any other symptoms of nervous system dysfunction (neurologic symptoms). The cause is unclear, but the tremor often runs in families.

Essential tremor usually begins during early adulthood but can begin at any age. The tremor slowly becomes more noticeable as people age. Thus, it is sometimes incorrectly called senile tremor. The tremor usually involves the arms and hands and sometimes affects the head. When it affects the head, people may look as if they are nodding yes or shaking their head no.

These tremors are usually worsened by holding a limb outstretched (against gravity) or by moving a limb.

Usually, essential tremor remains mild. However, it can be troublesome and embarrassing. It can affect handwriting and make using utensils difficult. In some people, the tremor gradually worsens over time, eventually resulting in disability. Symptoms may resemble those of Parkinson disease, and sometimes essential tremor is misdiagnosed as Parkinson disease.

EVALUATION

The following information can help people decide when a doctor's evaluation is needed and help them know what to expect during the evaluation.

WARNING SIGNS

The following symptoms are cause for concern:

- Tremors that start abruptly
- Other neurologic symptoms, such as a change in mental status, muscle weakness, changes in the way a person walks, and difficulty speaking
- A rapid heart rate and agitation

WHEN TO SEE A DOCTOR

People with warning signs should see a doctor immediately. People without warning signs should see a doctor as soon as possible, but a delay of a week or two (or slightly longer if the tremor has developed over months or years) is usually not harmful.

If people are under 50 years old and do not have a family history of tremor, being evaluated by a doctor is important to make sure that the cause is not another disorder or a drug.

WHAT A DOCTOR DOES

Doctors first ask questions about the person's symptoms and medical history and then do a physical examination. What doctors find during the history and physical examination often suggests a cause and the tests that may need to be done (see Table).

Doctors ask whether the tremor began gradually or suddenly, which body parts are affected, what triggers it (such as movement, rest, or standing), and what relieves or worsens it (such

SOME CAUSES AND FEATURES OF TREMOR

Cause	Features*	Tests
Postural tremor (tremor when a limb is held outstretched)		
Alcohol or a sedative (such as a benzodiazepine) when use is stopped	Agitation and a fine tremor starting 24–72 hours after the last use of alcohol or a benzodiazepine Sometimes high blood pressure, a rapid heart rate, or fever, especially in people who are hospitalized	A doctor's examination
Drugs such as ■ Amitriptyline ■ Beta-agonists (used to treat asthma) ■ Cocaine ■ Haloperidol ■ Lithium ■ SSRIs ■ Tamoxifen ■ Valproate	History of drug use	Stopping the drug to see whether the tremor goes away
Hormonal, metabolic, and toxic abnormalities that affect the brain: ■ Brain damage due to lack of oxygen (anoxic encephalopathy) ■ Liver failure (hepatic encephalopathy) ■ An overactive thyroid gland (hyperthyroidism) ■ Kidney failure ■ Overactive parathyroid glands (hyperparathyroidism) ■ Low blood sugar (hypoglycemia) ■ Poisons, including heavy metals such as lead	A tremor plus coma or lethargy and symptoms of an underlying disorder such as ■ For hyperthyroidism: Difficulty tolerating heat, excessive sweating, an increased appetite, weight loss, bulging eyes, and frequent bowel movements	Tests to help identify the cause, such as blood tests ■ To evaluate how well the liver, thyroid gland, kidneys, and parathyroid glands are functioning ■ To measure blood sugar levels ■ To identify poisons
Essential tremor	A coarse or fine, slow tremor that ■ Worsens slowly, over many years ■ Usually affects both arms and sometimes the head and voice ■ Often occurs in people with a family history of tremor No other symptoms of nervous system malfunction	A doctor's examination
Physiologic tremor	A fine, rapid tremor that ■ Occurs in otherwise healthy people ■ May become more noticeable when people take or stop taking certain drugs (see under Causes on page 392) or feel stressed, anxious, tired, or sleepy ■ Usually lessens when people drink small amounts of alcohol or take low doses of sedatives	A doctor's examination
Resting tremor		
Parkinsonism triggered by a drug, such as certain antipsychotic drugs and drugs used to relieve nausea	A history of drug use	Stopping the drug to see whether the tremor goes away *(continued)*

SOME CAUSES AND FEATURES OF TREMOR (continued)

Cause	Features*	Tests
Parkinson disease	A slow alternating tremor that ■ Often involves moving the thumb against the index finger as if moving small objects around (called pill rolling) ■ Sometimes also affects the chin or a leg ■ Usually starts on one side ■ Is accompanied by other symptoms, such as muscle stiffness, shaky and tiny handwriting, slow movements, and a shuffling walk Often no family history of Parkinson disease or tremor and no lessening of tremor after drinking alcohol	A doctor's examination Use of the drug levodopa to see whether improvement occurs
Intention tremor		
Cerebellar disorders: ■ Chronic alcoholism ■ Friedreich ataxia ■ Hemorrhage ■ Injury ■ Multiple sclerosis ■ Spinocerebellar ataxias ■ Stroke ■ Tumor	A slow tremor that ■ Usually occurs on one side of the body ■ Is accompanied by lack of coordination, especially when attempting to touch or grasp a targeted object or perform rapid alternating movements ■ Affects the muscles used in speech, making the voice tremble In some people, a family history of the disorder (as for Friedreich ataxia or spinocerebellar ataxias)	MRI of the brain
Drugs, such as ■ Alcohol ■ Anticonvulsants (such as phenytoin and valproate) ■ Beta-agonists ■ Cyclosporine ■ Lithium ■ Tacrolimus	A history of drug use	Stopping the drug to see whether the tremor goes away
Complex tremors		
Disorders that affect many of the nerves outside the brain and spinal cord (polyneuropathies): ■ Guillain-Barré syndrome ■ Diabetes	A tremor that ■ Varies in speed and width ■ Often occurs when people reach for an object and worsens as they get closer to the object ■ Often worsens when people hold a limb outstretched ■ Is accompanied by other symptoms of nerve damage, such as weakness, a pins-and-needles sensation, and loss of sensation	Electromyography (stimulating muscles and recording their electrical activity)
Psychogenic tremor (due to psychologic factors)	A tremor that ■ Begins suddenly or may stop just as suddenly ■ Varies in speed and width ■ Lessens when people are distracted	A doctor's examination

*Features include symptoms and results of the doctor's examination. Features mentioned are typical but not always present.
MRI = magnetic resonance imaging; SSRIs = selective serotonin reuptake inhibitors (a type of antidepressant).

as alcohol, caffeine, stress, or anxiety). If the tremor began suddenly, doctors ask about events that may have triggered it (such as a recent injury or use of a new drug).

Doctors review the person's past medical history, looking for conditions associated with tremor (see Table). They ask about tremors in close relatives. They review the drugs taken and ask about use of caffeine, alcohol, and recreational drugs (particularly whether the person recently stopped using such drugs).

Doctors do a physical examination, paying particular attention to the neurologic examination (including the way the person walks). Doctors note which body parts are affected by the tremor. They observe how fast the shaking movements are in various situations:

- When the affected body parts are at rest and when they are fully supported (for example, hands in the person's lap)
- While the person maintains certain positions (such as holding the arms outstretched)
- While the person is walking or doing tasks with the affected body part

The quality of the person's voice may be observed when holding a long note.

TESTING

Doctors can usually identify the type of tremor based on its characteristics and results of the medical history and physical examination. For example, if the tremor develops gradually, it is usually physiologic or essential tremor. If a postural tremor starts more suddenly, the cause may be psychologic factors, a poison, a disorder (such as hyperthyroidism), stopping use of alcohol or another drug (such as a sedative), or use of a drug known to cause tremor.

Brain imaging with magnetic resonance imaging (MRI) or computed tomography (CT) is done if

- The person has other neurologic symptoms.
- The tremor started suddenly or progresses rapidly.

For people with postural tremors, testing may also include blood tests to check for possible causes. Tests may include measurement of blood sugar and tests to evaluate how well the thyroid and parathyroid glands, liver, and kidneys are functioning.

TREATMENT

Any specific cause is treated when possible—for example, by stopping a drug that is causing the tremor or by treating hyperthyroidism. Parkinson disease can be treated with levodopa and other drugs.

For mild tremor, no treatment is needed. If tremors become bothersome, some simple measures can help:

- Grasping objects firmly and holding them close to the body to avoid dropping them
- Avoiding uncomfortable positions
- Not eating soup in public
- Using assistive devices, as instructed by an occupational therapist

Assistive devices may include rocker knives, utensils with large handles, and, particularly if the tremor is severe, button hooks, Velcro fasteners (instead of buttons or shoe laces), zipper pulls, straws, and shoe horns.

For physiologic or essential tremor, eliminating or minimizing the trigger may lessen the tremor. For example, avoiding caffeine, getting enough sleep, and minimizing stress may help. For some people, drinking alcohol in moderation may lessen the tremor, but doctors do not recommend this tactic as a treatment. Heavy drinking followed by suddenly stopping makes the tremor worse. If many daily activities (such as using utensils and drinking from a glass at mealtime) become difficult or if the person's work requires steady hands, drug therapy may help. It may include a beta-blocker (such as propranolol), the anticonvulsant primidone, or both. For physiologic tremor, occasionally taking a low dose of a benzodiazepine (a sedative), such as lorazepam, may help lessen the tremor.

Intention tremors are difficult to treat, but if the condition causing it can be corrected, the tremor may resolve. If the condition cannot be corrected, a therapist may put wrist and ankle weights on the affected limb to reduce the tremor. Or people may be taught to brace the limb during activity. These measures sometimes help.

DEEP BRAIN STIMULATION

Tiny electrodes are placed in the area of the brain involved in tremors. The electrodes deliver a painless shock to block the impulses causing tremors. Deep brain stimulation is sometimes done when drugs cannot control a severe, disabling tremor. Sometimes essential tremors or tremors due to Parkinson disease or another disorder require such treatment. Such treatments are available only at special centers.

or mental impairments. Physical and occupational therapists can provide simple coping strategies, and assistive devices may help older people maintain quality of life.

ESSENTIALS FOR OLDER PEOPLE

Many older people think that developing a tremor is a part of normal aging and may not seek medical attention. Nonetheless, older people should talk to their doctor, who can ask them questions and do a physical examination to check for possible causes of tremor. Doctors may then recommend strategies or possibly drugs to lessen the tremor.

Also, older people are more likely to be taking drugs that cause tremor and are more vulnerable to side effects of these drugs. Thus, when prescribing such drugs to older people, doctors try to prescribe the lowest effective dose. Such a dose may be lower than the doses used to treat younger adults.

Tremor can significantly affect quality of life in older people, interfering with their ability to function, especially if they have other physical

O⎯π KEY POINTS

- Tremors can be classified based on when they occur: when at rest (resting tremor), when moving toward a target (intention tremor), or when holding a limb outstretched (postural tremor).
- Most tremors are physiologic (normal) tremors, and some are essential tremor or are caused by other disorders.
- Tremors that occur during rest are often caused by Parkinson disease.
- Doctors can usually identify the cause based on the history and physical examination.
- If a tremor begins suddenly or is accompanied by other neurologic symptoms, people should see a doctor right away.
- People who are under 50 and have tremor should see a doctor.

URINARY INCONTINENCE IN ADULTS

Urinary incontinence is involuntary loss of urine. Incontinence can occur in both men and women at any age, but it is more common among women and older people, affecting about 30% of elderly women and 15% of elderly men. Although incontinence is more common among older people, it is not a normal part of aging. Incontinence may be sudden and temporary, as when a person is taking a drug that has a diuretic effect, or it may be long lasting (chronic). Even chronic incontinence may sometimes be relieved.

Urinary incontinence in children is discussed separately (see page 405).

There are several types of incontinence:

- **Urge incontinence** is uncontrolled urine leakage (of moderate to large volume) that occurs immediately after an urgent, irrepressible need to urinate. Getting up to urinate during the night (nocturia) and nocturnal incontinence are common.
- **Stress incontinence** is urine leakage due to abrupt increases in intra-abdominal pressure (for example, those that occur with coughing, sneezing, laughing, bending, or lifting). Leakage volume is usually low to moderate.
- **Overflow incontinence** is dribbling of urine from an overly full bladder. Volume is usually small, but leaks may be constant, resulting in large total losses.
- **Functional incontinence** is loss of urine because of a problem with thinking or a physical impairment unrelated to the control of urination. For example, a person with dementia due to Alzheimer disease may not recognize the need to urinate or not know where the toilet is. People who are bedridden may be unable to walk to the toilet or reach a bedpan.

Often, however, a person has more than one type of incontinence. People are then described as having mixed incontinence.

CAUSES

Several mechanisms can lead to urinary incontinence. Often, more than one mechanism is present:

- Weakness of the urinary sphincter or pelvic muscles (called bladder outlet incompetence)
- Something blocking the exit path of urine from the bladder (called bladder outlet obstruction)
- Spasm or overactivity of the bladder wall muscles (sometimes called overactive bladder)
- Weakness or underactivity of the bladder wall muscles
- Poor coordination of the bladder wall muscles with the urinary sphincter
- An increase in the volume of urine
- Functional problems

Weakness or underactivity of the bladder wall muscles, bladder outlet obstruction, or particularly both can lead to inability to urinate (urinary retention). Urinary retention can paradoxically lead to overflow incontinence because of leaking from an overly full bladder.

An increase in the volume of urine (for example, caused by diabetes, use of diuretics, or excessive intake of alcohol or caffeinated drinks) can increase the amount of urine lost to incontinence, trigger an episode of incontinence, or even cause temporary incontinence to develop. However, it should not cause chronic incontinence. Functional problems commonly increase the volume of urine lost among people who are incontinent. However, functional problems are rarely the only cause of permanent incontinence.

Overall, the **most common causes** of incontinence are

- Overactive bladder in children and young adults
- Pelvic muscle weakness in women as a result of childbirth
- Bladder outlet obstruction in middle-aged men
- Functional disorders such as stroke and dementia in older people

EVALUATION

Urinary incontinence usually does not indicate a disorder that is life threatening; nevertheless, incontinence may cause embarrassment or lead

SOME MECHANISMS OF INCONTINENCE

Mechanism	Examples
Weakness of the urinary sphincter or pelvic muscles (bladder outlet incompetence)	Atrophic urethritis, vaginitis, or both
	Drugs
	Pelvic muscle weakness (for example, caused by having had several vaginal deliveries or pelvic surgery)
	Prostate surgery
Blockage (bladder outlet obstruction)	Prostate enlargement (benign prostatic hyperplasia) or cancer
	Bladder stones
	Impacted stool
	Drugs
Overactivity of bladder wall muscles (overactive bladder)	Bladder irritation (for example, caused by infection, stones, or rarely cancer)
	Disorders that can affect brain centers that control urination (such as stroke, dementia, or multiple sclerosis)
	Cervical spondylosis or spinal cord dysfunction (which can put pressure on the spinal cord and thus impair bladder function)
	Bladder outlet obstruction
Underactivity of bladder wall muscles	Nerve damage (for example, by herniated disks, other spinal cord disorders, surgery, tumors, injury, diabetes, or alcoholism)
	Drugs
	Longstanding bladder outlet obstruction
	In women, often no identifiable cause
Poor coordination of the bladder wall with the sphincter muscles	Damage to spinal cord or brain nerve pathways to the bladder
Functional problems	Dementia
	Depression
	Psychoactive drugs that can decrease awareness of the need to urinate (for example, antipsychotic drugs, benzodiazepines, drugs that cause drowsiness such as sedatives and sleep aids, or tricyclic antidepressants)
	Restricted mobility (for example, caused by injury, weakness, restraints, stroke, other neurologic disorders, or musculoskeletal disorders)
	Situational limitations (such as not having a toilet nearby or traveling)
Increase in the volume of urine	Disorders such as diabetes mellitus or diabetes insipidus
	Use of diuretics (usually furosemide, bumetanide, or theophylline, but not thiazide diuretics)
	Excessive intake of caffeinated beverages (such as coffee, tea, cola, or some other soft drinks) or alcohol

people to restrict their activities unnecessarily, contributing to a decline in quality of life. Also, rarely, sudden incontinence can be a symptom of a spinal cord disorder. The following information can help people decide when a doctor's evaluation is needed and help them know what to expect during the evaluation.

WARNING SIGNS

In people with urinary incontinence, certain symptoms and characteristics are cause for concern. They include

- Symptoms of spinal cord damage (for example, weakness in the legs or loss of sensation in the legs or around the genitals or anus)

WHEN TO SEE A DOCTOR

People with warning signs should go to an emergency department at once. People without warning signs should call their doctor. The doctor will decide how quickly they need to be seen based on their other symptoms and other known conditions. In general, if incontinence is the only symptom, a delay of a week or so is not harmful.

Most people are embarrassed to mention incontinence to their doctors. Some people believe that incontinence is a normal part of aging. However, incontinence, even incontinence that has been present for some time or that occurs in an older person, may be helped by treatment. If symptoms of urinary incontinence are bothersome, interfere with activities of daily living, or cause people to curtail their social activities, people should see a doctor.

WHAT THE DOCTOR DOES

Doctors first ask questions about the person's symptoms and medical history. Doctors then do a physical examination. What they find during the history and physical examination often suggests a cause of the incontinence and the tests that may need to be done.

Doctors ask questions about the circumstances of urine loss, including amount, time of day, and any precipitating factors (such as coughing, sneezing, or straining). People are asked whether they can sense the need to urinate and, if so, whether the sensation is normal or comes with sudden urgency. Doctors may also ask the person to estimate the amount of urine leakage. Doctors will also ask whether the person has any additional problems with urination, such as pain or burning during urination, a frequent need to urinate, difficulty starting urination, or a weak urine stream. Sometimes doctors may ask people to keep a record of their urination habits over a day or two. This record is called a voiding diary. Each time the person urinates, the volume and time are recorded. After an episode of incontinence, the person also records any related activities, especially eating, drinking, drug use, or sleep.

SOME DRUGS THAT CAN CAUSE INCONTINENCE	
Mechanism	Examples
Weakness of the urinary sphincter or pelvic muscles (bladder outlet incompetence)	Alpha-adrenergic blockers (such as alfuzosin, doxazosin, prazosin, tamsulosin, or terazosin), which relax the urinary sphincter
	Hormone therapy (usually estrogen/progestin combination therapy taken by mouth), which can contribute to thinning of the pelvic muscles and supporting tissues
	Misoprostol, which relaxes the urinary sphincter
Blockage (bladder outlet obstruction)	Alpha-adrenergic agonists (such as pseudoephedrine), which can cause muscles in the bladder and prostate to contract
Underactivity of bladder wall muscles	Drugs with anticholinergic effects (such as antihistamines, antipsychotic drugs, benztropine, or tricyclic antidepressants), which inhibit bladder muscle contractions
	Calcium channel blockers (such as diltiazem, nifedipine, or verapamil), which inhibit bladder muscle contractions
	Opioids, which seem to inhibit bladder contractility

Doctors ask about whether the person has other disorders that are known to cause incontinence, such as dementia, stroke, urinary tract stones, spinal cord or other neurologic disorders, and prostate disorders. Doctors need to know what drugs a person is taking because some drugs cause or contribute to incontinence. Women are asked about number and types of deliveries and any complications. All are asked about previous pelvic and abdominal surgery, particularly prostate surgery in men.

The physical examination can help doctors narrow possible causes. Doctors test strength, sensation and reflexes in the legs, and sensation around the genitals and anus to detect nerve and muscle problems that may make it difficult for the person to remain continent.

In women, doctors do a pelvic examination to detect abnormalities that could cause incontinence, such as atrophic vaginitis or weakness of pelvic muscles. In men and women, doctors do a rectal examination to look for signs of constipation or damage to the nerves supplying the rectum. In men, the rectal examination allows doctors to check the prostate because an enlarged prostate or occasionally prostate cancer can contribute to incontinence. The person may be asked to cough with a full bladder to detect whether stress incontinence is present. Women may be asked to repeat this procedure during a pelvic examination, to see whether supporting some pelvic structures (with the doctor's fingers) eliminates the leak of urine.

TESTING

Often findings during the physical examination can help doctors determine the cause or identify factors that contribute to incontinence. However, some tests are often needed so doctors can make a firm diagnosis. Routinely obtained tests include

- Urinalysis and urine culture
- Blood tests of kidney function and sometimes others
- Postvoid residual volume (a catheter or ultrasonography probe is used to determine how much urine is left in the bladder after a person urinates)

Urodynamic testing includes cystometry, urinary flow rate testing, and cystometrography and is done when clinical evaluation and the above tests do not reveal the cause of incontinence.

- Cystometry is done to confirm urge incontinence and to determine whether the cause is overactive bladder. A bladder catheter is placed through the urethra. A doctor measures how much water can be injected into the bladder until the person develops a sense of urgency or bladder contractions.
- Peak urinary flow rate is measured in men to determine whether incontinence is caused by bladder outlet obstruction (usually caused by prostate disease). Men urinate into a special device (uroflowmeter) that measures the speed of urine flow and how much urine is released.
- Cystometrography is done if all other evaluation fails to reveal the cause of incontinence. Cystometrography is a test that measures bladder pressures when the bladder is filled with various volumes of water. Cystometrography is often done with electromyography, a test that can assess sphincter function. In certain centers with specialized equipment, bladder contraction strength can also be measured at the same time as sphincter and other bladder pressures.

Although urodynamic testing is important, results do not always predict response to drug treatment or assess the relative importance of multiple causes.

TREATMENT

The specific cause of incontinence can often be treated. There are also general measures that doctors may suggest to all people to reduce the inconvenience of incontinence. When a drug is causing a problem, doctors may be able to switch the person to a different drug or change the dosing schedule to provide relief (for example, a diuretic dose may be timed so that a bathroom is near when the drug takes effect). However, people should talk with their doctor before they stop taking a drug or change the amount or dosing schedule.

Drugs are often useful for some types of incontinence but should supplement rather than replace general measures. Drugs include those that relax the bladder wall muscle and those that increase sphincter tone. Drugs that relax the urinary sphincter may be used to treat outlet obstruction in men with urge or overflow incontinence.

GENERAL MEASURES

Regardless of the type and cause of incontinence, some general measures are usually helpful.

- Modifying fluid intake
- Bladder training
- Pelvic muscle exercises

Fluid intake can be limited at certain times (for example, before going out or 3 to 4 hours before bedtime). Doctors may suggest that people avoid fluids that irritate the bladder (such as caffeine-containing fluids). However, people should drink 48 to 64 oz (1500 to 2000 mL) of fluid a day because concentrated urine irritates the bladder.

Bladder training is a technique that involves having the person follow a fixed schedule for urination while awake. The doctor works with the person to establish a schedule of urinating every 2 to 3 hours and suppressing the urge to urinate at other times (for example, by relaxing and breathing deeply). As the person becomes better able to suppress the urge to urinate, the interval is gradually lengthened. A similar technique, called prompted voiding, can be used by people who care for a person with dementia or other cognitive problems. In this, the person is asked whether they need to urinate and whether they are wet or dry at specific intervals.

Pelvic muscle exercises (Kegel exercises) are often effective, especially for stress incontinence. People must be certain to exercise the correct muscles, the muscles around the urethra and rectum that stop the flow of urine. The muscles are tightly squeezed for 1 to 2 seconds and then relaxed for about 10 seconds. The exercises are repeated about 10 times three times each day. People are gradually able to increase the time the muscles are tightly squeezed until the contraction is held for about 10 seconds each time. Because it can be difficult to learn to control the correct muscles, doctors may need to provide instruction or recommend the use of biofeedback or electrical stimulation (an electronic version of pelvic floor exercises in which an electric current is used to stimulate the correct muscles).

URGE INCONTINENCE

The goal is to relax the bladder wall muscles. Bladder training, Kegel exercises, and relaxation techniques are tried first. Biofeedback also can be tried. With the urge to urinate, the person can try relaxing, standing in place or sitting down, or tightening the pelvic muscles. The most commonly used drugs are oxybutynin and tolterodine. Oxybutynin is available as a skin patch or skin gel as well as a pill. Newer drugs include myrabegron, fesoterodine, solifenacin, darifenacin, and trospium.

If other treatments are ineffective for urge incontinence, further treatments can be tried, such as gentle electrical stimulation of the sacral nerves by a device similar to a pacemaker, instillation of chemicals into the bladder (when the cause is a spinal cord or brain disorder), or, rarely, surgery.

STRESS INCONTINENCE

Treatment usually begins with bladder training and Kegel exercises. Avoiding physical stresses that cause loss of urine (for example, heavy lifting) and losing weight may help control incontinence. Pseudoephedrine may be useful in women with bladder outlet incompetence. Imipramine may be used for mixed stress and urge incontinence or for either separately. Duloxetine is also used for stress incontinence. If stress incontinence is caused by atrophic urethritis or vaginitis, estrogen cream is often effective. For people with stress incontinence, urinating frequently to avoid a full bladder is often helpful.

For stress incontinence that is not relieved with drugs and behavioral measures, surgery or devices such as pessaries may be helpful. The vaginal sling procedure creates a hammock of support to help prevent the urethra from opening during coughing, sneezing, or laughing. Most commonly, a sling is created from synthetic mesh. Mesh implants are effective, but a few people with mesh implants have serious complications. Alternatively, doctors can create a sling using tissue from the abdominal wall or leg. In men with stress incontinence, a mesh sling or an artificial urinary sphincter implant may be placed around the urethra to prevent leakage of urine.

OVERFLOW INCONTINENCE

Treatment depends on whether the cause is bladder outlet obstruction, weak bladder wall muscles, or both. For overflow incontinence caused by bladder outlet obstruction, specific

SOME DRUGS USED TO TREAT URINARY INCONTINENCE

Drug	How It Works	Comments
For weakness of the urinary sphincter or pelvic muscles (bladder outlet incompetence) causing stress incontinence		
Duloxetine	Helps strengthen contractions of the urinary sphincter	Somewhat limited experience with this drug
Imipramine (a tricyclic antidepressant)	Helps strengthen urinary sphincter contractions and relax an overactive bladder (an anticholinergic effect*)	Also used for overactive bladder and urge incontinence
Pseudoephedrine (an alpha-adrenergic agonist)	Helps strengthen urinary sphincter contractions	Can cause anxiety, insomnia, and, in men, inability to urinate
For bladder outlet obstruction in men causing urge or overflow incontinence		
Alpha-adrenergic blockers: ■ Alfuzosin ■ Doxazosin ■ Prazosin ■ Tamsulosin ■ Terazosin	Help relax the urinary sphincter	Tend to increase the speed of urine flow and help the bladder empty more completely May decrease blood pressure or cause fatigue
5-Alpha reductase inhibitors: ■ Dutasteride ■ Finasteride	Help shrink an enlarged prostate	Can take weeks or months to become effective Sometimes decrease sex drive or contribute to erectile dysfunction
For overactive bladder with urge or stress incontinence		
Darifenacin	Increases the bladder's filling capacity and decreases bladder wall muscle spasms (anticholinergic effects†)	—
Dicyclomine	Relaxes involuntary muscles Increases the bladder's filling capacity and decreases bladder wall muscle spasms (anticholinergic effects*)	Not as thoroughly studied as many other drugs
Fesoterodine	Increases the bladder's filling capacity and decreases bladder wall muscle spasms (anticholinergic effects†)	Not as thoroughly studied as many other drugs
Hyoscyamine	Increases the bladder's filling capacity and decreases bladder wall muscle spasms (anticholinergic effects*)	Not as thoroughly studied as many other drugs
Imipramine (a tricyclic antidepressant)	Helps strengthen urinary sphincter contractions Increases the bladder's filling capacity and decreases bladder wall muscle spasms (an anticholinergic effect*)	Particularly useful for nighttime incontinence
Myrabegron (a beta-adrenergic agonist)	Relaxes the bladder wall	Not as thoroughly studied as many other drugs May increase blood pressure
Oxybutynin	Many effects, such as relaxation of involuntary muscles and anticholinergic effects*, which include increasing the bladder's filling capacity and decreasing the bladder wall muscle spasms	May be the most effective drug Available as a tablet, skin patch, and gel *(continued)*

SOME DRUGS USED TO TREAT URINARY INCONTINENCE (continued)

Drug	How It Works	Comments
Solifenacin	Increases the bladder's filling capacity and decreases bladder wall muscle spasms (anticholinergic effects[†])	—
Tolterodine	Increases the bladder's filling capacity and decreases bladder wall muscle spasms (anticholinergic effects[†])	—
Trospium	Increases the bladder's filling capacity and decreases bladder wall muscle spasms (anticholinergic effects[*])	—
OnabotulinumtoxinA (a type of botulinum toxin)	Blocks the nerve activity in the bladder muscle that causes the bladder to contract involuntarily	Injected into the bladder wall through a cystoscope inserted in the bladder Used to treat incontinence in adults with overactive bladder caused by a neurologic disorder (such as multiple sclerosis) when other drugs are ineffective or have too many side effects
For weak bladder wall muscles with overflow incontinence		
Bethanechol	Helps bladder wall muscles contract	Usually ineffective Can cause flushing, abdominal cramps, and an increased heart rate

[*]Anticholinergic effects (such as dry mouth, constipation, and sometimes blurred vision or confusion) can be bothersome, particularly in older people.
[†]These drugs have anticholinergic effects that target the urinary system, so they tend to have fewer other anticholinergic side effects than other drugs with anticholinergic effects.

treatments may help relieve obstruction (for example, surgery or drugs for prostate disease, surgery for cystocele, and dilation or stenting for urethral narrowing).

For overflow incontinence caused by weak bladder wall muscles, treatments can include reducing the amount of urine in the bladder by intermittent insertion of a bladder catheter or, rarely, insertion of a catheter that remains in the bladder. The goal is to reduce the bladder's size, allowing its walls to regain some capacity to prevent it from overflowing. Other measures can help empty the bladder after urinating. These can include trying to urinate again after urination has ended (called double voiding), bearing down at the end of urination, and/or pressing over the lower abdomen at the end of urination. Occasionally, electrical stimulation can be used to help empty the bladder more completely.

ESSENTIALS FOR OLDER PEOPLE

Although incontinence is more common among older people, it is not a normal part of aging.

With aging, bladder capacity decreases, ability to delay urination declines, involuntary bladder contractions occur more often, and bladder contractions weaken. Thus, urination becomes more difficult to postpone and tends to be incomplete. The muscles, ligaments, and connective tissue of the pelvis weaken, contributing to incontinence. In postmenopausal women, decreased estrogen levels lead to atrophic urethritis and atrophic vaginitis and to decreasing the strength of the urethral sphincter. In men, prostate size increases, partially obstructing the urethra and leading to incomplete bladder emptying and strain on the bladder muscle. These changes occur in many normal, continent older people and may facilitate incontinence but do not cause it.

Incontinence greatly reduces quality of life, causing embarrassment, isolation, and depression. Incontinence is often a reason older people require care in a long-term care facility. Urine irritates the skin, contributing to the formation of pressure sores in people who are bedbound or chairbound. Older people with urge incontinence are at increased risk of falls and fractures as they rush to the toilet.

The most effective drugs for many kinds of incontinence have anticholinergic effects. These effects, such as constipation, dry mouth, blurred vision, and sometimes even confusion, can be particularly troublesome in older people.

KEY POINTS

- Incontinence is common and can greatly reduce a person's quality of life, so people should be evaluated by a doctor.
- Although incontinence is more common among older people, it is not a normal consequence of aging.
- Some causes are reversible, even if long-standing.

Urinary incontinence (enuresis) is defined as the involuntary release of urine occurring two or more times per month after toilet training. Incontinence may be present during the day (daytime incontinence), at night (nighttime incontinence or nocturnal enuresis), or both (combined incontinence). The duration of the process of toilet training, or the age at which children achieve urinary continence, varies greatly. However, more than 90% of children achieve daytime urinary continence by age 5. Nighttime continence may take longer to achieve. Bed-wetting or nighttime incontinence affects about 30% of children at age 4, 10% at age 7, 3% at age 12, and 1% at age 18. About 0.5% of adults continue to have nighttime incontinence. Doctors take these time lines into account when diagnosing urinary incontinence. Because the duration of the process of toilet training varies, young children are usually not considered to have daytime incontinence if they are under age 5 or 6 or nighttime incontinence if they are under age 7.

Daytime incontinence is more common among girls. Bed-wetting is more common among boys and among children who have a family history of nighttime incontinence. Both daytime and nighttime incontinence are symptoms—not diagnoses—and doctors look for an underlying cause.

CAUSES

The pattern of incontinence helps the doctor determine the likely cause. If the child has never had a consistent dry period during the day, the doctor considers the possibility of a birth defect, an anatomic abnormality, or certain behaviors that can lead to incontinence.

Several uncommon but important disorders affect the normal anatomy or function of the bladder, which can lead to urinary incontinence. For example, a spinal cord defect such as spina bifida can cause abnormal nerve function to the bladder and lead to incontinence. Some infants have a birth defect that prevents the bladder or urethra from developing completely, leading to nearly constant urine loss (total incontinence). Another type of birth defect causes the tubes that connect the kidneys to the bladder (ureters) to end in an abnormal location in the bladder or even outside the bladder (such as in the vagina or urethra or on the surface of the body), causing incontinence. Some children have an overactive bladder that easily spasms or contracts, causing incontinence, whereas others may have difficulty emptying their bladder.

Certain behaviors can lead to daytime incontinence, especially in girls. Such behaviors include urinating infrequently and urinating using an incorrect position (with legs too close together). With such positions, urine can accumulate in the vagina during urination, then dribble out after standing. Some girls experience bladder spasm when laughing, resulting in "giggle incontinence."

If the child has been dry for a long time and the incontinence is new, the doctor considers conditions that can cause loss of continence. These include constipation, infections, diet, emotional stress, and sexual abuse. Some medical conditions that the child develops can cause new urinary incontinence. Constipation, which is defined as difficult, hard, or infrequent stooling, is the most common cause of sudden changes in urinary continence in children. Bacterial urinary tract infections and viral infections causing bladder irritation (bacterial or viral cystitis) are common infectious causes.

To prevent urine from leaking, many children with incontinence learn to cross their legs or use other positions (holding maneuvers), such as squatting (sometimes with their hand or heel pressed between their legs). These holding maneuvers may increase the chance of developing a urinary tract infection. Sexually active adolescents can have urinary difficulties caused by certain sexually transmitted diseases. Dietary causes include caffeine and acidic juices, such as orange and tomato juice, which can irritate the bladder and lead to leakage of urine. Stressful events such as divorce or separation of the parents, moving, or loss of a family member can cause a child to develop urinary incontinence.

Similarly, children who are sexually abused may develop urinary incontinence. Children with diabetes mellitus or diabetes insipidus can develop incontinence because these disorders produce excessive amounts of urine.

COMMON CAUSES

Causes vary depending on whether incontinence occurs in the daytime or mainly at night.

In nighttime incontinence (nocturnal enuresis), most cases do not involve a medical disorder but result from a combination of factors, including

- Developmental delay
- Uncompleted toilet training
- A bladder that contracts before it is completely full
- Drinking too much before bedtime
- Problems waking up from sleep (for example, being a very deep sleeper)
- Family history (if one parent had nighttime incontinence, there is a 30% chance offspring will have it, increasing to 70% if both parents had it)

For daytime incontinence (diurnal enuresis), common causes include

- A bladder that is irritated because of a urinary tract infection or because something is pressing on it (such as a full rectum caused by constipation)
- An overactive bladder
- Urethrovaginal reflux (also called vaginal voiding), which can occur in girls who urinate in an incorrect position or who have extra skin folds, and can cause urine to back up into the vagina and then leak out when they stand up
- Anatomic abnormalities (for example, a misplaced ureter in girls or a congenital urinary tract obstruction)
- Weakness of the urinary sphincter, which controls the flow of urine out of the bladder (for example, because of a spinal cord abnormality)

In both types of incontinence, stress, attention-deficit/hyperactivity, or urinary tract infection can increase the risk of incontinence.

LESS COMMON CAUSES

For nighttime incontinence, an underlying medical disorder accounts for about 30% of cases. Contributing factors include some of the disorders that cause daytime incontinence along with disorders that increase the amount of urine. Such disorders include diabetes mellitus, diabetes insipidus, sickle cell disease (and sometimes sickle cell trait).

EVALUATION

Doctors first try to determine whether incontinence is simply a developmental issue or whether a disorder is involved.

WARNING SIGNS

In children with urinary incontinence, certain signs and characteristics are cause for concern. They include

- Signs or concerns of sexual abuse
- Excessive thirst, excessive volume of urine, and/or weight loss
- Incontinence during the day in children continuing beyond age 6
- Any signs of nerve damage, especially in the legs
- Signs of an abnormality of the spine

WHEN TO SEE A DOCTOR

Children who have any warning sign should immediately be brought to a doctor with experience in treating children unless the only warning sign is daytime incontinence continuing past age 6. Such children should see a doctor at some point, but a delay of a week or so is not harmful.

WHAT THE DOCTOR DOES

Doctors first ask questions about the child's symptoms and medical history. Doctors then do a physical examination. What they find during the history and physical examination often suggests a cause of the incontinence and the tests that may need to be done (see Tables on page 407 and on pages 408 to 409).

In the medical history, doctors ask about onset of symptoms, timing of symptoms, and whether symptoms are continuous (that is, constant dribbling) or intermittent. Having the parents record the timing, frequency, and volume of urine (a voiding diary) or stool (a stooling diary) in a journal can be helpful. Position while urinating and strength of urine steam are discussed.

SOME CAUSES AND FEATURES OF NIGHTTIME INCONTINENCE

Cause	Common Features*	Tests
Constipation	Infrequent, hard, pebblelike stools Sometimes abdominal discomfort In people who consume a constipating diet (for example, excessive milk and dairy products and few fruits and vegetables)	A doctor's examination Sometimes an x-ray of the abdomen Stooling diary
Increased urine output, which can have many causes, such as ■ Diabetes mellitus ■ Diabetes insipidus ■ Excessive water intake ■ Sickle cell disease or trait	Vary by the disorder	For diabetes mellitus, urine tests for glucose (sugar) and ketones and/or a blood test For diabetes insipidus or sickle cell disease, blood tests
Developmental delay	No daytime incontinence More common among boys and heavy sleepers Possibly family members who had wet the bed	A doctor's examination
Sleep apnea	Sometimes in children who snore and have pauses in breathing during sleep followed by loud snorts Excessive daytime sleepiness Enlarged tonsils	A sleep study test
Spinal defects (for example, spina bifida), leading to difficulty emptying the bladder (urinary retention)	Obvious spinal defects, a dimple or hair tuft in the lower back, and weakness or decreased sensation in the legs and feet	X-rays of the lower back Sometimes MRI of the spine
Stress	School problems, social isolation or problems, and family stress (such as divorce or separation of the parents)	A doctor's examination Voiding diary
Urinary tract infection	Pain while urinating, blood in the urine, the need to urinate frequently, and a sense of needing to urinate urgently Fever Abdominal pain	Urinalysis and urine culture

*Features include symptoms and the results of the doctor's examination. Features mentioned are typical but not always present.
MRI = magnetic resonance imaging.

SOME CAUSES AND FEATURES OF DAYTIME INCONTINENCE

Cause	Common Features*	Tests
Constipation	Infrequent, hard, pebblelike stools Sometimes abdominal discomfort Often in people who consume a constipating diet (for example, excessive milk and dairy products and few fruits and vegetables)	A doctor's examination Sometimes an x-ray of the abdomen Stooling diary
Dysfunctional voiding because the muscles involved in expelling urine from the bladder (the bladder muscle and urinary sphincter) are not coordinated	Sometimes stool incontinence and frequent urinary tract infections Possibly daytime and nighttime incontinence	Studies of urine flow Sometimes a voiding cystourethrogram (x-rays taken before, during, and after urination) Ultrasonography of the kidneys and bladder
Giggle incontinence	Urinating while laughing, almost exclusively in girls At other times, completely normal urination	A doctor's examination
Increased urine output, which can have many causes, such as ■ Diabetes mellitus ■ Diabetes insipidus ■ Excessive water intake ■ Sickle cell disease or trait	Vary by disorder	For diabetes mellitus, urine tests for glucose (sugar) and ketones and/or a blood test[†] For diabetes insipidus or sickle cell disease, blood tests
An overfull bladder	Waiting to the last minute to urinate Common among preschool children when they are absorbed in playing	Questions about when incontinence occurs Recording the timing, frequency, and volume of urine in a journal (voiding diary)
A bladder that does not empty completely (neurogenic bladder) because of a spinal cord or nervous system defect	Obvious abnormalities in the spine, a dimple or hair tuft in the lower back, and weakness and decreased sensation in the legs and feet	X-rays of the lower back Sometimes MRI of the spine Ultrasonography of the kidneys and bladder Studies of urine flow and pressure in the bladder (urodynamic studies)
Overactive bladder	A need to urinate urgently (essential for diagnosis) Commonly a frequent need to urinate during the day and night Sometimes use of holding maneuvers or body posturing (for example, children may squat)	A doctor's examination Sometimes studies of urine flow, voiding diary

(continued)

SOME CAUSES AND FEATURES OF DAYTIME INCONTINENCE *(continued)*

Cause	Common Features*	Tests
Sexual abuse	Sleep problems or school problems (such as delinquency or poor grades) Seductive behavior, depression, an unusual interest in or avoidance of all things sexual, and inappropriate knowledge of sexual things for age	Evaluation by sexual abuse experts
Stress‡	School problems, social isolation or problems, and family stress (for example, divorce or separation of the parents)	A doctor's examination
Anatomic abnormality (for example, a misplaced ureter in girls)	Complete daytime continence never achieved In girls, daytime and nighttime incontinence, a history of normal voiding but with continually wet underwear, and a discharge from the vagina Possibly a history of urinary tract infections and of other urinary tract abnormalities	Imaging studies of the kidneys and ureters, including sometimes CT of the abdomen and pelvis or MRI of the urinary tract
Urinary tract infection	Pain while urinating, blood in the urine, a need to urinate frequently, and a sense of needing to urinate urgently Sometimes fever, abdominal pain, and/or back pain	Urine culture and tests If results are positive, further evaluation
Back up of urine into the vagina (urethrovaginal reflux, or vaginal voiding)	Dribbling when standing after urination	A doctor's examination

*Features include symptoms and the results of the doctor's examination. Features mentioned are typical but not always present.
†Diabetes does not typically cause incontinence until blood sugar (glucose) levels are high enough to cause glucose to enter the urine.
‡Stress is a cause primarily when incontinence is sudden.
CT = computed tomography; MRI = magnetic resonance imaging.

Symptoms that suggest a cause include

- Decreased frequency of stools and/or hard stools (constipation)
- Fever, abdominal pain, pain while urinating, and increased urgency to pass urine (urinary tract infection)
- Itching around the anus and vagina (pinworm infection)
- Urinating frequently and producing a large volume of urine (diabetes insipidus or diabetes mellitus)
- Snoring or breathing pauses during sleep and being excessively sleepy during the day (sleep apnea)

Doctors also ask about any history of birth injuries or birth defects (such as spina bifida), nerve disorders, kidney disorders, and urinary tract infections. Doctors screen the child for the possibility of sexual abuse, which, although an uncommon cause, is too important to miss.

If there is a family history of bed-wetting or any urologic disorders, these should be brought to the doctors' attention. Doctors also ask questions about any stressors occurring near the start of symptoms, including difficulties at school, with friends, or at home (including questions about parents' marital difficulties). Although incontinence is not a psychologic disorder, a brief period of wetting may occur during times of psychologic stress.

Doctors then do a physical examination. Examination begins with the following:

- A review of vital signs for fever (urinary tract infection), signs of weight loss (diabetes), and hypertension (a kidney disorder)
- Examination of the head and neck for enlarged tonsils, mouth breathing, or poor growth (sleep apnea)
- Examination of the abdomen for any masses that suggest stool is being retained or for a full bladder
- Examination of the genitals in girls for any adhesions, scarring, or signs suggesting sexual abuse and in boys for any irritation or lesions on the penis or around the rectum
- Examination of the spine for any defects (for example, a tuft of hair or a dimple at the base of the spine)
- A neurologic examination to evaluate leg strength, sensation, deep tendon reflexes, and other reflexes (such as lightly touching the anus to see whether it constricts—called the anal wink—and, in boys, lightly stroking the inner thigh to see whether the testis is pulled up—called the cremasteric reflex)
- A rectal examination may be done during the physical examination to detect constipation or decreased rectal tone

TESTING

Sometimes doctors can diagnose the cause by the history, physical examination, a urinalysis, and a urine culture. Doctors may do other tests depending on what they find during their evaluation. For example, to help diagnose diabetes mellitus and diabetes insipidus, doctors do blood and/or urine tests to check sugar and electrolyte levels.

If a birth defect is suspected, an ultrasound examination of the kidneys and bladder and x-rays of the spine may be necessary. A special x-ray of the bladder and kidneys, called a voiding cystourethrogram, may also be necessary.

With this test, a dye is injected into the bladder using a catheter, which shows the anatomy of the urinary tract as well as the direction of urine flow.

TREATMENT

Learning about the cause and course of incontinence helps decrease the negative psychologic impact of urine accidents. Doctors ask how the child is being impacted by the incontinence because that could affect the treatment decision.

Treatment depends on the cause of the incontinence. For example, an infection is usually treated with antibiotics. Children with birth defects or anatomic abnormalities may need surgery. Nonspecific measures can be taken depending on whether incontinence is at night or during the day.

NIGHTTIME INCONTINENCE

The most effective long-term strategy is a bed-wetting alarm. Although labor intensive, the success rate can be as high as 70% when children are motivated to end the bed-wetting, and the family is able to follow the plan. It can take up to 4 months of nightly use for symptoms to completely resolve. Punishing children for bed-wetting is not helpful. It serves only to undermine treatment and cause poor self-esteem.

Drugs such as desmopressin (DDAVP) and imipramine can decrease the number of bed-wetting episodes. However, bed-wetting resumes in most children when the drug is stopped. Parents and children should be warned of this likelihood so that the child does not become devastated if bed-wetting starts again. Doctors prefer DDAVP to imipramine because of the rare potential of sudden death with imipramine use.

DAYTIME INCONTINENCE

General measures may include

- Trying urgency containment exercises (to strengthen the urinary sphincter)
- Gradually lengthening the time between visits to the bathroom (if the child is thought to have a weak bladder muscle or dysfunctional voiding)

- Changing behavior (for example, delaying urination) through positive reinforcement and scheduled urination
- Reminding children to urinate by a clock that vibrates or sounds an alarm (preferable to having a parent in the reminder role)
- Using methods that discourage retention of urine in the vagina (for example, sitting facing backward on the toilet or with the knees wide apart)

Urgency containment exercises involve telling children to go to the bathroom as soon as they feel the urge to urinate. But once in the bathroom, they are asked to hold the urine as long as they can. When they can hold it no longer they should start to urinate but then stop and start urinating every few seconds. This exercise strengthens the urinary sphincter and also gives children confidence that they can make it to the bathroom before they have an accident. This exercise should be taught after the child has been evaluated by a doctor.

The drugs oxybutynin and tolterodine can help if the problem is bladder spasm.

O—π KEY POINTS

- Understanding why the child is incontinent is essential to the child's outcome and well-being.
- Most often, incontinence is not caused by a medical disorder.
- Treatment includes behavioral changes, dietary changes, and sometimes drugs.
- Alarms are the most effective treatment for nighttime incontinence.
- Most nighttime incontinence improves as the child matures (15%/year resolve with no intervention).

Most people urinate about 4 to 6 times a day, mostly in the daytime. Normally, adults pass between 3 cups (700 milliliters) and 3 quarts (3 liters) of urine a day. Excessive urination can refer to

- An increased volume of urine (polyuria)
- A normal volume of urine with the need to go more often (urinary frequency)
- Both

Urinary frequency may be accompanied by a sensation of an urgent need to urinate (urinary urgency). Many people particularly notice polyuria because they have to get up to urinate during the night (nocturia). Nocturia also can occur if people drink too much fluid too close to bedtime, even if they drink no more than normal overall.

CAUSES

Some of the causes of increased urine volume differ from those of too-frequent urination. However, because many people who produce excessive amounts of urine also need to urinate frequently, these two symptoms are often considered together.

The most common causes of urinary frequency are

- Bladder infections (the most common cause in women and children)
- Urinary incontinence
- Noncancerous enlargement of the prostate gland (benign prostatic hyperplasia—the most common cause in men over 50)
- Stones in the urinary tract

The most common causes of polyuria in both adults and children are

- Uncontrolled diabetes mellitus (most common)
- Drinking too much fluid (polydipsia)
- Diabetes insipidus
- Taking diuretic drugs or substances (which increase the excretion of urine), such as alcohol or caffeine

Diabetes insipidus causes polyuria because of problems with a hormone called antidiuretic hormone (or vasopressin). Antidiuretic hormone helps the kidneys reabsorb fluid. If too little antidiuretic hormone is produced (a condition called central diabetes insipidus) or if the kidneys are unable to properly respond to it (nephrogenic diabetes insipidus), the person urinates excessively.

People with certain kidney disorders (such as interstitial nephritis or kidney damage resulting from sickle cell anemia) may also urinate excessively because these disorders also decrease the amount of fluid reabsorbed by the kidneys.

EVALUATION

Many people are embarrassed to discuss problems related to urination with their doctor. But because some disorders that cause excessive urination are quite serious, people who urinate excessively should be evaluated by a doctor. The following information can help people know when to see a doctor and what to expect during the evaluation.

WARNING SIGNS

In people with excessive urination, certain symptoms and characteristics are cause for concern. They include

- Weakness of the legs
- Fever and back pain
- Abrupt onset or onset during the first few years of life
- Night sweats, cough, and weight loss, especially in a person who has an extensive smoking history
- A mental health disorder

WHEN TO SEE A DOCTOR

People who have leg weakness should go to the hospital immediately because they may have a spinal cord disorder. People who have fever and back pain should see a doctor within a day because they may have a kidney infection. People who have other warning signs should see a doctor within a day or two. People without warning signs should schedule an appointment as soon as is convenient, usually within a few days to a week, although waiting longer is usually safe if symptoms have been developing over weeks or longer and are mild.

WHAT THE DOCTOR DOES

Doctors first ask questions about the person's symptoms and medical history and then do a physical examination. What they find during the history and physical examination often suggests a cause of excessive urination and the tests that may need to be done (see Table, below).

Doctors ask about

- Amounts of fluid drunk and urinated to determine whether the problem is related to urinary frequency or to polyuria
- How long symptoms have been present

SOME CAUSES AND FEATURES OF EXCESSIVE URINATION

Cause	Common Features*	Tests
Disorders that cause primarily frequent urination		
Cystitis (bladder infection)	Usually in women and girls A frequent and urgent need to urinate Burning or pain during urination Sometimes fever and pain in the lower back or side Sometimes blood in the urine or foul-smelling urine	Urinalysis and urine culture
Pregnancy	Typically during the last several months of pregnancy	A doctor's examination Sometimes urinalysis (to look for a urinary tract infection)
Prostate enlargement (benign or cancerous)	Mainly in men over 50 Slowly worsening urinary symptoms, such as difficulty starting urination, a weak urine stream, dribbling at the end of urination, and a sensation of incomplete urination Often detected during a digital rectal examination	Blood tests to measure the PSA level If the PSA level is elevated, biopsy of the prostate Sometimes ultrasonography
Prostatitis (prostate infection)	A tender prostate detected during a digital rectal examination Often fever, difficulty starting urination, and burning or pain during urination Sometimes blood in the urine In some cases, symptoms of a long-standing blockage in the urinary tract (including a weak urine stream, difficulty passing urine, or dribbling at the end of urination)	Urinalysis and urine culture and a digital rectal examination
Radiation cystitis (bladder damage caused by radiation therapy)	In people who have had radiation therapy of the lower abdomen, prostate, or perineum (the area between the genitals and anus) for treatment of cancer	A doctor's examination Sometimes insertion of a flexible viewing tube into the bladder (cystoscopy) and biopsy
Spinal cord dysfunction or injury	Weakness and numbness in the legs Retention of urine or uncontrollable loss of urine or stool (urinary or fecal incontinence) Sometimes an obvious injury	MRI of the spine

(continued)

SOME CAUSES AND FEATURES OF EXCESSIVE URINATION *(continued)*

Cause	Common Features*	Tests
Stones in the urinary tract (that do not block the flow of urine)	Occasional episodes of squeezing pain in the lower back, side (flank), or groin that comes and goes Depending on where the stone is, possibly frequent urination or sudden, severe urges to urinate	Urinalysis Ultrasonography or CT of the kidneys, ureters, and bladder
Substances that increase the excretion of urine, such as caffeine, alcohol, or diuretics	In otherwise healthy people shortly after they drink beverages containing caffeine or alcohol or in people who recently started taking a diuretic	Only a doctor's examination
Urinary incontinence	Unintentional passage of urine, most often when bending, coughing, sneezing, or lifting (called stress incontinence)	After water is inserted into the bladder, measurement of changes in pressure and the amount of urine in the bladder (cystometry)
Disorders that primarily increase the volume of urine		
Diabetes mellitus if uncontrolled	Excessive thirst Often in young children Sometimes in obese adults, who may already be known to have type 2 diabetes	Measurement of blood sugar (glucose) level
Diabetes insipidus, central	Excessive thirst that may appear suddenly or develop gradually Sometimes in people who have had a brain injury or brain surgery	Blood and urine tests, done before and after people are deprived of water, then given antidiuretic hormone (water deprivation test) Sometimes blood tests to measure the antidiuretic hormone level
Diabetes insipidus, nephrogenic	Excessive thirst that develops gradually In people who have a disorder that may affect the kidneys (such as sickle cell disease, Sjögren syndrome, cancer, hyperparathyroidism, amyloidosis, sarcoidosis, or certain inherited disorders) or who take a drug that may affect the kidneys (usually lithium, cidofovir, foscarnet, or ifosfamide)	Blood and urine tests Sometimes a water deprivation test
Diuretic use	In otherwise healthy people who recently started taking a diuretic Sometimes in people who take a diuretic surreptitiously (for example, competitive athletes or other people trying to lose weight)	Usually only a doctor's examination
Drinking too much fluid (polydipsia) often due to a mental health disorder	Sometimes in people known to have a mental health disorder	Similar to tests for central diabetes insipidus

*Features include symptoms and the results of the doctor's examination. Features mentioned are typical but not always present.

CT = computed tomography; MRI = magnetic resonance imaging; PSA = prostate-specific antigen.

- Whether any other urination problems are present
- Whether the person is taking diuretics, including beverages that contain caffeine

Some obvious findings may give clues to the cause of frequent urination. Pain or burning during urination, fever, and back or side pain may indicate an infection. In a person who drinks large amounts of beverages that contain caffeine or who has just started treatment with a diuretic, the diuretic substance is a likely cause. A man who has other problems with urination, such as difficulty starting urination, a weak urine stream, and dribbling at the end of urination, may have a prostate disorder.

Some obvious findings may also give clues to the cause of polyuria. For example, polyuria that starts during the first few years of life is likely caused by an inherited disorder such as central or nephrogenic diabetes insipidus or type 1 diabetes mellitus.

In women, the physical examination usually includes a pelvic examination and the taking of samples of cervical and vaginal fluid to check for sexually transmitted diseases. In men, the penis is examined for presence of a discharge, and doctors do a digital rectal examination to examine the prostate.

TESTING

Doctors do a urinalysis and often urine culture on most people. The need for other testing depends on what doctors find during the history and physical examination (see Table). If doctors are not sure whether the person is actually producing more urine than normal, they may collect and measure the amount of urine produced over 24 hours. If people actually have polyuria, doctors measure the blood glucose level. If diabetes mellitus is not the cause of polyuria and no other cause, such as excess intravenous fluids, is clearly responsible, other testing is necessary. The levels of electrolytes and concentration of certain salts (osmolarity) are measured in the blood, urine, or both, often after the person is deprived of water for a time and after the person is given antidiuretic hormone.

TREATMENT

The best way to treat excessive urination is to treat the underlying disorder. For example, diabetes mellitus is treated with diet and exercise plus insulin injections and/or drugs taken by mouth. In some cases, people can reduce excessive urination by decreasing their intake of coffee or alcohol. Doctors may also adjust the dosage of diuretics that may contribute to excessive urination.

ESSENTIALS FOR OLDER PEOPLE

Older men often urinate frequently because the prostate usually enlarges with age. In older women, frequent urination is also more common because of many factors, such as weakening of the pelvic supporting tissues after childbirth and the loss of estrogen after menopause. Both older men and older women may be more likely to take diuretics, so these drugs may contribute to excessive urination. Older people with excessive urination often need to urinate at night (nocturia). Nocturia can contribute to sleep problems and to falls, especially if a person is rushing to the bathroom or if the area is not well lit.

O— KEY POINTS

- Urinary tract infections are the most common cause of urinary frequency in children and women.
- Uncontrolled diabetes mellitus is the most common cause of polyuria.
- Benign prostatic hyperplasia is a common cause in men over 50.
- Excessive intake of caffeine can cause urinary frequency in all people.

URINATION, PAIN OR BURNING WITH (DYSURIA)

Burning or pain during urination may be felt at the opening of the urethra or, less often, over the bladder (in the pelvis, the lower part of the abdomen just above the pubic bone). Burning or pain during urination is an extremely common symptom in women, but it can affect men and can occur at any age.

CAUSES

Burning or pain during urination is typically caused by inflammation of the urethra or bladder. In women, inflammation in the vagina or in the region around the vaginal opening (called vulvovaginitis) can be painful when exposed to urine. Inflammation that results in burning or pain is usually caused by infection but sometimes by noninfectious conditions.

COMMON CAUSES

Overall, the most common causes of burning or pain during urination are

- Bladder infection (cystitis)
- Infection of the urethra (urethritis) due to a sexually transmitted disease (STD)

EVALUATION

Not every person who has pain or burning during urination needs to see a doctor right away. The following information can help people decide how quickly a doctor's evaluation is needed and help them know what to expect during the evaluation.

WARNING SIGNS

In people who have pain or burning during urination, certain symptoms and characteristics are cause for concern. They include

- Fever
- Pain in the back or side (flank pain)
- A recent history of insertion of a bladder catheter or other instrument
- Immune system disorders

- Repeat episodes (including frequent childhood infections)
- A known urinary tract abnormality

WHEN TO SEE A DOCTOR

People with immune system disorders and pregnant women with warning signs should see a doctor that day (or in the morning if symptoms develop overnight) because complications of a urinary tract infection can be serious in such people. Other people with warning signs should see a doctor in a day or two, as should those whose symptoms are particularly bothersome. For people without warning signs who have mild symptoms, a delay of 2 or 3 days is not harmful.

Women with frequent bladder infections may recognize characteristic symptoms that suggest another episode.

WHAT THE DOCTOR DOES

Doctors first ask questions about the person's symptoms and medical history and then do a physical examination. What they find during the history and physical examination often suggests a cause of the burning or pain during urination and the tests that may need to be done (see Table on pages 417 to 418).

Doctors may ask whether similar symptoms have occurred in the past. Doctors ask about symptoms that may accompany the pain and provide clues to the cause. For example, doctors may ask whether

- The urine is bloody, cloudy, or foul smelling
- Any discharge is noticed
- There has been any recent unprotected intercourse
- Potential irritants have been applied to the genitals
- A bladder catheter has recently been inserted or another urinary tract procedure has been done

Women are asked whether they might be pregnant.

In women, the physical examination usually includes a pelvic examination and the taking of

SOME CAUSES AND FEATURES OF PAINFUL URINATION

Cause	Common Features*	Tests
Infections†		
Cystitis (bladder infection)	Usually in women and girls A frequent and urgent need to urinate Getting up at night to urinate Sometimes blood in the urine or foul-smelling urine	A doctor's examination Usually urinalysis and urine culture
Epididymo-orchitis (infection of an epididymis and a testis)	Tenderness and swelling in a testis Possibly frequent urination or a discharge from the urethra Sometimes fever or nausea	A doctor's examination Sometimes urinalysis Sometimes STD testing
Prostatitis (infection of the prostate)	A tender prostate detected during a digital rectal examination Often fever, difficulty starting urination, frequent urination, the need to urinate during the night, and burning or pain during urination Sometimes blood in the urine Often symptoms of a long-standing blockage in the urinary tract (including a weak urine stream, difficulty passing urine, or dribbling at the end of urination)	Urinalysis and urine culture
Urethritis (infection of the urethra), typically due to an STD	Usually a visible discharge from the urethra in men Sometimes a discharge from the vagina in women In people who have recently had unprotected intercourse	STD testing
Vulvovaginitis (infection of the vulva and vagina)	A discharge from the vagina Often redness in the genital area	A doctor's examination, including examination of a sample of the discharge under a microscope
Disorders that cause inflammation		
Connective tissue disorders that cause inflammation (such as reactive arthritis or Behçet syndrome)‡	General or bodywide symptoms (including body pain and joint pain) that develop before urination becomes painful Sometimes sores on the skin, mouth, eyes, or genital area, including inside the vagina	STD testing Sometimes blood tests to check for these connective tissue disorders

(continued)

SOME CAUSES AND FEATURES OF PAINFUL URINATION (continued)

Cause	Common Features*	Tests
Contact with a substance that irritates the area or causes an allergic reaction (such as a spermicide, lubricant, or latex condom)	Sometimes redness in the genital area In people who have been exposed to a substance that could cause irritation or an allergic reaction	Only a doctor's examination
Interstitial cystitis (inflammation of the bladder without infection)	More common among women A frequent and urgent need to urinate Long-standing symptoms	Urinalysis and urine culture Examination of the interior of the bladder using a flexible viewing tube inserted through the urethra (cystoscopy), usually including removal of a sample of tissue for examination (biopsy of the bladder)
Other disorders		
Atrophic vaginitis or urethritis (thinning of tissues in the vagina or urethra)	In postmenopausal women Vaginal dryness Often pain during intercourse A discharge from the vagina Changes in the interior of the vagina (it becomes smooth and pale)	Only a doctor's examination
Tumors (usually bladder or prostate cancer)	Long-standing symptoms, such as a weak urine stream or difficulty starting urination Usually blood in the urine	If bladder cancer is suspected, cystoscopy If prostate cancer is suspected, a blood test to measure PSA levels If the PSA level is elevated, biopsy of the prostate

*Features include symptoms and the results of the doctor's examination. Features mentioned are typical but not always present.
†Infectious organisms that commonly cause painful urination include sexually transmitted organisms (such as those that cause gonorrhea, chlamydial infection, and trichomoniasis) and bacteria that are not sexually transmitted, mostly *Escherichia (E.) coli.*
‡This cause is rare.
PSA = prostate-specific antigen; STD = sexually transmitted disease.

samples of cervical and vaginal fluid to check for STDs. In men, the penis is examined for presence of a discharge, and doctors do a digital rectal examination to examine the prostate.

Doctors can sometimes get clues to the cause based on where symptoms are most severe. For example, if symptoms are most severe just above the pubic bone, a bladder infection may be the cause. If symptoms are most severe at the opening of the urethra, urethritis may be the cause. In men with a penile discharge, urethritis is often the cause. If burning affects mainly the vagina and the woman has a discharge, vaginitis may be the cause.

TESTING

Doctors do not always agree on the need for tests for certain adult women who have symptoms that suggest a bladder infection. Some doctors do urine tests, whereas others treat without doing any testing. All doctors do tests when the diagnosis is unclear. The first test is usually urinalysis. In many cases, doctors also do a urine culture to identify organisms causing infection and determine which antibiotics would be effective. For women of childbearing age who are not known to be pregnant, a pregnancy test is done. Testing for STDs is often done, for example, for men who have a discharge from the penis and for many women who have a vaginal discharge.

Cystoscopy and imaging of the urinary tract may be needed to check for anatomic abnormalities or other problems, especially if antibiotics have not been effective.

TREATMENT

The cause is treated. Often the cause is an infection, and antibiotics provide relief in a day or two. If pain is severe, doctors may give phenazopyridine for a day or two to relieve discomfort until antibiotics start to work. Phenazopyridine turns the urine a red-orange color.

KEY POINTS

- Although bladder infections are a common cause, many other disorders may cause painful urination.
- Burning or pain during urination may be a sign of an STD.
- Doctors may decide to treat women with an antibiotic and see whether symptoms resolve rather than do testing.

URINE, BLOOD IN

Blood in the urine (hematuria) can make urine appear pink, red, or brown, depending on the amount of blood, how long it has been in the urine, and how acidic the urine is. An amount of blood too small to change color of the urine (microscopic hematuria) may be found by chemical tests or microscopic examination. Microscopic hematuria may be found when a urine test is done for another reason.

People with hematuria may have other symptoms such as pain in the side or back (flank), lower abdominal pain, an urgent need to urinate, or difficulty urinating, depending on the cause of blood in the urine. If sufficient blood is present in the urine, the blood may form a clot. The clot can completely block the flow of urine, causing sudden extreme pain and inability to urinate. Bleeding severe enough to cause such a clot is usually caused by an injury to the urinary tract.

Red urine is not always caused by red blood cells. Red or reddish brown discoloration may also result from the following:

- Hemoglobin (which carries oxygen in red blood cells) in the urine due to the breakdown of red blood cells
- Muscle protein (myoglobin) in urine due to the breakdown of muscle cells
- Porphyria (a disorder caused by deficiencies of enzymes involved in the production of heme, a chemical compound that contains iron and gives blood its red color)
- Foods (for example, beets, rhubarb, and sometimes food coloring)
- Drugs (most commonly phenazopyridine, but sometimes cascara, diphenylhydantoin, methyldopa, rifampin, phenacetin, phenothiazines, and senna)

CAUSES

Blood in the urine may be caused by problems anywhere along the urinary tract from the kidneys to the ureters, bladder, or urethra. Some women at first mistake vaginal bleeding (see page 424) for blood in the urine.

COMMON CAUSES

The most common causes differ somewhat by the person's age but overall are

- Bladder infection (cystitis)
- Prostate infection (prostatitis)
- Urinary tract stones (in adults)

LESS COMMON CAUSES

Less common causes include

- Cancer (of the kidneys, bladder, or prostate)
- Noncancerous enlargement of the prostate (benign prostatic hyperplasia)
- Disorders of the small blood vessels of the kidneys (called kidney filtering disorders or glomerular disorders)
- Cysts in the kidneys (polycystic kidney disease)
- Narrowing scars (called strictures) or other abnormalities of the ureters

Cancer and benign prostatic hyperplasia may cause blood in the urine. These disorders are a concern mainly in people over 50, although younger people with risk factors (smoking, family history, or chemical exposures) may develop cancer.

Disorders of the microscopic blood vessels of the kidneys (glomeruli) can be a cause at any age. Kidney filtering disorders (glomerular disorders) may be part of a kidney disorder or may occur as a result of a disorder elsewhere in the body. Such disorders include infections (such as a heart valve infection), connective tissue disorders (such as systemic lupus erythematosus), blood disorders (such as serum sickness), or certain chronic disorders (such as diabetes). Also, almost any kind of kidney damage may cause small amounts of blood in the urine.

Severe injuries, such as from a fall or a motor vehicle crash, can injure the kidneys or bladder and cause bleeding.

Schistosoma haematobium, a parasitic worm that causes disease in Africa and, to a lesser extent, in India and parts of the Middle East, can invade the urinary tract, causing blood in the urine. Doctors consider schistosomiasis only if people have spent time in areas where the worm is found. Tuberculosis may cause blood in the urine.

EVALUATION

Doctors first try to establish that bleeding is the cause of red urine. Then they look for the cause of the bleeding, including where in the urinary tract (or occasionally elsewhere) the bleeding is originating. The following information can help people know when to see a doctor and what to expect during the evaluation.

WARNING SIGNS

In people with blood in the urine, certain symptoms and characteristics are cause for concern. They include

- Large amount of blood in the urine
- Age over 50
- Swelling of the feet or legs, plus high blood pressure

WHEN TO SEE A DOCTOR

People who notice blood in their urine should see their doctor within a day or two. However, people who are passing a large amount of blood, who are unable to urinate, or who have severe pain should see a doctor right away.

WHAT THE DOCTOR DOES

Doctors first ask questions about the person's symptoms and medical history and then do a physical examination. What they find during the history and physical examination often suggests a cause of the blood in the urine and the tests that may need to be done (see Table, below).

Doctors ask how long blood has been present and whether there have been any previous bleeding episodes. They ask about symptoms of urinary blockage, such as difficulty starting urination or inability to completely empty the bladder. Pain or discomfort is an important finding. Burning during urination or dull pain in the lower abdomen just above the pubic bone suggests a bladder infection. In men, mild to

SOME CAUSES AND FEATURES OF BLOOD IN THE URINE

Cause	Common Features*	Tests†
Benign prostatic hyperplasia (noncancerous enlargement of the prostate gland)	Mainly in men over 50 Often difficulty starting urination, a weak urine stream, a sensation of incomplete urination, or dribbling at the end of urination An enlarged prostate detected during a digital rectal examination	Blood tests to measure the PSA level Cystoscopy Often ultrasonography of the bladder to measure how much urine remains in the bladder after voiding (postvoid residual urine volume)
Bladder or kidney cancer	Mainly in people over 50 or with risk factors for these cancers (smoking, family members who have had cancer, or exposure to chemicals that may cause cancer) Sometimes burning or pain during urination or an urgent need to urinate Often symptoms that affect the whole body (such as fever, chills, weight loss or sweating)	Examination of the interior of the bladder using a flexible viewing tube inserted through the urethra (cystoscopy) Sometimes CT or MRI
Cystitis (bladder infection)	Usually in women and girls A frequent and urgent need to urinate Burning or pain during urination Getting up at night to urinate Sometimes blood in the urine or foul-smelling urine	A doctor's examination Usually urinalysis and urine culture

(continued)

SOME CAUSES AND FEATURES OF BLOOD IN THE URINE *(continued)*

Cause	Common Features*	Tests†
Injury	Usually an obvious injury	Usually CT of the abdomen and pelvis
Kidney filtering disorders (glomerular disorders, such as glomerulonephritis)	Sometimes high blood pressure and swelling in the feet or legs Possibly red or dark (cola-colored) urine Sometimes occurring after an infection Sometimes in people who have family members with a kidney or a connective tissue disorder	Urinalysis Blood tests Biopsy of the kidney
Polycystic kidney disease	Long-lasting pain in the flank or abdomen High blood pressure Sometimes enlarged kidneys detected on an imaging test done for another reason or during a doctor's examination	Ultrasonography Often CT or MRI of the abdomen
Prostate cancer	Mainly in men over 50 Sometimes a lump in the prostate detected during a digital rectal examination Occasionally a weak urine stream, difficulty starting urination, and dribbling at the end of urination	Blood tests to measure the PSA level If the PSA level is elevated, biopsy of the prostate
Prostatitis (infection of the prostate gland)	Often fever, difficulty starting urination, frequent urination, the need to urinate during the night, and burning or pain during urination Often symptoms of a long-standing blockage in the urinary tract (including a weak urine stream, difficulty passing urine, or dribbling at the end of urination) An enlarged, tender prostate detected during a digital rectal examination	A doctor's examination Urinalysis and urine culture Sometimes transrectal ultrasonography or cystoscopy
Sickle cell disease or trait	Usually in people already known to have sickle cell disease Mainly in people of African or Mediterranean descent Often in children and young adults	Blood tests to check for abnormal hemoglobin in red blood cells
Stones in the urinary tract	Severe pain in the lower back side (flank) that occurs suddenly or pain in the abdomen or groin that comes in waves Sometimes the urge to urinate but an inability to do so Sometimes vomiting	CT or ultrasonography of the kidneys, ureters, and bladder

*Features include symptoms and the results of a doctor's examination. Features mentioned are typical but not always present.
†Tests include urinalysis in all people, blood tests to evaluate renal function in most people, and imaging of the kidneys and pelvis in most older people.
CT = computed tomography; MRI = magnetic resonance imaging; PSA = prostate-specific antigen.

moderate pain in the lower back or pelvis is often the result of a prostate infection. Extremely severe pain is usually due to a stone or a blood clot blocking the flow of urine.

Doctors then do a physical examination. Usually, a pelvic examination is necessary in women. If women have blood in the vagina, a catheter may need to be inserted into the bladder to see whether the source of blood is the bladder or the vagina. In men, doctors usually do a digital rectal examination to check the prostate.

TESTING

Sometimes doctors can make a diagnosis based on the person's symptoms and the results of the physical examination. More often, because symptoms of many disorders overlap, testing is needed to determine the cause (or sometimes the presence) of blood in the urine. Urinalysis is the first test done. Urinalysis can detect blood (confirming that the red color of the urine is caused by blood) and may show evidence of a kidney filtering disorder. If infection is suspected, urine culture is usually done.

In all people over 50 and in people who have risk factors for cancer, doctors typically use a flexible viewing tube to look inside the bladder (cystoscopy) to determine the cause of bleeding.

People of any age who do not have an infection or a kidney filtering disorder as the cause of visibly bloody urine typically have imaging studies, such as computed tomography (CT), ultrasonography, or magnetic resonance imaging (MRI) of the abdomen and pelvis. For people under 50 who have only microscopic

hematuria and no other abnormalities detected during the physical examination, blood tests, or urinalysis, doctors may simply repeat the urinalysis in 6 or 12 months. If blood is still present, they will do further tests.

If doctors suspect a kidney filtering disorder (based of the results of urinalysis), they usually do blood tests to evaluate kidney function and sometimes a kidney biopsy. Blood tests for sickle cell disease may be needed in people of African or Mediterranean descent who are not known to have the disease.

In men who are 50 or older, doctors usually measure the level of prostate specific antigen (PSA) in the blood.

TREATMENT

Treatment is directed at the cause of the bleeding. Whatever the cause, if urine flow is blocked by blood clots, doctors usually insert a flexible tube in the bladder (urinary catheter) and try to flush out the blood clot.

O━╥ KEY POINTS

- Red urine is not always caused by blood.
- Many causes of blood in the urine are not serious.
- Risk of serious disease increases with age and the duration of the bloody urine.
- Testing for cancer is usually needed only for people over 50 or for younger people with risk factors for cancer.

VAGINAL BLEEDING

Abnormal vaginal bleeding includes any vaginal bleeding that occurs

- Before puberty
- During pregnancy
- After menopause
- Between menstrual periods

During the childbearing years, vaginal bleeding occurs normally as menstrual periods. However, menstrual periods are considered abnormal if they

- Become excessively heavy (saturating more than 1 or 2 tampons an hour)
- Last too long (more than 7 days)
- Occur too frequently (usually fewer than 21 days apart)
- Occur too infrequently (usually more than 90 days apart)

Typically, menstrual periods last from 3 to 7 days and occur every 21 to 35 days. In adolescents, the interval between periods varies more and may be as long as 45 days.

Vaginal bleeding may occur during early (see page 429) or late (see page 433) pregnancy and may result from problems (complications) related to the pregnancy.

Prolonged or excessive bleeding can result in iron deficiency, anemia, and sometimes dangerously low blood pressure (shock).

CAUSES

Vaginal bleeding may result from a disorder of the vagina, uterus, cervix, or another reproductive organ. It may also result from malfunction of the complex hormonal system that regulates the menstrual cycle or from bleeding disorders.

COMMON CAUSES

Likely causes of vaginal bleeding depend on the woman's age.

Newborn girls may have a small amount of vaginal bleeding. Before birth, they absorb estrogen through the placenta from their mother. After birth, these high levels of estrogen decrease rapidly, sometimes causing a little bleeding during the first 1 to 2 weeks of life.

During childhood, vaginal bleeding is abnormal and uncommon. When it occurs, it is most often caused by

- A foreign object (body), such as toilet paper or a toy, in the vagina or an injury

During the childbearing years, the most common cause is

- Dysfunctional uterine bleeding

Dysfunctional uterine bleeding results from changes in the hormonal control of the menstrual cycle that prevent the egg from being released. It is more likely to occur in adolescents (when menstrual periods are just starting) or in women in their late 40s (when periods are nearing an end).

Other common causes during the childbearing years include

- Complications of pregnancy in a woman who does not know she is pregnant
- Hormonal disorders, such as thyroid disorders
- Fibroids
- Bleeding when the egg is released (at ovulation) during the menstrual cycle
- Use of birth control pills (oral contraceptives), which can cause spotting or bleeding between periods (called breakthrough bleeding)

After menopause, the most common cause is

- Age-related thinning of the lining of the vagina (atrophic vaginitis) or uterus

LESS COMMON CAUSES

Cancer of the cervix, vagina, or lining of the uterus (endometrial cancer) can cause bleeding, usually after menopause. Cancer is an uncommon cause during the childbearing years. Excessively heavy menstrual periods may be the first sign of a bleeding disorder.

Children may have hormonal abnormalities that cause puberty to begin too early—a disorder called precocious puberty. In these children, menstrual periods start, breasts develop, and pubic and underarm hair appears too soon. Rarely, bleeding is caused by a tumor or an injury resulting from unsuspected child abuse.

EVALUATION

Doctors first focus on determining whether the cause is a serious disorder (such as an ectopic pregnancy) and whether the bleeding is excessive, possibly resulting in shock.

Doctors check for pregnancy in all women of childbearing age.

WARNING SIGNS

In women with vaginal bleeding, certain characteristics are cause for concern:

- Loss of consciousness, weakness, light-headedness, cold and sweaty skin, difficulty breathing, and a weak and rapid pulse (which indicate shock)
- Bleeding that occurs before menstrual periods start (before puberty) or after they stop (after menopause)
- Bleeding during pregnancy
- Excessive bleeding

Bleeding is considered excessive if women lose more than about a cup of blood, if more than 1 pad or tampon is saturated per hour for a few hours, or if the blood contains large clots.

WHEN TO SEE A DOCTOR

Women with warning signs should see a doctor immediately, as should those with large clots or clumps of tissue in the blood or with symptoms suggesting a bleeding disorder. These symptoms include easy bruising, excessive bleeding during toothbrushing or after minor cuts, and rashes of tiny reddish purple dots or larger splotches (indicating bleeding in the skin). However, if the only warning sign is vaginal bleeding before puberty or after menopause, a delay of a week or so is not harmful.

Women without warning signs should schedule a visit when practical, but a delay of several days is not likely to be harmful.

If vaginal bleeding continues in newborns for more than 2 weeks, they should be seen by a doctor.

WHAT THE DOCTOR DOES

Doctors first ask the woman questions about her symptoms and medical history. Doctors then do a physical examination. What they find during the history and physical examination often suggests a cause of the bleeding and the tests that may need to be done (see Table on pages 426 to 427).

Doctors ask about the bleeding:

- How many pads are used per day or hour
- How long bleeding lasts
- When it started
- When it occurs in relation to menstrual periods

They also ask about the woman's menstrual history:

- How old she was when menstrual periods started
- How long they last
- How heavy they are
- How long the interval between periods is
- Whether they are regular

The woman is asked whether she has had previous episodes of abnormal bleeding, has had a disorder that can cause bleeding (such as a recent miscarriage), or takes birth control pills or other hormones.

The physical examination includes a pelvic examination. During the examination, doctors can identify precocious puberty in children (based on the presence of pubic hair and breasts) and can sometimes identify disorders of the cervix, uterus, or vagina.

TESTING

If women are of childbearing age, doctors always do

- A urine test for pregnancy

If the urine pregnancy test is negative but doctors still suspect pregnancy, a blood test for pregnancy is done. The blood test is more accurate than the urine test when a pregnancy is very early (less than 5 weeks).

Tests commonly done include blood tests to measure thyroid hormone levels and, if bleeding has been heavy or lasted a long time, a complete blood cell count to check for anemia. Other blood tests are done depending on the disorder doctors suspect. For example, if a bleeding disorder is suspected, the blood's ability to clot is assessed. If polycystic ovary syndrome is suspected, blood tests to measure male hormone levels are done.

Ultrasonography is often used to look for abnormalities in the reproductive organs, particularly if women are over 35, if they have risk

SOME CAUSES AND FEATURES OF VAGINAL BLEEDING

Cause	Common Features*	Tests
During infancy		
Exposure to the mother's estrogen before birth	A small amount of bleeding during the first 1–2 weeks of life	A doctor's examination
During childhood		
A foreign object (body) in the vagina	Usually a foul-smelling discharge, often containing small amounts of blood Sometimes a history of having inserted an object into the vagina	A doctor's examination, sometimes done after the girl is sedated or given a general anesthetic
Early (precocious) puberty	Development of breasts and appearance of pubic and underarm hair (as occurs during puberty) at a young age	X-rays of the hand and wrist Blood tests to measure hormone levels
During the childbearing years		
Dysfunctional uterine bleeding	Usually bleeding that occurs frequently or irregularly or that lasts longer or is heavier than typical menstrual periods	Tests to rule out other possible causes, including blood tests and ultrasonography, often using a handheld ultrasound device inserted in the vagina
Endometriosis (abnormally located patches of tissue that is normally located only in the lining of the uterus)	Sharp or crampy pain that occurs before and during the first days of menstrual periods Often pain during sexual intercourse and/or bowel movements May eventually cause pain unrelated to the menstrual cycle Sometimes infertility	Insertion of a thin viewing tube (laparoscope) into the abdominal cavity to check for abnormal tissue and to obtain a sample for biopsy
Fibroids	Often no other symptoms With large fibroids, sometimes pain, pressure, or a feeling of heaviness in the pelvic area	A doctor's examination Often ultrasonography or sonohysterography (ultrasonography after fluid is infused into the uterus) If results are unclear, MRI
Polycystic ovary syndrome	Excess body hair (hirsutism) Irregular or no menstrual periods, acne, and excess fat in the torso Darkened and thickened skin in the underarm, on the nape of the neck, and in skinfolds	A doctor's examination Blood tests to measure levels of hormones, such as testosterone, luteinizing hormone, and follicle-stimulating hormone Ultrasonography of the pelvis
Pregnancy complications (of an unrecognized pregnancy) ■ A miscarriage (spontaneous abortion) or one that may occur (threatened abortion)	Crampy pelvic pain (in the lowest part of the torso) or back pain Sometimes passage of tissue through the vagina (usually occurs in a miscarriage)	A doctor's examination Ultrasonography of the pelvis For a suspected ectopic pregnancy: *(continued)*

SOME CAUSES AND FEATURES OF VAGINAL BLEEDING *(continued)*

Cause	Common Features*	Tests
Pregnancy complications *(continued)* ■ Ectopic pregnancy (an abnormally located pregnancy—not in its usual place in the uterus)	If an ectopic pregnancy ruptures, constant pelvic pain and sometimes light-headedness, fainting, or dangerously low blood pressure (shock)	■ Urine and blood tests to measure a hormone produced by the placenta (called human chorionic gonadotropin, or hCG) ■ Sometimes for a suspected ectopic pregnancy, laparoscopy or laparotomy (a large incision into the abdomen enabling doctors to directly view organs)
Spotting or bleeding between periods (breakthrough bleeding) during the first months that oral contraceptives are used	Often no other symptoms	A doctor's examination
After menopause		
Thinning of the lining of the vagina (atrophic vaginitis)	A scant discharge Pain during sexual intercourse	A doctor's examination Examination under a microscope and analysis of a sample of discharge
Thickening of the lining of the uterus (endometrial hyperplasia)	Often no other symptoms	Hysteroscopy (insertion of a viewing tube through the vagina to view the uterus) or sonohysterography Biopsy of tissue taken from the lining of the uterus
Cancer of the cervix or lining of the uterus (endometrium), which can occur but is much less common among younger women	Often no other symptoms until the cancer is advanced Sometimes vaginal bleeding or a bloody discharge Pain that develops gradually Sometimes weight loss	A Papanicolaou (Pap) test A biopsy Sometimes imaging tests of the pelvis such as ultrasonography, MRI, or CT of the pelvis
At any age		
Bleeding disorders	Easy bruising Excessive bleeding during toothbrushing or after minor cuts A rash of tiny reddish purple dots (petechiae) or larger splotches (purpura), indicating bleeding in the skin	A complete blood cell count, including the number of platelets Blood tests to assess the blood's ability to clot (prothrombin time and partial thromboplastin time) Examination of a sample of blood under a microscope
Injury (including that resulting from sexual abuse)	Sometimes a history of injuries Often vaginal discharge	A doctor's examination If sexual abuse is suspected: ■ Examination under a microscope and analysis of a sample of the discharge ■ Tests to detect sexually transmitted diseases using a sample of secretions taken from the cervix

*Features include symptoms and results of the doctor's examination. Features mentioned are typical but not always present.
CT = computed tomography; MRI = magnetic resonance imaging.

factors for endometrial cancer, or if bleeding continues despite treatment. For ultrasonography, a handheld ultrasound device is usually inserted into the vagina, but it may be placed on the abdomen.

If ultrasonography detects thickening of the uterine lining (endometrial hyperplasia), hysteroscopy or sonohysterography may be done to look for small growths in the uterus. For hysteroscopy, a viewing tube is inserted into the uterus through the vagina. For sonohysterography, fluid is infused into the uterus during ultrasonography to make abnormalities easier to identify. If results of these tests are abnormal or if they are inconclusive in women over 35 or with risk factors for cancer, doctors may take a sample of tissue from the lining of the uterus for analysis. The sample may be obtained by suction (through a tube) or by scraping—a procedure called dilation and curettage (D and C).

Other tests may be done, depending on which disorders seem possible. For example, a Papanicolaou (Pap) test or a biopsy of the cervix may be done to check for cancer of the cervix.

Dysfunctional uterine bleeding may be diagnosed if the examination and tests do not detect another cause.

TREATMENT

If women are in shock, they are given fluids intravenously and blood transfusions as needed to restore blood pressure.

When vaginal bleeding results from another disorder, that disorder is treated if possible. If bleeding has caused iron deficiency, women are given iron supplements.

Birth control pills or other hormones may be used to treat dysfunctional uterine bleeding.

Polyps, fibroids, cancers, and some benign tumors may be surgically removed from the uterus.

ESSENTIALS FOR OLDER WOMEN

Postmenopausal bleeding (occurring more than 6 months after menopause) is considered abnormal, even though it is relatively common. Such bleeding can indicate a precancerous disorder (such as thickening of the lining of the uterus) or cancer. Thus, if such bleeding occurs, older women should see a doctor promptly so that cancer can be ruled out. Older women should see a doctor promptly if they have

- Any vaginal bleeding
- A discharge that is pink or brown, possibly containing small amounts of blood

However, postmenopausal bleeding has many other causes. They include

- Thinning and drying of the lining of the uterus or vagina (the most common cause)
- Use of estrogen or other hormone therapy, particularly when use is stopped
- Polyps in the cervix or uterus
- Fibroids
- Infections

Because the tissues of the vagina may be thin and dry, examination of the vagina may be uncomfortable. Doctors may try using a smaller instrument (speculum) to make the examination less uncomfortable.

O—π KEY POINTS

- During the childbearing years, the most common cause of abnormal vaginal bleeding is dysfunctional uterine bleeding, which results from changes in the hormonal control of the menstrual cycle.
- In children, the cause is usually a foreign object or an injury, but sometimes sexual abuse is the cause.
- In women of childbearing age, a pregnancy test is done even when women do not think they could be pregnant.
- If any vaginal bleeding occurs after menopause, an evaluation to rule out cancer is necessary.

VAGINAL BLEEDING DURING EARLY PREGNANCY

During the first 20 weeks of pregnancy, 20 to 30% of women have vaginal bleeding. In about half of these women, the pregnancy ends in a miscarriage. If miscarriage does not occur immediately, problems later in the pregnancy are more likely. For example, the baby's birth weight may be low, or the baby may be born early (preterm birth), be born dead (stillbirth), or die during or shortly after birth. If bleeding is profuse, blood pressure may become dangerously low, resulting in shock.

The amount of bleeding can range from spots of blood to a massive amount. Passing large amounts of blood is always a concern, but spotting or mild bleeding may also indicate a serious disorder.

CAUSES

Vaginal bleeding during early pregnancy may result from disorders related to the pregnancy (obstetric) or not (see Table on pages 430 to 431). The **most common cause** is

■ A miscarriage

There are different degrees of miscarriage (also called spontaneous abortion). A miscarriage may be possible (threatened abortion) or certain to occur (inevitable abortion). All of the contents of the uterus (fetus and placenta) may be expelled (complete abortion) or not (incomplete abortion). The contents of the uterus may be infected before, during, or after the miscarriage (septic abortion). The fetus may die in the uterus and remain there (missed abortion). Any type of miscarriage can cause vaginal bleeding during early pregnancy.

The **most dangerous cause** of vaginal bleeding is

■ Rupture of an abnormally located (ectopic) pregnancy—one that is not in its usual place in the uterus—for example, one that is in a fallopian tube

Another possibly dangerous but less common cause is rupture of a corpus luteum cyst.

After an egg is released, the structure that released it (the corpus luteum) may fill with fluid or blood instead of breaking down and disappearing as it usually does. If an ectopic pregnancy or a corpus luteum cyst ruptures, bleeding may be profuse, leading to shock.

EVALUATION

Doctors first determine whether the cause is an ectopic pregnancy.

WARNING SIGNS

In pregnant women with vaginal bleeding during early pregnancy, the following symptoms are cause for concern:

■ Fainting, light-headedness, or a racing heart—symptoms that suggest very low blood pressure
■ Loss of large amounts of blood or blood that contains tissue or large clots
■ Severe abdominal pain that worsens when the woman moves or changes positions
■ Fever, chills, and a vaginal discharge that contains pus mixed with the blood

WHEN TO SEE A DOCTOR

Women with warning signs should see a doctor immediately. Women without warning signs should see a doctor within 48 to 72 hours.

WHAT THE DOCTOR DOES

Doctors ask about the symptoms and medical history (including past pregnancies, miscarriages, and abortions). Doctors then do a physical examination. What they find during the history and physical examination often suggests a cause and the tests that may need to be done (see Table).

Doctors ask about the bleeding:

■ How severe it is (for example, how many pads are used or soaked in an hour)
■ Whether clots or tissue were passed
■ Whether pain accompanies the bleeding

If pain is present, doctors ask when and how it started, where it occurs, how long it lasts, whether it is sharp or dull, and whether it is constant or comes and goes.

During the physical examination, doctors first check for fever and signs of substantial blood loss, such as a racing heart and low blood pressure. They then do a pelvic examination, checking to see whether the cervix (the lower part of the uterus) has started to open (dilate) to enable the fetus to pass through. If any tissue (possibly from a miscarriage) is detected, it is removed and sent to a laboratory to be analyzed.

Doctors also gently press on the abdomen to see whether it is tender when touched.

SOME CAUSES AND FEATURES OF VAGINAL BLEEDING DURING EARLY PREGNANCY

Cause	Common Features*	Tests†
Pregnancy-related (obstetric) disorders		
An ectopic pregnancy (an abnormally located pregnancy—not in its usual place in the uterus)	Sometimes only slight vaginal bleeding Abdominal or pelvic pain that ■ Is often sudden and constant (not crampy) ■ Begins in a specific spot ■ Is sometimes slight Usually tenderness when the pelvic examination is done If the ectopic pregnancy has ruptured, fainting, light-headedness, or a racing heart	Usually blood tests to measure a hormone produced by the placenta (human chorionic gonadotropin, or hCG) Ultrasonography of the pelvis Sometimes laparoscopy (insertion of a viewing tube through an incision in the abdomen) or laparotomy (surgery involving an incision into the abdomen)
A miscarriage that ■ Has occurred or is occurring ■ May occur (threatened abortion)	Crampy pain in the pelvis and often throughout the abdomen Often vaginal bleeding, sometimes with passage of tissue from the fetus	Tests as for ectopic pregnancy
Septic abortion (infection of the contents of the uterus)	Fever and chills, constant abdominal pain, vaginal discharge that contains pus Usually in women who have had an intentional abortion (often done by untrained practitioners or by the women themselves)	Cultures of samples taken from the cervix
A hydatidiform mole (overgrowth of tissue from the placenta) or another form of gestational trophoblastic disease	A uterus that is larger than expected No heartbeat or movement detected in the fetus Sometimes high blood pressure, swelling of the feet or hands, severe vomiting, or passage of tissue that resembles a bunch of grapes	Tests as for ectopic pregnancy A biopsy
Rupture of a corpus luteum cyst (which develops in the structure that releases the egg after the egg is released)	Abdominal or pelvic pain that ■ Begins in a specific spot ■ Sometimes causes nausea and vomiting ■ Usually begins suddenly Most common during the first 12 weeks of pregnancy	Ultrasonography of the pelvis

(continued)

SOME CAUSES AND FEATURES OF VAGINAL BLEEDING DURING EARLY PREGNANCY (continued)

Cause	Common Features*	Tests†
Disorders unrelated to the pregnancy		
Vaginitis (inflammation of the vagina, often due to infection)	Only spotting or slight bleeding A vaginal discharge Sometimes pain during sexual intercourse, pelvic pain, or both	A doctor's examination to rule out other causes Cultures of samples taken from the cervix
Cervicitis (infection of the cervix)	Only spotting or slight bleeding Sometimes tenderness when the pelvic examination is done, abdominal pain, or both	A doctor's examination to rule out other causes Cultures of samples taken from the cervix
Polyps (fingerlike growths) in the cervix, which are usually benign	Slight bleeding No pain Polyps sometimes seen protruding from cervix	A doctor's examination Follow-up visits to further evaluate the polyps

*Features include symptoms and results of the doctor's examination. Features mentioned are typical but not always present.
†A urine pregnancy test is typically done if women have had only a home pregnancy test. Because an ectopic pregnancy can be very dangerous, tests are done to look for ectopic pregnancy in most pregnant women with vaginal bleeding unless symptoms clearly point to another disorder.

TESTING

During the examination, doctors may use a handheld Doppler ultrasound device, placed on the woman's abdomen, to check for a heartbeat in the fetus.

If pregnancy has not been confirmed by a health care practitioner, a pregnancy test using a urine sample is done. Once pregnancy is confirmed, several tests are done:

- Blood type and Rh status (positive or negative)
- Usually ultrasonography
- Usually blood tests to measure a hormone (human chorionic gonadotropin, or hCG) produced by the placenta during early pregnancy

Rh status is determined because a pregnant woman with Rh-negative blood must be treated with $Rh_0(D)$ immune globulin if she has any vaginal bleeding. Treatment is needed to prevent her from producing antibodies that may attack the fetus's red blood cells in subsequent pregnancies. If bleeding is substantial (more than about a cup), doctors also do a complete blood cell count (CBC) and tests to check for abnormal antibodies or to cross-match blood (to determine whether the woman's blood type is compatible with a donor's). If blood loss is substantial or shock develops, tests are done to determine whether blood can clot normally.

Typically, ultrasonography is done using an ultrasound device inserted into the vagina unless the examination indicated that a complete miscarriage occurred. Ultrasonography can detect a pregnancy in the uterus and can detect a heartbeat after about 6 weeks of pregnancy. If no heartbeat is detected after this time, miscarriage is inevitable. If a heartbeat is detected, miscarriage is much less likely but may still occur. Ultrasonography can also help identify a miscarriage that is incomplete, is infected, or has been missed. It can detect any parts of the placenta or other pregnancy-related tissues that remain in the uterus. Ultrasonography can help identify a ruptured corpus luteum cyst and a hydatidiform mole or other forms of gestational trophoblastic disease. Sometimes ultrasonography can detect an ectopic pregnancy, depending on where it is located and how big it is.

Measuring hCG levels helps doctors interpret ultrasonography results and distinguish a normal pregnancy from an ectopic pregnancy. If the likelihood of an ectopic pregnancy is low, hCG levels are measured periodically. If the likelihood is moderate or high, doctors may make a small incision just below the navel and insert a viewing tube (laparoscope) to directly view the uterus and surrounding structures (laparoscopy) and thus determine whether an ectopic pregnancy is present.

TREATMENT

If bleeding is profuse, if shock develops, or if a ruptured ectopic pregnancy is likely, one of the first things doctors do is to place a large catheter in a vein so that blood can be quickly given intravenously.

When bleeding results from a disorder, that disorder is treated if possible. For example, surgery is done when an ectopic pregnancy has ruptured.

Although doctors have typically recommended bed rest when a miscarriage seems possible, there is no evidence that bed rest helps prevent miscarriage. Refraining from sexual intercourse is advised, although intercourse has not been definitely connected with miscarriages.

⊶ KEY POINTS

- The most common cause of bleeding during early pregnancy is a miscarriage.
- The most serious cause of vaginal bleeding is an ectopic pregnancy.
- A pregnant woman should see a doctor immediately if she has a racing heart, faints, or feels faint.
- Blood tests to determine whether blood is Rh-negative or Rh-positive are done because if a pregnant woman with Rh-negative blood has vaginal bleeding, she must be given $Rh_0(D)$ immune globulin to prevent her from producing antibodies that may attack the fetus's red blood cells in subsequent pregnancies.

VAGINAL BLEEDING DURING LATE PREGNANCY

During late pregnancy (after 20 weeks), 3 to 4% of women have vaginal bleeding. Such women are at risk of losing the baby or of bleeding excessively (hemorrhaging). Sometimes so much blood is lost that blood pressure becomes dangerously low (causing shock) or small blood clots form throughout the bloodstream (called disseminated intravascular coagulation).

CAUSES

The most common cause of bleeding during late pregnancy is

- The start of labor

Usually, labor starts with a small discharge of blood mixed with mucus from the vagina. This discharge, called the bloody show, occurs when small veins are torn as the cervix begins to open (dilate), enabling the fetus to pass through the vagina. The amount of blood in the discharge is small.

More serious but less common causes (see Table on page 435) include

- Placental abruption (abruptio placentae)
- Placenta previa
- Vasa previa
- Rupture of the uterus (rare)

In placental abruption, the placenta detaches from the uterus too soon. What causes this detachment is unclear, but it may occur because blood flow to the placenta is inadequate. Sometimes the placenta detaches after an injury, as may occur in a car crash. Bleeding may be more severe than it appears because some or most of the blood may be trapped behind the placenta and thus not be visible. Placental abruption is the most common life-threatening cause of bleeding during late pregnancy, accounting for about 30% of cases. Placental abruption may occur at any time but is most common during the 3rd trimester.

In placenta previa, the placenta is attached to the lower rather than the upper part of the uterus. When the placenta is lower in the uterus, it may partly or completely block the cervix (the lower part of the uterus), which the fetus must pass through. Bleeding may occur without warning, or it may be triggered when a practitioner examines the cervix to determine whether it is dilating or whether labor has started. Placenta previa accounts for about 20% of bleeding during late pregnancy and is most common during the 3rd trimester. It may occur during early pregnancy, but the placenta usually moves out of the way on its own before delivery.

In vasa previa, the blood vessels that provide blood to the fetus (through the umbilical cord) grow across the cervix, blocking the fetus's passageway. When labor starts, these small blood vessels may be torn, depriving the fetus of blood. Because the fetus has a relatively small amount of blood, loss of even a small amount can be serious, and the fetus may die.

Rupture of the uterus may occur during labor. It almost always occurs in women whose uterus has been damaged and contains scar tissue. Such damage may occur during a cesarean delivery or surgery or result from an infection or a severe abdominal injury.

Bleeding may also result from disorders unrelated to pregnancy.

RISK FACTORS

Various conditions (risk factors) increase the risk of disorders that can cause bleeding during late pregnancy.

For placental abruption, risk factors include

- High blood pressure
- Age over 35
- One or more previous pregnancies
- Cigarette smoking
- Use of cocaine
- Placental abruption in a previous pregnancy
- A recent abdominal injury

For placenta previa, risk factors include

- A cesarean delivery in a previous pregnancy
- One or more previous pregnancies
- A pregnancy with more than one fetus
- Placenta previa in a previous pregnancy
- Age over 35
- Cigarette smoking

For **vasa previa,** risk factors include

- A placenta located low in the uterus
- A placenta that is divided into sections
- A pregnancy with more than one fetus
- In vitro fertilization (fertilization of the egg in a laboratory and placement of the egg in the uterus)

For **rupture of the uterus,** risk factors include

- A cesarean delivery in a previous pregnancy
- Any surgery involving the uterus
- Age over 30
- Previous infections of the uterus
- Artificial starting (induction) of labor
- Injury, as may occur in a car crash

EVALUATION

Doctors focus on ruling out potentially serious causes of bleeding (such as placental abruption, placenta previa, vasa previa, and rupture of the uterus). If the evaluation rules out these more serious causes, doctors usually diagnose the most common cause—the start of labor, indicated by the bloody show.

WARNING SIGNS

Any vaginal bleeding late during pregnancy is considered a warning sign, except for the bloody show, which is only a small amount of blood mixed with mucus and which does not last long.

Doctors are particularly concerned about women with fainting, light-headedness, or a racing heart—symptoms that suggest very low blood pressure.

WHEN TO SEE A DOCTOR

A woman with vaginal bleeding late during pregnancy should go to the hospital immediately. However, if she suspects that the bleeding is the bloody show, she should call the doctor first. The doctor can determine how quickly she needs to be seen based on the amount and duration of bleeding and the presence of signs of labor.

WHAT THE DOCTOR DOES

Doctors first ask questions about the bleeding and other symptoms and about the medical history. Doctors then do a physical examination. What they find during the history and physical examination often suggests a cause of the pain and the tests that may need to be done (see Table on page 435).

Doctors ask about the bleeding:

- How long it lasts
- How severe it is
- What color the blood is
- Whether the woman has or has had other symptoms (such as abdominal pain, light-headedness, or fainting)

The woman is asked about her pregnancies: how many times she has been pregnant, how many children she has had, and whether she has had any miscarriages or abortions or any problems in previous pregnancies. The woman is asked whether the membranes have ruptured (whether her water broke), usually a sign that labor is starting or has started.

Doctors ask about conditions that increase the risk of the most common and serious causes of bleeding and about risk factors for these causes (see above), particularly a cesarean delivery in a previous pregnancy.

During the physical examination, doctors first check for signs of substantial blood loss, such as a racing heart and low blood pressure. They also check the heart rate of the fetus and, if possible, start monitoring the fetus's heart rate constantly (with electronic fetal heart monitoring). Doctors gently press on the abdomen to determine how large the uterus is, whether it is tender, and whether its muscle tone is normal. They then do a pelvic examination. They examine the cervix using an instrument that spreads the walls of the vagina apart (speculum).

Normally when delivery is near, doctors examine the cervix with a gloved hand to determine how dilated the cervix is and how the fetus is positioned. However, if bleeding occurs during late pregnancy, ultrasonography is done to check for placenta previa and vasa previa before this examination is done. If either disorder is present, the examination is not done because it may make the bleeding worse.

TESTING

The following tests are done:

- Ultrasonography
- A complete blood cell count
- Blood type and Rh status (positive or negative)

Ultrasonography using an ultrasound device placed in the vagina (transvaginal ultrasonography)

SOME CAUSES AND FEATURES OF VAGINAL BLEEDING DURING LATE PREGNANCY

Cause	Common Features*	Tests†
Labor	Passage of a discharge containing a small amount of blood mixed with mucus (bloody show) and no further bleeding Contractions in the lower abdomen at regular intervals plus opening (dilation) and thinning and pulling back (effacement) of the cervix Other typical signs of labor	A doctor's examination Sometimes ultrasonography
Placental abruption (premature detachment of the placenta from the uterus)	Pain or tenderness when the uterus is touched Passage of dark, clotted, or bright red blood but sometimes only slight bleeding Sometimes low blood pressure in the woman, with fainting, light-headedness, or a racing heart	A doctor's examination Ultrasonography
Placenta previa (an abnormally located placenta)	Painless vaginal bleeding with bright red blood Little or no tenderness when the uterus is touched	Ultrasonography or transvaginal ultrasonography (using an ultrasound device inserted into the vagina) by an experienced practitioner
Vasa previa (growth of the fetus's blood vessels across the cervix, blocking the fetus's passageway)	Painless vaginal bleeding Often signs of labor, such as contractions at regular intervals	Transvaginal ultrasonography using techniques to show blood flow (color Doppler ultrasonography)
Uterine rupture	Severe abdominal pain and tenderness when the abdomen is touched Stopping of contractions and often loss of muscle tone in the uterus Slight to moderate vaginal bleeding	A doctor's examination Laparotomy (surgery involving an incision into the abdomen)

*Features include symptoms and results of the doctor's examination. Features mentioned are typical but not always present.
†Ultrasonography is typically done in women with bleeding late in pregnancy, and a complete blood cell count, blood type, and Rh status (positive or negative) are usually done.

is often necessary to diagnose the cause of bleeding during late pregnancy. It can show the location of the placenta, umbilical cord, and blood vessels. Thus, it can help doctors rule out or identify placenta previa and vasa previa. However, ultrasonography cannot reliably distinguish placental abruption from rupture of the uterus. Doctors distinguish them based on results of the examination, including information about risk factors. Laparotomy is done to confirm a ruptured uterus. For this surgical procedure, doctors make an incision into the abdomen and pelvis so that they can directly view the uterus.

A complete blood cell count is done. Blood type and Rh status are determined so that a donor with a compatible blood type can be identified in case the woman needs a transfusion. If bleeding is profuse or if placental abruption is suspected, blood tests for disseminated intravascular coagulation are done. These tests include

- Prothrombin time and partial thromboplastin time (to determine whether blood can clot normally)
- Measurement of substances that help blood clot (clotting factors) and of proteins

produced when clots are broken up (fibrinogen and fibrin degradation products)

If the woman has Rh-negative blood, a blood test (Kleihauer-Betke test) may be done to measure how many of the fetus's red blood cells are in the woman's bloodstream. The results can help doctors determine how much $Rh_0(D)$ immune globulin the woman should be given to prevent her from producing antibodies that may attack the fetus's red blood cells in subsequent pregnancies.

TREATMENT

The disorder causing the bleeding is treated.

For placental abruption or placenta previa, bed rest in the hospital is usually recommended. There, the woman and fetus can be monitored, and treatment is readily available. If the bleeding stops, the woman is encouraged to walk and may be sent home. If bleeding continues or worsens or if the pregnancy is near term, the baby is delivered. Cesarean delivery is usually used if women have placenta previa and sometimes if women have placental abruption.

If vasa previa is diagnosed before labor starts, doctors schedule a cesarean delivery before labor starts, typically a few weeks before the due date. If placenta previa is diagnosed during labor, cesarean delivery is done. If the baby has lost a lot of blood, the baby may require a blood transfusion.

If the uterus has ruptured, the baby is delivered immediately. The uterus is repaired surgically.

If the woman has lost a lot of blood, she is given fluids intravenously. If this treatment is inadequate, she is given blood transfusions.

O—🔑 KEY POINTS

- Usually, a small vaginal discharge of blood mixed with mucus (bloody show) signals the start of labor.
- The severity of the bleeding does not always indicate the seriousness of the cause.
- Ultrasonography is done to help doctors identify serious disorders that can cause bleeding during late pregnancy.
- A woman with bleeding during late pregnancy may be hospitalized so that she and her fetus can be monitored and treated as needed.
- If bleeding is profuse, the woman may need to be given fluids intravenously or a blood transfusion.

A discharge from the vagina may occur normally or may result from inflammation of the vagina (vaginitis), which may be due to an infection. The genital area (vulva)—the area around the opening of the vagina—may also be inflamed. Depending on the cause of the discharge, other symptoms are often also present. They include itching, burning, irritation, redness, and sometimes pain during urination and sexual intercourse.

NORMAL DISCHARGE

A vaginal discharge can result from normal changes in estrogen levels. When levels are high, estrogen stimulates the cervix to produce secretions (mucus), and a small amount of mucus may be discharged from the vagina. Estrogen levels are high

- During menstrual cycles a few days before the egg is released
- In newborns for a week or two after birth because they absorb estrogen from their mother before birth
- A few months before girls have their first menstrual period
- During pregnancy

Typically, a normal discharge has no odor. It is usually milky white or thin and clear. During the childbearing years, the amount and appearance may vary during the menstrual cycle. For example, in the middle of the cycle when the egg is released (at ovulation), the cervix produces more mucus, and the mucus is thinner. Pregnancy, use of birth control pills (oral contraceptives), and sexual arousal also affect the amount and appearance of the discharge. After menopause, estrogen levels decrease, often reducing the amount of normal discharge.

ABNORMAL DISCHARGE

A vaginal discharge is considered abnormal if it is

- Heavier than usual
- Thicker than usual
- Puslike
- White and clumpy (like cottage cheese)
- Grayish, greenish, yellowish, or blood-tinged

- Foul- or fishy-smelling
- Accompanied by itching, burning, a rash, or soreness

CAUSES

An abnormal vaginal discharge is usually caused by vaginitis, which most often results from irritation by a chemical or from an infection.

COMMON CAUSES

Likely causes of a vaginal discharge depend on age.

During childhood, common causes include

- An infection due to bacteria from the digestive tract
- Chemicals in bubble baths or soaps
- A foreign object (body), such as a piece of toilet paper or sometimes a toy

An infection may occur when hygiene is poor. For example, young girls, especially those 2 to 6 years old, may transfer bacteria from the digestive tract to the genital area when they wipe from back to front or do not wash their hands after bowel movements.

If a foreign object is the cause, the discharge may contain small amounts of blood.

During the childbearing years, a discharge is usually caused by a vaginal infection. The most common are

- Bacterial vaginosis
- Candidiasis
- *Trichomonas* vaginitis (trichomoniasis of the vagina), which is usually sexually transmitted

Sometimes a discharge is caused by another infection, including sexually transmitted diseases (such as gonorrhea, a chlamydial infection, or trichomoniasis).

Vaginal infections are usually prevented by the protective bacteria (lactobacilli) that normally live in the vagina. These bacteria keep the acidity of the vagina in the normal range. When acidity in the vagina decreases, the number of protective bacteria decreases, and the number of harmful bacteria increases.

SOME CAUSES AND FEATURES OF A VAGINAL DISCHARGE

Cause	Common Features*	Tests
During childhood		
A foreign object (often toilet paper) in the vagina	A discharge, usually with a foul odor and often containing small amounts of blood	A doctor's examination, sometimes done after the girl is sedated or given a general anesthetic
Infections such as ■ Yeast (candidiasis) ■ Pinworm ■ Streptococcal ■ Staphylococcal	Itching, redness, and swelling Often pain during urination With pinworm infection, itching that worsens at night With streptococcal or staphylococcal infection, redness and swelling in the genital area	Examination under a microscope and analysis of a sample of the discharge to check for microorganisms that can cause vaginal infections Examination of the genital area and anus to check for pinworms
Sexual abuse	Soreness in the genital area Sometimes discharge that has a foul odor or contains blood Often vague symptoms (such as fatigue or abdominal pain) or changes in behavior (such as starting to have temper tantrums or to withdraw)	Examination under a microscope and analysis of a sample of the discharge Tests to detect sexually transmitted diseases using a sample of secretions taken from the cervix
During the childbearing years		
Bacterial vaginosis	A thin, white or gray cloudy discharge with a fishy odor Itching and irritation	Examination under a microscope and analysis of a sample of the discharge
Yeast infections	Irritation, itching, redness, and swelling in the genital area A thick, white, clumpy discharge that resembles cottage cheese Sometimes worsening of symptoms after intercourse and before menstrual periods Sometimes recent use of antibiotics or a history of diabetes	Examination under a microscope and analysis of a sample of the discharge
Trichomoniasis (a protozoan infection)	A usually profuse, yellow-green, frothy discharge with a fishy odor Itching, redness, swelling, and soreness in the genital area Sometimes pain during sexual intercourse and urination	Examination under a microscope and analysis of a sample of the discharge
Pelvic inflammatory disease	Aching pelvic pain that becomes increasingly severe and may be felt on one or both sides A discharge that sometimes has a foul odor and, as infection worsens, can become puslike and yellow-green Sometimes pain during sexual intercourse or urination, fever or chills, nausea, or vomiting	Tests to detect sexually transmitted diseases using a sample of secretions taken from the cervix Sometimes ultrasonography of the pelvis

(continued)

SOME CAUSES AND FEATURES OF A VAGINAL DISCHARGE *(continued)*

Cause	Common Features*	Tests
A foreign object (often a forgotten tampon) in the vagina	An often profuse discharge with an extremely foul odor	A doctor's examination
After menopause		
Thinning of the lining of the vagina (atrophic vaginitis)	A scant discharge Pain during sexual intercourse	A doctor's examination Examination under a microscope and analysis of a sample of the discharge
Irritation caused by urine or stool	General redness in the area around the genitals and anus Conditions that increase the risk of such irritation, such as being incontinent or bedbound	A doctor's examination
Cancer of the vagina, cervix, or lining of the uterus (endometrium)	A watery or bloody discharge Often no other symptoms until the cancer is advanced Pain that develops gradually and sometimes becomes chronic Sometimes weight loss	A Papanicolaou (Pap) test A biopsy Imaging tests such as ultrasonography, MRI, or CT
At any age		
Chemical irritation (such as that due to soaps, bubble baths, hygiene sprays, or vaginal creams and ointments)	Redness and soreness of the genitals	A doctor's examination
An abnormal opening (fistula) between the intestine and genital tract, which may result from ■ An injury during childbirth ■ Surgery ■ Inflammatory bowel disease ■ Cancer of the digestive tract or reproductive organs	A discharge with a foul odor Presence of stool in the vagina or in the vaginal discharge	A doctor's examination
Inflammation due to ■ Radiation therapy ■ Pelvic surgery ■ Certain chemotherapy drugs	Recent treatment of a disorder affecting the pelvis A discharge that contains pus Pain during urination and sexual intercourse Sometimes irritation, itching, redness, burning pain, and mild bleeding	A doctor's examination Usually examination under a microscope and analysis of a sample of the discharge

*Features include symptoms and results of the doctor's examination. Features mentioned are typical but not always present.
CT = computed tomography; MRI = magnetic resonance imaging.

The following make the growth of harmful bacteria more likely (and thus increase the risk of vaginal infections):

- Use of antibiotics (because they may reduce the number of protective bacteria)
- Menstrual blood or semen in the vagina (because they reduce the acidity of the vagina)
- Poor hygiene
- Frequent douching (because it can reduce the acidity of the vagina)
- Pregnancy
- Diabetes mellitus

After menopause, many women have an abnormal discharge. It occurs because the decrease in estrogen levels causes the vagina to thin and become drier. Moderate to severe thinning and drying is called atrophic vaginitis. A thin, dry vagina is more likely to become irritated and inflamed.

LESS COMMON CAUSES

During childhood, sexual abuse may be the cause. Such abuse can result in injury or a sexually transmitted disease.

During the childbearing years, the cause is sometimes a foreign object (such as a forgotten tampon). But in this age group, a discharge seldom results from inflammation alone (without infection).

In older women, urine or stool may irritate the area around the genitals and anus, resulting in a vaginal discharge. Such irritation may occur when women are incontinent (involuntarily pass stool or urine) or bedbound.

At any age, various products that come in contact with the genital area can irritate it, sometimes causing a discharge. Such products include hygiene sprays, perfumes, menstrual pads, laundry soaps, bleaches, fabric softeners, and sometimes spermicides, vaginal creams or lubricants, vaginal contraceptive rings, diaphragms, and, for women who are allergic to latex, latex condoms. Rarely, women have abnormal openings (fistulas) between the intestine and genital tract, resulting in a discharge from the vagina. This discharge sometimes contains stool. Fistulas may result from damage to the vagina during delivery (mainly in developing countries), Crohn disease, radiation therapy directed at the pelvis (the lowest part of the torso), injury during pelvic surgery, or tumors in the pelvis. Radiation therapy, pelvic surgery, and tumors can cause a vaginal discharge whether they cause fistulas or not.

EVALUATION

Often, doctors can identify the cause of an abnormal discharge based on characteristics of the discharge (such as appearance and odor), the woman's age, other symptoms, and simple tests that provide quick results.

WARNING SIGNS

In women with an abnormal discharge, certain characteristics are cause for concern:

- In girls, a fever or a yellow or green discharge with a fishy odor (because they may have a sexually transmitted disease resulting from sexual abuse)
- Severe abdominal or pelvic pain or pain that lasts more than 2 hours
- Drainage of pus, a fever, or other signs of infection in the reproductive organs
- Stool in the vaginal discharge

WHEN TO SEE A DOCTOR

Women or girls with warning signs should see a doctor within a day. However, if the only warning sign is stool in the discharge, a delay of several days is not likely to be harmful.

Women without warning signs should see a doctor within a few days.

If women recognize the symptoms of a yeast infection, are confident that what they have is a yeast infection, and have no other symptoms, they probably do not need to see a doctor every time they have a discharge. A discharge caused by a yeast infection is usually distinctive. It is thick, white, and often clumpy, resembling cottage cheese. However, sometimes yeast infections cause mainly itching and burning with only a small amount of discharge.

WHAT THE DOCTOR DOES

Doctors first ask the woman questions about her symptoms and medical history. Doctors then do a physical examination. What they find during the history and physical examination often suggests a cause of the pain and the tests that may need to be done (see Table on pages 438 to 439).

Doctors ask about the discharge:

- What it looks and smells like
- When it occurs in relation to menstrual periods and sexual intercourse
- Whether other symptoms (such as itching or pain) are present

Other questions include whether women use hygiene sprays or other products that may irritate the genital area and whether women have any conditions that can increase the risk of having a vaginal discharge.

The physical examination focuses on the pelvic examination.

TESTING

Simple tests, which can be done in or near the examination room, can provide quick results that often enable doctors to identify the cause. Additional tests are done to confirm or, if needed, to identify the cause.

Unless the cause is obvious (such as a foreign object or an allergic reaction), doctors use a cotton swab to take a sample of the discharge from the vagina or cervix. They examine the sample under a microscope to check for yeast infections, bacterial vaginosis, and *Trichomonas* vaginitis. They usually also send a sample to the laboratory to test for gonorrhea and chlamydial infections (which are sexually transmitted).

TREATMENT

The underlying condition is corrected or treated if possible. For example, bacterial vaginosis is treated with antibiotics.

Some general measures can help relieve symptoms, although they do not eliminate an infection.

GENERAL MEASURES

The genital area should be kept as clean as possible. Washing every day with a mild, unscented soap (such as glycerin soap) and rinsing and drying thoroughly are recommended. Changing underwear and bathing or showering once a day may help relieve symptoms. Improved hygiene is particularly useful if the cause is being incontinent or bedbound. Young girls should be taught good hygiene—to wipe from front to back, to wash their hands after bowel movements and urinating, and to avoid fingering the genital area.

If a product (such as a cream, powder, soap, or brand of condom) consistently causes irritation, it should not be used. Women are advised not to use feminine hygiene sprays and not to douche. These products do not eliminate the discharge and may make it worse. Douching may increase the risk of pelvic inflammatory disease.

Placing ice packs on the genital area or sitting in a warm sitz bath (with or without baking soda) may reduce soreness and itching. A sitz bath is taken in the sitting position with water covering only the genital and rectal area. Flushing the genital area with lukewarm water squeezed from a water bottle may also provide relief.

DRUGS

If symptoms are moderate or severe or do not respond to general measures, drugs may be needed. For example, a corticosteroid cream (such as hydrocortisone) or sometimes antihistamines taken by mouth can relieve itching.

ESSENTIALS FOR OLDER WOMEN

After menopause, estrogen levels decrease markedly. As a result, the amount of normal discharge usually decreases. However, because the lining of the vagina thins and becomes drier (called atrophic vaginitis), the vagina is more likely to become irritated, often resulting in an abnormal discharge from the vagina. This discharge may be watery and thin or thick and yellowish.

Thinning also makes certain vaginal infections more likely to develop. The thin, dry vaginal tissues are more easily damaged, allowing usually harmless bacteria from the skin to enter tissues under the skin and cause infection there. Such infections are usually not serious but can cause discomfort.

Older women are more likely to have treatments that can reduce estrogen levels and thus make the vagina more likely to become irritated. Such treatments include removal of both ovaries, radiation therapy directed at the pelvis, and certain chemotherapy drugs.

Problems that make good hygiene difficult, such as being incontinent or bedbound, are more common among older women. Poor hygiene can result in chronic inflammation of the genital area due to irritation by urine or stool.

Vaginal infections, such as bacterial vaginosis, yeast infections, and *Trichomonas* vaginitis are uncommon after menopause but may occur in women with risk factors for these infections. Risk factors for yeast infections include diabetes and incontinence. Risk factors for bacterial vaginosis and *Trichomonas* vaginitis include new or several sex partners.

If older women are sexually active, condoms should be used to reduce the risk of sexually transmitted diseases. However, because condoms can irritate the vaginal tissues, particularly in older women, using lubricants is essential. Only water-based lubricants should be used with latex condoms. Oil-based lubricants (such as petroleum jelly) can weaken latex and cause the condom to break.

Because the risk that vaginal bleeding is due to cancer increases after menopause, older women should see a doctor promptly if they have a discharge, particularly if the discharge contains blood or is brown or pink (possibly indicating a small amount of blood). A blood-tinged, pink, or brown discharge after menopause can be a warning sign of a precancerous disorder (such as thickening of the lining of the uterus) or cancer and should not be ignored.

⊶ KEY POINTS

- A vaginal discharge may be accompanied by itching, redness, burning, and soreness.
- Likely causes depend on age.
- Usually, doctors examine a sample of the discharge to check for microorganisms that can cause infections.
- Treatment depends on the cause, but applying cold packs or sitting in a warm sitz bath can help relieve symptoms.
- Any discharge that occurs after menopause requires prompt evaluation by a doctor.

VAGINAL ITCHING

Vaginal itching may involve the vagina or the genital area (vulva), which contains the external genital organs. Itching is an unpleasant sensation that seems to require scratching for relief.

Many women occasionally have short episodes of vaginal itching that resolve without treatment. Itching is considered a problem only when it persists, is severe, recurs, or is accompanied by a discharge (see page 437).

CAUSES

The most common causes of vaginal itching include the following:

- Infections: Bacterial vaginosis, candidiasis (a yeast infection), and trichomoniasis (a protozoan infection)
- Irritation or allergic reactions: Chemicals that come in contact with the vagina or genital area, such as those in laundry detergents, bleaches, fabric softeners, synthetic fibers, bubble baths, soaps, feminine hygiene sprays, perfumes, menstrual pads, fabric dyes, toilet tissue, vaginal creams, douches, condoms, and contraceptive foams
- After menopause, atrophic vaginitis: Thinning and drying of the lining of the vagina due to decreased estrogen levels

Less common causes include skin disorders such as psoriasis and lichen sclerosus. Lichen sclerosus is characterized by thin white areas on the vulva around the opening of the vagina. If untreated, lichen sclerosus can cause scarring and may increase the risk of cancer of the vulva.

EVALUATION

Doctors can usually determine the cause by asking about symptoms and by examining the genital area and vagina.

WARNING SIGNS

There are no warning signs for vaginal itching unless it is accompanied by pain and/or discharge. Then, the warning signs are the same as those for pelvic pain (see page 324) and/or vaginal discharge (see page 437).

WHEN TO SEE A DOCTOR

Women should see a doctor if itching lasts more than a few days or if other symptoms suggesting an infection (such as pain or discharge) develop.

WHAT THE DOCTOR DOES

Doctors first ask the woman questions about her symptoms, particularly whether she has any symptoms of infection, and about her medical history. She is also asked whether she uses any products that may irritate the area. Doctors then do a physical examination, which focuses on the pelvic examination.

If women have a discharge, a sample of the discharge is taken, examined, and analyzed.

TREATMENT

The underlying condition is corrected or treated when possible. General measures can help relieve symptoms.

GENERAL MEASURES

Changing underwear and bathing or showering once a day help keep the vagina and genital area clean. More frequent washing may cause excessive dryness, which can increase itching. Using a cornstarch-based unscented body powder can help keep the genital area dry. Women should not use talc-based powders. A nonallergenic soap should be used. Other products (such as creams, feminine hygiene sprays, or douches) should not be applied to the vaginal area. These general measures may minimize exposure to irritants that cause itching.

If a medical product (such as a prescription cream) or a brand of condom appears to cause irritation and itching, it should not be used. Women should talk to their doctor before they stop using prescription products.

DRUGS

Applying a mild (low-strength) corticosteroid cream such as hydrocortisone to the genital area may provide temporary relief. The cream should not be put into the vagina and should be used for only a short period of time. For severe itching, an antihistamine taken by mouth may help temporarily. Antihistamines also cause drowsiness and may be useful if symptoms interfere with sleep.

Lichen sclerosus is treated with a cream or an ointment containing a high-strength corticosteroid (such as clobetasol), available by prescription.

O━π KEY POINTS

- Itching is a problem only when it persists, is severe, recurs, or is accompanied by pain or by a discharge that looks or smells abnormal, suggesting an infection.
- Keeping the genital area clean and dry and not using products that can irritate it can help.
- Sometimes a mild corticosteroid cream relieves itching temporarily.

VISION, BLURRED

Blurred vision is the most common vision symptom. When doctors talk about blurred vision, they typically mean a decrease in sharpness or clarity that has developed gradually. Sudden, complete loss of vision in one or both eyes (blindness) is considered something different—see Vision Loss, Sudden on page 455.

CAUSES

Blurred vision has four general mechanisms:

- Disorders affecting the retina, the light-sensing structure at the back of the eye
- Clouding of normally transparent eye structures (cornea, lens, and vitreous humor—the jellylike substance that fills the eyeball) that light rays must pass through to reach the retina
- Disorders affecting the pathways of nerves that carry visual signals from the eye to the brain (such as the optic nerve)
- Imperfect focusing of light rays on the retina (refractive errors)

Certain disorders can have more than one mechanism. For example, refraction can be impaired by early cataracts or by the reversible lens swelling caused by poorly controlled diabetes.

Some disorders that cause blurred vision are more likely to cause other symptoms that prompt people to seek medical attention, such as eye pain and eye redness (for example, acute corneal disorders such as abrasions, ulcers, herpes simplex keratitis, or herpes zoster ophthalmicus).

COMMON CAUSES

The most common causes of blurred vision include

- Refractive errors (such as nearsightedness, farsightedness, or astigmatism), the most common cause overall
- Age-related macular degeneration
- Cataracts
- Damage of the retina resulting from diabetes (diabetic retinopathy)
- Glaucoma

LESS COMMON CAUSES

Rare disorders that can cause blurred vision include

- Inherited disorders affecting the optic nerve, called hereditary optic neuropathies (for example, dominant optic atrophy and Leber hereditary optic neuropathy)
- Corneal scarring due to vitamin A deficiency (rare in developed nations)

EVALUATION

The following information can help people decide when a doctor's evaluation is needed and help them know what to expect during the evaluation.

WARNING SIGNS

In people with blurred vision, certain symptoms and characteristics are cause for concern. They include

- Sudden change in vision
- Severely reduced vision, particularly in only one eye, even if the symptoms began gradually
- Eye pain (with or without eye movement)
- Loss of a specific area in the field of vision (called a visual field defect)
- Human immunodeficiency virus (HIV) infection or AIDS or other disorder affecting the immune system

WHEN TO SEE A DOCTOR

People who have warning signs should usually go to an emergency department right away. People who have a bodywide disorder that sometimes causes retinal damage (for example, diabetes, high blood pressure, or sickle cell disease) should see an eye doctor as soon as is practical, usually within a few days. However, if vision has been deteriorating gradually for months or years but has not been severely impaired and there are no warning signs, waiting a week or longer is usually not harmful. Eye examinations should be done by an ophthalmologist or optometrist. Ophthalmologists are medical doctors who specialize in the evaluation and treatment (surgical and nonsurgical) of all types of eye disorders. Optometrists are health care practitioners who specialize in the diagnosis and treatment of refractive errors (which are treated by prescribing glasses or contact lenses). However, optometrists can often diagnose certain other eye problems and then refer people to an ophthalmologist for treatment. People should usually see an ophthalmologist if they have warning signs.

WHAT THE DOCTOR DOES

Doctors first ask questions about the person's symptoms and medical history. Doctors then do a physical examination. What they find during the history and physical examination often suggests a cause of the blurred vision and the tests that may need to be done (see Table, below).

Doctors ask many questions about the person's symptoms because it is important to understand exactly what the person means by blurred vision. For example, people who have actually lost vision in part of their visual field (visual field defect) may describe this sensation only as blurred vision. The presence of other eye symptoms, such as eye redness, sensitivity to light, floaters, a sensation of sudden flashes of light that can look like lightning, spots, or stars (photopsias), and pain at rest or with eye movement, helps doctors determine the cause. Doctors also ask about the effects of darkness (night vision) and bright lights (for example, causing blur, star bursts, or halos) and whether the person wears corrective lenses.

Doctors also ask questions about symptoms of possible causes and about the presence of disorders that are known to be risk factors for eye

SOME CAUSES AND FEATURES OF BLURRED VISION

Cause	Common Features*	Tests
Clouding of normally transparent eye structures		
Cataracts	Symptoms that begin gradually	A doctor's examination
	Loss of the ability to distinguish between light and dark (loss of contrast) and glare (seeing halos and star bursts around lights)	
	Often in people with risk factors (such as older age or use of corticosteroids)	
Corneal scarring after an injury or an infection	Usually in people with a previous injury or infection	A doctor's examination
Disorders that affect the retina		
Age-related macular degeneration	Usually symptoms that begin gradually	Sometimes an eye imaging test
	Loss of central vision (what a person is looking at directly) much more than peripheral vision (what is seen out of the corner of the eye)	
Infection of the retina (as may be caused by *Toxoplasma* parasites)	Usually in people who have HIV infection or another disorder that weakens the immune system	Tests to check for organisms suspected to be causing the infection
	Often eye redness or pain	
Retinitis pigmentosa (progressive deterioration of the retina)	Symptoms that begin gradually	Specialized testing (such as measuring the retina's responses to light in various conditions), done by an ophthalmologist *(continued)*
	Primarily night blindness	

SOME CAUSES AND FEATURES OF BLURRED VISION (continued)

Cause	Common Features*	Tests
Retinopathy (damage of the retina) associated with a bodywide disorder such as high blood pressure, systemic lupus erythematosus (lupus), diabetes, Waldenström macroglobulinemia, and multiple myeloma or other disorders that can cause thickening of the blood (hyperviscosity syndrome)	Often in people known to have such disorders Usually other symptoms in addition to loss of vision	Tests to check for disorders suspected to be causing retinopathy

Disorders that affect the optic nerve or its connections in the brain

Open-angle glaucoma	Missing stairs and not seeing parts of written or typed words	Measurement of pressure inside the eye (tonometry), examination of the angles between eye structures such as the cornea and iris (gonisocopy), and optic nerve testing, done by an ophthalmologist
Optic neuritis (inflammation of the optic nerve), which can be related to multiple sclerosis	Usually mild pain that may worsen when one eye (often) or both eyes are moved Partial or complete loss of vision Symptoms that can become severe in hours or days No effect on the eyelids and cornea	Often MRI with a radiopaque dye

Disorders that affect focus

Refractive errors (such as nearsightedness, farsightedness, and astigmatism)	Sharpness of vision (visual acuity) that varies with distance from objects Decreased acuity that can be corrected by using glasses or a pinhole device	Testing of refraction by an optometrist or ophthalmologist

*Features include symptoms and the results of the doctor's examination. Features mentioned are typical but not always present.
HIV = human immunodeficiency virus; MRI = magnetic resonance imaging.

disorders (for example, high blood pressure, diabetes, HIV infection or AIDS, and sickle cell disease).

Examination of the eyes may be all that is necessary.

Testing **visual acuity** (sharpness of vision) is the first step. Ideally, acuity is measured while the person stands about 20 feet (6 meters) from a standard eye chart (Snellen chart) posted or projected on a wall. Each eye is measured separately while the other eye is covered. Visual acuity is measured with and without the person's own glasses. Sometimes the doctor has the person look through a device that has a pinhole. This device can usually correct refractive errors almost completely but does not correct vision that is blurred due to other causes.

The **eye examination** is also important. The doctor carefully examines the entire eye using an ophthalmoscope (a light with magnifying lenses that shines into the back of the eye), slit lamp (an instrument that enables a doctor to examine the eye under high magnification), or both. Often the eyes are dilated

WHAT IS ASTIGMATISM?

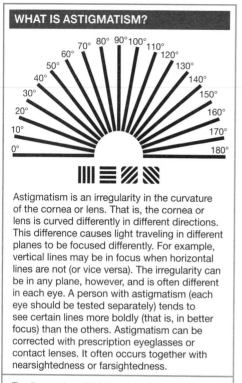

Astigmatism is an irregularity in the curvature of the cornea or lens. That is, the cornea or lens is curved differently in different directions. This difference causes light traveling in different planes to be focused differently. For example, vertical lines may be in focus when horizontal lines are not (or vice versa). The irregularity can be in any plane, however, and is often different in each eye. A person with astigmatism (each eye should be tested separately) tends to see certain lines more boldly (that is, in better focus) than the others. Astigmatism can be corrected with prescription eyeglasses or contact lenses. It often occurs together with nearsightedness or farsightedness.

The diagram above is of a standard chart used to test for astigmatism in one eye at a time.

for ophthalmoscopy with eye drops. Pressure inside the eye (intraocular pressure) is measured (called tonometry).

Symptoms and findings during the eye examination often help suggest a cause. For example, if visual acuity returns while corrective lenses or a pinhole device is used, simple refractive error is usually the cause of blurring.

TESTING

Testing depends on the suspected cause of the blurred vision. People with symptoms of bodywide disorders should have appropriate testing. For example, testing might include blood tests for diabetes, systemic lupus erythematosus, or HIV infection, blood pressure monitoring, and possibly electrocardiography if high blood pressure or a kidney disorder is suspected.

TREATMENT

Underlying disorders are treated. Corrective lenses or surgery may be used to improve visual acuity, sometimes even when the cause is not just refractive error (for example, for early cataracts).

ESSENTIALS FOR OLDER PEOPLE

Although some decrease in visual acuity normally occurs with aging, acuity normally is correctable to 20/20 with refraction, even in very old people.

O—π KEY POINTS

- Refractive error is the most common cause of blurred vision.
- If refractive error is the problem, corrective lenses or surgery (particularly if cataracts are the cause of the change in refractive error) can usually correct the blurriness.
- Doctors check visual acuity and determine whether glasses or a pinhole device corrects the problem, and if it does not, they dilate the eye with drops and carefully examine the retina.

VISION, DOUBLE

Double vision (diplopia) is seeing two images of one object. Double vision may occur when only one eye is open (monocular diplopia) or, more commonly, when both eyes are open (binocular diplopia). Binocular double vision disappears when either eye is closed. Other symptoms, such as eye pain, bulging eye, or muscle weakness, can be present depending on the cause of double vision.

CAUSES

Monocular double vision can occur when something distorts light transmission through the eye to the retina (the light-sensing structure at the back of the eye). There may be more than two images. One of the images is of normal quality (for example, in brightness, contrast, and clarity). The other image or images are of inferior quality.

The most common causes of monocular double vision are

- Clouding of the lens of the eye (cataract)
- Problems with the shape of the cornea (for example, keratoconus, in which the cornea changes from its normal round shape to a conelike shape)
- Uncorrected refractive error, usually astigmatism

Refractive error is imperfect focusing of light rays on the retina. Astigmatism (see art box on page 448) is refractive error caused by abnormal curvature of the cornea (the clear layer in front of the iris and pupil).

Other causes of monocular double vision include corneal scarring and a dislocated lens.

Binocular double vision suggests the eyes are not pointing at the same object. People normally see an object as a single image even though each eye receives its own separate image of that object. To perceive single images, the eyes must be aligned so that both point to the same object at the same time (called conjugate alignment). When the eyes are not properly aligned, people see two images, both of equal quality. Sometimes binocular double vision becomes apparent only when people move their eyes to an extreme in a certain direction (for example, to the far right or left, or up or down).

There are many possible causes of binocular double vision. The most common are

- Paralysis of one of the nerves that controls the muscles that move the eye (called the 3rd, 4th, and 6th cranial nerves)
- Myasthenia gravis
- Mechanical blockage of eye movement

Most commonly, the eyes are misaligned because of a disorder affecting the cranial nerves supplying the muscles that move the eyes, called extraocular muscles. The paralysis may be isolated and the cause may be unknown. Known causes include disorders that typically interfere with the ability of the nerves to control muscles. For example, myasthenia gravis, botulism, and Guillain-Barré syndrome can affect muscles throughout the body, including the muscles that move the eyes.

Anything that mechanically interferes with eye motion can keep the eyes from aligning properly and cause double vision. Examples include entrapment of an eye muscle in a fracture of the eye socket and deposition of abnormal tissue in the eye socket as can occur with the form of hyperthyroidism called Graves disease.

EVALUATION

Some causes of double vision are minor, but some can be very serious. The following information can help people know when to see a doctor and what to expect during the evaluation.

WARNING SIGNS

In people with double vision, certain symptoms and characteristics are cause for concern. They include

- Any symptoms besides double vision that could represent nervous system dysfunction (for example, weakness or paralysis, loss of sensation, speech or language problems, trouble swallowing or walking, vertigo, headache, incontinence, or clumsiness)

- Eye pain
- Bulging of the eye (proptosis)
- Recent injury to the eye or head

Double vision should always be evaluated by a doctor even if it is temporary. People who have warning signs should be evaluated by a doctor right away, usually in an emergency department. All people who have double vision, even if it has resolved, should see a doctor as soon as convenient, usually within a few days.

Doctors first ask questions about the person's symptoms and medical history. Doctors then do a physical examination. What they find during the medical history and physical examination helps suggest a cause of the double vision and any tests that need to be done (see Table, below).

Doctors want to know whether double vision involves one or both eyes and whether it is constant or comes and goes. They also ask whether the images are side by side or on top of one another and whether double vision tends to

SOME CAUSES OF DOUBLE VISION WHEN BOTH EYES ARE OPEN

Cause	Common Features*	Tests
Disorders that affect control of eye muscles by the nervous system†		
Certain strokes or transient ischemic attacks	Often in older people and in people with risk factors for these disorders (such as high blood pressure, atherosclerosis, and diabetes) Sometimes slurred speech, weakness, and/or difficulty walking	MRI or CT
A mass that presses on a nerve, such as a bulge in an artery (aneurysm) or a tumor	Often pain (sudden if caused by an aneurysm) and often other symptoms of nervous system dysfunction (such as muscle weakness, loss of coordination, and abnormal sensations in the skin)	MRI or CT of the brain (done immediately)
Inflammation or infection of the eye or surrounding structures (for example, abscess, sinusitis, and, rarely, with a blood clot in the cavernous sinus at the base of the skull)	Constant pain Sometimes fever, chills, fatigue, loss of sensation in the face, and/or bulging eyes	CT or MRI
Multiple sclerosis	Usually periods of relatively good health alternating with episodes of worsening symptoms Weakness that comes and goes from day to day Abnormal sensations such as tingling, numbness, pain, burning, and itching Clumsiness Loss of strength or dexterity in a leg or hand, which may become stiff As the disorder progresses, shakiness, partial or complete paralysis, and involuntary muscle contractions (spasticity), sometimes causing painful cramps Slowed, slurred speech Problems with urination and/or bowel function	MRI of the brain and spinal cord

(continued)

SOME CAUSES OF DOUBLE VISION WHEN BOTH EYES ARE OPEN (continued)

Cause	Common Features*	Tests
Myasthenia gravis	Double vision that comes and goes Difficulty speaking or swallowing Weakness Muscles that weaken when they are used repeatedly	Strength testing after a drug that relieves symptoms of myasthenia gravis is injected (edrophonium test)
Wernicke syndrome	History of long-term alcohol abuse Clumsiness, poor coordination, and confusion	A doctor's examination
Disorders that block eye motion		
Graves disease (an overactive thyroid gland that causes muscles and tissues around the eye to thicken—called infiltrative ophthalmopathy)	Bulging of the eyes, often eye pain or irritation, watering, sensitivity to light, an enlarged thyroid gland (goiter), and thickened skin on the shins	Blood tests to evaluate thyroid function
Injury, such as a fracture of the eye socket (orbit) or a collection of blood (hematoma)	Pain In people who have obviously had a recent eye injury	CT or MRI
Tumors (near the base of the skull, the sinuses, or the eye socket)	Often pain unrelated to eye movement, bulging of one eye, and sometimes other symptoms of nervous system dysfunction	MRI or CT

*Features include symptoms and the results of the doctor's examination. Features mentioned are typical but not always present.
†Whether pain is present varies by cause.
CT = computed tomography; ECG = electrocardiography; MRI = magnetic resonance imaging.

occur only when the person is gazing in a particular direction. Doctors ask about any pain, numbness of the forehead or cheek, facial weakness, vertigo, and swallowing or speech problems because these symptoms may indicate a cranial nerve problem. Doctors also ask about symptoms of other nervous system problems and symptoms of other disorders.

The most important part of the physical examination is the eye examination. Doctors check the person's vision. They also carefully look for bulging of one or both eyes and a drooping eyelid and check how the pupils respond to light. They check the eyes' movements by asking the person to follow their finger as it moves up and down and far to the right and to the left. Doctors then use a slit lamp (an instrument that enables a doctor to examine the eye under high magnification) and ophthalmoscopy to examine the internal structures of the eyes.

Symptoms and examination findings can provide helpful information about which causes are most likely. For example, if double vision comes and goes and there are other symptoms of possible nervous system dysfunction, myasthenia gravis and multiple sclerosis are among the likely causes. If the eyes do not point in the same direction, the direction of gaze in which double vision occurs sometimes indicates which cranial nerve is dysfunctional.

TESTING

People with double vision in one eye usually are referred to an ophthalmologist (a medical doctor who specializes in the evaluation and treatment—surgical and nonsurgical—of eye disorders). Testing is not needed before the person is referred. The ophthalmologist examines the person's eyes carefully for eye disorders.

In people with double vision affecting both eyes, more testing is often needed because many disorders may cause binocular double vision. Tests depend on what doctors find during the history and physical examination.

Most people require imaging with magnetic resonance imaging (MRI) or computed tomography (CT) to detect abnormalities of the eye socket (orbit), skull, brain or spinal cord. Imaging may need to be done right away if doctors think an infection, an aneurysm, or a stroke is the cause of double vision.

In people with symptoms of Graves disease (such as bulging of the eyes, eye pain, watering, and an enlarged thyroid gland), thyroid tests (serum thyroxine [T_4] and thyroid-stimulating hormone [TSH] levels) are done. Testing for myasthenia gravis and multiple sclerosis may be needed, particularly if double vision comes and goes.

Not all people require testing. Some cases of double vision clear up without treatment. If symptoms and examination findings suggest no serious cause, doctors may recommend that the person's eyes be checked regularly for a few weeks to see whether the vision clears up before they recommend any testing.

TREATMENT

The best way to treat double vision is to treat the underlying disorder.

KEY POINTS

- People with double vision plus sudden or severe pain, injury, or symptoms of nervous system dysfunction should usually go to an emergency department.
- Double vision may go away on its own, but people should still see a doctor.
- The most important part of the examination is the eye examination, but usually imaging is needed.

VISION LOSS, SUDDEN

Loss of vision is considered sudden if it develops within a few minutes to a couple of days. It may affect one or both eyes and all or part of a field of vision. Loss of only a small part of the field of vision (for example, as a result of a small retinal detachment) may seem like blurred vision. Other symptoms, for example eye pain, may occur depending on the cause of vision loss.

CAUSES

Sudden loss of vision has three general causes:

- Clouding of normally transparent eye structures
- Abnormalities of the retina (the light-sensing structure at the back of the eye)
- Abnormalities of the nerves that carry visual signals from the eye to the brain (the optic nerve and the visual pathways)

Light must travel through several transparent structures before it can be sensed by the retina. First, light passes through the cornea (the clear layer in front of the iris and pupil), then the lens, and then the vitreous humor (the jellylike substance that fills the eyeball). Anything that blocks light from passing through these structures, for example, a corneal ulcer or bleeding into the vitreous humor, can cause loss of vision.

Most of the disorders that cause total loss of vision when they affect the entire eye may cause only partial vision loss when they affect only part of the eye.

COMMON CAUSES

The most common causes of sudden loss of vision are

- Blockage of a major artery of the retina (central retinal artery occlusion)
- Blockage of an artery to the optic nerve (ischemic optic neuropathy)
- Blockage of a major vein in the retina (central retinal vein occlusion)
- Blood in the jellylike vitreous humor near the back of the eye (vitreous hemorrhage)
- Eye injury

Sudden retinal artery blockage can result from a blood clot or small piece of atherosclerotic material that breaks off and travels into the artery. The artery to the optic nerve can be blocked in the same ways and can also be blocked by inflammation (such as may occur with giant cell [temporal] arteritis). A blood clot can form in the retinal vein and block it, particularly in older people with high blood pressure or diabetes. People with diabetes are also at risk of bleeding into the vitreous humor.

Sometimes what seems like a sudden start of symptoms may instead be sudden recognition. For example, a person with long-standing reduced vision in one eye (possibly caused by a dense cataract) may suddenly become aware of the reduced vision in the affected eye after covering the unaffected eye.

LESS COMMON CAUSES

Less common causes of sudden loss of vision (see Table on pages 456 to 457) include stroke or transient ischemic attack (TIA), acute glaucoma, retinal detachment, inflammation of the structures in the front of the eye between the cornea and the lens (anterior uveitis, sometimes called iritis), certain infections of the retina, and bleeding within the retina as a complication of age-related macular degeneration.

EVALUATION

Sudden loss of vision is an emergency. Most causes are serious.

WHEN TO SEE A DOCTOR

All people who experience a sudden loss of vision should see an ophthalmologist (a medical doctor who specialize in the evaluation and treatment—surgical and nonsurgical—of eye disorders) or go to the emergency department right away.

WHAT THE DOCTOR DOES

Doctors first ask questions about the person's symptoms and medical history. Doctors then do a physical examination. What they find during the history and physical examination often suggests a cause and the tests that may need to be done (see Table on pages 456 to 457).

WHEN THE VISUAL PATHWAYS ARE DAMAGED

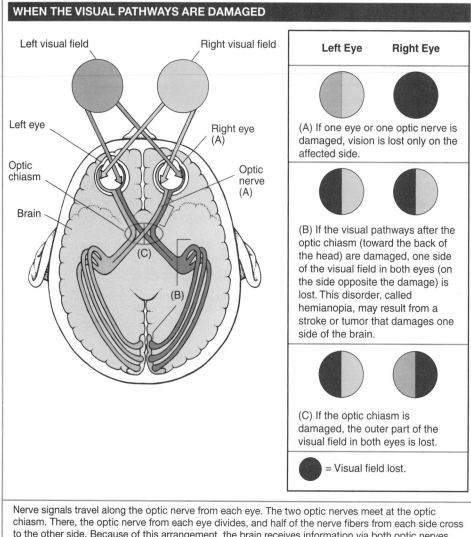

Nerve signals travel along the optic nerve from each eye. The two optic nerves meet at the optic chiasm. There, the optic nerve from each eye divides, and half of the nerve fibers from each side cross to the other side. Because of this arrangement, the brain receives information via both optic nerves for the left visual field and for the right visual field. Damage to an eye or the visual pathway causes different types of vision loss depending on where the damage occurs.

Doctors ask the person to describe when loss of vision occurred, how long it has been present, and whether if has progressed. People are asked whether loss affects one or both eyes and whether loss is total or affects only a specific part of the field of vision. Doctors also ask about other vision symptoms such as floaters, flashing lights, halos around lights, distorted color vision, jagged or mosaic patterns, or eye pain. Doctors ask about symptoms that are not related to the eyes and risk factors for disorders that may cause eye problems.

The physical examination concentrates primarily on the eyes, but doctors may also do a general physical examination, including, for example, examination of the skin and the nervous system.

For the eye examination, doctors first carefully check sharpness of vision (visual acuity), usually by having the person read letters on a chart, first while one eye is covered and then with both uncovered. Doctors check how the pupils narrow (constrict) in response to light and how well the eyes can follow a moving

HOW AND WHY BLINDNESS DEVELOPS

Anything that blocks the passage of light from the environment to the back of the eye or disrupts the transmission of nerve impulses from the back of the eye to the brain will interfere with vision. Legal blindness is defined as a visual acuity of 20/200 or worse in the better eye, even after correction with eyeglasses or contact lenses, or a visual field restricted to less than 20° in the better eye. Many people who are considered legally blind can distinguish shapes and shadows but not normal detail.

Blindness can occur under the following circumstances:

Light cannot reach the retina.

- Damage to the cornea caused by infections such as herpes keratoconjunctivitis or an infection that follows contact lens overwearing, which results in an opaque corneal scar
- Damage to the cornea caused by vitamin A deficiency (keratomalacia), which causes dry eyes and results in an opaque corneal scar (rare in developed nations)
- Damage to the cornea caused by a severe injury that results in an opaque corneal scar
- A cataract, which causes loss of clarity of the lens

Light rays do not focus on the retina clearly.

- Imperfect focusing of light rays on the retina (refraction errors) that cannot be fully corrected with eyeglasses or contact lenses (such as from certain types of cataracts)

The retina cannot sense light rays normally.

- Detached retina
- Diabetes mellitus
- Macular degeneration
- Retinitis pigmentosa
- Inadequate blood supply to the retina, usually due to a blockage of the retinal artery or vein, which may be caused by inflammation of the blood vessel wall (such as that caused by giant cell arteritis), or due to a blood clot that travels to the eye from somewhere else (such as from the carotid artery in the neck)
- Infection of the retina (such as from *Toxoplasma*, parasites, or fungi) in people who have AIDS

Nerve impulses from the retina are not transmitted to the brain normally.

- Disorders affecting the optic nerve or its pathways inside the brain, such as brain tumors, strokes, infections, and multiple sclerosis
- Glaucoma
- Inflammation of the optic nerve (optic neuritis)

The brain cannot interpret information sent by the eye.

- Disorders that affect the areas of the brain that interpret visual impulses (visual cortex), such as strokes and tumors

---

object. Color vision may be tested. Doctors examine the eyes and eyelids using a slit lamp (an instrument that enables a doctor to examine the eye under high magnification) and measure pressure in the eye. Ophthalmologists, after instilling drops that dilate the pupils, examine the retina thoroughly with a slit lamp or light that is shone from a head lamp through a hand-held instrument.

TESTING

The presence or absence of pain helps narrow the list of possible causes considerably. If vision returns quickly on its own, transient ischemic attack and ocular migraine are among the likely causes.

Often findings during the eye examination provide enough information for doctors to diagnose the cause of loss of vision. Sometimes, however, testing is needed depending on what disorders are suspected (see Table on pages 456 to 457). The following tests are of particular importance:

- Ultrasonography is done to view the retina if the retina is not clearly visible during an ophthalmoscopic examination.

SOME CAUSES AND FEATURES OF SUDDEN LOSS OF VISION

Cause	Common Features*	Tests
Sudden loss of vision without eye pain		
Blockage of the central retinal artery (the artery that carries blood to the retina)	Almost instantaneous, complete loss of vision in one eye In people with risk factors for atherosclerosis (such as high blood pressure, abnormal blood lipids, or cigarette smoking)	A doctor's examination
Blockage of the central retinal vein (the vein that carries blood away from the retina)	In people with risk factors for this disorder (such as diabetes, high blood pressure, a tendency for blood to clot excessively, or sickle cell disease)	A doctor's examination
Vitreous hemorrhage (bleeding into the vitreous humor—the jellylike substance that fills the back of the eyeball)	In people who have had specks, strings, or cobwebs in their field of vision (floaters) or who have risk factors for vitreous hemorrhage (such as diabetes, a tear in the retina, sickle cell disease, or an eye injury) Usually loss of the entire field of vision (not in just one or more spots)	Examination by an ophthalmologist Sometimes ultrasonography of the retina
Giant cell (temporal) arteritis (inflammation of the large arteries of the head, neck, and upper body), which can block blood flow to the optic nerve	Sometimes headache, pain while combing the hair, or pain in the jaw or tongue when chewing Sometimes aches and stiffness in the large muscles of the arms or legs (polymyalgia rheumatica)	Erythrocyte sedimentation rate (a blood test) Biopsy of the temporal artery
Ischemic optic neuropathy (damage of the optic nerve caused by blockage of its blood supply)	In people with risk factors for this disorder (such as diabetes or high blood pressure) or in people who have had an episode of very low blood pressure, which sometimes causes fainting	A doctor's examination
Macular hemorrhage (bleeding around the macula—the most sensitive part of the retina) resulting from age-related macular degeneration	Usually in people known to have age-related macular degeneration or in people with risk factors for blood vessel disorders (such as high blood pressure, cigarette smoking, or abnormal blood lipids)	A doctor's examination
Ocular migraine (migraines that affect vision)	Shimmering, irregular spots that drift slowly across the field of vision of one eye for about 10 to 20 minutes Sometimes blurring of central vision (what a person is looking at directly) Sometimes a headache after the disturbances in vision Often in young people or in people known to have migraines	A doctor's examination
Migraine aura	A blind spot, sometimes with a shimmering spot that drifts across the field of vision, and that lasts usually 10 to 60 minutes Usually a headache after the disturbances in vision Usually in people known to have migraines	A doctor's examination

(continued)

SOME CAUSES AND FEATURES OF SUDDEN LOSS OF VISION *(continued)*

Cause	Common Features*	Tests
Detachment of the retina	Sudden, spontaneous flashes of light that can look like lightning, spots, or stars (photopsias) that occur repeatedly	A doctor's examination
	Loss of vision that affects one area, usually what is seen out of the corners of the eye (peripheral vision)	
	Loss of vision that spreads across the field of vision like a curtain	
	Sometimes in people with risk factors for detachment of the retina (such as a recent eye injury, recent eye surgery, or severe nearsightedness)	
Strokes or transient ischemic attack	Usually loss of the same parts of the field of vision in both eyes	MRI or CT
	In people with risk factors for these disorders (such as high blood pressure, atherosclerosis, diabetes, abnormal blood lipids, and cigarette smoking)	
	Sometimes slurred speech, impaired eye movements, muscle weakness, and/or difficulty walking	
Sudden loss of vision with eye pain		
Closed-angle glaucoma	Severe eye ache and redness	Measurement of pressure inside the eye (tonometry)
	Headache, nausea, vomiting, and sensitivity to light	
	Disturbances in vision such as seeing halos around lights	Examination of eye's drainage channels with a special lens (gonioscopy), done by an ophthalmologist
Corneal ulcer	Often a grayish patch on the cornea that later becomes an open, painful sore	A doctor's examination
	Eye ache or a foreign object (body) sensation	Culture of a sample taken from the ulcer, done by an ophthalmologist
	Eye redness and watering	
	Sensitivity to light	
	Sometimes in people who have had an eye injury or who have slept with their contact lenses in	
Optic neuritis (inflammation of the optic nerve), which can be related to multiple sclerosis	Usually mild pain that may worsen when the eyes are moved	Often MRI
	Partial or complete loss of vision	
	Eyelids and corneas that appear normal	

*Features include symptoms and the results of the doctor's examination. Features mentioned are typical but not always present.
CT = computed tomography; ECG = electrocardiography; MRI = magnetic resonance imaging.

- Gadolinium-enhanced MRI is done for some people with eye pain and certain other symptoms and when optic nerve swelling is seen during the eye examination.
- Erythrocyte sedimentation rate (ESR—a blood test that indirectly measures inflammation in the body) is done, particularly in people over age 50 or who have headache, and C-reactive protein is often measured as well.

TREATMENT

The disorder causing the loss of vision is treated as rapidly as possible, although treatment may not be able to save or restore vision. However, prompt treatment may decrease the risk of the same process occurring in the other eye.

O—π KEY POINTS

- Sudden loss of vision is an emergency, so people should go directly to a hospital.
- The presence or absence of pain helps indicate which causes are most likely.
- If vision returns quickly on its own, transient ischemic attack and ocular migraine are among the likely causes.

WEAKNESS

Weakness refers to loss of muscle strength. That is, people cannot move a muscle normally despite trying as hard as they can. However, the term is often misused. Many people with normal muscle strength say feel weak when they feel tired (see Fatigue on page 143) or when their movement is limited because of pain or joint stiffness.

For a person to intentionally move a muscle (called a voluntary muscle contraction), the brain must generate a signal that travels a pathway from

- The brain
- Through nerve cells in the brain stem and spinal cord
- Through nerves from the spinal cord to the muscles (called peripheral nerves)
- Across the connection between nerve and muscle (called a neuromuscular junction)

Also, the amount of muscle tissue must be normal, and the tissue must be able to contract in response to the signal from the nerves. Therefore, true weakness results only when one part of this pathway—brain, spinal cord, nerves, muscles, or the connections between them—is damaged or diseased.

Weakness may develop suddenly or gradually. Weakness may affect all of the muscles in the body (called generalized weakness) or only one part of the body. For example, depending on where the spinal cord is damaged, spinal cord disorders may cause weakness only of the legs.

Symptoms depend on which muscles are affected. For example, when weakness affects muscles of the chest, people may have difficulty breathing. When weakness affects muscles that control the eyes, people may have double vision. Complete muscle weakness causes paralysis. People may have other symptoms depending on what is causing the weakness. Weakness is often accompanied by abnormalities in sensation, such as tingling, a pins-and-needles sensation, and numbness.

CAUSES

Because malfunction in the same part of the signal pathway causes similar symptoms regardless of cause, the many causes of muscle weakness are usually grouped by the location of the cause (see Table on pages 461 to 465). That is, causes are grouped as those that affect the brain, spinal cord, peripheral nerves, muscles, or connections between nerves and muscles. However, some disorders affect more than one location.

COMMON CAUSES

Causes differ depending on whether weakness is generalized or affects only specific muscles.

The most common causes of generalized weakness are

- A decrease in general physical fitness (called deconditioning), which may result from illness and/or a decrease in physical reserves (frailty), such as muscle mass, bone density, and the heart's and lungs' ability to function, especially in older people
- Loss of muscle tissue (wasting, or atrophy) due to long periods of inactivity or bed rest, as occurs in an ICU
- Damage to nerves due to a severe illness or injury, such as severe or extensive burns
- Certain muscle disorders, such as those due to a low level of potassium (hypokalemia), consumption of too much alcohol, or use of corticosteroids
- Drugs used to paralyze muscles—for example, to keep people from moving during surgery or while on a ventilator

The most common causes of weakness in specific muscles are

- Strokes (the most common cause of weakness affecting one side of the body)
- A pinched nerve, as occurs in carpal tunnel syndrome
- A ruptured or herniated disk in the spine
- Pressure on (compression of) the spinal cord, as can result from cancer that has spread to the spinal cord
- Multiple sclerosis

LESS COMMON CAUSES

Many other conditions sometimes cause weakness (see Table on pages 461 to 465). For example, electrolyte abnormalities (such as a low level of magnesium or calcium) can cause weakness that sometimes comes and goes, as well as muscle cramping and twitches.

FATIGUE

Many people report weakness when their problem is actually fatigue (see page 143). Common causes of fatigue include a severe illness, cancer, a chronic infection (such as HIV infection, hepatitis, or mononucleosis), heart failure, anemia, chronic fatigue syndrome, fibromyalgia, and mood disorders (such as depression).

EVALUATION

First, doctors try to determine whether people are weak or simply tired. If people are weak, doctors then determine whether the weakness is severe enough or worsening quickly enough to be life threatening.

WARNING SIGNS

In people with weakness, the following symptoms are cause for concern:

- Weakness that develops over a few days or less
- Difficulty breathing
- Difficulty raising the head while lying down
- Difficulty chewing, talking, or swallowing
- Loss of the ability to walk

WHEN TO SEE A DOCTOR

People who have any warning sign should go to an emergency department immediately. Immediate medical attention is crucial because weakness accompanied by a warning sign can worsen quickly and cause permanent disability or be fatal. People without warning signs should call their doctor. The doctor can decide how quickly they need to be seen based on their symptoms and other disorders they have. For most of these people, a delay of a few days is not harmful.

If the weakness worsens gradually (over months to years), people should discuss the problem with their doctor at their next routine visit.

WHAT THE DOCTOR DOES

Doctors first ask questions about the person's symptoms and medical history. Doctors then do a physical examination. What they find during the history and physical examination often suggests a cause and the tests that may need to be done (see Table on pages 461 to 465).

Doctors ask people to describe in detail what they are experiencing as weakness. Doctors ask

- When the weakness began
- Whether it began suddenly or gradually
- Whether it is constant or is worsening
- Which muscles are affected
- Whether and how the weakness affects the ability to do certain activities, such as breathing, brushing their teeth or hair, speaking, swallowing, standing up from a seated position, climbing stairs, and walking
- Whether they have other symptoms that indicate malfunction of the nervous system, such as speech or vision problems, loss of sensation or memory, or seizures

What seems to be sudden weakness is sometimes gradual weakness, but people do not notice it until they can no longer do something, such as walking or tying their shoes.

Based on the description of weakness, doctors can often identify the most likely causes, as for the following:

- A muscle disorder: Weakness beginning in the hips and thighs or the shoulders (that is, people have difficulty standing up or lifting their arms overhead) and no effect on sensation
- A peripheral nerve disorder: Weakness beginning in the hands and feet (that is, people have difficulty lifting a cup, writing, or stepping over a curb) and loss of sensation

Doctors also ask about other symptoms, which may suggest one or more possible causes. For example, if people with back pain and a history of cancer report weakness in a leg, the cause may be cancer that has spread and put pressure on the spinal cord.

People are asked about symptoms that suggest fatigue or another problem, rather than true muscle weakness. People with true muscle weakness often report difficulty doing specific tasks, and the weakness follows a pattern (for example, becomes worse after walking). Fatigue tends to cause more general symptoms and does not follow a particular pattern. That is, it is present all the time and affects the whole body. Doctors ask about recent or current disorders that commonly cause fatigue, such as any recent severe illness or a mood disorder (such as depression).

Doctors ask about past and current use of drugs, including alcohol and recreational drugs. Whether family members have had similar symptoms can help doctors determine whether the cause is hereditary.

During the physical examination, doctors focus on the nervous system (neurologic examination) and muscles. Doctors test the cranial nerves (which connect the brain with the eyes, ears, face, and various other parts of the body), for example, by checking eye movements, the ability to speak clearly, and the ability to rotate the head.

Doctors observe how the person walks and check for other signs that the nervous system is malfunctioning, such as loss of coordination or sensation. Muscles are checked for size and unusual unintended movements (such as involuntary twitches and shaking). Doctors note how smoothly muscles move and whether there is involuntary resistance to movement (detected when doctors try to move a muscle that they have asked the person to relax).

Reflexes are checked. Reflexes are automatic responses to a stimulus. For example, doctors test the knee jerk reflex by gently tapping the muscle tendon below the kneecap with a rubber hammer. Normally, the knee then jerks involuntarily. This evaluation helps doctors identify which part of the nervous system is probably affected, as for the following:

- The brain or spinal cord: If reflexes are very easy to trigger and are strong
- The nerves: If reflexes are hard to trigger and are slow or absent

Muscle strength is tested by asking the person to push or pull against resistance or to do maneuvers that require strength, such as walking on the heels and tiptoes or standing up.

A general physical examination is done to look for other symptoms that may suggest a cause, such as difficulty breathing.

SOME CAUSES AND FEATURES OF MUSCLE WEAKNESS

Cause	Common Features*	Tests
Brain disorders		
Brain tumors	Headaches, personality changes, confusion, difficulty concentrating, drowsiness, loss of balance and coordination, and paralysis or numbness Sometimes seizures	MRI or CT of the brain
Multiple sclerosis (affects the brain, spinal cord or both)	Usually other symptoms of nervous system malfunction (such as loss of sensation, loss of coordination, and vision problems) Weakness that - Tends to come and go - Sometimes affects different parts of the body - Is worse in hot weather	MRI of the brain Sometimes a spinal tap (lumbar puncture)
Stroke	Symptoms that occur suddenly: - Weakness or paralysis, usually on one side of the body - Abnormalities in or loss of sensation on one side of the body - Difficulty speaking, sometimes with slurred speech - Confusion - Dimness, blurring, or loss of vision, particularly in one eye - Dizziness or loss of balance and coordination	A doctor's examination CT or MRI of the brain

(continued)

SOME CAUSES AND FEATURES OF MUSCLE WEAKNESS *(continued)*

Cause	Common Features*	Tests
Spinal cord disorders†		
Acute transverse myelitis (sudden spinal cord inflammation), often due to ■ Multiple sclerosis ■ Inflammation of blood vessels ■ Certain infections such as Lyme disease or syphilis	Tingling, numbness, and muscle weakness that ■ Occur rapidly (over hours to a few days) ■ Start in the feet and move upward Usually a bandlike tightness around the chest or abdomen Often difficulty passing urine When an injury is severe, loss of bowel and bladder control and/or reduced sexual response, including erectile dysfunction in men	MRI of the spinal cord A spinal tap
Compression of the spinal cord that develops suddenly (acute), as may result from ■ Abscesses (pockets of pus) ■ Hematomas (pockets of blood) ■ Injuries of the neck or back ■ Some cancers	For acute, symptoms that develop in hours or days For chronic, symptoms that are present for weeks to months Weakness or paralysis of the legs and sometimes arms and loss of sensation With abscesses, infections, or tumors, tenderness to the touch over the compressed area	MRI of the spinal cord
Compression that develops slowly (chronic), as may result from ■ Cervical spondylosis (degeneration of the vertebral disks due to arthritis) ■ Spinal stenosis (narrowing of the passageway for the spine) due to arthritis ■ Some tumors	When an injury is severe, loss of bowel and bladder control and/or reduced sexual response, including erectile dysfunction in men	MRI of the spinal cord
Compression of a spinal nerve root by a ruptured disk	Weakness, numbness, or both in one leg or arm Usually back or neck pain that shoots down the leg or arm	Usually MRI or CT of the spinal cord Usually electromyography (stimulating muscles and recording their electrical activity) Sometimes nerve conduction studies (measuring how fast nerves transmit signals)
Cauda equina syndrome, caused by pressure on several spinal nerve roots, as may result from ■ A ruptured or herniated disk ■ Spread of cancer to the spine	Weakness in both legs Loss of feeling in the upper inner part of the thighs, the buttocks, bladder, genitals, and the area between them (saddle area) Usually pain in the lower back Loss of bowel and bladder control and/or reduced sexual response, including erectile dysfunction in men	MRI of the spinal cord

(continued)

SOME CAUSES AND FEATURES OF MUSCLE WEAKNESS *(continued)*

Cause	Common Features*	Tests
Multiple sclerosis (affects the brain, spinal cord, or both)	Usually other symptoms of nervous system malfunction (such as loss of sensation, loss of coordination, and vision problems) Weakness that ■ Tends to come and go ■ Sometimes affects different parts of the body ■ Is worse in hot weather	MRI of the brain and spinal cord Sometimes a spinal tap

Disorders that affect the peripheral nerves and the brain or spinal cord‡

Cause	Common Features*	Tests
Amyotrophic lateral sclerosis (ALS)	Progressive muscle weakness that ■ Often starts in the hands ■ Sometimes affects one side more than the other Clumsiness, involuntary muscle contractions, and muscle cramps Drooling and difficulty speaking and swallowing As the disorder progresses, difficulty breathing and eventually death	Electromyography and sometimes nerve conduction studies Often MRI of the spinal cord to rule out spinal cord disorders that can cause similar symptoms
Postpolio syndrome	Muscles that tire easily and progressive muscle weakness Sometimes muscle twitching and loss of muscle tissue In people who have had polio	Electromyography and sometimes nerve conduction studies

Disorders that simultaneously affect many nerves (polyneuropathies)

Cause	Common Features*	Tests
Guillain-Barré syndrome	Weakness and often loss of sensation that ■ Usually begin in both legs ■ Then progress upward to the arms When severe, difficulty swallowing and breathing	Electromyography and nerve conduction studies A spinal tap
Nerve damage caused by ■ Excessive use of alcohol ■ Diabetes ■ Drugs (such as vincristine, cisplatin, or statins) ■ Infections (such as diphtheria, hepatitis C, HIV infection, Lyme disease, or syphilis) ■ Sarcoidosis ■ Severe illness (especially in the intensive care unit) ■ Toxic substances (such as lead or mercury) ■ Vitamin deficiency (such as thiamin, vitamin B₆, or vitamin B₁₂ deficiency)	Muscle weakness that ■ Often begins in both feet ■ Then affects the hands ■ Then progresses up the legs and arms Loss of sensation, typically before muscles become weak	Electromyography and nerve conduction studies Other tests depending on the disorder suspected, such as ■ Urine tests to check for toxins ■ Blood tests to check for certain antibodies or to measure sugar, vitamin, or drug levels ■ Sometimes a spinal tap

(continued)

SOME CAUSES AND FEATURES OF MUSCLE WEAKNESS *(continued)*

Cause	Common Features*	Tests
Disorders that affect the connections between nerves and muscles (neuromuscular junction disorders)		
Botulism (due to the bacteria *Clostridium botulinum*)	At first, often a dry mouth, drooping eyelids, vision problems (such as double vision), difficulty swallowing and speaking, and rapidly progressive muscle weakness, often beginning in the face and moving down the body When contaminated food is the source, nausea, vomiting, stomach cramps, and diarrhea No changes in sensation	Blood or stool tests to check for toxins produced by the bacteria Sometimes electromyography or examination of a stool sample to check for bacteria
Myasthenia gravis	Weak and drooping eyelids, double vision, difficulty speaking and swallowing, and weakness in the arms and legs Excessive weakness of affected muscles that ■ Occurs after muscles are used ■ Disappears when they are rested ■ Recurs when they are used again	Use of a drug (edrophonium test) to see whether it improves muscle strength after muscles are used Blood tests to check for certain antibodies and/or electromyography
Organophosphate (insecticide) poisoning	Tearing of the eyes, blurred vision, increased salivation, sweating, coughing, vomiting, frequent bowel movements and urination, and weak muscles that twitch	A doctor's examination Sometimes blood tests to identify the toxin
Disorders that affect muscles (myopathies)‡		
Muscle malfunction due to use of alcohol, corticosteroids, or various other drugs	Weakness that tends to first cause difficulty lifting the arms overhead or standing up Use of a drug that can cause muscle damage When due to use of alcohol or certain other drugs, muscle aches and pains	A doctor's examination Stopping any drug that can cause muscle malfunction Sometimes electromyography Blood tests to measure levels of muscle enzymes that leak from damaged muscles into the blood
Viral infections that cause muscle inflammation	Muscle aches and pains that are worsened by movement, especially walking Sometimes fever, a runny nose, cough, sore throat, and/or fatigue	Sometimes only a doctor's examination Muscle biopsy (removal of a piece of muscle tissue for examination under a microscope)
Conditions that cause generalized muscle wasting: ■ Burns ■ Cancer ■ Lack of use due to prolonged bed rest or immobilization in a cast ■ Sepsis (infection of the bloodstream) ■ Starvation	Loss of muscle tissue In people with obvious evidence of the problem	A doctor's examination

(continued)

SOME CAUSES AND FEATURES OF MUSCLE WEAKNESS *(continued)*

Cause	Common Features*	Tests
Electrolyte abnormalities (including a low level of potassium, magnesium, or calcium) due to certain disorders or use of diuretics	Weakness that ■ Affects the whole body ■ May come and go ■ Is often accompanied by muscle cramping and twitches	Blood tests to measure the level of potassium and other electrolytes
Muscular dystrophies (such as Duchenne muscular dystrophy and limb-girdle muscular dystrophy)	Progressive muscle weakness that ■ May start during infancy, childhood, or adulthood ■ Depending on the type, may progress rapidly, causing early death In some types, an abnormally curved spine (scoliosis) and weakness of the spinal muscles, which often develop during childhood	A thorough family history to determine whether any family members have had a similar disorder Genetic testing Muscle biopsy X-rays of the spine to check for scoliosis

*Features include symptoms and results of the doctor's examination. Features mentioned are typical but not always present.
†Symptoms vary depending on the location (level) of the damage. Areas that are supplied by the parts of the spinal cord below the damaged part are affected.
‡Sensation is usually not affected.
CT = computed tomography; MRI = magnetic resonance imaging.

Generally, if the history and physical examination do not detect specific abnormalities that suggest a brain, spinal cord, nerve, or muscle disorder, the cause is likely to be fatigue.

TESTING

If people have severe or rapidly progressing generalized weakness or any problems breathing, doctors first do tests to evaluate the strength of the respiratory muscles (pulmonary function tests). Results of these tests help doctors estimate the risk of sudden, severe malfunction of the lungs (acute respiratory failure).

Other testing is done based on where doctors think the problem is:

■ A brain disorder: Magnetic resonance imaging (MRI) or, if MRI is not possible, computed tomography (CT)
■ A spinal cord disorder: MRI or, when MRI is not possible, CT myelography and sometimes a spinal tap (lumbar puncture)
■ A peripheral nerve disorder (including polyneuropathies) or a neuromuscular junction disorder: Electromyography and usually nerve conduction studies
■ A muscle disorder (myopathy): Electromyography, usually nerve conduction studies,

and possibly MRI, measurement of muscle enzymes, muscle biopsy, and/or genetic testing.

Occasionally, MRI is not available or cannot be done—for example, in people who have a pacemaker, another implanted metal device, or other metal (such as shrapnel) in their body. In such cases, another test is substituted.

For CT myelography, CT is done after a needle is inserted into the lower back to inject a radiopaque dye into the fluid that surrounds the spinal cord. For electromyography, small needles are inserted into a muscle to record its electrical activity when the muscle is at rest and when it is contracting. Nerve conduction studies use electrodes or small needles to stimulate a nerve. Then doctors measure how fast the nerve transmits signals.

If people have no symptoms besides weakness and no abnormalities are detected during the examination, test results are usually normal. However, doctors sometimes do certain blood tests, such as

■ A complete blood cell count (CBC)
■ Measurement of levels of electrolytes (such as potassium, calcium, and magnesium), sugar (glucose), and thyroid-stimulating hormone

- Erythrocyte sedimentation rate (ESR), which can detect inflammation

Blood tests are sometimes done to evaluate kidney and liver function and to check for the hepatitis virus.

TREATMENT

If the cause is identified, it is treated if possible. If weakness began suddenly and causes difficulty breathing, a ventilator may be used.

Physical and occupational therapy can help people adapt to permanent weakness and compensate for loss of function. Physical therapy can help people maintain and sometimes regain strength.

ESSENTIALS FOR OLDER PEOPLE

As people age, the amount of muscle tissue and muscle strength tend to decrease. These changes occur partly because older people may become less active but also because the production of the hormones that stimulate muscle development decreases. Thus, for older people, bed rest during an illness can have a devastating effect. Compared with younger people, older people start out with less muscle tissue and strength at the beginning of the illness and lose muscle tissue more quickly during the illness.

Drugs are another common cause of weakness in older people because older people take more drugs and are more susceptible to side effects of drugs.

When evaluating older people who report weakness, doctors also focus on conditions that do not cause weakness but interfere with balance, coordination, vision, or mobility or that make movement painful (such as impaired vision or arthritis). Older people may mistakenly describe the effects of such conditions as weakness.

O—π KEY POINTS

- Many people mistakenly say they feel weak when they really mean they are tired or their movement is limited because of pain and/or stiffness.
- True muscle weakness results only when one part of the pathway necessary for voluntary muscle movement (from brain to muscles) malfunctions.
- If weakness becomes severe over a few days or less or if people have any warning sign, they should see a doctor immediately.
- Often, doctors can determine whether the problem is true muscle weakness and can identify the cause based on the pattern of symptoms and results of the physical examination.
- Physical therapy is usually helpful in maintaining strength no matter what the cause of weakness is.

WEIGHT LOSS

Involuntary weight loss refers to weight loss that occurs when a person is not dieting or otherwise trying to lose weight. Because everyone's weight goes up and down slightly over time (such as during an illness), doctors typically become concerned only when people lose more than about 10 pounds (4 to 5 kilograms) or, in smaller people, 5% of their body weight. Such weight loss can be a sign of a serious physical or mental disorder. In addition to weight loss, people may have other symptoms, such as loss of appetite, fever, pain, or night sweats, due to the underlying disorder.

CAUSES

Most often, weight loss occurs because people take in fewer calories than their body needs. They may take in fewer calories because their appetite has decreased or because they have a disorder that prevents their digestive tract from absorbing nutrients (called malabsorption). Less often, people have a disorder that causes them to use more calories (for example, an overactive thyroid gland). Sometimes, both mechanisms are involved. For example, cancer tends to decrease appetite but also increases caloric expenditure, leading to rapid weight loss.

Almost any long-term illness of sufficient severity can cause weight loss (for example, severe heart failure or emphysema). However, these disorders have usually been diagnosed by the time weight loss occurs. This discussion focuses on weight loss as the first sign of illness. Causes can be divided into those in people who have increased appetite and those in people who have a decreased appetite.

With increased appetite, the most common unrecognized causes of involuntary weight are

- An overactive thyroid gland (hyperthyroidism)
- Uncontrolled diabetes
- Disorders that cause malabsorption

With decreased appetite, the most common unrecognized causes of involuntary weight are

- Mental disorders (for example, depression)
- Cancer

- Drug adverse effects
- Drug abuse

EVALUATION

The following information can help people decide when a doctor's evaluation is needed and help them know what to expect during the evaluation.

Because many disorders can cause involuntary weight loss, doctors usually need to do a thorough evaluation.

WARNING SIGNS

In people with involuntary weight loss, certain symptoms and characteristics are cause for concern. They include

- Fever and night sweats
- Bone pain
- Shortness of breath, cough, and coughing up blood
- Excessive thirst and increased urination
- Headache, jaw pain when chewing, and/or new vision disturbances (for example, double vision, blurred vision, or blind spots) in a person over 50

WHEN TO SEE A DOCTOR

People who have warning signs should see a doctor right away. People who have no warning signs should see a doctor when possible. Typically a delay of a week or so is not harmful.

WHAT THE DOCTOR DOES

Doctors first ask questions about the person's symptoms and medical history. Doctors then do a physical examination. What they find during the history and physical examination often suggests a cause of the weight loss and the tests that may need to be done (see Table on pages 468 to 469).

Doctors first ask about how much weight the person has lost and over what time period. Doctors may ask about

- Changes in clothing size, appetite, and food intake

- Whether the person has difficulty swallowing
- Whether bowel patterns have changed
- What other symptoms the person has, such as fatigue, malaise, fevers, and night sweats
- Whether the person has a history of a disorder that causes weight loss
- What drugs, including prescription, over-the-counter, and recreational drugs and herbal products, the person is taking
- Whether there are any changes in the person's living situation (for example, loss of a loved one, loss of independence or job, loss of a communal eating routine)

SOME COMMON CAUSES AND FEATURES OF INVOLUNTARY WEIGHT LOSS

Cause	Common Features*	Tests
Adrenal gland underactivity	Abdominal pain, fatigue, abnormal areas of skin darkening, and light-headedness	Blood tests
Alcoholism	History of excessive alcohol consumption In men, feminization, with loss of muscle tissue, decrease in armpit hair, smooth skin, breast growth In men and women, sometimes a distended abdomen due to fluid (ascites) and small purple spots on the skin (spider angiomas)	A doctor's examination Sometimes liver function tests and/or liver biopsy
Anorexia nervosa	Inappropriate fear of weight gain in an emaciated young woman or adolescent female and lack of normal periods	Only a doctor's examination
Cancer	Often night sweats, fatigue, and fever Sometimes bone pain at night or other organ-specific symptoms	Organ-specific evaluation
Depression	Sadness, fatigue, loss of sexual desire and/or pleasure, and sleep disturbance	Only a doctor's examination
Diabetes mellitus, type 1 (newly developed or poorly controlled)	Increased appetite Excessive thirst and increased urination	Measurement of the amount of sugar (glucose) in the blood
Drugs - Drugs of abuse: Amphetamines, cocaine, and opioids - Herbal and OTC products: Aloe, caffeine, cascara, chitosan, chromium, dandelion, ephedra, 5-hydroxytryptophan, garcinia, guarana, guar gum, glucomannan, herbal diuretics, ma huang, pyruvate, St. John's wort, and yerba mate - Prescription: Antiretroviral drugs, cancer chemotherapy drugs, digoxin, exenatide, levodopa, liraglutide, metformin, NSAIDs, SSRIs, topiramate, and zonisamide	History of use	A doctor's examination Sometimes stopping the drug

(continued)

SOME COMMON CAUSES AND FEATURES OF INVOLUNTARY WEIGHT LOSS (continued)

Cause	Common Features*	Tests
Fungal infections (in the lungs or bodywide)	Fever, night sweats, fatigue, cough, and shortness of breath Often a history of living in or visiting an area where a specific fungus is common	Usually cultures and stains Sometimes blood tests Sometimes biopsy
Giant cell (temporal) arteritis	Headache, muscle pains, jaw pain when chewing, fever, and/or visual disturbances in a person over 50	Blood tests Sometimes temporal artery biopsy
Worm infections in the digestive tract	Fever, abdominal pain, bloating, flatulence, and diarrhea Usually residence in or travel to developing countries	Microscopic examination of stool
HIV/AIDS	Fever, shortness of breath, cough, swollen lymph nodes throughout the body, diarrhea, and fungal infections	Blood tests
Kidney disease	Limb swelling, fatigue, itching, and sometimes frothy urine	Blood tests and urine tests
Loss of taste	Usually risk factors (for example, cranial nerve dysfunction, use of certain drugs, and aging)	Only a doctor's examination
Malabsorption	Diarrhea, flatulence, and sometimes greasy or oily stools	Stool testing
Dental problems	Tooth or gum pain Bad breath, gum disease, and missing and/or decayed teeth	Only a doctor's examination
Sarcoidosis	Cough and shortness of breath Fever, fatigue, and swelling of lymph nodes throughout the body	Chest x-ray Sometimes chest CT Biopsy
Heart valve infection (bacterial endocarditis)	Fever, night sweats, joint pain, shortness of breath, and fatigue Often in people with heart valve disorders or who inject drugs intravenously	Blood cultures Echocardiography
Thyroid gland overactivity (hyperthyroidism)	Increased appetite Heat intolerance, sweating, tremor, anxiety, rapid heart beat, and diarrhea	Blood tests to evaluate thyroid function
Tuberculosis	Fever, night sweats, cough, and coughing up blood Sometimes risk factors (for example, exposure to people with tuberculosis or residence in poor living conditions)	Sputum culture and smear

*Features include symptoms and the results of the doctor's examination. Features mentioned are typical but not always present.

CT = computed tomography; HIV = human immunodeficiency virus; NSAIDs = nonsteroidal anti-inflammatory drugs, OTC = over-the-counter; SSRIs = selective serotonin reuptake inhibitors.

During the physical examination, doctors check vital signs for fever, a rapid heart beat, rapid breathing, and low blood pressure. The general physical examination is very thorough because many disorders can cause involuntary weight loss. Doctors examine the heart, lungs, abdomen, head and neck, breasts, nervous system, rectum (including a prostate examination for men and testing for blood in the stool), genitals, liver, spleen, lymph nodes, joints, and skin. Doctors also assess the person's mood.

Weight is measured, and body mass index is calculated.

TESTING

People's symptoms and doctors' findings on physical examination suggest the cause of weight loss in about half of people, including many people eventually diagnosed with cancer.

Screening for common cancers (for example, colonoscopy for colon cancer or mammography for breast cancer) is often done. Other testing is done depending on what disorders the doctor suspects. When the history and physical examination do not suggest specific causes, some doctors do a series of tests, including a chest x-ray, blood tests, and urinalysis, to narrow down a cause. These tests are followed by more specific tests as needed.

If all test results are normal, doctors usually reevaluate the person within a few months to see if new symptoms or findings have developed.

TREATMENT

The underlying disorder is treated. To help people eat more, doctors often try behavioral measures, such as encouraging people to eat, assisting them with eating, providing favorite or strongly flavored foods, and offering only small portions. If behavioral measures are ineffective, high-nutrition food supplements can be tried. Feedings through a tube inserted into the stomach are a last resort and are worthwhile only in certain specific situations. For example, tube feedings can be worthwhile if a person has a disorder that will eventually be cured or resolve, whereas tube feedings may not be worthwhile if a person stops eating because of severe Alzheimer disease.

ESSENTIALS FOR OLDER PEOPLE

Incidence of involuntary weight loss increases with aging, often reaching 50% among nursing home residents. Older people are more likely to have involuntary weight loss because disorders that cause weight loss are more common among older people. There are also normal age-related changes that contribute to weight loss. Typically, many factors are involved.

Normal age-related changes that can contribute to weight loss include the following:

- Decreased sensitivity to certain appetite-stimulating mediators and increased sensitivity to certain inhibitory mediators
- A decreased rate of gastric-emptying (prolonging the feeling of fullness)
- Decreased sensitivities of taste and smell
- Loss of muscle mass (sarcopenia)

In addition, social isolation is common in older people, which tends to decrease food intake. Depression and dementia are very common contributing factors, particularly among nursing home residents. It is often difficult to sort out the exact contribution of specific factors.

Older people may benefit from nutritional supplements. However, supplements should be given between meals and at bedtime. Otherwise, supplements might decrease the appetite at mealtime. Feeding and shopping assistance may also help some people.

O━┬ KEY POINTS

- Involuntary weight loss exceeding 10 pounds or 5% of body weight over a period of a few months is cause for concern.
- Tests are done based on the person's symptoms and findings on physical examination.
- Extensive testing is not usually needed to identify the cause of weight loss.

WHEEZING

Wheezing is a whistling sound that occurs during breathing when the airways are partially blocked.

CAUSES

Wheezing results from a narrowing or blockage (obstruction) somewhere in the airways. The narrowing may be widespread (as occurs in asthma, chronic obstructive pulmonary disease [COPD], and some severe allergic reactions) or only in one area (as may result from a tumor or a foreign object lodged in an airway).

COMMON CAUSES

Overall, the most common causes are

- Asthma
- COPD

LESS COMMON CAUSES

Wheezing may occur in other disorders that affect the small airways, including heart failure, a severe allergic reaction (anaphylaxis), and inhalation of a toxic substance. Wheezing caused by heart failure is called cardiac asthma.

Sometimes, otherwise healthy people wheeze during a bout of acute bronchitis. In children, wheezing may be caused by bronchiolitis (infection of the lower respiratory tract) or inhalation (aspiration) of a foreign object (see Table on pages 472 to 473).

EVALUATION

A person with severe breathing problems (respiratory distress) is evaluated and treated at the same time.

The following information can help people decide when a doctor's evaluation is needed and help them know what to expect during the evaluation.

WARNING SIGNS

In people with wheezing, the following symptoms are of particular concern:

- Labored breathing, weakening efforts to breathe, or a decreased level of consciousness
- Swelling of the face and tongue

WHEN TO SEE A DOCTOR

People with warning signs or shortness of breath should go to the hospital emergency department immediately, by ambulance if necessary. People who have wheezing that comes and goes and are not short of breath can usually wait a day or two.

WHAT THE DOCTOR DOES

Doctors first ask questions about the person's symptoms and medical history and then do a physical examination. What doctors find during the history and physical examination often suggests a cause and the tests that may need to be done (see Table).

Doctors determine whether the wheezing is occurring for the first time or has occurred before. If the person has had wheezing before, they determine whether current symptoms are different in nature or severity.

Important clues to a diagnosis are

- Whether the wheezing started suddenly or gradually
- Whether it comes and goes
- Whether any conditions (such as an upper respiratory infection, exposure to an allergen, particular seasons of the year, cold air, exercise, or feeding in infants) trigger it or make it worse

Other symptoms that can provide clues to the diagnosis include shortness of breath, fever, cough, and sputum production. Doctors ask about the person's history of smoking and exposure to secondhand smoke.

During the physical examination, doctors check the person's temperature and heart and breathing rates. Doctors look for signs of respiratory distress and examine the lungs, particularly how well air moves in and out and whether wheezing seems to affect all of the lungs or only part. A doctor is usually able to detect wheezing by listening with a stethoscope as the person breathes. Loud wheezing can be heard easily, sometimes even without a stethoscope. To hear mild wheezing, doctors may need to listen with a stethoscope while the person exhales

SOME CAUSES AND FEATURES OF WHEEZING

Cause	Common Features*	Tests†
Acute bronchitis	Cough	A doctor's examination
	Sometimes symptoms of an upper respiratory infection (such as a stuffy nose)	
	Usually no known history of a lung disorder	
Allergic reactions	Wheezing that starts suddenly, usually within 30 minutes of exposure to a known or potential allergen such as pollen	A doctor's examination
	Often a stuffy nose, hives, itchy eyes, and sneezing	
Asthma	Usually a history of asthma	A doctor's examination
	Wheezing that starts spontaneously or after exposure to specific stimuli (such as pollen or another allergen, an upper respiratory infection, cold, or exercise)	Sometimes one or more of the following tests: ■ Tests to evaluate how well the lungs are functioning (pulmonary function tests) ■ Measurement of peak air flow (how fast air can be exhaled) ■ Measurement of lung function before and after exercise or administration of methacholine (a drug that narrows airways) ■ Sometimes use of bronchodilators (drugs that widen airways) to see whether symptoms go away
Bronchiolitis (infection of the lower respiratory tract)	In children under 18 months old	A doctor's examination
	Usually occurring from November to April in the Northern Hemisphere	
	Usually symptoms of an upper respiratory infection (such as a stuffy nose and fever) and rapid breathing	
A chronic obstructive pulmonary disease (COPD) flare-up	In middle-aged or older people	A chest x-ray
	In people who already have COPD	Pulmonary function tests
	Usually a history of extensive smoking	
	Labored breathing	
Drugs (such as ACE inhibitors, beta-blockers, aspirin, and other NSAIDs)	In people who have recently started using a new drug, most often in those with a history of airway obstruction (as occurs in asthma)	A doctor's examination
Lung tumors	Wheezing while inhaling and exhaling, especially in people with risk factors for or signs of cancer (such as a history of smoking, night sweats, weight loss, and coughing up blood)	A chest x-ray or CT of the chest Bronchoscopy

(continued)

SOME CAUSES AND FEATURES OF WHEEZING *(continued)*

Cause	Common Features*	Tests†
A foreign object that has been inhaled	High-pitched wheezing or cough that starts suddenly in people (typically infants or young children) without any symptoms of an upper respiratory infection, fever, or other symptoms of illness	A chest x-ray or CT of the chest Bronchoscopy
GERD with repeated reflux of stomach contents into the lungs (chronic aspiration)	Chronic or recurring wheezing Often burning pain in the chest (heartburn) or abdomen that tends to worsen after eating certain foods, while exercising, or while lying flat A sour taste, particularly after awakening Hoarseness A cough that occurs in the middle of the night or early morning No symptoms of an upper respiratory infection or allergy	Sometimes only a doctor's examination Sometimes use of drugs that suppress acid, such as a histamine-2 (H_2) blocker or proton pump inhibitor, to see whether symptoms go away Sometimes insertion of a flexible viewing tube into the esophagus and stomach (endoscopy) Sometimes placement of a sensor in the esophagus to monitor acidity (pH) for 24 hours
Heart failure	Usually swelling (edema) of the legs Shortness of breath that worsens while lying flat or that appears 1–2 hours after falling asleep Sounds suggesting fluid in the lungs, heard through a stethoscope	A chest x-ray Sometimes a blood test to measure a substance that is produced when the heart is strained called brain natriuretic peptide (BNP) Sometimes echocardiography
Irritants that are inhaled	Wheezing that starts suddenly after exposure to irritants at work (occupational exposure) or inappropriate use of cleaning products	A doctor's examination

*Features include symptoms and results of the doctor's examination. Features mentioned are typical but not always present.
†Doctors usually measure the oxygen level in blood with a sensor placed on a finger (pulse oximetry). A chest x-ray is usually taken unless the person's symptoms are clearly a flare-up of an already diagnosed chronic disorder.
ACE = angiotensin-converting enzyme; COPD = chronic obstructive pulmonary disease; CT = computed tomography; GERD = gastroesophageal reflux disease; NSAIDs = nonsteroidal anti-inflammatory drugs.

forcefully. A persistent wheeze that occurs in one location in smokers may be due to lung cancer. Doctors also examine the heart, nose and throat, limbs, hands, feet, and skin.

TESTING

Tests are done to assess severity, determine diagnosis, and identify complications. They usually include the following:

- Measurement of oxygen levels in the blood with a sensor placed on a finger (pulse oximetry)

- A chest x-ray (if the diagnosis is unclear)
- Sometimes measurement of gases (oxygen and carbon dioxide) and acidity (pH) in an artery (arterial blood gas analysis)
- Sometimes tests to evaluate how well the lungs are functioning (pulmonary function testing)

If wheezing has occurred for the first time, a chest x-ray may help in the diagnosis. In people with persistent, repeated, or undiagnosed episodes of wheezing, pulmonary function tests may be needed to help measure the extent of airway narrowing and to assess the benefits of treatment. If asthma seems possible but is not confirmed by pulmonary function tests, people may be asked to exercise or be given a drug that triggers wheezing in people with asthma. If airway obstruction occurs, asthma can be confirmed.

If doctors suspect a tumor or a foreign object lodged in an airway, they can insert a flexible viewing tube (bronchoscope) into the airway to identify the problem and, if it is an object, remove it.

TREATMENT

The main goal of treatment is to treat the underlying disorder.

Bronchodilators (which widen the airways), such as inhaled albuterol, can relieve wheezing. Corticosteroids, taken by mouth for a week or two, can often help relieve an acute episode of wheezing if it is due to asthma or chronic obstructive pulmonary disease. Long-term control of persistent wheezing due to asthma may require inhaled corticosteroids, mast cell stabilizers, and leukotriene inhibitors.

Histamine-2 (H_2) blockers (such as diphenhydramine) given intravenously, corticosteroids (such as methylprednisolone), albuterol taken through a nebulizer, and epinephrine injected under the skin (subcutaneously) are given to people with a severe allergic reaction.

O━π KEY POINTS

- Asthma is the most common cause, but not all wheezing is caused by asthma.
- Wheezing that starts suddenly in people without a lung disorder may be due to inhalation of a foreign object or a toxic substance, an allergic reaction, or heart failure.
- Pulmonary function tests can identify and measure airway narrowing.
- Inhaled bronchodilators can help relieve wheezing, but the disorder causing wheezing must also be treated.

COMMON MEDICAL TESTS

A large number of tests are widely available. Many tests are specialized for a particular disorder or group of related disorders. Other tests are commonly used for a wide range of disorders.

Tests are done for a variety of reasons, including

- Screening
- Diagnosing a disorder
- Evaluating the severity of a disorder so that treatment can be planned
- Monitoring the response to treatment

Sometimes a test is used for more than one purpose. A blood test may show that a person has too few red blood cells (anemia). The same test may be repeated after treatment to determine whether the number of red blood cells has returned to normal. Sometimes a disorder can be treated at the same time a screening or diagnostic test is done. For example, when colonoscopy (examination of the inside of the large intestine with a flexible viewing tube) detects growths (polyps), they can be removed before colonoscopy is completed.

TYPES OF TESTS

There are different types of medical tests but the lines that separate them often become blurred. For example, endoscopy of the stomach enables the examiner to view the inside of the stomach as well as obtain tissue samples for examination in a laboratory. Tests are usually one of the six following types.

ANALYSIS OF BODY FLUIDS

The most commonly analyzed fluids are

- Blood
- Urine
- Fluid that surrounds the spinal cord and brain (cerebrospinal fluid)
- Fluid within a joint (synovial fluid)

Less often, sweat, saliva, and fluid from the digestive tract (such as gastric juices) are analyzed. Sometimes the fluids analyzed are present only if a disorder is present, as when fluid

collects in the abdomen, causing ascites, or in the space between the two-layered membrane covering the lungs and lining the chest wall (pleura), causing pleural effusion.

IMAGING

These tests provide a picture of the inside of the body—in its entirety or only of certain parts. Ordinary x-rays are the most common imaging tests. Others include ultrasonography, radioisotope (nuclear) scanning, computed tomography (CT), magnetic resonance imaging (MRI), positron emission tomography (PET), and angiography.

ENDOSCOPY

A viewing tube (endoscope) is used to directly observe the inside of body organs or spaces (cavities). Most often, a flexible endoscope is used, but in some cases, a rigid one is more useful. The tip of the endoscope is usually equipped with a light and a camera, so the examiner watches the images on a television monitor rather than looking directly through the endoscope. Tools are often passed through a channel in the endoscope. One type of tool is used to cut and remove tissue samples.

Endoscopy usually consists of passing the viewing tube through an existing body opening, such as the following:

- Nose: To examine the voice box (laryngoscopy) or the lungs (bronchoscopy)
- Mouth: To examine the esophagus (esophagoscopy), stomach (gastroscopy), and small intestine (upper gastrointestinal endoscopy)
- Anus: To examine the large intestine, rectum, and anus (coloscopy)
- Urethra: To examine the bladder (cystoscopy)
- Vagina: To examine the uterus (hysteroscopy)

However, sometimes an opening in the body must be created. A small cut (incision) is made through the skin and the layers of tissue beneath the skin, so that the endoscope can be passed into a body cavity. Such incisions are used to view the inside of the following:

- Joints (arthroscopy)
- Abdominal cavity (laparoscopy)
- Area of the chest between the lungs (mediastinoscopy)
- Lungs and pleura (thoracoscopy)

MEASUREMENT OF BODY FUNCTIONS

Often, body functions are measured by recording and analyzing the activity of various organs. For example, electrical activity of the heart is measured with electrocardiography (ECG), and electrical activity of the brain is measured with electroencephalography (EEG). The lungs' ability to hold air, to move air in and out, and to exchange oxygen and carbon dioxide is measured with pulmonary function tests.

BIOPSY

Tissue samples are removed and examined, usually with a microscope. The examination often focuses on finding abnormal cells that may provide evidence of inflammation or of a disorder, such as cancer. Tissues that are commonly examined include skin, breast, lung, liver, kidney, and bone.

ANALYSIS OF GENETIC MATERIAL (GENETIC TESTING)

Usually, cells from skin, blood, or bone marrow are analyzed. Cells are examined to check for abnormalities of chromosomes, genes (including DNA), or both. Genetic testing may be done in the following:

- Fetuses: To determine whether they have a genetic disorder
- Children and young adults: To determine whether they have a disorder or are at risk of developing a disorder
- Adults: Sometimes to help determine the likelihood that their relatives, such as children or grandchildren, will develop certain disorders

RISKS AND RESULTS

Every test has some risk. The risk may be the possibility of injury during the test, or it may be the need for further testing if the result is abnormal. Further testing is often more expensive, dangerous, or both. Doctors weigh the risk of a test against the usefulness of the information it will provide.

Normal test values are expressed as a range, which is based on the average values in a healthy population. That is, 95% of healthy people have values within this range. However, average values are slightly different for women and men and may vary by age. For some tests, these values also vary among laboratories. Thus, when doctors get a laboratory test result, the laboratory also gives them its own normal range for that test. The table below lists some typical normal results. However, because values vary by laboratory, people should consult their doctor about the significance of their own test results rather than refer to this table.

BLOOD TESTS*	
Test	**Reference Range or Threshold (Conventional Units†)**
Acidity (pH)	7.35–7.45
Alcohol (ethanol)	0 mg/dL (more than 0.1 mg/dL usually indicates intoxication)
Ammonia	15–50 units/L
Amylase	53–123 units/L
Antinuclear antibodies (ANA)‡	0 (negative result)
Ascorbic acid	0.4–1.5 mg/dL
Bicarbonate (carbon dioxide content)	18–23 mEq/L
Bilirubin	*Direct:* Up to 0.4 mg/dL
	Total: Up to 1.0 mg/dL
Blood volume	8.5–9.1% of body weight
Calcium	8.5–10.5 mg/dL (slightly higher in children) *(continued)*

BLOOD TESTS* *(continued)*

Test	Reference Range or Threshold (Conventional Units†)
Carbon dioxide pressure (expressed as a comparison with how high the level of mercury [Hg] rises in a tube due to air pressure at sea level)	35–45 mm Hg
Carboxyhemoglobin (carbon monoxide in hemoglobin)	Less than 5% of total hemoglobin
CD4 cell count	500–1500 cells/µL
Ceruloplasmin	15–60 mg/dL
Chloride	98–106 mEq/L
Complete blood cell count (CBC)	See individual tests: Hemoglobin, hematocrit, mean corpuscular hemoglobin, mean corpuscular hemoglobin concentration, mean corpuscular volume, platelet count, and white blood cell count
Copper	70–150 µg/dL
Creatine kinase (CK), also called creatine phosphokinase (CPK)	*Male:* 38–174 units/L *Female:* 96–140 units/L
Creatine kinase (CK) in its different forms (isoenzymes)	5% or less of CK-MB (the form that occurs mainly in heart muscle)
Creatinine	0.6–1.2 mg/dL
Electrolytes	See individual tests: Calcium, chloride, magnesium, potassium, and sodium (which are routinely tested)
Erythrocyte sedimentation rate (ESR)	*Male:* 1–13 mm/hour *Female:* 1–20 mm/hour
Glucose	*Fasting:* 70–110 mg/dL
Hematocrit	*Male:* 45–52% *Female:* 37–48%
Hemoglobin	*Male:* 13–18 g/dL *Female:* 12–16 g/dL
Iron	60–160 µg/dL (higher in males)
Iron-binding capacity	250–460 µg/dL
Lactate (lactic acid)	*Venous:* 4.5–19.8 mg/dL *Arterial:* 4.5–14.4 mg/dL
Lactic dehydrogenase	50–150 units/L
Lead	20 µg/dL or less (much lower in children)
Lipase	10–150 units/L
Lipids:	
Cholesterol, total	Less than 225 mg/dL (for age 40–49 yr; increases with age)
High-density lipoprotein (HDL)	30–70 mg/dL
Low-density lipoprotein (LDL)	60 mg/dL
Triglycerides	40–200 mg/dL (higher in males)
Liver function tests	Include bilirubin (total), phosphatase (alkaline), protein (total and albumin), transaminases (alanine and aspartate), prothrombin
Magnesium	1.5–2.0 mg/dL *(continued)*

BLOOD TESTS* *(continued)*

Test	Reference Range or Threshold (Conventional Units†)
Mean corpuscular hemoglobin (MCH)	27–32 pg/cell
Mean corpuscular hemoglobin concentration (MCHC)	32–36% hemoglobin/cell
Mean corpuscular volume (MCV)	76–100 cubic μm
Osmolality	280–296 mOsm/kg plasma
Oxygen pressure (expressed as a comparison with the level of mercury [Hg] in a tube, which results from air pressure at sea level)	83–100 mm Hg
Oxygen saturation (arterial)	96–100%
Partial thromboplastin time (PTT)	30–45 seconds
Phosphatase (alkaline)	50–160 units/L (higher in infants and adolescents, lower in females)
Phosphorus	3.0–4.5 mg/dL
Platelet count	150,000–350,000/mL
Potassium	3.5–5.0 mEq/L
Prostate-specific antigen (PSA)	0–4 ng/mL (increases with age)
Protein:	
Total	6.0–8.4 g/dL
Albumin	3.5–5.0 g/dL
Globulin	2.3–3.5 g/dL
Prothrombin time (PT)	10–13 seconds
Red blood cell (RBC) count	4.2–5.9 million/mL
Sodium	135–145 mEq/L
Thyroid-stimulating hormone (TSH)	0.5–5.0 m units/L
Transaminases (liver enzymes):	
Alanine (ALT)	1–21 units/L
Aspartate (AST)	7–27 units/L
Troponin in its different forms:	
I	Less than 1.6 ng/mL
T	Less than 0.1 ng/mL
Urea nitrogen (BUN)	7–18 mg/dL
Uric acid	3.0–7.0 mg/dL
Vitamin A§	30–65 μg/dL
White blood cell (WBC) count	4,300–10,800 /mL

*Blood can be tested for many other substances as well.
†Conventional units can be converted to international units by using a conversion factor. International units (IU), a different system, are sometimes used by laboratories.
‡Other antibodies can also be identified.
§Other vitamins can also be measured.

DIAGNOSTIC PROCEDURES

Procedure	Body Area or Sample Tested	Description
Amniocentesis	Fluid from the sac surrounding the fetus	Analysis of fluid, removed by a needle inserted through the abdominal wall, to detect an abnormality in the fetus
Arteriography (angiography)	Any artery in the body, commonly in the brain, heart, kidneys, aorta, or legs	X-ray study using radiopaque dye injected through a thin tube (catheter), which is threaded to the artery being studied, to detect and outline or highlight a blockage or defect in an artery
Audiometry	Ears	Assessment of the ability to hear and distinguish sounds at specific pitches and volumes using headphones
Auscultation	Heart	Listening with a stethoscope for abnormal heart sounds
Barium x-ray studies	Esophagus, stomach, intestine, or rectum	X-ray study to detect ulcers, tumors, or other abnormalities
Biopsy	Any tissue in the body	Removal and examination of a tissue sample under a microscope to check for cancer or another abnormality
Blood pressure measurement	Usually an arm	Test for high or low blood pressure, usually using an inflatable cuff wrapped around the arm
Blood tests	Usually a blood sample from an arm	Measurement of substances in the blood to evaluate organ function and to help diagnose and monitor various disorders
Bone marrow aspiration	Hipbone or breastbone	Removal of a bone marrow sample by a needle for examination under a microscope to check for abnormalities in blood cells
Bronchoscopy	Airways of the lungs	Direct examination with a viewing tube to check for a tumor or other abnormality
Cardiac catheterization	Heart	Study of heart function and structure using a catheter inserted into a blood vessel and threaded to the heart
Chorionic villus sampling	Placenta	Removal of a sample for examination under a microscope to check for abnormalities in the fetus
Chromosomal analysis	Blood	Examination under a microscope to detect a genetic disorder or to determine a fetus's sex
Colonoscopy	Large intestine	Direct examination with a viewing tube to check for a tumor or other abnormality

(continued)

DIAGNOSTIC PROCEDURES *(continued)*

Procedure	Body Area or Sample Tested	Description
Colposcopy	Cervix	Direct examination of the cervix with a magnifying lens
Computed tomography (CT)	Any part of the body	Computer-enhanced x-ray study to detect structural abnormalities
Cone biopsy	Cervix	Removal and examination of a cone-shaped piece of tissue, usually using a heated wire loop or a laser
Culture	A sample from any area of the body (usually a fluid such as blood or urine)	Growth and examination of microorganisms from the sample to identify infection with bacteria or fungi
Dilation and curettage (D and C)	Cervix and uterus	Examination of a sample under a microscope to check for abnormalities in the uterine lining using a small, sharp instrument (curet).
Dual x-ray absorptiometry (DEXA)	Skeleton, focusing on specific regions, usually the hip, spine, and wrist	Low-dose x-ray study to determine the thickness of bones
Echocardiography	Heart	Study of heart structure and function using sound waves
Electrocardiography (ECG)	Heart	Study of the heart's electrical activity using electrodes attached to the arms, legs, and chest
Electroencephalography (EEG)	Brain	Study of the brain's electrical function using electrodes attached to the scalp
Electromyography	Muscles	Recording of a muscle's electrical activity using small needles inserted into the muscle
Electrophysiologic testing	Heart	Test to evaluate rhythm or electrical conduction abnormalities using a catheter inserted into a blood vessel and threaded to the heart
Endoscopic retrograde cholangiopancreatography (ERCP)	Biliary tract	X-ray study of the biliary tract done after injection of a radiopaque dye and using a flexible viewing tube
Endoscopy	Digestive tract	Direct examination of internal structures using a flexible viewing tube
Enzyme-linked immunosorbent assay (ELISA)	Usually blood	Test that involves mixing the sample of blood with substances that can trigger allergies (allergens) or with microorganisms to test for the presence of specific antibodies
Fluoroscopy	Digestive tract, heart, or lungs	A continuous x-ray study that enables a doctor to see the inside of an organ as it functions
Hysteroscopy	Uterus	Direct examination of the inside of the uterus with a flexible viewing tube

(continued)

DIAGNOSTIC PROCEDURES *(continued)*

Procedure	Body Area or Sample Tested	Description
Intravenous urography	Kidneys and urinary tract	X-ray study of the kidneys and urinary tract after a radiopaque dye is injected into a vein (intravenously)
Joint aspiration	Joints, especially those of the shoulders, elbows, fingers, hips, knees, ankles, and toes	Removal and examination of fluid from the space within joints to check for blood cells, crystals formed from minerals, and microorganisms
Laparoscopy	Abdomen	Direct examination using a viewing tube inserted through an incision in the abdomen to diagnose and treat abnormalities in the abdomen
Magnetic resonance imaging (MRI)	Any part of the body	Imaging test using a strong magnetic field and radio waves to check for structural abnormalities
Mammography	Breasts	X-ray study to check for breast cancer
Mediastinoscopy	Chest	Direct examination of the area of the chest between the lungs using a viewing tube inserted through a small incision just above the breastbone
Myelography	Spinal column	Simple or computer-enhanced x-ray study of the spinal column after injection of a radiopaque dye
Nerve conduction study	Nerves	Test to determine how fast a nerve impulse travels using electrodes or needles inserted along the path of the nerve
Occult blood test	Large intestine	Test to detect blood in stool
Ophthalmoscopy	Eyes	Direct examination using a handheld device that shines light into the eye to detect abnormalities inside the eye
Papanicolaou (Pap) test	Cervix	Examination of cells scraped from the cervix under a microscope to detect cancer
Paracentesis	Abdomen	Insertion of a needle into the abdominal cavity to remove fluid for examination
Percutaneous transhepatic cholangiography	Liver and biliary tract	X-ray study of the liver and biliary tract after a radiopaque dye is injected into the liver
Positron emission tomography (PET)	Brain and heart	Imaging test using particles that release radiation (positrons) to detect abnormalities in function
Pulmonary function tests	Lungs	Tests to measure the lungs' capacity to hold air, to move air in and out of the body, and to exchange oxygen and carbon dioxide as people blow into a measuring device *(continued)*

DIAGNOSTIC PROCEDURES (continued)

Procedure	Body Area or Sample Tested	Description
Radionuclide imaging	Many organs	Imaging test using particles that release radiation (radionuclides) to detect abnormalities in blood flow, structure, or function
Reflex tests	Tendons	Tests using a physical stimulus (such as a light tap) to detect abnormalities in nerve function
Retrograde urography	Bladder and ureters	X-ray study of the bladder and ureters after a radiopaque dye is inserted into the ureter
Sigmoidoscopy	Rectum and last portion of the large intestine	Direct examination using a viewing tube to detect tumors or other abnormalities
Skin allergy tests	Usually an arm or the back	Tests for allergies done by placing a solution containing a possible allergen on the skin, then pricking the skin with a needle
Spinal tap (lumbar puncture)	Spinal canal	Removal of spinal fluid, using a needle inserted into the hipbone, to check for abnormalities in spinal fluid
Spirometry	Lungs	Test of lung function that involves blowing into a measuring device
Stress testing	Heart	Test of heart function during exertion using a treadmill or other exercise machine and electrocardiography (if people cannot exercise, a drug is used to simulate exercise's effects)
Thoracentesis	The space between the pleura, a two-layered membrane that covers the lungs and lines the chest wall (pleural space)	Removal of fluid from this space with a needle to detect abnormalities
Thoracoscopy	Lungs	Examination of the lung surfaces, pleura, and pleural space through a viewing tube
Tympanometry	Ears	Measurement of the resistance to pressure (impedance) in the middle ear using a device inserted in the ear and sound waves to help determine the cause of hearing loss
Ultrasonography (ultrasound scanning)	Any part of the body	Imaging using sound waves to detect structural or functional abnormalities
Urinalysis	Kidneys and urinary tract	Chemical analysis of a urine sample to detect protein, sugar, ketones, and blood cells
Venography	Veins	X-ray study using a radiopaque dye (similar to arteriography) to detect blockage of a vein

THE ONE-PAGE MERCK MANUAL OF HEALTH

People think healthy living involves rare treasures and dark secrets—the exotic plant from a Tibetan meadow, the secret advice from a sage in a remote village—or years of intense study and practice. Actually, the truth is hidden in plain sight, and it's pretty simple (though seldom easy). That's why The Merck Manual of Health requires only *one* sheet of paper.

DIET AND NUTRITION

- Eat less (yes, this means you), particularly less sugars, simple carbohydrates, trans fats, and saturated fats.
- Eat more fruits, vegetables, and whole grains
- Vary your diet
- If your medical condition requires a special diet, *follow it*

VITAMINS AND SUPPLEMENTS

- If you're a breastfed baby, take vitamin D; if you're a bottle-fed baby, use formula with iron
- If you're over 50 years old, take calcium and vitamin D
- If you're pregnant (or thinking of becoming pregnant), take prenatal vitamins

SUBSTANCE USE

- Don't smoke (and if you do, *don't* smoke in bed)
- Drink alcohol only in moderation (if that's hard for you, don't drink at all)
- Don't take any drugs that aren't intended to treat a medical problem

EXERCISE AND SLEEP

- Do 30 to 60 minutes of structured exercise (aerobic *and* resistance) that is appropriate for your age and medical condition (fun is good) *at least* 3 times per week
- Walk more—and take the stairs
- Keep as regular a sleep schedule as possible

INFECTIONS

- Wash your hands before eating and cooking
- Store, prepare, and cook foods (particularly meats) appropriately
- Drink only clean or treated water
- Practice safe sex
- Wash minor wounds with soap and water and keep covered
- Use appropriate clothing and insect repellent when mosquito or tick exposure is likely
- Don't do intravenous drugs, and if you do, don't share needles

INJURIES AND GENERAL SAFETY

- Wear a seatbelt; if you're a child, use a car seat
- Wear a helmet while riding a bicycle or motorcycle and use other protective gear as appropriate for the activity (recreation or occupation)
- Store and handle firearms safely
- Follow the accepted safety procedures for your job and recreational activities
- Don't operate vehicles or power equipment while intoxicated, overly sleepy, or distracted
- Look before crossing or entering a road, changing lanes, or merging
- Wear a life vest while boating, don't dive into shallow water, and learn to swim
- Have working smoke and carbon monoxide detectors in your home

MENTAL HEALTH

- Treat others as you would be treated
- Accept responsibility for your actions; also take responsibility for someone or something besides yourself
- Make *and keep* friends
- Act nicer: Don't speak ill to or about others
- Practice mind-calming techniques (for example, meditation or prayer)
- Don't sweat the small stuff and be sensible about what's small
- With adversity, change what you can, live with what you can't, and try to know the difference

- When you do something, do your best (but don't expect more from yourself than your best)
- Do something useful for your family and community
- Understand that you will die (yes, you) and you will experience pain and loss

HEALTH CARE

- Brush your teeth at least twice a day
- See a dentist regularly for cleaning and examination
- See a health care practitioner regularly for age-appropriate and sex-appropriate screening (blood pressure, glucose, and lipid levels; Pap smears, mammograms, and colon cancer screening; prenatal screening) and vaccinations

- Be cautious about sun exposure and wear sunscreen
- If something feels wrong physically or mentally, see appropriate practitioners: If you trust them, do what they advise; if you don't trust them, or if what they say seems too good to be true or doesn't make sense, don't ignore the issue, get another opinion

If you do all of these things but think yo need something more, take the time, effort, an money you'd spend looking for a better supple ment, diet, or exercise and instead read a boo to a child or help those in your community wh are in need.

Yours in Good Health,

Robert S. Porter, MD

Editor-in-Chief, The Merck Manuals

Note: Page numbers followed by *t* indicate tables; those followed by *f* indicate figures (art boxes); those followed by *sb* indicate sidebars.

The Merck Manual Go-To Home Guide for Symptoms is set in 9.5 Minion Pro, with heads set in Helvetica Neue. The original drafts were produced using a web-based content management system hosted by Vasont Systems. Book composition services were provided by Cenveo Publisher Services in Fort Washington, Pennsylvania. The book was printed by the web offset printing process on 50-pound Finch Opaque Vellum paper at Courier Printing in Westford, Massachusetts.

NOTES

NOTES